Mayo Clinic
Medical Manual

Mayo Clinic
Medical Manual

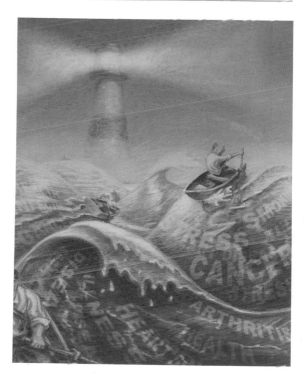

Editors

Guilherme H. M. Oliveira, M.D.
Gillian C. Nesbitt, M.D.
Joseph G. Murphy, M.D.

MAYO CLINIC SCIENTIFIC PRESS
TAYLOR & FRANCIS GROUP

PREFACE

The urge to write this book—and it was indeed an urge—arose because of two reasons. The first was the lack of a book that approached patient care from the viewpoint of on-call medical residents. New residents faced with admitting a sick patient in the middle of the night have three priorities: one, a working diagnosis; two, a management plan that will get the patient through the night; and three, deciding when to call for help from the attending physician. This on-call manual seeks to empower residents to reach a working diagnosis and to develop a short-term management plan using the clinical history, physical examination, and essential on-call investigations. The layout of the book allows the reader to look up signs, symptoms, and laboratory abnormalities; to develop a list of differential diagnoses; and to formulate a management plant. Residents were recruited to write all the chapters in conjunction with the attending staff.

In conclusion, this Manual intends to be a uniquely useful tool for young doctors. We hope we have been able to blend the simplicity and focus essential to the the neophyte with the knowledge and precision required by the expert.

LIST OF CONTRIBUTORS

Andrea C. Adams, M.D.
Consultant, Department of Neurology, Mayo Clinic; Assistant Professor of Neurology, Mayo Clinic College of Medicine; Rochester, Minnesota

Timothy R. Aksamit, M.D.
Consultant, Division of Pulmonary and Critical Care Medicine, Mayo Clinic; Assistant Professor of Medicine, Mayo Clinic College of Medicine; Rochester, Minnesota

Robert C. Albright, Jr., D.O.
Consultant, Division of Nephrology and Hypertension, Mayo Clinic; Assistant Professor of Medicine, Mayo Clinic College of Medicine; Rochester, Minnesota

Amindra S. Arora, M.B.B.Chir.
Consultant, Division of Gastroenterology and Hepatology, Mayo Clinic; Assistant Professor of Medicine, Mayo Clinic College of Medicine; Rochester, Minnesota

Rendell W. Ashton, M.D.
Fellow in Pulmonary and Critical Care Medicine, Mayo School of Graduate Medical Education and Instructor in Medicine, Mayo Clinic College of Medicine, Rochester, Minnesota

Rebecca S. Bahn, M.D.
Consultant, Division of Endocrinology, Diabetes, Metabolism, Nutrition, Mayo Clinic; Professor of Medicine, Mayo Clinic College of Medicine; Rochester, Minnesota

Kiran M. Bambha, M.D.
Fellow in Gastroenterology and Hepatology, Mayo School of Graduate Medical Education and Instructor in Medicine, Mayo Clinic College of Medicine, Rochester, Minnesota

J. D. Bartleson, M.D.
Consultant, Department of Neurology, Mayo Clinic; Associate Professor of Neurology, Mayo Clinic College of Medicine; Rochester, Minnesota

T. Jared Bunch, M.D.
Fellow in Cardiovascular Diseases, Mayo School of Graduate Medical Education and Assistant Professor of Medicine, Mayo Clinic College of Medicine, Rochester, Minnesota

John B. Bundrick, M.D.
Consultant, Division of General Internal Medicine, Mayo Clinic; Assistant Professor of Medicine, Mayo Clinic College of Medicine; Rochester, Minnesota

Kevin A. Bybee, M.D.
Resident in Cardiovascular Diseases, Mayo School of Graduate Medical Education and Instructor, Mayo Clinic College of Medicine, Rochester, Minnesota

Casey R. Caldwell, M.D.
Consultant, Division of Primary Care Internal Medicine, Mayo Clinic; Instructor in Medicine, Mayo Clinic College of Medicine; Rochester, Minnesota

Sean M. Caples, D.O.
Senior Associate Consultant, Division of Pulmonary and Critical Care Medicine, Mayo Clinic; Assistant Professor of Medicine, Mayo Clinic College of Medicine; Rochester, Minnesota

Paul E. Carns, M.D.
Consultant, Department of Anesthesiology, Mayo Clinic; Assistant Professor of Anesthesiology, Mayo Clinic College of Medicine; Rochester, Minnesota

Gregory D. Cascino, M.D.
Consultant, Department of Neurology, Mayo Clinic; Professor of Neurology, Mayo Clinic College of Medicine; Rochester, Minnesota

Yoon-Hee K. Cha, M.D.
Formerly, Student, Mayo Medical School, Mayo Clinic College of Medicine, Rochester, Minnesota; presently, Chief Resident in Neurology, UCSF, San Francisco, California

Suresh T. Chari, M.D.
Consultant, Division of Gastroenterology and Hepatology, Mayo Clinic; Associate Professor of Medicine, Mayo Clinic College of Medicine; Rochester, Minnesota

Lin Y. Chen, M.D.
Resident in Internal Medicine, Mayo Graduate School of Medicine; Instructor in Medicine, Mayo Clinic College of Medicine; Rochester, Minnesota

Lisa S. Chow, M.D.
Fellow in Endocrinology, Diabetes, Metabolism, Nutrition, Mayo School of Graduate Medical Education and Instructor in Medicine, Mayo Clinic College of Medicine, Rochester, Minnesota

David Allan Cook, M.D.
Resident in Gastroenterology and Hepatology, Mayo School of Graduate Medical Education, Mayo Clinic College of Medicine, Rochester, Minnesota

Douglas J. Creedon, M.D.
Senior Associate Consultant, Division of Obstetrics, Mayo Clinic, Rochester, Minnesota

Arjun Deb, M.D.
Resident in Cardiovascular Diseases, Mayo School of Graduate Medical Education, Mayo Clinic College of Medicine, Rochester, Minnesota

Ives R. De Chazal, M.D.

Fellow in Critical Care Medicine, Mayo School of Graduate Medical Education, Mayo Clinic College of Medicine, Rochester, Minnesota

Ramona S. deJesus, M.D.

Senior Associate Consultant, Division of Primary Care Internal Medicine, Mayo Clinic; Instructor in Medicine, Mayo Clinic College of Medicine; Rochester, Minnesota

Shamina Dhillon, M.D.

Fellow in Gastroenterology and Hepatology, Mayo School of Graduate Medical Education and Instructor in Medicine, Mayo Clinic College of Medicine, Rochester, Minnesota

Lisa A. Drage, M.D.

Consultant, Department of Dermatology, Mayo Clinic; Assistant Professor of Dermatology, Mayo Clinic College of Medicine; Rochester, Minnesota

William F. Dunn, M.D.

Consultant, Division of Pulmonary and Critical Care Medicine, Mayo Clinic; Associate Professor of Medicine, Mayo Clinic College of Medicine; Rochester, Minnesota

Grace K. Dy, M.D.

Fellow in Pulmonary and Critical Care Medicine, Mayo School of Graduate Medical Education, Mayo Clinic College of Medicine, Rochester, Minnesota

Jon O. Ebbert, M.D., M.Sc.

Consultant, Division of Primary Care Internal Medicine, Mayo Clinic; Assistant Professor of Medicine, Mayo Clinic College of Medicine; Rochester, Minnesota

Randall S. Edson, M.D.

Consultant, Division of Infectious Diseases, Mayo Clinic; Professor of Medicine, Mayo Clinic College of Medicine; Rochester, Minnesota

Scott D. Eggers, M.D.

Senior Associate Consultant, Department of Neurology, Mayo Clinic; Assistant Professor of Neurology, Mayo Clinic College of Medicine; Rochester, Minnesota

Lynn L. Estes, Pharm.D.

Infectious Disease Pharmacist Specialist, Mayo Clinic; Assistant Professor of Pharmacy, Mayo Clinic College of Medicine; Rochester, Minnesota

Luke T. Evans, M.D.

Resident in Gastroenterology and Hepatology, Mayo School of Graduate Medical Education, Mayo Clinic College of Medicine, Rochester, Minnesota

Fernando C. Fervenza, M.D.

Consultant, Division of Nephrology, Mayo Clinic; Associate Professor of Medicine, Mayo Clinic College of Medicine; Rochester, Minnesota

Javier D. Finkielman, M.D.
Fellow in Nephrology and Hypertension, Mayo School of Graduate Medical Education and Instructor in Medicine, Mayo Clinic College of Medicine, Rochester, Minnesota

Matthew L. Flaherty, M.D.
Resident in Neurology, Mayo School of Graduate Medical Education, Mayo Clinic College of Medicine, Rochester, Minnesota

Rafael Fonseca, M.D.
Consultant, Division of Hematology, Mayo Clinic; Associate Professor of Medicine, Mayo Clinic College of Medicine; Rochester, Minnesota

David A. Froehling, M.D.
Consultant, Division of General Internal Medicine, Mayo Clinic; Assistant Professor of Medicine, Mayo Clinic College of Medicine; Rochester, Minnesota

Apoor S. Gami, M.D.
Fellow in Cardiovascular Diseases, Mayo School of Graduate Medical Education and Assistant Professor of Medicine, Mayo Clinic College of Medicine, Rochester, Minnesota

Gunjan Y. Gandhi, M.D.
Fellow in Endocrinology, Diabetes, Metabolism, Nutrition and Instructor in Medicine, Mayo Clinic College of Medicine, Rochester, Minnesota

Dennis A. Gastineau, M.D.
Consultant, Division of Hematology, Mayo Clinic; Associate Professor of Medicine, Mayo Clinic College of Medicine; Rochester, Minnesota

Anna M. Georgiopoulos, M.D.
Chief Resident Associate in Primary Care Internal Medicine, Mayo School of Graduate Medical Education, Mayo Clinic College of Medicine, Rochester, Minnesota

Karin F. Giordano, M.D.
Fellow in Hematology, Mayo School of Graduate Medical Education, Mayo Clinic College of Medicine, Rochester, Minnesota

John W. Graves, M.D.
Consultant, Division of Nephrology and Hypertension, Mayo Clinic; Associate Professor of Medicine, Mayo Clinic College of Medicine; Rochester, Minnesota

Stephen F. Grinton, M.D.
Consultant, Division of Pulmonary Medicine, Mayo Clinic, Jacksonville, Florida; Associate Professor of Medicine, Mayo Clinic College of Medicine, Rochester, Minnesota

Geeta G. Gyamlani, M.D.
Fellow in Pulmonary and Critical Care Medicine, Mayo School of Graduate Medical Education, Mayo Clinic College of Medicine, Rochester, Minnesota

Thomas M. Habermann, M.D.
Consultant, Division of Hematology, Mayo Clinic; Professor of Medicine, Mayo Clinic College of Medicine; Rochester, Minnesota

J. Eileen Hay, M.B.Ch.B.
Consultant, Division of Gastroenterology and Hepatology, Mayo Clinic; Professor of Medicine, Mayo Clinic College of Medicine; Rochester, Minnesota

John A. Heit, M.D.
Consultant, Division of Cardiovascular Diseases, Mayo Clinic; Professor of Medicine, Mayo Clinic College of Medicine; Rochester, Minnesota

Robert W. Hoel, Pharm.D.
Pharmacist, Hospital Pharmacy Services, Mayo Clinic, Rochester, Minnesota

Jonathan M. Holmes, B.M., B.Ch.
Chair, Department of Ophthalmology, Mayo Clinic; Professor of Ophthalmology, Mayo Clinic College of Medicine; Rochester, Minnesota

Arshad Jahangir, M.D.
Consultant, Division of Cardiovascular Diseases, Mayo Clinic; Associate Professor of Medicine, Mayo Clinic College of Medicine, Rochester, Minnesota

Constance Jennings, M.D.
Senior Associate Consultant, Division of Pulmonary and Critical Care Medicine, Mayo Clinic; Assistant Professor of Medicine, Mayo Clinic College of Medicine; Rochester, Minnesota

Garvan C. Kane, M.D.
Resident in Cardiovascular Diseases, Mayo School of Graduate Medical Education and Instructor in Medicine, Mayo Clinic College of Medicine, Rochester, Minnesota

A. Scott Keller, M.D.
Senior Associate Consultant, Division of General Internal Medicine, Mayo Clinic; Instructor in Medicine, Mayo Clinic College of Medicine; Rochester, Minnesota

Kurt A. Kennel, M.D.
Senior Associate Consultant, Division of Endocrinology, Diabetes, Metabolism, Nutrition, Mayo Clinic; Assistant Professor of Medicine, Mayo Clinic College of Medicine; Rochester, Minnesota

Peter D. Kent, M.D.
Fellow in Rheumatology, Mayo School of Graduate Medical Education, Mayo Clinic College of Medicine, Rochester, Minnesota

Stephen L. Kopecky, M.D.
Consultant, Division of Cardiovascular Diseases, Mayo Clinic; Associate Professor of Medicine, Mayo Clinic College of Medicine; Rochester, Minnesota

Stephen M. Lange, M.D.
Consultant, Division of Gastroenterology and Hepatology, Mayo Clinic, Jacksonville, Florida; Assistant Professor of Medicine, Mayo Clinic College of Medicine, Rochester, Minnesota

Augustine S. Lee, M.D.
Senior Associate Consultant, Division of Pulmonary Medicine, Mayo Clinic, Jacksonville, Florida; Assistant Professor of Medicine, Mayo Clinic College of Medicine, Rochester, Minnesota

Kaiser G. Lim, M.D.
Consultant, Division of Pulmonary and Critical Care Medicine, Mayo Clinic; Assistant Professor of Medicine, Mayo Clinic College of Medicine; Rochester, Minnesota

Lionel S. Lim, M.D.
Fellow in Primary Care Internal Medicine, Mayo School of Graduate Medical Education, Mayo Clinic College of Medicine, Rochester, Minnesota

Adam J. Locketz, M.D.
Fellow in Pain Medicine, Mayo School of Graduate Medical Education, Mayo Clinic College of Medicine, Rochester, Minnesota

Conor G. Loftus, M.D.
Senior Associate Consultant, Division of Gastroenterology and Hepatology, Mayo Clinic; Assistant Professor of Medicine, Mayo Clinic College of Medicine; Rochester, Minnesota

Edward V. Loftus, Jr., M.D.
Consultant, Division of Gastroenterology and Hepatology, Mayo Clinic; Associate Professor of Medicine, Mayo Clinic College of Medicine; Rochester, Minnesota

William F. Marshall, M.D.
Consultant, Division of Infectious Diseases, Mayo Clinic; Assistant Professor of Medicine, Mayo Clinic College of Medicine; Rochester, Minnesota

Stanley I. Martin, M.D.
Resident in Endocrinology, Diabetes, Metabolism, Nutrition, Mayo School of Graduate Medical Education, Mayo Clinic College of Medicine, Rochester, Minnesota

Matthew W. Martinez, M.D.
Resident in Cardiovascular Diseases, Mayo School of Graduate Medical Education and Instructor in Medicine, Mayo Clinic College of Medicine, Rochester, Minnesota

Thomas G. Mason, M.D.
Consultant, Division of Rheumatology, Mayo Clinic; Assistant Professor of Medicine and of Pediatrics, Mayo Clinic College of Medicine; Rochester, Minnesota

Kathleen M. McEvoy, M.D.
Consultant, Department of Neurology, Mayo Clinic; Assistant

Professor of Neurology, Mayo Clinic College of Medicine; Rochester, Minnesota

Lawrence K. McKnight, M.D.

Resident in Nephrology and Hypertension, Mayo School of Graduate Medical Education, Mayo Clinic College of Medicine, Rochester, Minnesota

M. Molly McMahon, M.D.

Consultant, Division of Endocrinology, Diabetes, Metabolism, Nutrition, Mayo Clinic; Professor of Medicine, Mayo Clinic College of Medicine; Rochester, Minnesota

Victor M. Montori, M.D.

Senior Associate Consultant, Division of Endocrinology, Diabetes, Metabolism, Nutrition, Mayo Clinic, Rochester, Minnesota

Paul S. Mueller, M.D.

Consultant, Division of General Internal Medicine, Mayo Clinic; Assistant Professor of Medicine, Mayo Clinic College of Medicine; Rochester, Minnesota

William C. Mundell, M.D.

Consultant, Division of General Internal Medicine, Mayo Clinic; Instructor in Medicine, Mayo Clinic College of Medicine; Rochester, Minnesota

Joseph G. Murphy, M.D.

Consultant, Division of Cardiovascular Diseases, Mayo Clinic; Associate Professor of Medicine, Mayo Clinic College of Medicine; Rochester, Minnesota

Gillian C. Nesbitt, M.D.

Resident in Internal Medicine, Mayo Clinic College of Medicine, Rochester, Minnesota

Guilherme H. M. Oliveira, M.D.

Senior Resident Associate in Internal Medicine, Mayo School of Graduate Medical Education, Mayo Clinic College of Medicine, Rochester, Minnesota

Amy S. Oxentenko, M.D.

Fellow in Gastroenterology and Hepatology, Mayo School of Graduate Medical Education and Assistant Professor of Medicine, Mayo Clinic College of Medicine, Rochester, Minnesota

Darrell S. Pardi, M.D.

Consultant, Division of Gastroenterology and Hepatology, Mayo Clinic; Assistant Professor of Medicine, Mayo Clinic College of Medicine; Rochester, Minnesota

Miguel A. Park, M.D.

Senior Associate Consultant, Division of Allergic Diseases, Mayo Clinic; Instructor in Medicine, Mayo Clinic College of Medicine; Rochester, Minnesota

Sanjay V. Patel, B.M., B.Ch.

Senior Associate Consultant, Department of Ophthalmology, Mayo

Clinic; Assistant Professor of Ophthalmology, Mayo Clinic College of Medicine, Rochester, Minnesota

Jason Persoff, M.D.
Senior Associate Consultant, Division of Hospital Internal Medicine, Mayo Clinic, Jacksonville, Florida; Assistant Professor of Medicine, Mayo Clinic College of Medicine; Rochester, Minnesota

Steve G. Peters, M.D.
Consultant, Division of Pulmonary and Critical Care Medicine, Mayo Clinic; Professor of Medicine, Mayo Clinic College of Medicine; Rochester, Minnesota

David H. Pfizenmaier II, M.D., D.P.M.
Senior Resident in Cardiovascular Diseases, Mayo School of Graduate Medical Education, Mayo Clinic College of Medicine, Rochester, Minnesota

Axel Pflueger, M.D.
Fellow in Infectious Diseases, Mayo School of Graduate Medical Education and Instructor in Medicine, Mayo Clinic College of Medicine, Rochester, Minnesota

Udaya B. S. Prakash, M.D.
Consultant, Division of Pulmonary and Critical Care Medicine, Mayo Clinic; Professor of Medicine, Mayo Clinic College of Medicine; Rochester, Minnesota

Rajiv K. Pruthi, M.B.B.S.
Consultant, Division of Hematology, Mayo Clinic; Assistant Professor of Medicine, Mayo Clinic College of Medicine; Rochester, Minnesota

Jeffrey T. Rabatin, M.D.
Consultant, Division of Pulmonary and Critical Care Medicine, Mayo Clinic; Assistant Professor of Medicine, Mayo Clinic College of Medicine; Rochester, Minnesota

Otis B. Rickman, D.O.
Senior Associate Consultant, Division of Pulmonary and Critical Care Medicine, Mayo Clinic; Assistant Professor of Medicine, Mayo Clinic College of Medicine; Rochester, Minnesota

Douglas L. Riegert-Johnson, M.D.
Resident in Pulmonary and Critical Care Medicine, Mayo School of Graduate Medical Education, Mayo Clinic College of Medicine, Rochester, Minnesota

Vanessa Z. Riegert-Johnson
Student, Mayo Medical School, Mayo Clinic College of Medicine, Rochester, Minnesota

Charanjit S. Rihal, M.D.
Consultant, Division of Cardiovascular Diseases, Mayo Clinic; Professor of Medicine, Mayo Clinic College of Medicine; Rochester, Minnesota

Thom W. Rooke, M.D.
Consultant, Division of Cardiovascular Diseases, Mayo Clinic;

Professor of Medicine, Mayo Clinic College of Medicine; Rochester, Minnesota

Edward C. Rosenow III, M.D.
Emeritus Consultant, Division of Pulmonary and Critical Care Medicine, Mayo Clinic; Emeritus Professor of Medicine, Mayo Clinic College of Medicine; Rochester, Minnesota

Andrew D. Rule, M.D.
Fellow in Nephrology and Hypertension, Mayo School of Graduate Medical Education and Instructor in Medicine, Mayo Clinic College of Medicine, Rochester, Minnesota

William Sanchez, M.D.
Fellow in Gastroenterology and Hepatology, Mayo School of Graduate Medical Education and Instructor of Medicine, Mayo Clinic College of Medicine, Rochester, Minnesota

Paul D. Scanlon, M.D.
Consultant, Division of Pulmonary and Critical Care Medicine, Mayo Clinic; Professor of Medicine, Mayo Clinic College of Medicine; Rochester, Minnesota

Nicola E. Schiebel, M.D.
Consultant, Department of Emergency Medicine, Mayo Clinic; Assistant Professor of Emergency Medicine, Mayo Clinic College of Medicine; Rochester, Minnesota

Alexander Schirger, M.D.
Consultant, Division of Cardiovascular Diseases, Mayo Clinic; Professor of Medicine, Mayo Clinic College of Medicine; Rochester, Minnesota

James B. Seward, M.D.
Consultant, Division of Cardiovascular Diseases, Mayo Clinic; Professor of Medicine, Mayo Clinic College of Medicine; Rochester, Minnesota

Tait D. Shanafelt, M.D.
Senior Associate Consultant, Division of Hematology, Mayo Clinic; Assistant Professor of Medicine, Mayo Clinic College of Medicine; Rochester, Minnesota

Clarence Shub, M.D.
Consultant, Division of Cardiovascular Diseases, Mayo Clinic; Professor of Medicine, Mayo Clinic Collge of Medicine, Rochester, Minnesota

Marina G. Silvelra, M.D.
Resident in Gastroenterology and Hepatology, Mayo School of Graduate Medical Education, Mayo Clinic College of Medicine, Rochester, Minnesota

Ripudamanjit Singh, M.D.
Senior Associate Consultant, Division of Cardiovascular Diseases, Mayo School of Graduate Medical Education and Assistant Professor of Medicine, Mayo Clinic College of Medicine, Rochester, Minnesota

Kirby D. Slifer, D.O.
Resident in Pulmonary and Critical Care Medicine, Mayo School of Graduate Medical Education, Mayo Clinic College of Medicine, Rochester, Minnesota

Jay Smith, M.D.
Consultant, Department of Physical Medicine and Rehabilitation, Mayo Clinic; Associate Professor of Physical Medicine and Rehabilitation, Mayo Clinic College of Medicine; Rochester, Minnesota

Cacia V. Soares-Welch, M.D.
Resident in General Internal Medicine, Mayo School of Graduate Medical Education, Mayo Clinic College of Medicine, Rochester, Minnesota

Thomas C. Sodeman, M.D.
Advanced Fellow in Gastroenterology and Hepatology, Mayo School of Graduate Medical Education, Mayo Clinic College of Medicine, Rochester, Minnesota

Paul Y. Takahashi, M.D.
Consultant, Division of Primary Care Internal Medicine, Mayo Clinic; Assistant Professor of Medicine, Mayo Clinic College of Medicine; Rochester, Minnesota

Dariush S. Takhtehchian, M.D.
Resident in Cardiovascular Diseases, Mayo School of Graduate Medical Education, Mayo Clinic College of Medicine, Rochester, Minnesota

Pierre Theuma, M.D.
Resident in Endocrinology, Diabetes, Metabolism, Nutrition, Mayo School of Graduate Medical Education, Mayo Clinic College of Medicine, Rochester, Minnesota

Rochelle R. Torgerson, M.D., Ph.D.
Fellow in Dermatology, Mayo School of Graduate Medical Education, Mayo Clinic College of Medicine, Rochester, Minnesota

Santhi Swaroop Vege, M.D.
Consultant, Division of General Internal Medicine, Mayo Clinic; Professor of Medicine, Mayo Clinic College of Medicine; Rochester, Minnesota

K. L. Venkatachalam, M.D.
Fellow in Cardiovascular Diseases, Mayo School of Graduate Medical Education, Mayo Clinic College of Medicine, Rochester, Minnesota

Thomas R. Viggiano, M.D.
Consultant, Division of Gastroenterology and Hepatology, Mayo Clinic; Professor of Medicine, Mayo Clinic College of Medicine; Rochester, Minnesota

Stacey A. R. Vlahakis, M.D.
Senior Associate Consultant, Division of Infectious Diseases, Mayo

Clinic; Assistant Professor of Medicine, Mayo Clinic College of Medicine; Rochester, Minnesota

Kenneth J. Warrington, M.D.

Fellow in Rheumatology, Mayo School of Graduate Medical Education, Mayo Clinic College of Medicine, Rochester, Minnesota

Edwin G. Wells III, M.D.

Formerly, Student, Mayo Medical School, Mayo Clinic College of Medicine, Rochester, Minnesota; presently, Resident Physician in Emergency Medicine, Loma Linda, California

John W. Wilson, M.D.

Consultant, Division of Infectious Diseases, Mayo Clinic; Assistant Professor of Medicine, Mayo Clinic College of Medicine; Rochester, Minnesota

Walter R. Wilson, M.D.

Consultant, Division of Infectious Diseases, Mayo Clinic; Assistant Professor of Microbiology and Professor of Medicine, Mayo Clinic College of Medicine; Rochester, Minnesota

Nina Wokhlu, M.D.

Senior Resident Associate in Cardiovascular Diseases, Mayo School of Graduate Medical Education, Mayo Clinic College of Medicine, Rochester, Minnesota

Thomas P. Worley, M.D.

Resident in Hematology, Mayo School of Graduate Medical Education, Mayo Clinic College of Medicine, Rochester, Minnesota

Gregory A. Worrell, M.D.

Consultant, Department of Neurology, Mayo Clinic; Assistant Professor of Neurology, Mayo Clinic College of Medicine; Rochester, Minnesota

R. Scott Wright, M.D.

Consultant, Division of Cardiovascular Diseases, Mayo Clinic; Associate Professor of Medicine, Mayo Clinic College of Medicine; Rochester, Minnesota

William F. Young, Jr., M.D.

Consultant, Division of Endocrinology, Diabetes, Metabolism, Nutrition, Mayo Clinic; Professor of Medicine, Mayo Clinic College of Medicine; Rochester, Minnesota

Steven J. Younger, M.D.

Resident in Nephrology and Hypertension, Mayo School of Graduate Medical Education, Mayo Clinic College of Medicine, Rochester, Minnesota

Steven R. Ytterberg, M.D.

Consultant, Division of Rheumatology, Mayo Clinic; Associate Professor of Medicine, Mayo Clinic College of Medicine; Rochester, Minnesota

TABLE OF CONTENTS

Signs and Symptoms

Therapy

Insights

ABBREVIATIONS

The following abbreviations are used in the text, tables, and figure legends and are defined only here:

AIDS	acquired immunodeficiency syndrome
ALT	alanine aminotransferase
aPTT	activated partial thromboplastin time
AST	aspartate aminotransferase
BUN	blood urea nitrogen
CBC	complete blood count
CK	creatine kinase
CK-MB	creatine kinase, muscle & brain subunits
COPD	chronic obstructive pulmonary disease
CSF	cerebrospinal fluid
CT	computed tomography
ECG	electrocardiography
EEG	electroencephalography
EMG	electromyography
ESR	erythrocyte sedimentation rate
HIV	human immunodeficiency virus
ICU	intensive care unit
IM	intramuscular
INR	international normalized ratio
IV	intravenous
LDH	lactate dehydrogenase
MRI	magnetic resonance imaging
NPO	nothing by mouth
NSAID	nonsteroidal antiinflammatory drug
PMN	polymorphonuclear neutrophil
PO	by mouth, orally
PT	prothrombin time
PTT	partial thromboplastin time
RBC	red blood cell
SQ	subcutaneous
TB	tuberculosis
WBC	white blood cell

Other, less frequent abbreviations are defined when first used in each chapter.

ABDOMINAL PAIN

Shamina Dhillon, M.D.
Thomas R. Viggiano, M.D.

IS THE PATIENT'S LIFE AT RISK?

- Abdominal pain is a common sign encountered by interns.
- Vital signs and general appearance are clues to urgency of the underlying problem.
- Pain in conjunction with the abnormalities below often points to certain conditions that indicate imminent danger.

Hypotension and/or Tachycardia

- Bleeding—perforated viscus, ruptured aortic aneurysm, aortic dissection, ruptured spleen or solid organ (kidney, liver)
- Inflammatory response syndrome or sepsis—necrotizing fasciitis, secondary peritonitis, spontaneous bacterial peritonitis, acute pancreatitis
- Volume depletion—bowel obstruction, acute pancreatitis
- Tissue hypoperfusion—acute myocardial infarction, severe heart failure, mesenteric infarction

Altered Mental Status

- Cerebral hypoperfusion—aortic hypoperfusion, ruptured aortic aneurysm, myocardial infarction, advanced sepsis
- Severe metabolic derangement—spontaneous bacterial peritonitis, advanced sepsis, necrotizing panniculitis, mesenteric infarction
- Hypoxemia—pulmonary embolism, myocardial infarction, sepsis

Tachypnea and Low Oxygen Saturation

- Pulmonary embolism
- Heart failure
- Myocardial infarction

In addition to the above, certain clinical observations and physical examination findings point to specific life-threatening diagnoses in patients with abdominal pain. The presence of these findings should alert interns to a potentially harmful situation for the patient.

Worrisome Physical Findings
- Abdominal rigidity—perforated viscus
- Hypoactive or absent bowel sounds—perforated viscus, bowel obstruction, ischemic gut
- Patient's position
  - ▲ Lying still—perforated viscus, myocardial infarction
  - ▲ Restless/writhing—bowel obstruction, ischemic bowel

Character of Pain
- Burning—perforated ulcer and myocardial infarction
- Dull—acute appendicitis and myocardial infarction
- Tearing—aortic dissection
- Constricting—acute cholecystitis, myocardial infarction
- Boring—acute pancreatitis, expanding abdominal aortic aneurysm
- Crampy—bowel obstruction
- Diffuse—ruptured abdominal aortic aneurysm, bowel obstruction, peritonitis, heart failure

Onset of Pain
- Sudden—perforated ulcer, ruptured abdominal aortic aneurysm, aortic dissection, ruptured ectopic pregnancy, bowel ischemia
- Rapid—acute pancreatitis, acute cholecystitis
- Gradual—acute appendicitis, bowel obstruction

Radiation of Pain
- Back/flank—abdominal aortic dissection, pancreatitis
- Scapula—acute cholecystitis
- Right lower quadrant—acute appendicitis

ADDRESSING THE RISK
- Serial abdominal exams are essential when managing patients with abdominal pain. The following measures are indicated

for monitoring patients with abdominal pain and the associated condition listed below.

Hypotension

- Check orthostatic blood pressure as the patient tolerates.
- Establish large-bore IV access.
- Place Foley catheter to monitor urine output and adjust fluids.
- If blood pressure is not responding to fluid challenge, transfer to ICU for monitoring and initiate pressors.
- Involve surgery *early* if vascular catastrophe is suspected.
- Type and crossmatch 2-4 RBC units.
- ECG

Tachycardia

- Large-bore IV access
- Normal saline IV initially to increase intravascular volume maximally
- Consider type and crossmatch early.

Oliguria

- Foley catheter for accurate urine output
- Remember: urine is liquid gold, keep it flowing.
- Fluid challenge to meet urine output goal of 0.5 mL/kg per hour

Altered Mental Status

- Check arterial blood gas values early.
- Replace volume to ensure adequate blood pressure and perfusion to vital organs.
- Check electrolyte panel early because certain imbalances such as hypercalcemia can mimic abdominal pain and altered mental status.
- Check ECG and chest X-ray to rule out potential sources of hypoxia or hypercarbia.

DIFFERENTIAL DIAGNOSIS

- The differential diagnosis by anatomical location is listed in Table 1 and the extra-abdominal causes of pain are listed in Table 2.

Table 1. Differential Diagnosis by Anatomical Location

Left upper quadrant
Empyema
Gastritis
Myocardial infarction
Pancreatitis
Pneumonia
Pulmonary infarction
Splenic artery aneurysm
Splenic infarct
Splenomegaly

Left lower quadrant
Colon cancer
Diverticulitis
Ectopic pregnancy
Endometriosis
Intestinal obstruction
Ovarian cyst
Pelvic inflammatory disease
Renal calculi
Ulcerative colitis

Diffuse abdominal pain
Abdominal aortic aneurysm
Appendicitis
Colitis
Gastroenteritis
Inflammatory bowel disease
Intestinal ischemia
Mesenteric venous thrombosis
Spontaneous bacterial peritonitis

Right upper quadrant
Cholangitis
Cholecystitis
Choledochal cyst
Choledocholithiasis
Hepatic abscess
Hepatic metastasis
Hepatitis
Hepatomegaly
Pancreatitis
Peptic ulcer
Pneumonia
Pulmonary infarction
Subphrenic abscess

Right lower quadrant
Appendicitis
Crohn disease
Diverticulitis
Ectopic pregnancy
Endometriosis
Gastroenteritis
Meckel diverticulitis
Mesenteric lymphadenitis
Ovarian cyst
Pelvic inflammatory disease
Renal calculi
Ruptured peptic ulcer
Salpingitis
Ulcerative colitis

Epigastrium
Cholecystitis
Myocardial ischemia
Pancreatitis
Peptic ulcer
Reflux esophagitis

Table 2. Extra-abdominal Causes of Pain

Cardiac
  Myocardial ischemia or
    infarction
  Congestive heart failure
  Endocarditis
  Myocarditis
Thoracic
  Pneumonitis
  Pleurodynia
  Pulmonary embolism
  Pneumothorax
  Empyema
  Esophagitis
  Esophageal spasm
  Esophageal rupture
Neurologic
  Radiculitis —spinal cord or
    peripheral
  Nerve tumors
  Arthritis of spine
  Abdominal epilepsy
  Tabes dorsalis

Metabolic
  Uremia
  Diabetes mellitus
  Porphyria
  Acute adrenal insufficiency
  Hyperlipidemia
  Hyperparathyroidism
    (hypercalcemia)
Hematologic
  Sickle cell anemia
  Hemolytic anemia
  Acute leukemia
  Henoch-Schönlein purpura
Toxic
  Hypersensitivity reaction—
    insect bites, reptile venoms
  Lead poisoning
Infectious
  Herpes zoster
  Osteomyelitis
  Typhoid fever
Miscellaneous
  Muscular contusion, hema
    toma, or tumor
  Narcotic withdrawal
  Familial Mediterranean fever
  Psychiatric disorders

DIFFERENTIATING THE DIFFERENTIAL

- After first managing any immediate threat to a patient with abdominal pain, the history and physical exam can lead to the diagnosis.
- The history and physical findings that should be ascertained when considering various causes of abdominal pain are listed in Table 3.
- The history and physical findings that may be helpful in localizing the problem to a specific organ are listed in Table 4.

Table 3. Differentiating by Etiology

Vascular	Infectious	Mechanical obstruction	Metabolic	Gynecologic causes
History	**History**	**History**	**History**	**History**
Postprandial pain	NVD before pain	Previous surgical procedures	Polyuria	Date of last menstrual period
Coronary artery disease	Detailed food history	Weight loss from malignancy	Polydipsia	Previous cesarean section
Atherosclerosis	Travel history	Fever from lymphoma	Change in urine output	or TAH
Claudication	Fever	Change in bowel habits	Fatigue	Dysfunctional uterine bleeding
Physical	**Physical**	Bilious emesis	Lead exposure	Alteration in menstrual cycle
Atrial fibrillation	Bloody diarrhea	**Physical**	**Physical**	STD history
Cardiac arrhythmia	Diffuse tenderness	Abdominal scars	Dry mucous mem-	Vaginal discharge
Pulsatile mass		Abdominal wall mass	branes	Dysuria
Diminished peripheral		Abdominal distension	Hypotension	**Physical**
pulses		Hypoactive bowel sounds		Cervical motion tenderness
Abdominal bruits		Inguinal hernia		Adnexal tenderness
Pain out of proportion				Vaginal discharge
to physical findings				

NVD, nausea, vomiting, diarrhea; STD, sexually transmitted disease; TAH, total abdominal hysterectomy.

Table 4. Differentiating by Organ System

Esophagus	Stomach	Small intestine	Colon	Biliary tract	Pancreas
History	**History**	**History**	**History**	**History**	**History**
Excessive emesis (Boerhaave)	NSAID use	Flatus	History of inflammatory bowel disease	Drug/alcohol use	Alcohol use
Alcohol abuse	Relief with antacid use	Last bowel movement	History of diverticulosis	Change in stool/urine color	History of gallstones
Heartburn	Smoking	**Physical**	Tenesmus	History of transfusions	Steatorrhea
Dysphagia	Alcohol	Abdominal distension	**Physical**	Alcohol use	**Physical**
Physical	**Physical**	Visible peristaltic wave	Distension	History of gallstones	Epigastric tenderness
Subcutaneous emphysema	Epigastric tenderness			**Physical**	Cullen sign
				Jaundice	Grey Turner sign

DIAGNOSTIC TEST ORDERING

- For all patients with abdominal pain, the following lab tests should be ordered:
  - ▲ CBC with differential
  - ▲ Electrolytes
  - ▲ Urinalysis
  - ▲ Pregnancy test in women of childbearing age
  - ▲ CT of abdomen with and without contrast
- The appropriate tests for various signs and symptoms are given in Table 5.
- Diagnostic tests for specific disease states are listed in Table 6.

INITIAL MANAGEMENT

Abdominal Aortic Aneurysm Rupture

- *Surgical emergency!*
- Type and crossmatch at least 4 units of blood immediately.
- Resuscitate with fluids and blood as needed until operating room is ready.
- Preoperative antibiotic prophylaxis

Acute Cholecystitis

- Start fluids—0.9 normal saline for replacement, initial fluid bolus if hypovolemic

Table 5. Appropriate Tests According to Signs and Symptoms

Signs/symptoms	Appropriate tests
Fever, abdominal pain	CBC, blood cultures, paracentesis if ascites, CT
Peritoneal signs	Abdominal film—flat and upright, CT
RUQ pain	Ultrasound, AST, ALT, alkaline phosphatase, total/direct bilirubin, CT
Epigastric pain	Amylase, lipase, AST, ALT, ultrasound, CT
Diarrhea, fever	Fecal WBCs, stool bacterial & parasite cultures, *Clostridium difficile* toxin if recent antibiotic use
Pulsatile mass	Abdominal ultrasound, CT
Diffuse pain, athero-sclerosis risk	LDH, ABG to assess acidosis, ECG, angiography with contrast CT

ABG, arterial blood gases; RUQ, right upper quadrant.

Table 6. Diagnostic Tests for Specific Disease States

Suspected diagnosis	Diagnostic modalities
Ruptured abdominal aortic aneurysm, aortic dissection	CT Ultrasound
Perforated viscus	Plain *upright* film (pneumoperitoneum in 75% of patients) CT with water-soluble contrast to localize perforation
Bowel obstruction	Plain abdominal films CT
Acute pancreatitis	Lipase (sensitivity, 60%; specificity, 80%-99%), CT if complications suspected
Appendicitis	Ultrasound
Cholecystitis	Ultrasound (positive predictive value of Murphy sign, 90%)
Ruptured ectopic pregnancy	Transvaginal ultrasound (sensitivity, 84.4%; specificity, 98.9% if positive pregnancy test)

- NPO except oral medication
- Start antibiotics—piperacillin-tazobactam (Zosyn)* 3.375 mg IV every 6 hours if renal function is preserved
- Surgical consult
- Nasogastric suctioning if persistent emesis

Acute Appendicitis
- NPO
- Start fluids
- Ampicillin-sulbactam (Unasyn)* 3 g IV every 6 hours
- Surgical consult
- Antipyretics

Acute Pancreatitis
- NPO
- Nasogastric tube if emesis

---

*These antibiotics are suggestions and can be modified as indicated by the clinical scenario.

- Aggressive fluid therapy because fluid depletion is usually between 1 and 3 L
- Foley catheter to monitor urine output, at least 0.5 mL/kg per hour
- Oxygen
- Alcohol withdrawal prophylaxis
- H_2-blockers
- Imipenem if necrosis is suspected
- Monitor calcium and magnesium levels.
- Analgesia for pain control
- Think ahead for nutritional support if long-term NPO status.

Small-Bowel Obstruction
- NPO
- H_2-blockers
- Nasogastric tube
- Fluid therapy
- Analgesia for pain control
- Serial abdominal exams every 6 hours
- Piperacillin-tazobactam* 3.375 mg IV every 6 hours if renal function preserved

Acute Diverticulitis
- Metronidazole (Flagyl)* 500 mg 4 times daily and levofloxacin (Levaquin)* 500 mg PO once daily
- Bowel rest
- NPO
- IV fluids
- Analgesia for pain control

---

*These antibiotics are suggestions and can be modified as indicated by the clinical scenario.

ANEMIA

Miguel A. Park, M.D.
Paul S. Mueller, M.D.

IS THE PATIENT'S LIFE AT RISK?

- Several clinical situations involving anemic patients warrant immediate evaluation and treatment.
  - ▲ Active bleeding, especially if hypovolemia or shock is present
  - ▲ Evidence of myocardial ischemia (e.g., angina pectoris, myocardial infarction) and/or ischemia of other tissues
  - ▲ Evidence of new-onset hemolysis

ADDRESSING THE RISK

Active Bleeding, Especially if Hypovolemia or Shock Is Present

- Obtain IV access with 2 large-bore (16-gauge if possible) catheters for rapid fluid resuscitation and/or transfusion. Resistance to flow is determined by both the length and diameter of the catheter. A short peripheral IV catheter causes less resistance to flow than a long central line of the same diameter. Hence, peripheral IV catheters may be better suited for rapid fluid resuscitation and/or transfusion than a central line.
- If the clinical situation allows, type and crossmatch the patient's blood. Otherwise, give type O-negative blood.
- Closely monitor for evidence of hypovolemia and shock (e.g., blood pressure, jugular venous pressure, urine output).
- Identify and address the source of bleeding.

Evidence of Myocardial Ischemia and/or Ischemia of Other Tissues

- Appropriately evaluate and treat myocardial ischemia,

Special abbreviation used in this chapter: RI, reticulocyte index.

- If hemoglobulin is <10 g/dL and/or hematocrit is ≤30%, some evidence suggests that RBC transfusions may be beneficial.

Evidence of New-Onset Hemolysis
- Assess for myocardial and other tissue ischemia (see above).
- Request an immediate hematology consult.
- If evidence of thrombotic thrombocytopenic purpura, prepare for possible plasma exchange.

DIFFERENTIAL DIAGNOSIS
Definition
- Anemia is defined by the World Health Organization as hemoglobin <12 g/dL in women and <13 g/dL in men

DIFFERENTIATING THE DIFFERENTIAL
A history and physical exam are the first steps in the evaluation of anemia.

History
- Is there a personal and/or family history of anemia (e.g., sickle cell, thalassemia, hereditary spherocytosis)?
- Are there any past or present medical conditions that can cause anemia (e.g., rheumatoid arthritis, systemic lupus erythematosus, chronic renal failure, gastroesophageal reflux disease with Cameron erosions, liver disease, endocrine disease)?
- Review for medications that may cause anemia (e.g., NSAIDs, anticoagulants, alcohol, chemotherapy agents).
- Is there a history of blood loss (e.g., menorrhagia, bloody or black stools, hematemesis, blood-tinged urine, retroperitoneal hemorrhage)?
- What is the patient's general nutritional state (e.g., involuntary weight loss)?
- Is there a history of a recent viral illness (which is associated with aplastic anemia)?
- If female, is the patient of childbearing age (e.g., pregnancy, HELLP syndrome)? Note: HELLP is hemolytic anemia, elevated liver function tests, low platelets.

Physical Exam
- Skin, nails, and eyes

- ▲ Jaundice (hemolysis)
- ▲ Bruising and ecchymoses (e.g., aplastic anemia, myelodysplastic syndrome)
- ▲ Koilonychia, or "spooning" of the nails (iron deficiency)
- ▲ Atrophic glossitis and angular stomatitis (iron deficiency)
- ▲ Pallor
- ▪ Lymphadenopathy
- ▪ Cardiovascular
  - ▲ Malfunctioning mechanical valve (hemolysis)
  - ▲ Murmur
- ▪ Abdominal/rectal
  - ▲ Hepatosplenomegaly
  - ▲ Rectal exam for blood and mass
- ▪ Musculoskeletal
  - ▲ Bone tenderness or pain (e.g., leukemia, multiple myeloma, metastatic cancer)
- ▪ Pelvic examination, especially if child-bearing age (ruptured ectopic pregnancy)
- ▪ Neurologic
  - ▲ Loss of vibration and position sense (vitamin B_{12} deficiency)
- ▪ Any site of biopsy or surgical wound
- ▪ Figures 1-3 and Tables 1-9 assist in evaluating patients who have common causes of anemia.

Table 1. Microcytic Anemia— Mean Corpuscular Volume <80 fL

Iron deficiency (see Table 4)
Thalassemia syndromes
Anemia of chronic disease
Lead poisoning
Sideroblastic anemia
Celiac sprue
Vitamin B_6 deficiency

Table 2. Macrocytic Anemia—Mean Corpuscular Volume >100 fL

Alcohol abuse
Vitamin B_{12}/folate deficiency
Liver disease
Hypothyroidism
Chemotherapy/drugs (see Table 5)
Myelodysplasia
Reticulocytosis
Cell-counter artifact

Table 3. Normocytic Anemia—Mean Corpuscular Volume 80-100 fL

Decreased production (see Table 6)
Increased destruction (see Table 7)
Early blood loss

Table 4. Iron Deficiency Anemia

Blood loss	Increased requirement	Decreased absorption
Gastrointestinal ulcers, malignancies, sprue, esophagitis, etc.	Pregnancy	Partial gastrectomy
Menstruation		Malabsorption syndromes
Phlebotomy, surgery, trauma		Sprue
Genitourinary: renal cell cancer, paroxysmal nocturnal hemoglobinuria, etc.		
Infections: schistosomiasis, hookworm, etc.		

Table 5. Medications Associated With Macrocytosis

Alcohol	Phenobarbital
Azathioprine	Phenytoin
Cytosine arabinoside (cytarabine)	Primidone
5-Fluorouracil	Sulfamethoxazole
Hydroxyurea	Sulfasalazine
Methotrexate	Triamterene
Oral contraceptives	Zidovudine

Table 6. Differential Diagnosis of Decreased Production in Normocytic Anemias

Inflammatory states/ anemia of chronic disease	Renal disease	Hypometabolic/hypermeta- bolic states	Bone marrow failure/infiltration
Collagen vascular disease	End-stage renal disease	Protein deprivation	Chemotherapy, radiation, medications, toxins
Acute/chronic infections	Nephritis	Endocrine deficiency states	Infections
Bacterial		Hypothyroidism	TB
TB		Hypopituitarism	Epstein-Barr virus
Hepatitis C		Adrenal insufficiency	HIV
HIV		Hyperthyroidism	Parvovirus
Malignancies		Hyperparathyroidism	Malignancies
Chronic granulomatous diseases (e.g., sarcoidosis)			Metastatic (e.g., breast, prostate, lung)
			Leukemia/lymphoma
			Multiple myeloma
			Myelofibrosis
			Paroxysmal nocturnal hemoglobinuria, which can present as myelofibrosis or acute leukemia

Table 6 (continued)

Inflammatory states/ anemia of chronic disease	Renal disease	Hypometabolic/hypermetabolic states	Bone marrow failure/infiltration
			Aplastic anemia:
			Idiopathic
			Fanconi anemia (autosomal recessive disorder presenting with severe pancytopenia in 1st 2 decades of life)
			Pure RBC aplasia, including Diamond-Blackfan anemia (congenital form of pure RBC aplasia appearing in childhood)
			Graft-versus-host disease

Modified from Hillman RS, Ault KA. Hematology in clinical practice: a guide to diagnosis and management. 2nd ed. New York: McGraw-Hill; 1998. p. 62. Used with permission.

Table 7. Intravascular and Extravascular Hemolysis for Normocytic Anemia

Intravascular	Extravascular
Blood transfusion: ABO mismatched transfusion	Autoimmune hemolysis
	Warm-reacting (IgG) AIHA
Bacterial/parasitic infections	Cold-reacting (IgM) AIHA
Bartonellosis	Bacterial and viral infections
Clostridial sepsis	Infectious mononucleosis
Malaria	Malaria
Mycoplasma pneumonia	*Mycoplasma* pneumonia
Paroxysmal hemoglobinuria	Drug-induced hemolysis
Paroxysmal nocturnal hemoglobinuria	Glucose-6-phosphate dehydrogenase deficiency
Paroxysmal cold hemoglobinuria	Autoimmune drug reactions
	Hemoglobinopathies
Mechanical heart valves	Thalassemia syndromes
Snake bites	Sickle cell disease
Thermal burns	Membrane structural defects
	Hereditary spherocytosis
	Hereditary elliptocytosis
	Acanthocytosis
	Others
	Disseminated intravascular coagulation
	Thrombotic thrombocytopenic purpura
	Hemolytic uremic syndrome
	Eclampsia (HELLP syndrome)

AIHA, autoimmune hemolytic anemia; HELLP, hemolytic anemia, elevated liver function tests, low platelets.

Modified from Hillman RS, Ault KA. Hematology in clinical practice: a guide to diagnosis and management. 2nd ed. New York: McGraw-Hill; 1998. p. 187-8. Used with permission.

Table 8. Serum Profiles of Selected Anemias

	Marrow damage	Acute/chronic inflammatory	Renal disease	Hypometabolic states	Thalassemia	Iron deficiency	Hemoglobinopathy	Macrocytic anemia	Dysplastic	Sideroblastic	Chronic hemolytic
RBC morphology	Normolytic/normochromic	Normocytic/microcytic	Normocytic	Variable	Microcytic/hypochromic	Normocytic/microcytic hypochromic	Normocytic/normochromic	Macrocytic/normochromic	Mixed	Mixed	Normocytic/normochromic
RI	<2	<2	<2	<2	<2	<2	>3-5	<1	<2	<2	>3-5
Serum iron	N1/increased	Decreased	N1	N1	N1/increased	Decreased	N1/increased	Increased	N1	Increased	N1
TIBC	N1	Decreased	N1	N1	N1	Increased	N1	N1	N1	N1	N1
Serum ferritin	Increased	Increased	N1	N1	>100 µg/L	<10 µg/L	>100 µg/L	Increased	N1	N1/increased	N1/increased
% Saturation	30-50	10-20	N1	N1	>20	<10	NA	>50	NA	NA	NA

NA, not applicable; N1, normal; RI, reticulocyte index; TIBC, total iron-binding capacity.

Table 9. Clues in the Peripheral Smear to the Diagnosis of Anemia

Peripheral smear finding	Differential diagnosis
Basophilic stippling	Lead poisoning, β-thalassemia, megaloblastic anemia, sideroblastic anemia
Bite cells	G6PD
Blasts	Leukemia
Burr cells	Uremia
Heinz bodies	G6PD
Howell-Jolly bodies	Hyposplenism, megaloblastic anemia
Hypersegmented neutrophils	Vitamin B_{12} and/or folate deficiency
Rouleau formation	Multiple myeloma
Schistocytes	TTP, HUS, HELLP syndrome, DIC, collagen vascular disease, heart valve hemolysis
Spherocytes	Hereditary spherocytosis, autoimmune hemolytic anemia, severe burns
Spur cells (acanthrocytes)	Chronic liver disease
Target cells	Liver disease, thalassemia
Teardrop cells (dacrocytes)	Myelofibrosis

DIC, disseminated intravascular coagulation; G6PD, glucose-6-phosphate dehydrogenase deficiency; HELLP, hemolytic anemia, elevated liver function tests, low platelets; HUS, hemolytic uremic syndrome; TTP, thrombotic thrombocytopenic purpura.

TESTS AND WORK-UP

- After a thorough history and physical exam, all anemia evaluations should include hemoglobin level, hematocrit, mean cell volume, reticulocyte count, and a peripheral blood smear. Specimens for a peripheral blood smear and reticulocyte count should be drawn before blood transfusions unless the clinical situation warrants emergent transfusion.
- The reticulocyte count should be converted to the reticulocyte index (RI).

    RI = % reticulocyte × (patient hematocrit/normal hematocrit)
- The RI is divided by 2 if nucleated RBCs are present.
- Most cases of anemia are diagnosed with this basic approach. If not, this approach usually suggests the next steps.

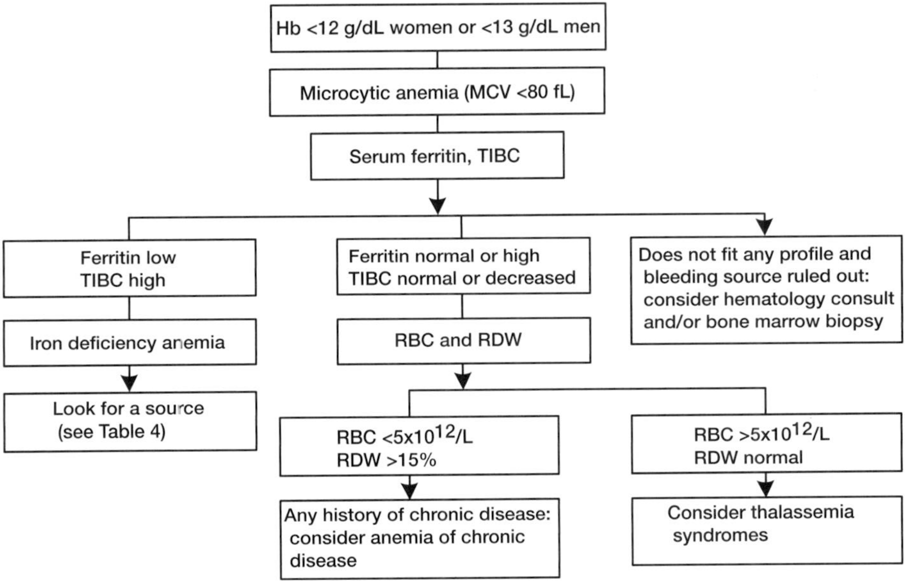

Fig. 1. Algorithm for the diagnosis of microcytic anemia. Hb, hemoglobin; MCV, mean corpuscular volume; TIBC, total iron-binding capacity; RDW, red cell distribution width.

MANAGEMENT

Management of anemia includes the treatment of the underlying cause of the anemia. Two special circumstances are considered.

Iron Deficiency Anemia

- After the underlying source of iron deficiency anemia is addressed, oral supplement with iron is the treatment of choice.

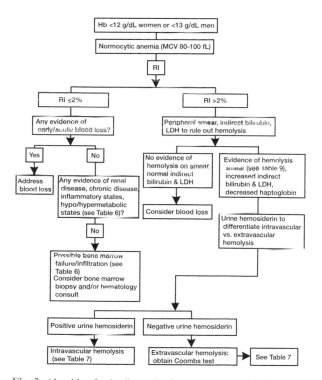

Fig. 2. Algorithm for the diagnosis of normocytic anemia. Hb, hemoglobin; MCV, mean corpuscular volume; RI, reticulocyte index.

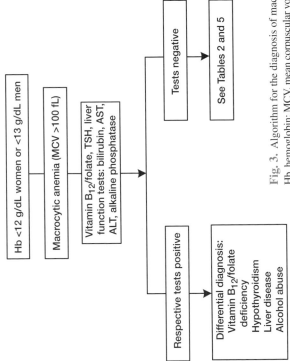

Fig. 3. Algorithm for the diagnosis of macrocytic anemia. Hb, hemoglobin; MCV, mean corpuscular volume; TSH, thyroid-stimulating hormone.

- Ferrous sulfate, 325 mg orally 3 times daily, is given 1 hour before or 2 hours after a meal.
- For better absorption, ascorbic acid 250 mg can be given with the ferrous sulfate.
- Check CBC in 4 weeks.
- Six months of treatment should replenish the iron stores.

Indications for RBC Transfusion
- In most cases, RBC transfusion is not indicated for hemoglobin >10 g/dL.
- RBC transfusion is indicated for hemoglobin <7 g/dL. Two units of RBCs should be given to those who are stable. Some patients may need more units of RBCs depending on the rate of ongoing blood loss.
- It is unclear if RBC transfusion is warranted for patients with hemoglobin of 7-10 g/dL. RBC transfusions may be beneficial for patients with myocardial ischemia who have hemoglobin <10 g/dL and/or hematocrit ≤30%.
- Patients >65 years and/or who have cardiovascular or respiratory disease (e.g., COPD) may not tolerate anemia. These patients may benefit from RBC transfusions if hemoglobin <8 g/dL.

BACK PAIN

A. Scott Keller, M.D.
Jay Smith, M.D.

IS THE PATIENT'S LIFE AT RISK?

- Rapidly assess the patient: vital signs, history (predisposing factors), physical exam.

Abdominal Aortic Aneurysm Rupture

- Classic triad of abdominal or back pain, hypotension, and pulsatile abdominal mass (usually left of midline and above umbilicus)
  - ▲ Signs and symptoms of shock—hypotension, tachycardia, mental status change
  - ▲ May lead to spinal cord infarction or death if rupture occurs
- Pulses or blood pressure may be unequal in upper vs. lower extremities or in left vs. right lower limb.
- Consider the history—age, hypertension, atherosclerosis, peripheral vascular disease, known abdominal aortic aneurysm with recent expansion and/or diameter >5 cm, spontaneous symptom onset, use of anticoagulants.

Aortic Dissection

- Spontaneous onset of acute, severe, tearing pain in the chest and/or interscapular region
  - ▲ Pain may last hours and often requires high doses of analgesia.
  - ▲ Pain is unrelated to position, but it may wax and wane.
  - ▲ Patient may have associated syncope, weakness, or paralysis from spinal cord ischemia.
- Patient may have hypertension or hypotension and pulses or blood pressure may be unequal in upper vs. lower or left vs. right extremities
  - ▲ Pulses may be absent.
  - ▲ Patient may have new-onset aortic regurgitation, pulmonary

edema, or neurologic deficits.
- Consider the history—spontaneous onset, age, hypertension, cystic medial necrosis, Marfan syndrome, congenital bicuspid valve, coarctation, third-trimester pregnancy, history of blunt chest trauma (e.g., motor vehicle accident).

Cord Compression (Due to Trauma, Tumor, or Infection)
- Pain is localized to back and/or lower limb, worsens with movement, coughing, sneezing, or straining (Valsalva effect).
  - ▲ Patient may have Lhermitte phenomenon, a shock-like sensation along the spinal cord precipitated by head flexion.
  - ▲ Exam often reveals spinal percussion tenderness, upper motor neuron signs, and possibly a sensory level.
  - ▲ If the conus medullaris or cauda equina is involved, lower motor neuron findings may be present, including dermatomal deficits.
  - ▲ Patient may have bladder/bowel difficulties
- Pain from trauma—caused by contact or heavy lifting; may involve disk herniation, fracture with bony impingement (e.g., osteoporosis), or epidural hematoma
- Pain from tumor
  - ▲ History of cancer suggests metastatic spine involvement until proved otherwise.
  - ▲ Tumor is suggested by lack of comfortable position or by increased pain when supine or at nighttime.
- Pain from infection (epidural abscess)
  - ▲ Classic triad of pain (along spine or leg), fever, and weakness; rapidly progressive
  - ▲ Consider the history of immune system compromise—diabetes mellitus, renal failure, alcoholism, malignancy, IV drug abuse, HIV, prolonged steroid use.
  - ▲ Also consider other infections (skin, vertebral osteomyelitis, decubitus ulcer, spinal surgery, pyelonephritis); most are due to *Staphylococcus aureus*; streptococcal organisms and gram-negative bacilli are other common causes.

ADDRESSING THE RISK
See Table 1.

DIFFERENTIAL DIAGNOSIS
See Table 2.

Table 1. Addressing the Risk

Condition	Vital signs	Symptoms	Exam findings	Treatment
Abdominal aortic aneurysm rupture	Hypotension, unequal pulse/blood pressure upper vs. lower limbs	Severe pain in abdomen, back, flank(s), shock	Pulsatile abdominal mass	Two large-bore IVs of normal saline, blood, emergency surgery consult Don't waste time on tests!
Aortic dissection	Hypertension or hypotension, loss of pulses	Acute tearing pain in chest and/or interscapular area	Loss of or unequal pulses/blood pressure Aortic regurgitation, pulmonary edema, neurologic findings	If hypertensive, give IV β-blocker (pulse 60), sodium nitroprusside If hypotensive, IV fluid & blood, TEE, CT Emergency surgical consult
Cord compression (trauma, tumor, epidural abscess)	Fever (if infection or tumor), otherwise may be normal	Back pain, usually aggravated by coughing or straining Weakness/numbness of legs, bladder or bowel disturbances	Localized spinal tenderness, lower motor neuron & dermatomal deficits	Emergency spine surgery consult and analgesics CT, MRI, possibly lumbar puncture Surgery if trauma, dexamethasone and surgery if tumor, IV antibiotics & surgery if infection

TEE, transesophageal echocardiography.

27

Table 2. Differential Diagnosis

Gastrointestinal	Rheumatologic
Bowel disorder	Ankylosing spondylitis
Gallbladder disease	Polymyalgia rheumatica
Pancreatic disease	Psoriatic arthritis
Peptic ulcer	Reiter syndrome
Gynecologic	Rheumatoid arthritis
Ectopic pregnancy	Spinal
Endometriosis	Arachnoiditis
Ovarian cyst or tumor	Disk herniation
Ovarian torsion	Osteoarthritis
Pregnancy	Spinal stenosis
Tubo-ovarian abscess	Spondylolysis
Hematologic	Spondylolisthesis
Sickle cell crisis	Primary tumor
Infectious	Metastatic tumor
Diskitis	Trauma
Epidural abscess	Vertebral fracture
Herpes zoster	Traumatic spondylolysis
Meningitis	Osteoporotic compression
Myelitis	fracture
Osteomyelitis	Musculoskeletal/ligamentous
Pneumonia	strain
Prostatitis	Vascular disease
Sacroiliitis	Abdominal aortic aneurysm
TB (Pott disease)	rupture
Urinary	Aortic dissection
Metabolic	Myocardial infarction
Hyperparathyroidism	Pulmonary embolism
Osteomalacia	Spinal cord infarction
Osteoporosis	(anterior spinal artery)
Paget disease	Other
Psychiatric	Diffuse idiopathic skeletal
Anxiety	hyperostosis
Depression	Fibromyalgia
Functional/malingering	Pericarditis
Substance abuse	Pleural effusion
Renal	Pyriformis syndrome
Infection	Retroperitoneal fibrosis,
Polycystic kidney	hemorrhage, or mass
Renal vein thrombosis	
Stone	
Tumor	

DIFFERENTIATING THE DIFFERENTIAL

Gastrointestinal

- Bowel disorders
  - ▲ Abdominal pain, possible radiation to back, nausea/vomiting, diarrhea or constipation, possible hematochezia or melena
  - ▲ Abdominal X-ray, CBC, electrolytes, CT
  - ▲ May need upper and lower barium studies, colonoscopy
- Gallbladder disease
  - ▲ Right upper quadrant pain (colicky postprandial if stones, constant if cholecystitis), can be referred to right shoulder (diaphragm irritation)
  - ▲ Altered bowel sounds, nausea/vomiting, Murphy sign
  - ▲ CBC, liver function tests, alkaline phosphatase, ultrasound
- Pancreatitis or pancreatic cancer
  - ▲ Pain is epigastric and can radiate to back, often worse when the patient is supine.
  - ▲ Nausea, vomiting, shock
  - ▲ Patient may have fever.
  - ▲ CBC, lipase, amylase, liver function tests, calcium, LDH, lipids
  - ▲ Abdominal X-ray may show calcifications, CT most helpful
- Peptic ulcer perforation
  - ▲ Usually associated with epigastric pain
  - ▲ Can cause acute upper abdominal and back pain, shock, peritoneal signs, decreased bowel sounds, rectal bleeding (may be occult)
  - ▲ Abdominal X-ray to check for free air, CBC, amylase, esophagogastroduodenoscopy, gastric lavage

Gynecologic

- Usually low abdominal and/or pelvic pain
  - ▲ Pain may radiate to back if uterosacral ligament is involved.
  - ▲ Obtain history of sexual activity, sexually transmitted diseases (including salpingitis), birth control, and menstruation.

- ▲ Perform gynecologic and abdominal exam.
- ▲ Fever can indicate infection.
- ■ Hypotension/shock, vaginal bleeding, and amenorrhea can imply ruptured ectopic pregnancy.
- ■ CBC, β-human chorionic gonadotropin, blood cultures if infection, pelvic/transvaginal ultrasound or pelvic CT

Hematologic (Sickle Cell Disease)
- ■ Back pain may be due to acute sickle crisis with bone ischemia/infarct, osteomyelitis (*S. aureus*, *E. coli*, *Salmonella*), or vertebral compression from bone marrow hyperplasia with cortical thinning.
- ■ CBC, blood cultures, X-rays
- ■ Fluid hydration, analgesia, oxygen as needed, appropriate antibiotics as necessary

Infectious
- ■ History of IV drug use, urinary tract infection, skin infection (including herpetic lesions), previous back surgery
  - ▲ Back pain plus fever; patient may have progressive neurologic involvement
  - ▲ CBC, ESR, C-reactive protein, blood cultures, empiric IV antibiotics (vancomycin, nafcillin)
  - ▲ CT/MRI, plain X-rays
  - ▲ May need biopsy to confirm organism
- ■ Infectious or inflammatory myelitis can present with focal neck or back pain with progressive neurologic involvement.
  - ▲ Causes include herpes zoster, Cytomegalovirus, herpes simplex, Epstein-Barr virus, rabies, or schistosomiasis.
  - ▲ Can be associated with systemic lupus erythematosus, Sjögren disease, Behçet disease, and sarcoidosis
  - ▲ MRI of spine and brain with gadolinium
  - ▲ CSF usually shows mononuclear pleocytosis, PMNs may be present, protein levels may be elevated.

Metabolic
- ■ May be chronic pain or acute onset from fracture
  - ▲ Patient may have radicular symptoms or signs if there is neural compression.
  - ▲ Check X-rays, alkaline phosphatase, calcium, phosphate, and 25-hydroxyvitamin D. May check parathyroid hormone.

  ▲ Check creatinine, sodium, and potassium
- Osteomalacia = poor quality bone—25-hydroxyvitamin D is low, alkaline phosphatase is increased, calcium is low or normal, phosphate may be low, urinary calcium is low; bone biopsy is diagnostic
- Osteoporosis = low-density bone—serum calcium and phosphate generally normal
  ▲ Phosphate can be increased if postmenopausal; alkaline phosphatase can be increased if recent fracture.
  ▲ Check bone density and metabolic screen for reversible causes.
- Paget disease = chaotic bone resorption and formation—alkaline phosphatase is increased, but calcium and phosphate are normal; urinary pyridinoline collagen cross links are increased.
  ▲ X-rays show mixed areas of sclerosis and lysis (also seen in some bone tumors).

Psychiatric

- Past history of mental illness (depression, anxiety, psychosis), substance abuse, or childhood abuse. Always rule out true pathology!
- Waddell signs suggest significant psychologic distress rather than true pathology; consider psychologic/psychiatric referral if 3 of 5 tests are positive, although some may be seen in neuropathic pain.
- Waddell signs can be remembered by acronym TORDS: tenderness, overreaction, regionalization, distraction, and simulated tests.
  ▲ Superficial tenderness or deep pain over entire lumbar area when skin is lightly pinched/rolled.
  ▲ Overreaction is disproportionate verbalization and expression.
  ▲ Regionalization involves nonanatomic pain, weakness, or give-way weakness during test but normal strength spontaneously.
  ▲ Distracting tests produce discordant findings, such as no back pain when patient is sitting and knee is extended,

but severe back pain with supine straight leg raise.

▲ Simulated tests give the appearance of checking for pathology but should not elicit back pain. Two such tests are axial loading (pressing downward on standing patient's head) and rotation (when the shoulders and pelvis are passively rotated in the same plane while the patient stands relaxed with feet together).

Renal

- Can cause abdominal, flank, or back pain along with hematuria
- Stones and infections can cause urinary frequency, urgency, and dysuria.
  - ▲ Stone pain is usually colicky and may radiate into groin.
  - ▲ Ultrasound or pelvic CT, CBC, urinalysis, and urine culture
  - ▲ Blood cultures if fever
- Infection and renal vein thrombosis can cause fever.
  - ▲ Thrombosis can lead to hemorrhagic infarct, causing hypovolemia, shock, and poor renal function.
  - ▲ Check for elevated LDH and alkaline phosphatase.
  - ▲ Hypertension occurs in cases of bilateral thrombosis.
  - ▲ Elderly patients may have pulmonary emboli.
- Tumors may cause back pain from local invasion or spinal metastasis; tumor mass and polycystic kidneys may be palpable.

Rheumatologic

- All may have elevated ESR, most respond to NSAIDs and/or corticosteroids.
- Rheumatoid arthritis
  - ▲ Symmetric, deforming joint involvement, prolonged morning stiffness
  - ▲ Anemia, usually positive rheumatoid factor, may have rheumatoid nodules
  - ▲ Treat with guided exercise, rest, NSAIDs; may need azathioprine, hydroxychloroquine, or methotrexate
- Reiter syndrome
  - ▲ Low back pain from sacroiliitis, tenderness of Achilles tendon insertion, uveitis, urethritis, and sausage digits
  - ▲ Ask about recent bowel or genitourinary infections (*Campylobacter, Chlamydia, Salmonella, Shigella, Yersinia*).

- Psoriatic arthritis
  - ▲ Asymmetric arthritis, psoriasis, sausage digits
  - ▲ May precede or follow skin lesions
  - ▲ Check scalp, gluteal cleft, and umbilicus.
- Ankylosing spondylitis
  - ▲ Young adults, M>F
  - ▲ Gradual onset low back pain that limits mobility because of sacroiliitis
  - ▲ Prolonged morning stiffness that improves with exercise
  - ▲ "Bamboo spine" and sacroiliac erosions (fusion in later stages) on X-ray
  - ▲ Patient may have elevated ESR, usually has HLA-B27 (but so do 7%-8% of normal population).
- Polymyalgia rheumatica
  - ▲ Painful muscles worse with movement, leading to apparent (not true) weakness. CK is usually normal.
  - ▲ Morning stiffness and inexplicable shoulder and hip girdle pain, may have headache, jaw claudication, visual changes if associated with temporal arteritis
  - ▲ If visual changes occur, treat immediately with steroids to prevent blindness.
  - ▲ May have systemic symptoms such as fever, malaise, and weight loss

Spinal Disorders
- Arachnoiditis
  - ▲ Inflammation and fibrosis of arachnoid layer of spinal meninges
  - ▲ Severe back and radicular pain; may fluctuate in intensity and distribution and result in weakness
  - ▲ May be idiopathic or follow subarachnoid hemorrhage, meningitis, trauma, surgery, intrathecal injections; limited treatment options
  - ▲ Exam consistent with mixed mechanical-radicular syndrome
  - ▲ MRI shows clumping of nerve roots in cauda equina or empty thecal sac (nerve roots stuck to periphery of thecal sac).

- Disk herniation
  - ▲ Usually, but not always, related to traumatic event
  - ▲ Pain often begins in lower back and radiates to buttocks and into leg(s) below knee.
  - ▲ S1 radiculopathy may manifest as buttock pain only, without distal radiation.
  - ▲ Pain may be worse in leg than back; it is increased with sitting, straining, coughing, and forward flexion.
  - ▲ Patient may lean ("sciatic scoliosis") and have muscle spasm, myotomal weakness, dermatomal sensory deficit, and reflex loss.
  - ▲ Straight leg raise may be positive—*leg pain* produced when extended lower limb is passively raised while patient is supine. It is more specific if symptoms occur at <60° of straight leg raise.
  - ▲ Crossed straight-leg raise occurs when contralateral leg is raised and symptoms are reproduced in the symptomatic leg; this is not sensitive but very specific for mass lesions (e.g., lumbar disk) causing radiculopathy.
  - ▲ Cauda equina syndrome is a surgical emergency and manifests as asymmetric leg weakness or sensory loss (including perianal area), variable areflexia, and bowel/bladder dysfunction; X-rays usually show osteoarthritis, MRI is test of choice when necessary.
- Osteoarthritis
  - ▲ Pain worsens with activity, resolves with rest
  - ▲ Brief morning stiffness, gelling, local tenderness, crepitus
  - ▲ X-rays exclude other important osseous problems, but radiographic osteoarthritis is not always symptomatic.
- Spinal stenosis
  - ▲ Low back pain, motor weakness, and pseudoclaudication (leg numbness or aching when walking, relieved with rest, but normal pedal pulses)
  - ▲ Pain is aggravated by extension of lumbar spine and relieved by flexion and rest.
  - ▲ Spinal stenosis may occur centrally (as described above) or laterally, causing radicular symptoms with pseudoclaudicatory features.
  - ▲ X-rays usually show osteoarthritis; MRI is diagnostic of structural stenosis, but structural stenosis not always symptomatic.

- Spondylolysis (stress fracture of the pars interarticularis, usually at L5-S1)
  - ▲ Low back pain, worse with standing or extending
  - ▲ Stork test—standing on one leg and extending may produce pain on that side.
  - ▲ X-ray may show fracture up to 70% of time; oblique views are more sensitive.
  - ▲ Bone scans and CT (thin cut with contiguous slices) are very sensitive; MRI is less sensitive.
  - ▲ If bilateral, spondylolysis may develop into spondylolisthesis.
- Spondylolisthesis (forward slippage of one vertebra over another)
  - ▲ Low back pain, typically worse with extension and standing
  - ▲ May result in lumbar or sacral radiculopathy because of stenosis caused by the slippage
  - ▲ May present as radiculopathy similar to disk herniation or root level pseudoclaudication as in stenosis
  - ▲ Symptoms typically are relieved with flexion, sitting, or lying supine.
  - ▲ Exam may show step-off deformity at spinous process because of forward slip, muscle hypertonicity, positive stork test (see spondylolysis), or neurologic signs if radiculopathy is present.
  - ▲ Can be isthmic (result from spondylolysis) or degenerative (usually at L4-5 and result from disk degeneration and facet joint laxity allowing slippage)
  - ▲ X-rays are diagnostic of spondylolisthesis; MRI may be needed to determine if stenosis exists; flexion-extension X-rays may show instability if the segment is hypermobile.

Trauma
- Suggested by history, local tenderness
- Musculoskeletal or ligamentous strain is the most common cause of acute low back pain. Patient may have paraspinal muscle tenderness and spasm but not radicular signs or neurologic deficits.

- Osteoporotic compression fracture is seen most commonly in elderly white women. It is often seen with minimal trauma, such as opening a window. X-rays confirm the diagnosis.
- Vertebral fracture is usually from significant fall or motor vehicle accident. X-rays confirm the diagnosis.

Tumor
- Multiple myeloma is most common primary tumor.
  - ▲ Look for Bence Jones proteins in urine, check serum protein electrophoresis.
  - ▲ Other primary bone tumors, both benign and malignant, are rare and primarily observed in younger patients (10-30 years).
  - ▲ Most metastatic tumors are in older patients.
- If cauda equina or conus medullaris, treat urgently.
- Cancer risk factors include age ≥ 50 years, history of cancer, unexplained weight loss, or failure to improve after 4-6 weeks of conservative therapy.
  - ▲ If none of these four risk factors is present, cancer can be ruled out with virtually 100% sensitivity.
- Main cancers that metastasize to bone are breast, lung, lymphoma, thyroid, kidney, and prostate.
  - ▲ If metastatic cancer, usually elevated ESR and alkaline phosphatase (also acid phosphatase if prostate), calcium may be elevated.

Vascular Disease
- Ruptured aneurysm or dissection—hypotension, severe pain, pulsatile midline mass, and loss of or unequal pulses; patient may have new-onset aortic regurgitation.
- Myocardial infarction—substernal chest tightness/pressure radiating to left arm/axilla or jaw, diaphoresis, nausea, dyspnea
- Pulmonary embolism—acute dyspnea, tachycardia, pleuritic pain
- Spinal cord infarction (anterior spinal artery)—acute-onset pain, sparing of posterior columns, sharply demarcated cord level

Other
- Diffuse idiopathic skeletal hyperostosis causes spinal stiffness

and mild pain; X-rays show osteophyte formation and calcification of anterior longitudinal ligament and peripheral disk margins.

- Fibromyalgia is characterized by widespread musculoskeletal pain, stiffness, paresthesia, easy fatigability, nonrestorative sleep, and multiple symmetric tender points; it mainly affects women.
- Pericarditis may cause chest pain or pain radiating to back; it typically improves when patient leans forward.
- Pleural effusion may cause back or pleuritic pain.
- Pyriformis syndrome typically has pain and tenderness in buttock, may radiate down leg, but back pain is rare; worse when sitting; may be confused with L5-S1 radiculopathy
- Retroperitoneal fibrosis or hemorrhage
  - ▲ Fibrosis may be the cause of back pain in patients with a history of retroperitoneal injury, surgery, methysergide use, or radiation.
  - ▲ Consider hemorrhage in a patient with acute-onset lumbar pain who takes anticoagulants.

TEST ORDERING

- Urgent assessment required if fever >38°C for 48 hours, unrelenting night pain, pain with weakness or numbness below knee, leg weakness, loss of bowel or bladder control, progressive neurologic deficit, hypotension/shock; consult the appropriate service.
- Back pain with fever and rapidly progressive weakness
  - ▲ CBC, ESR, C-reactive protein, urinalysis, blood cultures, amylase, lipase, lipids
  - ▲ CT or MRI
- Back pain, hypotension
  - ▲ Call surgery
  - ▲ Chest/abdominal X-ray (free air), ultrasound, CT, or aortogram
- Tearing back pain in chest radiating to interscapular region
  - ▲ CBC, chest X-ray, ECG
  - ▲ Transesophageal echocardiogram or CT, possible aortogram

- History of cancer, age >50 years, insidious onset of pain, weight loss, pain at rest
  - Spinal/chest X-rays, mammogram
  - CBC, ESR, alkaline phosphatase, calcium, phosphate, prostate-specific antigen, thyroid-stimulating hormone, vitamin D, Bence Jones protein, serum protein electrophoresis
  - CT or MRI, possible bone scan
- Back pain with recent trauma
  - Spinal X-rays
  - Possible CT or MRI
- Back pain with radicular pain
  - MRI
  - Possible EMG

MANAGEMENT OF THE MOST COMMON CAUSES OF ACUTE BACK PAIN

Musculoskeletal

- Gentle range-of-motion exercises (bedrest 1-2 days if not able to ambulate because of pain)
- NSAIDs
- Gradual resumption of daily activities
- Muscle relaxants (e.g., cyclobenzapine [Flexeril] or baclofen) may be used initially but may cause sedation.
- Narcotics are rarely indicated.

Osteoarthritis

- NSAIDs
- Intra-articular (facet joint) corticosteroid injections may be useful.
- Regular exercise is beneficial (avoid overuse), as are heating pads or warm baths, weight reduction, and physical therapy.
- Lumbosacral corset may provide symptomatic relief.
- Can lead to radicular symptoms, cauda equina compression syndrome, spinal stenosis, disk herniation, and spondylolisthesis

Disk Herniation

- If nonprogressive radicular pain, initial nonsurgical treatment for 6 weeks allows inflammation to subside: pain resolves in 90% of patients.

- Treatment is same as for musculoskeletal pain.
- Epidural injections of corticosteroids can provide temporary relief.
- If pain does not resolve or if rapidly progressive neurologic deficits occur, surgery is indicated.

BLEEDING DISORDERS

Thomas P. Worley, M.D.
John A. Heit, M.D.
Rajiv K. Pruthi, M.B.B.S.

IS THE PATIENT'S LIFE AT RISK?

- If the following abnormalities exist, call for backup and do not let the diagnostic work-up delay stabilization of the patient:
  - ▲ Vital signs—tachycardia, hypotension
  - ▲ General appearance—pallor, cold and clammy appearance
  - ▲ Mental status changes or confusion
  - ▲ Obvious large bleeding site
  - ▲ Bleeding from numerous sites

ADDRESSING THE RISK

- For serious or life-threatening bleeding
  - ▲ Secure the airways.
  - ▲ Obtain venous access—two large-bore peripheral IVs.
  - ▲ Start fluid resuscitation with 0.9 isotonic saline, and order emergency RBCs.
  - ▲ Give nasal oxygen if intubation is not necessary.
  - ▲ Obtain a priority type and crossmatch, CBC, aPTT, PT, and fibrinogen to assess the degree of bleeding and to screen for coagulopathy.
- Evaluation
  - ▲ Mental status changes, thrombocytopenia, hemolytic anemia, fever, and renal failure are indicative of thrombotic thrombocytopenic purpura.
    - • Confirm with a peripheral blood smear (presence of schistocytes).
    - • Treatment should be started immediately (see below).
  - ▲ In a bleeding patient, specific-component replacement therapy depends on the underlying coagulation abnormality.

Special abbreviation used in this chapter: IVIg, intravenous immunoglobulin.

- Results of laboratory tests are not always available immediately; thus, it is important to assess the patient clinically, taking into account the patient's previous history (e.g., liver disease, malignancy) and medication use.
- In the absence of signs and symptoms for thrombotic thrombocytopenic purpura, replenishment with fresh frozen plasma, cryoprecipitate, and platelets should be considered.
▲ In a patient with bleeding from multiple sites, an increase in aPTT and PT, and thrombocytopenia, consider acute disseminated intravascular coagulopathy.
- Initiate a diagnostic work-up for potential causes.
▲ For patients receiving anticoagulation (heparin or warfarin) or with a known plasma coagulation disorder, attend to the following potential life-threatening issues:
- New neurologic deficits—rule out central nervous system bleeding (CT of head).
- New onset of back pain or radicular pain—rule out retroperitoneal hematoma (CT of abdomen).

DIFFERENTIAL DIAGNOSIS
- Bleeding disorders can be classified into the following four main categories:
  ▲ Platelet disorders (Table 1)
  ▲ Vascular disorders (Table 2)
  ▲ Plasma coagulation disorders (Table 3)
  ▲ Mixed disorders (Table 4)

DIFFERENTIATING THE DIFFERENTIAL
- In the hospital, abnormal bleeding is often due to the patient's underlying disease or treatment of the disease. The history and physical exam should focus on identifying the following common causes:
  ▲ Liver disease, splenomegaly, uremia
  ▲ Anticoagulation, chemotherapy administration
  ▲ Recent procedure (surgery, biopsy) that would be a source of bleeding
- Common reasons for initiating a bleeding disorder work-up
  ▲ History indicative of more bleeding than expected for a hemostatic challenge
  ▲ Spontaneous bleeding

- ▲ Physical manifestations of bleeding
- ▲ Lab abnormalities
- ▲ Determine the type of bleeding (Table 5) and the onset of bleeding (Table 6) to formulate a suggested abnormality.
- ■ Physical exam findings will suggest a diagnostic category and guide further testing (Table 7).

Table 1. Platelet Disorders

Quantitative platelet disorders (thrombocytopenia)
    Decreased production or bone marrow failure
        Aplastic anemia
        Myelofibrosis
        Leukemia
        Metastatic marrow infiltration
        Viral infection—influenza, hepatitis, rubella, HIV
        Myelosuppression—radiation, toxic agents, drugs, chemotherapy
        Vitamin B_{12}, folate deficiency
        Congenital thrombocytopenias
    Decreased survival and increased destruction
        Immune mediated
            Idiopathic thrombocytopenic purpura
            Autoimmune secondary to rheumatic disease, infection, malignancy
            Drug-induced immune thrombocytopenia—heparin, quinine
            Post-transfusion thrombocytopenia
        Nonimmune mediated
            Thrombotic thrombocytopenic purpura
            Hemolytic uremic syndrome
            HELLP syndrome
            Disseminated intravascular coagulation
            Extracorporeal circulation
            Prosthetic intravascular devices
            Paroxysmal nocturnal hemoglobinuria
            Cavernous hemangioma
    Splenic sequestration
    Dilutional thrombocytopenia (after large amounts of fluid or RBCs)
    Artifactual thrombocytopenia (platelet clumping)
    Type 2B von Willebrand disease

Table 1 (continued)

Qualitative platelet disorders
    Congenital qualitative disorders
        Bernard-Soulier syndrome (giant platelets)
        Glanzmann thrombasthenia
Paraproteinemias
    Uremia
    Liver failure
    Thrombocytosis
    Medications
        Antiplatelet drugs—aspirin/NSAIDs, clopidogrel,
          glycoprotein IIb/IIIa inhibitors
        ω-3 fatty acids
        Semisynthetic penicillins or cephalosporins

HELLP, hemolysis, elevated liver enzymes, low platelet count.

Table 2. Vascular Disorders

Congenital disorders
    Hereditary hemorrhagic telangiectasia (Rendu-Osler-Weber
      syndrome)
    Cavernous hemangioma
    Connective tissue disorders
        Ehlers-Danlos syndrome
        Osteogenesis imperfecta
        Pseudoxanthoma elasticum
Acquired disorders
    Structural abnormalities—surgical or procedural disruption,
      ulcerations, polyps, bladder or uterine abnormalities
    Scurvy
    Immunoglobulin disorders
        Cryoglobulinemia
        Benign hyperglobulinemia
        Waldenström macroglobulinemia
        Amyloidosis
        Henoch-Schönlein purpura
    Glucocorticoid excess

Table 3. Plasma Coagulation Disorders

Hereditary disorders
    Afibrinogenemia
    Dysfibrinogenemia
    Factor II deficiency
    Factor VII deficiency
    Factor XIII deficiency
    Hemophilia A (factor VIII deficiency)
    Hemophilia B (factor IX deficiency, Christmas disease)
    Hemophilia C (factor XI deficiency)
    von Willebrand disease
Acquired disorders
    Anticoagulants
    Disseminated intravascular coagulation
    Factor X deficiency (seen in amyloidosis)
    Factor VIII inhibitor (or other factor inhibitor)
    Liver disease
    Primary fibrinolysis
    Uremia
    Vitamin K deficiency

Table 4. Mixed Disorders

Liver failure
Uremia
Disseminated intravascular coagulation

Table 5. History of Bleeding Type and Associated General Abnormalities*

Type of bleeding	Disorder suggested
Mucocutaneous bleeding (i.e., epistaxis), petechiae	Platelet disorder or vasculitis
Delayed, recurrent oozing from a cut or surgical site; hematoma formation, hemarthrosis	Plasma coagulation disorder
Menorrhagia, gastrointestinal bleeding, hematuria, or central nervous system bleeding	Both platelet & coagulation defects; also must consider structural abnormality

*Note: Epistaxis and menorrhagia are classically associated with von Willebrand disease. Hemarthrosis is classically associated with hemophilia.

Table 6. History of Onset of Bleeding: Congenital Versus Acquired Bleeding Disorders

Duration of bleeding	Disorder suggested
Lifelong	Congenital defect; often of a single factor; confirm with family history (bleeding or consanguinity), personal history of bleeding with trauma, tooth extractions, circumcision, menses, surgical procedures, history of iron responsive anemia
Recent onset	Acquired disorder; usually affecting multiple coagulation factors; confirm with history of no lifelong excessive bleeding
	Inquire about concurrent symptoms or medical conditions, new medications (NSAIDs, aspirin, semisynthetic penicillins, warfarin) & dietary habits (vitamin K deficiency, ethanol use)

Table 7. Associated Physical Exam Findings

Physical exam finding	General disorder suggested
Dependent asymptomatic petechiae	Thrombocytopenia
Palpable, pruritic petechiae in clusters	Vasculitis
Palpable purpura	Vasculitis
Superficial bleeding	Thrombocytopenia or vascular defect
Deep hematoma	Coagulation disorder
Hemarthrosis	Coagulation disorder (classically hemophilia)
Extensive superficial purpura	Coagulation disorder
Splenomegaly	Platelet sequestration
Skin or joint laxity	Connective tissue disorder
Telangiectasias	Vascular disorder
Palmar erythema, asterixis, spider angiomata, gynecomastia	Coagulopathy secondary to liver disease

TEST ORDERING

- All patients being evaluated for a bleeding disorder should have the following:
  - ▲ CBC with differential
  - ▲ aPTT and PT
  - ▲ von Willebrand factor
  - ▲ Peripheral blood smear
- Other more specific tests include thrombin time, fibrin degradation products, D-dimer, platelet aggregation studies, specific coagulation factor/inhibitor assays, and mixing studies.
- Algorithms for evaluating patients with bleeding disorders and findings suggestive of platelet or vessel wall abnormality, or suggestive of an acquired plasma coagulation disorder, or suggestive of a congenital plasma coagulation disorder are given in Figures 1, 2, and 3, respectively.

INITIAL MANAGEMENT

Idiopathic Thrombocytopenic Purpura

- Confirmation
  - ▲ Thrombocytopenia—check peripheral blood smear for clumping
  - ▲ Rule out other causes of thrombocytopenia.
    - Normal PT, aPTT, and fibrin degradation products
    - Lack of hemolyzed red cells on peripheral blood smear
  - ▲ Discontinue any drugs that may be causative.
- *No role for platelet transfusions* unless patient is actively bleeding or has platelet count <10,000/μL (<10 × 10^9/L).
- If bleeding—prednisone, 1-2 mg/kg daily, and follow platelet count
- If refractory to corticosteroids or rapid correction of platelet count is needed—IVIg 0.4 g/kg daily infused 3-5 consecutive days
  - ▲ In cases of emergency—IVIg 1 g/kg and repeat in 24 hours.
- If no response after 2-3 weeks of corticosteroids, consider splenectomy.

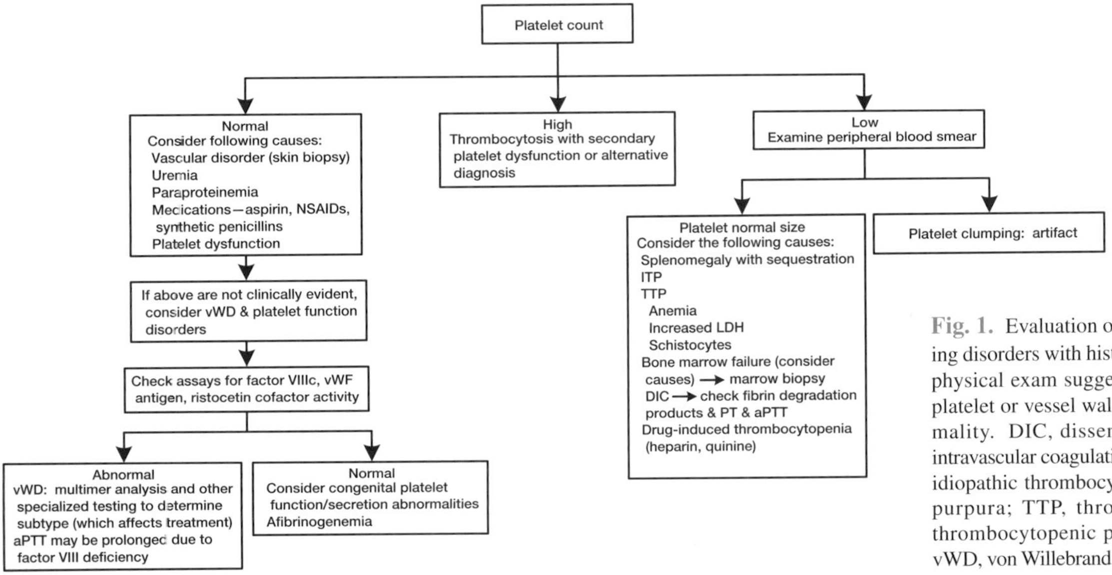

Fig. 1. Evaluation of bleeding disorders with history and physical exam suggestive of platelet or vessel wall abnormality. DIC, disseminated intravascular coagulation; ITP, idiopathic thrombocytopenic purpura; TTP, thrombotic thrombocytopenic purpura; vWD, von Willebrand disease; vWF, von Willebrand factor.

Platelet count

High
Thrombocytosis with secondary platelet dysfunction or alternative diagnosis

Low
Examine peripheral blood smear

Platelet clumping: artifact

Platelet normal size
Consider the following causes:
Splenomegaly with sequestration
ITP
TTP
Anemia
Increased LDH
Schistocytes
Bone marrow failure (consider causes) → marrow biopsy
DIC → check fibrin degradation products & PT & aPTT
Drug-induced thrombocytopenia (heparin, quinine)

Normal
Consider following causes:
Vascular disorder (skin biopsy)
Uremia
Paraproteinemia
Medications—aspirin, NSAIDs, synthetic penicillins
Platelet dysfunction

If above are not clinically evident, consider vWD & platelet function disorders

Check assays for factor VIIIc, vWF antigen, ristocetin cofactor activity

Abnormal
vWD: multimer analysis and other specialized testing to determine subtype (which affects treatment) aPTT may be prolonged due to factor VIII deficiency

Normal
Consider congenital platelet function/secretion abnormalities
Afibrinogenemia

48

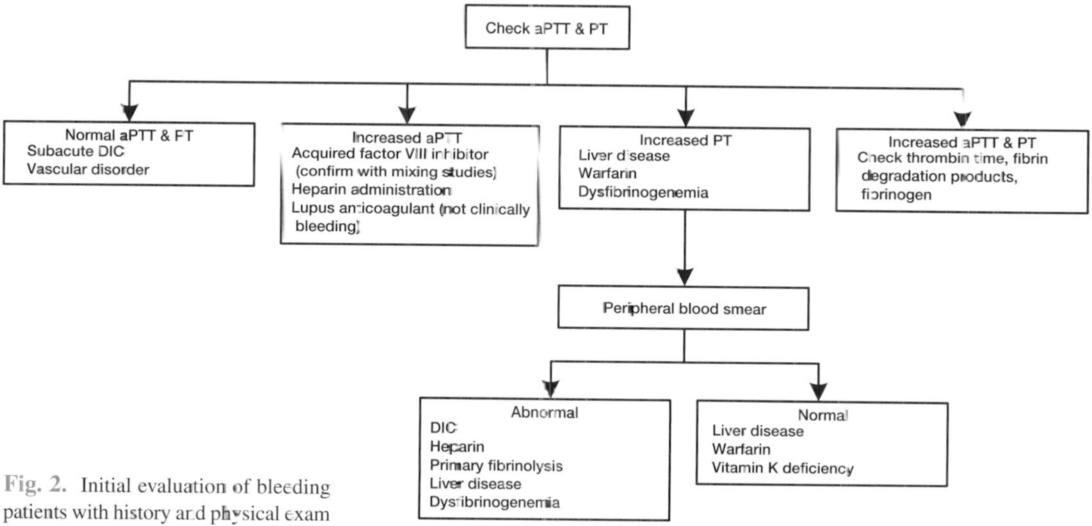

Fig. 2. Initial evaluation of bleeding patients with history and physical exam suggestive of an acquired plasma coagulation disorder. DIC, disseminated intravascular coagulation.

49

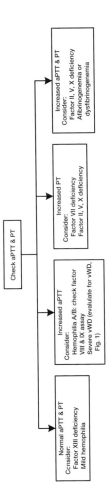

Fig. 3. Evaluation of bleeding patients with history and physical exam suggestive of a congenital plasma coagulation disorder. vWD, von Willebrand disease.

Thrombotic Thrombocytopenic Purpura
- Confirmation—thrombocytopenia, anemia, schistocytes, increased LDH, with/without mental status changes, fever.
- Methylprednisolone, 1-2 mg/kg daily, in combination with
  - ▲ Plasma exchange—should be initiated without delay, 2-3 L exchange/day with fresh frozen plasma
  - ▲ If plasma exchange is not immediately available—transfusion with fresh frozen plasma until plasma exchange is possible
- *Platelet transfusions are contraindicated.*
- Consider possible causes—infection, drugs, malignancy, chemotherapy, bone marrow transplant, pregnancy, idiopathic

von Willebrand Disease
- Most common congenital bleeding abnormality
- Confirmation
  - ▲ With/without abnormal bleeding time
  - ▲ Decreased or normal von Willebrand factor antigen
  - ▲ Decreased or normal factor VIIIc
  - ▲ Decreased ristocetin cofactor activity
- Specialized testing is needed to establish type of von Willebrand disease, and *treatment should be based on the type.*
- On diagnosis, a trial of desmopressin acetate (DDAVP) should be considered except for patients with type 2B von Willebrand disease (in whom it is contraindicated) or type 3 (in whom it is ineffective).
- Without previously established efficacy for the individual patient, desmopressin acetate should not be the first therapy of choice for management of bleeding in von Willebrand disease.
- von Willebrand disease type 1 and types 2A, 2N, and 2M (spontaneous bleeding or surgery)
  - ▲ Desmopressin acetate 0.3 µg/kg infusion in 50 mL of saline over 30 minutes, may be repeated every 12 to 24 hours (note that rapid tachyphylaxis and syndrome of inappropriate antidiuretic hormone with hyponatremia and seizures can develop with subsequent doses if repeated within 24 hours)

- ▲ If desmopressin acetate is ineffective, treat with factor VIII–von Willebrand factor concentrate as below.
- ■ von Willebrand disease types 2A, 2B, 2M, and 3 (spontaneous bleeding)
  - ▲ Factor VIII–von Willebrand factor concentrate 20-30 IU/kg
  - ▲ Cryoprecipitate should be avoided, but it can be used in case of emergency if factor VIII–von Willebrand factor concentrate is not available.
  - ▲ Monitor factor VIII coagulant levels—goal factor VIIIc, >30 IU/dL
  - ▲ Before a major operation, increase dose to 40-60 IU/kg per day with a goal factor VIIIc >50 IU/dL until healing is complete.

Hemophilia A (Factor VIII Deficiency)
- ■ Confirmation
  - ▲ Male patient
  - ▲ With/without a bleeding history or family history
  - ▲ Increased aPTT
  - ▲ Decreased factor VIII assay (<0.5 U/mL)

Life-Threatening Bleeding
- ■ Replace the deficient factor VIII, available as recombinant products (rFVIII) or as purified plasma-derived products (FVIII), 30-40 U/kg infusion repeated every 12 hours
- ■ Goal plasma factor VIII level, 80%-100%
- ■ Up to 50% of patients with hemophilia A may have factor VIII inhibiting antibodies, treatment then must be recombinant activated factor VII (rFVIIa), activated prothrombin coagulant complex (aPCC), or porcine factor VIII.

Minor Bleeding
- ■ Replace factor VIII, as above, with rFVIII or FVIII, 25 U/kg.
- ■ Goal plasma factor VIII level, 50%
- ■ In patients with mild hemophilia A, desmopressin acetate, 0.3 µg/kg infusion over 30 minutes, may be sufficient to stop minor bleeding.

Warfarin-Induced Coagulopathy
- ■ Confirmation—history of warfarin use and increased INR

Life-Threatening Bleeding
- Fresh frozen plasma, 15 mL/kg (goal INR, <1.5) for immediate and temporary correction of coagulopathy

or

- Prothrombin complex concentrate, 25 U/kg
  - ▲ Requires less volume and has more rapid onset
  - ▲ Associated with slight risk of thrombosis
- Vitamin K, 5-10 mg PO or by nasogastric tube
  - ▲ If unable to give enterally or malabsorption is present, then vitamin K 1 mg IV over 60 minutes
  - ▲ Because of small risk of anaphylaxis, epinephrine should be kept at the bedside.

Non–Life-Threatening Bleeding or Asymptomatic Increased INR
- Vitamin K, 5-10 mg PO
  - ▲ If unable to take enterally or malabsorption is present, give IV, as above.
- If INR <5.0 and no evidence of bleeding, hold warfarin and allow INR to correct without treatment while monitoring closely.
- Note: After vitamin K administration and resumption of warfarin therapy, it will take a longer time for INR to increase to the targeted therapeutic range. Use of higher doses of warfarin may result in overshooting target INR.

Acute Disseminated Intravascular Coagulation
- Confirmation
  - ▲ Increase in PT, aPTT, thrombin time, fibrin degradation products, D-dimer
  - ▲ Decrease in fibrinogen
  - ▲ Thrombocytopenia complexes
  - ▲ Increased soluble fibrin monomer complexes
- Diagnose and treat the underlying cause (sepsis, hypoxia, acidosis, malignancy).
- Supportive care
- Replacement of consumed coagulation factors (fresh frozen plasma), fibrinogen (cryoprecipitate), and platelets

Liver Failure

- Confirmation
  - ▲ Acute fulminant liver failure—extreme prolongation of PT, aPTT, and thrombin time, along with clinical scenario
  - ▲ Chronic liver failure—variable prolongation of PT, aPTT, and thrombin time
  - ▲ Often associated with disseminated intravascular coagulation
- If the patient is not actively bleeding, give vitamin K, 5 mg PO daily.
- For acute bleeding episodes, give fresh frozen plasma, 20-30 mL/kg; however, use judiciously to avoid fluid overload.
- For procedures (liver biopsy), give 2 units of fresh frozen plasma immediately before the procedure.
  - ▲ Replace platelets if $<50 \times 10^9$/L and fibrinogen if <75 mg/dL.

CHEST PAIN

Guilherme H. M. Oliveira, M.D.
Joseph G. Murphy, M.D.
R. Scott Wright, M.D.

IS THE PATIENT'S LIFE AT RISK?

- Evaluate the general status of the patient:
  - ▲ Confusion and agitation suggest decreased cerebral perfusion.
  - ▲ Profuse diaphoresis signals adrenergic discharge as seen in myocardial infarction, unstable angina, dissection, and major catastrophes.
  - ▲ Hypotension, cyanosis, and low pulse oxymetry levels suggest life-threatening conditions.
  - ▲ Tachycardia and tachypnea in the setting of pain are nonspecific.
- If an abnormality is detected with this approach, consider myocardial infarction, unstable angina, pulmonary embolism, tension pneumothorax, aortic dissection, or arrhythmia.
- Before proceeding with further evaluation, call for backup.

ADDRESSING THE RISK

- Immediately rule out conditions whose treatment will most imminently avert death:
  - ▲ Tension pneumothorax
  - ▲ Arrhythmia with hemodynamic instability
- Tension pneumothorax—blood pressure measurement and chest X-ray (see chapter on Chest X-ray)
- Arrhythmia—ECG (see chapter on ECG)
- Tachyarrhythmias with hemodynamic instability require immediate electrical cardioversion.
- If patient is not coding, general measures to be undertaken initially include
  - ▲ Oxygen—try to ensure oxygen saturation of at least 90%.
  - ▲ Venous access—make sure patient has a large-bore access for eventual fluid resuscitation.

▲ Monitor cardiac rhythm and blood pressure.

▲ Let ICU know about the patient.

Differential Diagnosis
See Table 1.

Table 1. Causes of Chest Pain

Cardiovascular	Musculoskeletal
Angina	Costochondritis (Tietze syndrome)
Myocardial infarction	Radicular syndromes
Aortic dissection	Inflammatory syndromes
Pericarditis	Sternum osteomyelitis
Aortic stenosis	Rib fractures
Mitral valve prolapse	Metastatic bone disease
Tachyarrhythmias	Psychogenic
Pulmonary	Panic attack
Pulmonary embolism	Conversion disorders
Pneumonia	Other
Pneumothorax	Herpes zoster
Pleuritis	Syndrome X
Gastrointestinal	Intrathoracic tumors
Esophageal spasm	Mondor disease
Esophagitis	
Esophageal cancer	
Hiatal hernia	
Peptic ulcer disease	
Gallbladder disease	
Aerophagia	

Differentiating the Differential

■ Classify chest pain as typical angina, atypical angina, noncoronary chest pain:

▲ Typical angina—deep, crushing retrosternal discomfort (usually not described as pain) of moderate to severe intensity; predictable with exertion, cold, or emotion; recurrent, lasting 3-20 minutes; relieved by rest or nitroglycerin; with or without radiation to neck, arm, or jaw; may be accompanied by nausea and diaphoresis

▲ Atypical angina—a variation of the above in which the pain may have a burning quality, may not always occur with the same degree of effort or at rest, and may be referred to other parts of the chest, such as left side; more common in women

▲ Noncoronary chest pain—usually well localized, sharp or tearing in quality, lasts <3 minutes or several hours or days, is unpredictable, nonreproducible with exertion, varying severity, not usually relieved by nitroglycerin or rest

Risk factors, symptoms, and signs are listed in Tables 2, 3, and 4, respectively.

Ordering Tests

■ All patients in the hospital with chest pain should have ECG, chest X-ray, and oxymetry level (Table 5).

Initial Management of 7 Causes of Chest Pain

Uncomplicated Myocardial Infarction

(see chapter on Acute Coronary Syndromes)

■ Confirmation— >1-mm ST-segment elevation on contiguous ECG leads ± troponin rise ± CK-MB and CK enzyme curve
■ Management
  ▲ Oxygen intranasally at 2-5 L/min
  ▲ Aspirin 325 mg PO
  ▲ Morphine 2-4 mg IV as needed for pain
  ▲ Metoprolol 5 mg IV every 15 minutes until heart rate <60 beats/min
  ▲ Thrombolysis or percutaneous coronary intervention
  ▲ Troponin, CK, CK-MB, ECG every 6 hours

Unstable Angina

■ Confirmation—new chest pain or pain at rest ± wave inversion T wave or new ST-segment depressions
■ Management
  ▲ Oxygen intranasally at 2-5 L/min
  ▲ Aspirin 325 mg PO
  ▲ Nitroglycerin (patch, paste, or IV)
  ▲ Heparin 5,000 IU IV bolus + infusion to target aPTT of 50-75 seconds
  ▲ Metoprolol 5 mg IV every 15 minutes until heart rate <60 beats/min
  ▲ Atorvastatin 80 mg PO or simvastatin 40 mg PO

- ▲ Troponin, CK, CK-MB, aPTT, ECG every 6 hours
- ▲ Emergency angiography and percutaneous coronary intervention of culprit flow-limiting lesion
- ▲ Clopidogrel 300 mg PO unless emergency coronary artery bypass graft is planned.

Pulmonary Embolism
- ■ Confirmation—high-probability ventilation-perfusion scan, thrombus seen on spiral CT or pulmonary angiography
- ■ Management
  - ▲ Oxygen intranasally at 2-5 L/min
  - ▲ Heparin 5,000 IU IV bolus + infusion to target aPTT of 50-75 seconds (if clinical suspicion is high, should not await confirmation)
  - ▲ Thrombolysis if hemodynamically unstable
  - ▲ Thrombolysis if massive pulmonary embolism with right ventricle failure and shock
  - ▲ aPTT every 6 hours
  - ▲ Chest X-ray daily
  - ▲ Arterial blood gases daily

Aortic Dissection
- ■ Confirmation—flap seen on transesophageal echocardiography or chest CT

Table 2. **Risk Factors**

Age >60: MI, PE, aortic dissection, pneumonia, herpes zoster, malignancy

Age <40: psyche, musculoskeletal, pneumothorax, pericarditis, GERD

Hypertension: aortic dissection, MI

Female: psyche, gallbladder, aerophagia, syndrome X

Male: MI, PUD, aortic dissection

Tobacco: pneumonia, MI, PUD, malignancy

Postoperative: MI, PE, pneumonia, musculoskeletal

Alcohol: PUD, pneumonia, GERD

Obesity: PE, GERD, MI

Diabetes mellitus: MI, UA

Dyslipidemia: MI, UA, aortic dissection

Marfan syndrome: aortic dissection

GERD, gastroesophageal reflux disease; MI, myocardial infarction; PE, pulmonary embolism; PUD, peptic ulcer disease; UA, unstable angina.

Table 3. **Symptoms**

Quality of the pain
> Constrictive: MI, esophageal spasm, psyche
> Burning: MI, UA, herpes zoster, GERD, PUD
> Tearing: aortic dissection, esophageal rupture
> Pleuritic: pleuritis, pneumonia, PE, pneumothorax, pericarditis
> Sharp: musculoskeletal, Tietze syndrome, psyche, aortic
>   dissection, PUD, pneumothorax, rib fracture
> Dull, steady: MI, UA, musculoskeletal, esophageal spasm,
>   PUD, pericarditis

Location
> Retrosternal: MI, UA, esophageal spasm, GERD, aortic dissection
> Sides: psyche, pneumonia, pleuritis, pneumothorax
> Back: aortic dissection, pneumonia, pleuritis, pneumothorax

Duration
> <1 min: probably nothing, psyche
> 5 min-20 min: stable angina, esophageal spasm, pneumo-
>   thorax
> >20 min-2 h: UA, MI, musculoskeletal, aortic dissection, PE
> Several hours to days: musculoskeletal, GERD, pneumonia,
>   pericarditis, PUD, cancer

Radiation
> Arms: MI, UA, stable angina, psyche
> Neck: MI, UA, carotid dissection, cervical radiculopathy
> Jaw: MI, UA
> Back: aortic dissection, PE, pneumothorax, gallbladder
>   disease

Provocative factors
> Exertion with lag: angina, UA, MI, aortic dissection
> Exertion without lag: musculoskeletal, PE, esophageal spasm
> Emotion: UA, MI, psyche
> Breathing: pneumonia, pneumothorax, PE, pleuritis,
>   pericarditis
> Vomiting: esophageal rupture
> Chest palpation: Tietze syndrome, Mondor disease, rib
>   fracture, metastasis, osteomyelitis
> Eating: esophageal spasm, GERD, PUD

Relieving factors
> Rest with lag: angina
> Rest without lag: musculoskeletal
> Nitroglycerin: angina, UA, esophageal spasm
> Antacids: GERD, PUD
> Leaning forward: pericarditis
> Shallow breathing: pneumonia, pleuritis
> No relief: MI, PE, aortic dissection, pneumothorax

GERD, gastroesophageal reflux disease; MI, myocardial infarction; PE, pulmonary
embolus; PUD, peptic ulcer disease; UA, unstable angina.

Table 4. Signs

Hypotension	Pericardial rub
MI	Pericarditis
Massive pulmonary embolism	Pleural rub
Pneumonia with sepsis	Pneumonia
Tension pneumothorax	Pulmonary embolism
Hypertension	Hamman sign
Aortic dissection	Esophageal rupture
Cyanosis	Subcutaneous emphysema
Pulmonary embolism	Esophageal rupture
Pneumothorax	Abolished breath sounds
Myocardial infarction with	Pneumothorax with effusion
cardiogenic shock	Hyperresonant percussion
Pneumonia	Pneumothorax
S_3	Low oxygen saturation
Unstable angina	Pulmonary embolism
Myocardial infarction	Pneumothorax
Aortic stenosis	Shock
Murmur	Pneumonia
Unstable angina	Vesiculopapular rash
Myocardial infarction	Herpes zoster
Aortic stenosis	Profuse diaphoresis
Distended neck veins	Myocardial infarction
Right ventricular myocardial	Aortic dissection
infarction	Pulmonary embolism
Tension pneumothorax	Pulse asymmetry
Superior vena cava	Aortic dissection
syndrome	

- ▲ Oxygen intranasally at 2-5 L/min
- ▲ Labetalol IV infusion at 2 mg/min, titrate to systolic blood pressure <110 mm Hg (initiation should not await confirmation)

or

- ▲ Nitroprusside IV 2.5-5 µg/kg per minute + propranolol 1 mg IV every 4-6 hours
- ▲ Consult emergency cardiovascular surgery.

Pericarditis
- ▪ Confirmation—transthoracic echocardiography with thickened pericardium and fluid
- ▪ Management
  - ▲ NSAIDs PO
  - ▲ Pericardiocentesis for tamponade

Pneumothorax

- Confirmation—chest X-ray with air in the pleura
- Management
  - ▲ Oxygen intranasally at 2-5 L/min
  - ▲ Thoracocentesis or chest tube

Table 5. **Diagnostic Test Ordering for Chest Pain (CP)**

Findings	Diagnosis	Tests ordered
CP + diaphoresis + S_3 ± murmur	MI, unstable angina, aortic stenosis	ECG, enzyme curve, echo, CXR
Sharp/pleuritic pain + low O_2 sat + dyspnea	Pneumothorax, PE, esophageal rupture	CXR, ABGs, spiral CT or V/Q scan
CP + dyspnea ± distended neck veins + hypotension	Pneumothorax, right ventricle MI, massive PE	CXR, ECG, enzyme curve, echo, spiral CT or V/Q scan
Severe back pain + hypertension	Aortic dissection, MI	CXR, ECG, enzyme curve, TEE or CT thorax
Retrosternal CP + vomiting + diaphoresis	MI, unstable angina	ECG, enzyme curve
Retrosternal CP related to meals	Esophageal causes, PUD	EGD, barium swallow
Any CP + CAD risk factors	MI, unstable angina	ECG, enzymes
Acute dyspnea + bilateral crackles	MI with CHF, unstable angina, PE	ECG, CXR, enzyme curve
Pericardial rub ± distended neck veins	Pericarditis, pleuritis	CXR, ECG, echo
Hypertension + pulse asymmetry	Aortic dissection, coarctation	CXR, TEE, CT thorax
CP + fixed distended neck veins ± Horner syndrome	Superior vena cava syndrome, Pancoast syndrome	CXR, CT thorax

ABG, arterial blood gas; CAD, coronary artery disease; CHF, congestive heart failure; CXR, chest X-ray; echo, echocardiography; EGD, esophagogastroduodenoscopy; MI, myocardial infarction; O_2 sat, oxygen saturation; PE, pulmonary embolus; PUD, peptic ulcer disease; TEE, transesophageal echocardiography; V/Q, ventilation-perfusion.

Esophageal Spasm/Reflux

- Confirmation—barium swallow or esophagogastroduo-denoscopy
- Management
  - ▲ Omeprazole 40 mg PO
  - ▲ Maalox 20 mL PO
  - ▲ Esophagogastroduodenoscopy in AM

COUGH, HEMOPTYSIS, AND HICCUP

Douglas L. Riegert-Johnson, M.D.
Vanessa Z. Riegert-Johnson
Constance Jennings, M.D.

COUGH AND HEMOPTYSIS

IS THE PATIENT'S LIFE AT RISK?

- Cough not associated with other comorbidities—rarely life threatening
- Potentially life-threatening situations include
  - ▲ Massive hemoptysis— >600 mL/24-48 hours or amount sufficient to cause hemodynamic or respiratory compromise
    - Medical emergency (mortality rate, 38%)
    - Differential diagnosis: bronchiectasis, bronchogenic pneumonia, TB, aspergillosis, necrotizing gram-negative pneumonia, endobronchial mass
  - ▲ Pneumothorax

ADDRESSING THE RISK

Massive Hemoptysis
- Determine that blood has originated from the chest and not the gastrointestinal or upper respiratory tract.
- Ensure hemodynamic stability.
- Position the patient semiupright with bleeding side down.
- Consider emergent pulmonology consultation for emergent bronchoscopy.
- Consider emergent radiology consultation for emergent bronchial artery embolization.
- Consider chest CT if patient is stabilized.
- Consider emergent thoracic surgery consultation if embolization is not successful.
- Assess adequacy of airway; admister oxygen.

Special abbreviation used in this chapter: ACE, angiotensin-converting enzyme.

- Order CBC, aPTT, PT, crossmatch; reverse anticoagulation as needed.
- Volume replacement as needed
- Conservative management if due to bronchiectasis

Pneumothorax
- Establish airway patency, hemodynamic stability, and adequate oxygenation.
- If tension pneumothorax is suspected based on clinical findings—no breath sounds, hyperresonance, no tactile fremitus on affected side, and possibly a shift in trachea away from affected side—immediately insert a 14-16–gauge needle in 2nd intercostal space midclavicular line.

DIFFERENTIAL DIAGNOSIS

The differential diagnosis of cough is listed in Table 1 and that for hemoptysis in Table 2. The symptoms and signs of common causes of cough and hemoptysis are listed in Table 3.

Table 1. Differential Diagnosis of Cough

Acute (<3 weeks)	Chronic (≥3 weeks)
Common	Common
Postnasal drip due to common cold (most common), acute bacterial sinusitis or rhinitis	ACE inhibitor
COPD exacerbation	Postnasal drip due to common cold, acute bacterial sinusitis or rhinitis
Bronchitis	Cough-variant asthma
Less common	GERD-induced bronchitis, asthma, or laryngeal inflammation
Pneumonia	Postinfectious, following bronchitis
Aspiration	Chronic bronchitis
Pulmonary embolism	*Bordetella pertussis*
Postoperative atelectasis	Less common
Congestive heart failure	Eosinophilic bronchitis
All causes of chronic cough	Bronchiectasis
	Cystic fibrosis
	Interstitial lung disease
	Bronchogenic carcinoma

ACE, angiotensin-converting enzyme; GERD, gastroesophageal reflux disease.

DIFFERENTIATING THE DIFFERENTIAL

- Evaluation of cough and/or hemoptysis should include posteroanterior and lateral chest X-rays.
- Purulent sputum (thick green or yellow) suggests bronchitis, pneumonia, bronchiectasis, or lung abscess.
- A "dry" cough may implicate laryngeal inflammation or habit cough.

Table 2. Differential Diagnosis of Hemoptysis

Massive (>600 mL/24 hours)	Mild and moderate
Common	Common
Bronchiectasis	Bronchitis, acute and chronic
TB	Pneumonia
Less common	Bronchogenic carcinoma
Invasive aspergillosis	Less common
Bronchogenic carcinoma	Lung abscess
	Mitral stenosis
	Pulmonary embolus

Table 3. Symptoms, Signs, and Radiographic Findings in Common Causes of Cough and Hemoptysis

Symptoms (Sx) and signs	Chest X-ray	Diagnosis
Sx: Nasal congestion/discharge, feeling of drainage in throat, underlying Sx of sinusitis or vasomotor rhinitis Signs: Drainage in posterior pharynx, nasal discharge, cobblestoning of oropharyngeal mucosa, mucus in oropharynx	Normal	Postnasal drip
Sx: Acute onset, throat clearing, nasal discharge, nasal obstruction, throat irritation	Normal	Common cold
Sx: Sneezing, clear nasal drainage, seasonal Sx	Normal	Allergic rhinitis

Table 3 (continued)

Symptoms (Sx) and signs	Chest X-ray	Diagnosis
Sx: Sinus pain & tenderness, purulent nasal discharge, tooth pain	Normal	Acute sinusitis
Sx: Excessive watery discharge associated with temperature changes	Normal	Vasomotor rhinitis
Sx: Dyspnea, purulent sputum, history of COPD or smoking Signs: Fever, hypoxemia	Hyperinflation bullae, examine for infiltrates	COPD exacerbation
Sx: Cough, purulent sputum, no history of smoking Signs: Fever, coarse rhonchi (may clear with cough)	Normal	Bronchitis
Sx: Following upper respiratory tract illness Signs: No physical exam findings, diagnosis of exclusion, self-limited	Postinfectious Normal	cough
Sx: Dyspnea, expiratory wheezing, prolonged expiration, nighttime Sx Signs: Decreased peak expiratory flow, expiratory wheeze	Hyperventilation, look for signs of underlying cause	Asthma exacerbation
Sx: Dyspnea, cough with purulent sputum Signs: Fever, bronchial breathing, inspiratory crackles	Consolidation	Pneumonia
Sx: Dyspnea, hemoptysis, chest pain (especially pleuritic), risk factors* Signs: Tachycardia, tachypnea, pleural rub, loud P_2, right ventricle heave	Normal or subtle peripheral consolidation & atelectasis	Pulmonary embolism
Sx: Substantial smoking history, hemoptysis, dyspnea, chest wall pain, hoarseness Signs: Wheezing, lymphadenopathy, Horner syndrome, signs consistent with pneumonitis due to obstruction, clubbing, hypercalcemia	If normal, NPV of 100% for bronchogenic carcinoma in patients with cough	Bronchogenic carcinoma
Sx: Copious sputum production, history of recurrent infections	"Tram tracking" of bronchi	Bronchiectasis

Table 3 (continued)

Symptoms (Sx) and signs	Chest X-ray	Diagnosis
Sx: Chronic cough, night sweats, weight loss, HIV+ or risk factors, positive PPD, TB risk factors	Upper lobe abnormalities, Ghon complex[‡]	TB[†]
Sx: Dyspnea, orthopnea Signs: Bilateral basal inspiratory crackles, S$_3$, increased jugular venous pressure	Cephalization, Kerley B lines, pleural effusions	Congestive heart failure exacerbation

NPV, negative predictive value; P$_2$, second pulmonic sound; S$_3$, third heart sound.
*Risk factors: personal/family history of pulmonary embolism, deep venous thrombosis, malignancy, postoperative immobility, oral contraceptive pills, trauma.
[†]If TB is considered, patient must be isolated.
[‡]Small parenchymal infiltrate and enlarged hilar lymph nodes.

TEST ORDERING

- Posteroanterior and lateral chest X-rays for all patients; tests suggested according to diagnosis are listed in Table 4.

INITIAL MANAGEMENT

Disease-Specific Therapy

- Angiotensin-converting enzyme (ACE) inhibitor suspected
  - ▲ Discontinue ACE inhibitor for 4 weeks and reevaluate
  - ▲ Consider angiotensin II receptor blocker
  - ▲ If ACE inhibitor is needed, may treat cough with cromolyn 2 puffs 4 times daily
- Postnasal drip—Symptomatic treatment consists of first-generation antihistamines and decongestants; most likely causes and treatment include
  - ▲ Sinusitis—antibiotics (amoxicillin, if contraindicated use trimethoprim-sulfamethoxazole [Bactrim]), nasal steroids
  - ▲ Allergic rhinitis—nasal steroids, second-generation antihistamines
  - ▲ Vasomotor rhinitis—first-generation antihistamines, ipratropium (Atrovent)
- Postinfectious cough—by definition, a diagnosis of exclusion, is self-limited

Table 4. Testing According to Diagnosis

Diagnosis	Suggested tests
Acute cough (<3 weeks)	
Postnasal drip	
Sinusitis	May treat empirically, consider sinus CT
Allergic rhinitis	Allergy testing
Vasomotor rhinitis	None
COPD exacerbation	Arterial blood gases
	Evaluate for underlying cause such as pneumonia, pulmonary embolus, or neoplasm
Bronchitis	Chest X-ray, CBC, sputum Gram stain, C/S
Pneumonia	CBC, sputum Gram stain, blood & sputum C/S
TB*	PPD, 3 serial sputums for AFB & Cx, rapid PCR testing, gastric aspirate if no sputum for AFB/Cx, consider HIV test
Pulmonary embolism	D-dimer, spiral CT, V/Q scan
Chronic cough (≥3 weeks)	
Cough-variant asthma	Methacholine challenge
GERD	Empiric trial of proton pump inhibitors, 24-hour pH probe

AFB, acid-fast bacillus; C/S, culture and sensitivities; Cx, cultures; GERD, gastroesophageal reflux disease; PCR, polymerase chain reaction; V/Q, ventilation-perfusion.

    ▲ If symptoms are severe, may attempt therapy with ipratropium and inhaled and oral corticosteroids
- TB
  - ▲ Isolate patient
  - ▲ Therapy is isoniazid (INH), rifampin, pyrazinamide, ethambutol
  - ▲ Regimen adjusted according to susceptibility
  - ▲ Consult infectious diseases if extrapulmonary TB, drug-resistant, or coinfection with HIV
- Bronchitis
  - ▲ No treatment if viral cause is suspected.
  - ▲ For prolonged symptoms, consider azithromycin or tetracycline.

- Bronchiectasis
  - ▲ Bronchial hygiene, antibiotics directed at predominant pathogen
  - ▲ If fever, antipseudomonal coverage pending sputum culture
- *Bordetella pertussis*—erythromycin

Symptomatic Therapy

- Antitussive therapy—dextromethorphan, codeine, and ipratropium aerosol are only widely available agents
- Protussive therapy
  - ▲ Cough associated with retained mucus secretions (e.g., due to bronchiectasis, cystic fibrosis, or chronic bronchitis) should not be treated with antitussive agents.
  - ▲ In chronic bronchitis, mucolytics have not been proved to be effective.

HICCUP (SINGULTUS)

DIFFERENTIAL DIAGNOSIS

More than 100 causes of hiccup have been reported. The most common are listed in Table 5.

DIFFERENTIATING THE DIFFERENTIAL

The signs and symptoms of hiccup and the corresponding diagnosis are listed in Table 6.

TEST ORDERING

- The most important diagnostic tool is a thorough history and physical exam.
- Initial recommended tests are CBC with differential, electrolytes, and chest X-ray.
- Additional testing is directed by history and physical exam findings and could include calcium, creatinine, liver function tests, toxicology screen, and MRI or CT of head, chest, or abdomen.

MANAGEMENT

- Identify and treat the underlying cause if possible.

Table 5. Common Causes of Hiccup

Benign causes
Idiopathic gastric distension: aerophagia, carbonated beverages, endoscopic insufflation
Excitement, emotion
Temperature change: hot/cold beverages, hot/cold showers, tobacco use

Malignant causes
Anatomical: consider lesion from brainstem along course of phrenic and vagus nerves to level of diaphragm
CNS: neoplasms, trauma, ischemia, hemorrhage
Chest: pericarditis, pneumonia, bronchitis, lung cancer
Abdomen: liver or spleen abscesses, peptic ulcer disease, gastritis, gastric or pancreatic cancer
Medications: alcohol, anesthetics, dexamethasone, methyldopa, sulfonamides, antiepileptics, chlordiazepoxide
Metabolic: uremia, fever, electrolyte disturbances (especially hyponatremia)

CNS, central nervous system.

- The following stepwise algorithm can be used for hiccups of any cause:
  - ▲ Nonpharmacologic
    - • Breath holding
    - • Valsalva maneuver
    - • Granulated sugar 2 g swallowed dry with little moisture
    - • Hyperventilating into a paper bag
    - • Direct stimulation of nasal or oral pharynx with a plastic catheter
    - • "Lifting" of the uvula with tongue blade
    - • Nasogastric tube if gastric distension is present
  - ▲ Pharmacologic
    - • Chlorpromazine—patient may develop orthostatic hypotension and bradycardia and should be monitored
    - • Metoclopramide
    - • Nifedipine

Table 6. Signs and Symptoms of Hiccup and Corresponding Diagnosis

Signs and symptoms	Diagnosis
Hiccups resolve with sleep, no organic findings	Psychogenic or idiopathic
Postoperative	Anesthetics, irritation of phrenic or vagus nerve
Transient paralysis, dysarthria, visual loss, headache	Stroke
Seizures, fever, mental status changes, headache	Encephalitis
Anxiety, abdominal bloating, abdominal pain, abdominal gas on KUB	Aerophagia

KUB, kidney, ureter, bladder X-ray.

DELIRIUM AND DEMENTIA

Lionel S. Lim, M.D.
Paul Y. Takahashi, M.D.

IS THE PATIENT'S LIFE AT RISK?

Rule Out the Following Life-Threatening Conditions:

- Hypoxia due to any cardiopulmonary process
- Hypercarbia
- Hypoglycemia
- Intracranial process (e.g., bleeding, infarction, infection, tumor)
- Infection and/or sepsis
- Myocardial ischemia
- Drug effect or withdrawal

Distinguish Between Delirium and Dementia by Recognizing the Following:

- Consciousness
  - ▲ Determine if the level of consciousness has changed.
  - ▲ Change of consciousness characterized by "negative" symptoms such as drowsiness or lethargy or "positive" symptoms such as agitation
- Cognition
  - ▲ Alteration in mental functioning and thought processes
  - ▲ This alteration may be present in both delirium and dementia.
  - ▲ Inattention and disorganized thinking are key features of delirium.
- Course
  - ▲ Delirium—characterized by acute changes in which the delirium may fluctuate
  - ▲ Dementia—more insidious and tends to be slowly progressive
- Cause
  - ▲ Delirium—a consequence of an underlying medical condition or medication

▲ Dementia—not a consequence of an underlying medical condition or medication

Delirium, dementia, and depression are compared in Table 1.

ADDRESSING THE RISK

Obtain the Following Information:

- Temperature, pulse, blood pressure
- Respiratory rate—is respiratory distress or failure present? What is the oxygen saturation? Obtain arterial blood gases.
- Obtain a glucometer reading immediately.

Stabilize the Patient

- Ensure the patient is hemodynamically stable. Otherwise, get help!

Table 1. Comparison of Delirium, Dementia, and Depression

Feature	Delirium	Dementia	Depression
Onset	Acute	Insidious	Variable
Course	Fluctuating	Steadily progressive	Diurnal variation
Consciousness & orientation	Clouded, disoriented	Clear until late stages	Generally unimpaired
Attention & memory	Poor short-term memory, inattention	Poor short-term memory without marked inattention	Poor attention but memory intact
Psychosis	Common (psychotic ideas are fleeting & simple in content)	Less common	Occurs in small number of patients (psychotic symptoms are complex & in keeping with prevailing mood)
EEG	Abnormal in 80%-90%, generalized diffuse slowing in 80%	Abnormal in 80%-90%, generalized diffuse slowing in 80%	Generally normal

- Maintain a patent airway; supplement breathing with oxygen.
- Establish IV access, and start fluids if patient is hypotensive.

Brief History and Focused Physical Exam
- Determine the patient's previous and existing medical problems.
- Do you suspect drug or alcohol abuse?
- What are the patient's current medications?
- What is the patient's code status?
- Perform a focused neurologic, cardiopulmonary, and abdominal exam.

DELIRIUM

DIFFERENTIAL DIAGNOSIS
See Tables 2 and 3.

Table 2. Pharmacologic Causes of Delirium*

Sedatives or hypnotics (intoxication or withdrawal)
  Benzodiazepines
    Alprazolam
    Chlordiazepoxide
    Diazepam
    Flurazepam
    Triazolam
  Barbiturates
  Chloral hydrate
  Ethanol
Analgesics
  Opioids & opioid agonists
    Meperidine (Demerol)
    Methadone
    Pentazocine (Talwin)
    Propoxyphene (Darvon)
Antipsychotics
  Low potency, highly anticholinergic drugs
  Atypical antipsychotics—clozapine

Table 2 (continued)

Antidepressants
  Lithium
  Tricyclic antidepressants
    Amitriptyline
    Doxepin
    Imipramine
  Selective serotonin reuptake inhibitors (less common)
Cardiac medications
  Antiarrhythmics—lidocaine
  Antihypertensives
  Digitalis
Gastrointestinal tract medications—histamine (H_2) blockers
Neurologic medications
  Anticonvulsants—phenytoin (Dilantin)
  Antiparkinsonian drugs
Antiflammatory agents
  Corticosteroids
  NSAIDs—indomethacin (Indocin)
Antihistamines (especially first generation with sedating properties)
  Diphenhydramine (Benadryl)
Other anticholinergics
  Atropine
  Baclofen
  Benztropine mesylate (Cogentin)
  Cyclobenzaprine (Flexeril)
  Oxybutynin (Ditropan)
  Scopolamine

*Specifically mentioned medications have a high association with delirium.

DIFFERENTIATING THE DIFFERENTIAL

Medical History

- What are the symptoms, duration of delirium, and course (gradual or stepwise progression, rapidity of progression)?
- What was previous and present functional and cognitive status?
- Any recent changes in the medical history?
- Any illicit drug or alcohol use?
- Any previous episodes of delirium?
- In older patients, how is bowel and bladder function, i.e., constipation and urinary obstruction?

Table 3. Nonpharmacologic Causes of Delirium

Metabolic disorders
- Hypoglycemia or hyperglycemia
- Hypothyroidism or hyperthyroidism
- Acid-base imbalance
- Anemia
- Vitamin deficiencies or malnutrition
- Fluid & electrolyte imbalances
  - Hyponatremia
  - Hypernatremia
  - Hypercalcemia

Cardiovascular disorders
- Congestive heart failure
- Myocardial infarction
- Cardiac arrhythmia
- Shock
- Hypertensive encephalopathy

Central nervous system disorders
- Head trauma
- Seizures
- Cerebrovascular diseases
- Infections
- Space-occupying lesions (tumor, subdural hematoma, abscess)
- Vasculitis

Pulmonary (hypoxia) disorders
- Pulmonary embolism
- Pneumonia
- COPD
- Fat embolism

Gastrointestinal disorders
- Hepatic encephalopathy
- Severe fecal impaction

Genitourinary disorders
- Uremia
- Urinary tract infection
- Severe urinary retention

Infections

Sleep deprivation

Postoperative state

- Any history of the following:
  - ▲ Infections (including HIV and AIDS)
  - ▲ Central nervous system disorder (e.g., stroke)
  - ▲ Hepatic or renal impairment
  - ▲ Recent surgical procedure
  - ▲ Trauma
  - ▲ Diabetes mellitus
  - ▲ Thyroid dysfunction
  - ▲ Chronic cardiopulmonary conditions (e.g., coronary artery disease, congestive heart failure, COPD)
  - ▲ Head injury

Physical Exam
- Perform a mental status exam.
- Pay special attention to cardiopulmonary and abdominal exams.
- Examine the skin to assess hydration status, and check orthostatics.
- Look for signs of hypo- or hyperthyroidism.
- Look for focal neurologic deficits.
- Delirium + Fever, Tachycardia, Tremors, Agitation, Hypertension = Delirium Tremens (ethanol withdrawal)
- Fever + Meningism = Meningitis or Subarachnoid Hemorrhage
- If patient is severely obtunded, consider diffuse encephalitis, metabolic encephalopathy, or brainstem stroke.
- Metabolic encephalopathies are manifested by asterixis (arrhythmic flapping tremor of outstretched wrists).

Special Circumstances
The elderly are at high risk for delirium because of age-related reduced physiologic reserve, underlying medical comorbidity, possible preexisting cognitive defects, polypharmacy, and altered drug metabolism.

TEST ORDERING
Lab Tests
- Routine
  - ▲ Chemistry panel—electrolytes (sodium, potassium, calcium, magnesium), bicarbonate, BUN and creatinine, glucose

- ▲ Liver function tests
- ▲ CBC
- ▲ Arterial blood gases
- ▲ Urinalysis
- ▪ Selected patients
  - ▲ Osmolarity
  - ▲ Ammonia (NH_3) (hepatic dysfunction and hepatic encephalopathy)
  - ▲ Serum/urine toxicology (especially if comatose and/or diagnosis is unclear)
  - ▲ Ethanol
  - ▲ Sensitive thyroid-stimulating hormone
  - ▲ Cultures (blood, urine, sputum)
  - ▲ ESR
  - ▲ HIV testing

TEST ORDERING
Lab Tests (to Rule Out Reversible Forms of Dementia)
- ▪ Routine
  - ▲ CBC
  - ▲ ESR
  - ▲ Electrolytes (sodium, potassium, calcium, magnesium) & glucose
  - ▲ Renal function tests (BUN, creatinine)
  - ▲ Liver function tests
  - ▲ Vitamin B_{12} & folate
  - ▲ Syphilis serology (fluorescent treponemal antibody, absorbed test)
  - ▲ Urinalysis
  - ▲ Thyroid screen (sensitive thyroid-stimulating hormone)
- ▪ Selected patients
  - ▲ HIV testing
  - ▲ Lyme serology
  - ▲ Urinary heavy metals
  - ▲ Toxicology screen
  - ▲ Paraneoplastic antibodies
  - ▲ Antinuclear antibody
  - ▲ Extractable nuclear antigen

Neuroimaging

- CT of brain—preferably performed with and without contrast medium
- MRI of brain
  - ▲ May be needed to identify strokes or ischemic changes not detectable with CT
  - ▲ Preferably performed with and without contrast medium, with sagittal, axial, and coronal views

Neuropsychometric Testing

- Helpful in differentiating depression from dementia
- In cases of false-positive or negative Mini-Mental State Examination scores because of low educational level or high baseline intelligence, respectively

Others (Not Routinely Used)

- Genetic testing (familial forms of Alzheimer and frontotemporal dementia, parkinsonism, Creutzfeldt-Jakob disease)
- Apolipoprotein E (Alzheimer dementia)
- EEG (Creutzfeldt-Jakob disease, metabolic encephalopathy, encephalitis)

ECG—Cardiac Ischemia or Arrhythmias

Chest X-ray—Congestive Heart Failure, Pneumonia, or Other Pulmonary Processes

Neuroimaging

- CT of head with and without contrast as a screen if localized intracranial process is suspected (e.g., hemorrhage, tumor, infarction, subarachnoid hemorrhage, abscess)
- If meningitis is suspected and papilledema, focal neurologic findings, or unconsciousness is present, it may be reasonable to perform CT of the head before performing lumbar puncture. Blood specimens must be drawn for cultures and empiric antibiotic therapy be given while CT is pending.
- In the elderly, consider performing CT of the head if there is a history of falling, even if head injury was not reported.

CSF Exam

- Perform if at least 1 of the following is suspected:

- ▲ Meningitis
- ▲ Encephalitis
- ▲ Subarachnoid hemorrhage (even if CT of the head is "negative"); check for xanthochromia

EEG
- ▪ Consider an EEG if the patient is comatose and any of the following is suspected:
  - ▲ Clinically unrecognized seizures
  - ▲ Herpes encephalitis
  - ▲ Creutzfeldt-Jakob disease
- ▪ May be useful in diagnosing metabolic or drug-induced delirium

INITIAL MANAGEMENT
- ▪ Three components to managing delirium:
  - ▲ Identify and treat the underlying cause.
  - ▲ Use nonpharmacologic measures to ameliorate symptoms (Table 4).
  - ▲ Initiate pharmacologic therapy for severe agitation and behavioral disturbance (Table 5).

DEMENTIA

DIFFERENTIAL DIAGNOSIS
Common and other causes of dementia are listed in Table 6.

DIFFERENTIATING THE DIFFERENTIAL
Medical History
- ▪ Avoid relying solely on the patient's history; obtain information from caregiver or close relative.
- ▪ Localize the lesion by directing questions toward the various domains of cognitive function (Table 7).
- ▪ Neurologic syndromes associated with dementia are listed in Table 8.

Physical Exam
- ▪ Signs to look for—nuchal rigidity, papilledema, focal facial

Table 4. Nonpharmacologic Interventions to Ameliorate Symptoms Associated With Delirium

Environmental interventions
    Optimize sensorineural input: eyeglasses, hearing aids, dentures
    Overcome barriers to communication
        Visual aids & alternative means of communication (e.g., pen & paper) for verbally impaired patient (e.g., because of intubation, stroke)
        Provide interpreter if necessary
    Room modifications
        Quiet environment with gentle music or television
    Preserve diurnal rhythm
        Lights on during day, night-lights at night
        Provide a window view for day-night orientation
        In-room clocks
    Room near nursing station to facilitate close observation
    Place familiar objects in patient's room
    Constant room temperature
Patient comfort measures
    Adequate analgesia for pain relief while avoiding over-medication
    Early mobility & physical activity
    Minimize sleep interruptions
    Adequate nutritional intake
    Reduce unnecessary physical restraints
Psychosocial support
    Maintain interaction with family & friends
    Consistency in staff caring for the patient (e.g., a key nurse)
    Provide regular verbal reminders to orient patient to time, location, & people involved in patient's care

or limb weakness or asymmetric deep tendon reflexes, parkinsonism, frontal release signs (glabellar, grasp, snout), gait impairment, fasciculations

- Parkinsonian signs may indicate either dementia with Lewy bodies or frank Parkinson disease.
- Hypertension and other cardiovascular findings and focal neurologic signs favor diagnosis of multi-infarct dementia.
- Perform a screening mental status exam such as Mini-Mental State Examination (Table 9).
- Alternatively, the clock-drawing test may be performed—ask patient to draw a clock face with the hands at 11:10.

Table 5. Pharmacologic Therapy for Severe Agitation and Behavioral Disturbance

Haloperidol (Haldol)

    0.5-10 mg IM or IV (1-2 mg PO or 0.5-1 mg IM or IV in elderly) depending on level of disturbance and likely tolerance (consider age, physical status, risk of side effects)

    Observe patient for 20-30 minutes

    If patient remains unmanageable but has no adverse effects, double the dose & continue monitoring

    Although occurrence of extrapyramidal side effects is low, use caution if prescribing for patient with known Parkinson disease

    Repeat the cycle until acceptable response or side effects occur

    Patient should be manageable & not obtunded

Lorazepam (Ativan)

    Mild to moderate agitation: 1-2 mg PO or 0.5-1 mg IM initially

    Moderate to severe agitation: 1-2 mg IM or 0.5 mg IV initially

    May be given every 4 hours as needed

    Beneficial for reducing antipsychotic medications when extrapyramidal side effects occur

    Monitor respiratory functions & level of sedation carefully

    Consider giving flumazenil if toxicity occurs

Table 6. Causes of Dementia

Common

    Mild cognitive impairment

    Alzheimer dementia

    Dementia with Lewy bodies

    Frontotemporal dementia

    Vascular dementia

    Normal-pressure hydrocephalus*

Other

    Vitamin deficiencies

        Thiamine (B_1) (Wernicke encephalopathy)*

        B_{12} (pernicious anemia) or folate deficiency*

    Endocrine & other organ failure

        Hypothyroidism

        Adrenal insufficiency & Cushing syndrome*

        Hypo- or hyperparathyroidism*

        Renal failure*

        Liver failure*

        Pulmonary failure*

Table 6 (continued)

Chronic infections
 HIV
 Neurosyphilis*
 Papovavirus (progressive multifocal leukoencephalopathy)
 Prion (Creutzfeldt-Jakob disease)
 TB, fungal, or protozoal*
 Sarcoidosis*
 Whipple disease*
 Lyme disease*
 Brain abscess*
Head trauma or diffuse brain damage
 Chronic subdural hematoma*
 Postanoxia
 Postencephalitis
Neoplastic
 Primary brain tumor*
 Metastatic brain tumor*
 Paraneoplastic limbic encephalitis
Psychiatric
 Depression (pseudodementia)*
Sleep disorder
 Obstructive sleep apnea*
 Central sleep apnea*
 Restless legs syndrome*
 Periodic limb movement disorder*
Degenerative disorders
 Parkinson disease
 Huntington disease
 Progressive supranuclear palsy
 Multiple sclerosis
Toxic
 Numerous (highly anticholinergic) prescription drugs*
 Illicit drugs*
 Heavy metals*
Miscellaneous
 Vasculitis*
 Acute intermittent porphyria*
 Recurrent nonconvulsive seizures*

*Potentially treatable dementia.

Table 7. Localization of Cognitive Domain

Cognitive domain	Location	"Does patient..."
Memory	Mesial temporal lobe	Recall the details of recent events? Tend to repeat questions?
Executive functions	Frontal lobe	Demonstrate poor judgment? Have difficulty planning & reasoning? Behave in inappropriate, overly joyful, overly tearful, or markedly sedentary manner?
Language	Dominant hemisphere (usually left) in frontotemporoparietal area	Struggle to recall names of persons or objects? Struggle to express his/her thoughts? Struggle to understand oral or written information?
Calculations	Dominant hemisphere (usually left) in parietal area Can be impaired when attention poor, e.g., frontal lobe dysfunction	Balance the checkbook without errors? Struggle to make correct change?
Limb praxis	Dominant hemisphere (usually left) in parietal or mesial frontal area	Operate a car with difficulty? Use eating utensils or tools correctly?
Dressing praxis	Nondominant hemisphere (usually right) in parietal area	Have trouble getting dressed?
Visuospatial function	Nondominant hemisphere (usually right) in parietal area	Get lost in the home, in stores, or while driving?

Table 8. Neurologic Syndromes Associated With Dementia[*][†]

Associated syndrome	Likely diagnosis
Impairment in memory only	Mild cognitive impairment
Impairment in memory & other cognitive domain(s)	Alzheimer dementia
Visual hallucinations, parkinsonism, visuospatial abnormalities	Dementia with Lewy bodies
"Acting out dreams"	REM sleep behavior disorder
Restless legs	Restless legs syndrome
Leg twitching	Periodic limb movement disorder
Episodes of frequent arousals & gasping for air	Obstructive sleep apnea
Personality/behavioral change and/or language disturbance	Frontotemporal dementia
Stroke + stepwise cognitive decline	Vascular dementia
Cognitive decline, ataxic gait, urinary incontinence	Normal-pressure hydrocephalus

[*]All prescription and nonprescription drugs should be scrutinized for potential cognitive side effects.
[†]Alcohol intake and nutrition screening for possible thiamine deficiency.

(Score—5, perfect; 4, minor visuospatial error; 3, "10" inaccurately placed; 2, moderate disorganization of numbers; 1, fails to draw a basic representation of a clock)
- Physical exam and history clues to the diagnosis are given in Table 10.

INITIAL MANAGEMENT
Basic Principles
- Treat any correctable cause of dementia.
- Ensure that infections, hypoxia, dehydration, metabolic disturbances, pain, and constipation are treated effectively.
- Correct hearing or visual loss to extent possible.
- Avoid agents with anticholinergic properties.
- Minimize psychoactive medications with possible adverse cognitive side effects to the fewest agents at the lowest effective doses.
- Nonpharmacologic interventions (see Table 4)

Table 9. Mini-Mental State Examination

	Points
1. Orientation	
Name: season, date, day, month, year	5 (1 for each name)
Name: hospital, floor, town, state, country	5 (1 for each name)
2. Registration	
Identify 3 objects by name and ask patient to repeat	3 (1 for each object)
3. Attention and calculation	
Serial 7s—subtract from 100 (e.g., 93, 86, 79, 72, 65)	5 (1 for each subtraction)
4. Recall	
Recall the 3 objects presented earlier	3 (1 for each object)
5. Language	
Name pencil & watch	2 (1 for each object)
Repeat "No ifs, ands, or buts"	1
Follow a 3-step command (e.g., "Take this paper, fold it in half, and place it on the table")	3 (1 for each command)
Write "close your eyes," and ask patient to obey written command	1
Ask patient to write a sentence	1
Ask patient to copy a design (e.g., intersecting pentagons)	1
Total	30*

*Score <24 is abnormal.

Pharmacologic Therapy
- Alzheimer dementia
  - ▲ Vitamin E 1,000 IU twice daily
  - ▲ Donepezil (Aricept), galantamine (Reminyl), rivastigmine (Exelon), or tacrine (Cognex—this is rarely used because of side effects, especially hepatotoxicity)
- Dementia with Lewy bodies
  - ▲ Donepezil or rivastigmine for behavioral symptoms
  - ▲ Use carbidopa-levodopa (Sinemet) for cognitive or motor symptoms; avoid if psychosis is present.

Table 10. Physical Exam and History Clues to the Diagnosis

Presentation	Possible causes

Atypical course
  Rapidly progressive
  Waxing and waning
  Series of abrupt changes in
    clinical course
	Vascular, infectious, toxic/
	metabolic processes, vasculitis, multiple sclerosis, dementia with Lewy bodies, frontotemporal dementia, vascular dementia, Creutzfeldt-Jakob disease

Systemic symptoms
  Headache
  Fever
  Dry eyes/mouth
  Myalgias
  Arthralgias
  Weight loss
  Skin lesions
	Infection, vasculitis, neoplastic, paraneoplastic processes

Sleep disorder
  Excessive daytime somnolence
  Loud snoring
  Observed apnea
  Motor restlessness/insomnia
  Leg jerks while sleeping
	Obstructive sleep apnea, central sleep apnea, restless legs syndrome, periodic limb movement disorder

Neuropsychiatric symptoms
  Behavioral/personality change
  Apathy
  Visual hallucinations
  Delusions
  Agitation
	Dementia with Lewy bodies, frontotemporal dementia, infection, vasculitis, toxic/metabolic processes

Neurologic symptoms or signs
  Diplopia
  Dysphagia
  Face or limb weakness or
    numbness
  Gait unsteadiness
	Brain tumor, abscess

Parkinsonian signs
  Masked facies
  Abnormal gait
  Stooped posture
  Tremor
  Rigidity
	Parkinson disease, dementia with Lewy bodies, normal-pressure hydrocephalus

▲ Avoid conventional neuroleptic agents because parkinsonism can worsen.

▲ Delusions, hallucinations, agitation may respond to selective serotonin reuptake inhibitors, carbamazepine, valproic acid, or newer neuroleptic agents (e.g., quetiapine).

▲ Treat underlying depression.

■ Frontotemporal dementia

▲ Donepezil, rivastigmine, carbidopa-levodopa, and psychostimulants can help cognitive symptoms.

▲ Behavioral dyscontrol may respond to selective serotonin reuptake inhibitors, carbamazepine, or valproic acid.

■ Vascular dementia

▲ Control hypertension and diabetes.

▲ Aspirin, clopidogrel (warfarin for selected causes)

■ Normal-pressure hydrocephalus

▲ Consider ventriculoperitoneal shunt, especially if symptoms have been present <2 years.

▲ Carbidopa-levodopa may be helpful in some patients.

Nonpharmacologic Therapy

■ Promote establishment of a daily routine.

■ Regular light exercise

■ Support groups (Alzheimer Association)

■ Address safety issues.

▲ Driving assessment

▲ Home environment

▲ Wandering

DIARRHEA

David Allan Cook, M.D.
Darrell S. Pardi, M.D.

DEFINITION
- Stool weight >250 g/day

ACUTE DIARRHEA
Is the Patient's Life at Risk?
- Risk can be from underlying disease process or secondary effects.

Potentially Dangerous Diseases
- Invasive infection: *Salmonella*, *Shigella*, other
- Toxin: hemolytic uremic syndrome from *Escherichia coli* O157:H7
- Ischemia: ischemic bowel
- Poisoning: organophosphate exposure
- Gastrointestinal bleed (is this really melena?)
- Impaction, early obstruction, toxic megacolon

Secondary Effects
- Hypovolemia: dehydration
- Electrolyte abnormalities: sodium, potassium, bicarbonate
- Anemia (if blood loss)

Immediate Evaluation
History
- Frequency and volume of stool, e.g., large volume—dehydration?

Special abbreviations used in this chapter: EGD, esophagogastroduodenoscopy; O&P, ova and parasites; SBFT, small-bowel follow-through; VIP, vasoactive intestinal peptide.

- Character of stool, e.g., black tar—melena?
- Abdominal pain: severe pain in ischemia, cramping relieved with defecation in infection, dull ache with impaction
- Past history: abdominal surgery, HIV-positive
- Recent hospitalization or antibiotic use (*Clostridium difficile*?)
- Medications

Examination
- Vital signs: fever >38.3°C, hypotension, tachycardia, orthostasis
- Dehydration (physical exam is unreliable in adults—in evaluation, consider skin turgor, orthostasis, flat jugular venous pressure, tachycardia, hypotension)
- Abdomen: peritoneal signs
- Rectal: frank blood or melena indicates gastrointestinal bleed; occult or streaked blood suggests inflammatory diarrhea.

Further Evaluation Directed by History and Exam Findings
- CBC, electrolytes, and renal function
- Consider abdominal X-ray.
- Consider fecal WBCs, *Clostridium difficile* toxin, and bacterial culture. Blood culture if severely ill or known HIV-positive

Addressing the Risk
Is There Hypovolemia/Dehydration?
- IV access
- Normal saline
- Record volume input and output.
- Type and screen for transfusion if possible bleeding.
- Assess electrolytes and renal function.

Is There Severe Abdominal Pain?
- Consider surgical consult
- Check liver chemistry values (ALT, alkaline phosphatase, bilirubin), amylase, serum lactate.
- NPO
- IV fluids
- Abdominal X-ray; consider abdominal CT.

Is There Question of Severe Infection?
- Consider antibiotics after obtaining stool cultures.

Differential Diagnosis
Infectious
- Acute diarrhea is nearly always infectious in outpatients, less so in inpatients.
- Invasive bacteria: *Campylobacter jejuni*, some *E. coli*, *Salmonella* spp., *Shigella* spp., *Yersinia enterocolitica*
- Toxigenic bacteria: *Clostridium difficile*, *Vibrio cholerae*, some *E. coli*
- Parasitic: amebae, *Giardia*, *Cryptosporidium*, *Cyclospora*
- Virus: adenovirus, *Rotavirus*, Norwalk virus
- Food poisoning: *Bacillus cereus*, *Clostridium perfringens*, *Staphylococcus aureus*, other *Vibrio* spp., *Listeria monocytogenes*

Medications
- Antibiotics, antacids (magnesium), laxatives, quinine, digoxin, NSAIDs, sorbitol, colchicine, tube feedings, herbal remedies

Toxins
- Organophosphates

Diet
- Undigested sugars (lactose in milk, sweeteners like sorbitol, fructose from fruit or juice), fiber

Ischemia

Impaction

Differentiating the Differential
Key Distinction—Inflammatory vs. Noninflammatory
- Inflammatory
  - ▲ Usually arises from the colon = low volume, may be mucoid
  - ▲ "Dysentery" = abdominal pain/cramp, fever, WBCs and RBCs in stool
- Noninflammatory
  - ▲ Usually from the small bowel = large volume, watery
  - ▲ No WBCs or RBCs in stool
- The history provides the majority of information.

Onset, Duration
- More than 3 weeks is "chronic"

Frequency, Volume, and Form of Stool; Nighttime Stool; Incontinence
- Is this true diarrhea (>250 mL) or simply loose stool or frequent defecation?
- Absence of nighttime stool suggests condition is *not* organic.
- Incontinence may imply an anatomic (or neurologic) abnormality.

Blood, Pus, Mucus, Oil/Grease
- Mucus suggests irritable bowel syndrome or infection.
- Oil (steatorrhea) suggests fat malabsorption (see "Chronic").

Pain, Fever, Weight Loss
- "Pain more impressive than exam" suggests ischemia.
- Rectal pain and urgency = tenesmus, suggests inflammation.
- Fever suggests inflammation.

Recent Travel, Camping, Swimming, Eating
- Trip to Mexico, for example, suggests "traveler's diarrhea" or parasite.
- Camping suggests *Giardia* infection.
- Eating history may suggest food poisoning.

Diet
- Dairy: lactose intolerance is common.
- Sorbitol (included in many diet foods) and fructose (fruits, juices) can cause diarrhea.
- Ethanol in excess

Medications
- New medications, laxatives, antibiotics; self-treatment for constipation

Abdominal Operations, HIV Status, Other Medical Conditions
- Previous surgery may suggest partial obstruction.
- AIDS has its own differential (not discussed here).

Test Ordering
- Usually not necessary in acute diarrhea in an outpatient setting without dysentery

Further Evaluation Is Indicated If
- Significant pain
- Fever (>38.3°C)
- Dehydration
- Bloody stool
- Extended duration (>5 days)

Further Evaluation Includes
- Stool WBC, ova and parasites (O&P), *Clostridium difficile* toxin; consider bacterial culture
  - ▲ Cultures are rarely positive (<10%) *unless* WBCs are present (then 75% positive) or other red flags are present.
  - ▲ Stool cultures or O&P for *new* diarrhea after *3 days of hospitalization* is virtually useless (but check *C. difficile* toxin).
  - ▲ When checking O&P or *C. difficile* toxin, 3 negative tests are required to reliably rule out infection.
- CBC, electrolytes, creatinine/BUN
- Consider abdominal X-ray.
- Consider flexible sigmoidoscopy.

Management
- Nearly all acute diarrhea is mild, self-limited, and resolves in <5 days.
- Hydration (PO preferred with balanced rehydration solution; IV if needed)
- Specific treatment if cause is known
- Bismuth subsalicylate (Pepto-Bismol)

Antidiarrheal (If Not Inflammatory)
- Loperamide (Imodium)
- Diphenoxylate with atropine (Lomotil)

Antibiotics
- Often not indicated

- Treat (only if not improving spontaneously)
  - ▲ Antibiotic resistance is often a problem and varies geographically.
  - ▲ *Shigella* (ampicillin), *Vibrio parahaemolyticus* (erythromycin), *Yersinia enterocolitica* (trimethoprim-sulfamethoxazole [Bactrim]), *Campylobacter jejuni* (ciprofloxacin), *V. vulnificus* (tetracycline)
  - ▲ Fluoroquinolones are also effective.
  - ▲ Do *not* treat *Salmonella* (except if severe or systemic, then with ciprofloxacin) because it may prolong carriage state.
  - ▲ Do *not* treat *E. coli* O157:H7 because it may increase the risk of hemolytic uremic syndrome.

CHRONIC DIARRHEA (>3 WEEKS)
Differential Diagnosis
Osmotic
- Medications including laxatives
- Undigested sugars
  - ▲ Carbohydrate malabsorption: sorbitol, lactulose, mannitol, fiber
  - ▲ Enzyme dysfunction: lactose, fructose

Fatty (Subset of Osmotic)
- Maldigestion
  - ▲ Decreased bile salts: cirrhosis, bile duct obstruction, ileal resection
  - ▲ Pancreatic dysfunction: chronic pancreatitis, cystic fibrosis, duct obstruction
- Malabsorption
  - ▲ Celiac sprue, tropical sprue
  - ▲ Short-bowel syndrome
  - ▲ Bacterial overgrowth: diabetes mellitus, scleroderma, previous bowel surgery
  - ▲ Lymphatic obstruction
  - ▲ Infection: *Giardia*, *Isospora*, *Mycobacterium avium-intracellulare*, *Tropheryma whippelii* (Whipple disease)

Secretory
- Endocrine
  - ▲ Gastrointestinal: vasoactive intestinal peptide (VIP)-secreting tumor (VIPoma), carcinoid tumor, gastrinoma, medullary thyroid cancer

▲ Systemic: Addison disease, hyperthyroidism
- Stimulant laxatives, other medications
- Villous adenoma, lymphoma
- Connective tissue diseases: vasculitis, systemic lupus erythematosus, mixed connective tissue disease
- Bile salt malabsorption (ileal resection)

Inflammatory
- Inflammatory bowel disease: ulcerative colitis, Crohn disease, lymphocytic or collagenous colitis
- Malignancy: colon cancer, lymphoma
- Radiation colitis or enteritis
- Infection (see below)
- Ischemia

Motility
- Postsurgical: vagotomy, sympathectomy
- Scleroderma
- Diabetes mellitus
- Hyperthyroidism
- Irritable bowel syndrome

Infection
- Parasite: *Giardia*, ameba
- HIV-related: *Cyclospora*, Microsporida, *Cryptosporidium, Isospora, Mycobacterium avium-intracellulare* complex
- TB
- *Clostridium difficile*
- Viral: cytomegalovirus, herpes simplex virus—usually immunocompromised host

Differentiating the Differential
History
- Same as for acute diarrhea

Examination
- Same as for acute diarrhea, plus signs of systemic illness
- Skin: flushing (serotonin syndrome), rash, erythema nodosum

- Oral: inflammatory bowel disease, celiac sprue
- Ocular: inflammatory bowel disease, Reiter syndrome
- Joints: inflammatory bowel disease, Whipple disease, connective tissue disease
- Lymphadenopathy

Test Ordering
Stage I—Classify Diarrhea
- Stool: WBCs, *Clostridium difficile* toxin, occult blood, pH, electrolytes (sodium, potassium, ± osmolality), 72-hour fecal fat (on a high fat diet), laxative screen (magnesium, sulfate [SO_4], phosphate [PO_4])
  - ▲ WBCs or RBCs = inflammatory
  - ▲ Low pH = sugar malabsorption
  - ▲ Osmolar gap = $290 - [(\text{sodium} + \text{potassium}) \times 2]$
    - Gap <50, sodium >90 = secretory
    - Gap >100, sodium <60 = osmotic
    - If possibility of dilution (urine, water), check osmolality.
      - \>375 = urine (sodium usually >150)
      - <200 = water
  - ▲ >14 g fat/24 hours = steatorrhea (malabsorptive)
    - 7-14 g indeterminate
- Blood: CBC, ESR, electrolytes, albumin, INR, thyroid-stimulating hormone
  - ▲ Anemia: consider inflammatory bowel disease, malabsorption, malignancy.
  - ▲ Eosinophils: consider parasite (*Strongyloides*), eosinophilic enteritis, malignancy.
  - ▲ High ESR: consider inflammatory bowel disease, malignancy, connective tissue disease.
  - ▲ Low sodium, high potassium: consider Addison disease.
  - ▲ Low albumin, high INR: consider malabsorption.
  - ▲ Note: If long-standing diarrhea, consider nutrition evaluation (25-OH vitamin D, zinc, iron, vitamin B_{12}, folate in addition to INR and albumin).

Stage II—Evaluate According to Class
- **Secretory** diarrhea
  - ▲ Increased secretion of electrolytes, normal osmolar gap
  - ▲ Large volume, no change with fast
  - ▲ Infection?: bacterial culture, O&P × 3, *Giardia* antigen, HIV

- If HIV-positive, must check (in addition to above) for *Cyclospora* (modified acid-fast stain), *Cryptosporidium* (ELISA preferred to modified acid fast), and Microsporida
  - ▲ Structural defect?: small-bowel follow-through (SBFT), colonoscopy, abdominal CT, upper endoscopy esophago-gastroduodenoscopy (EGD) with small-bowel biopsy
  - ▲ Endocrine?: serum gastrin, VIP, calcitonin, somatostatin; urine 5-hydroxyindoleacetic acid, metanephrine/cate-cholamines, histamine; consider adrenocorticotropic hormone stimulation test
  - ▲ Bile acid malabsorption?: consider trial of cholestyramine
  - ▲ Consider serum protein electrophoresis
- **Osmotic** diarrhea
  - ▲ Improves with fasting
  - ▲ Increased osmolar gap
  - ▲ Low pH (<6)
    - Undigested sugars?: review diet and medications (sorbitol)
    - Hydrogen breath (H_2) test
  - ▲ High stool magnesium, SO_4, PO_4: laxative or antacid use
- **Fatty** (subset of osmotic) diarrhea
  - ▲ Weight loss, nutrition deficiency, steatorrhea
  - ▲ Small-bowel disorder?: SBFT, EGD with small-bowel biopsy (including Congo red stain for amyloid)
  - ▲ Pancreatic insufficiency?: secretin stimulation test, chole-cystokinin stimulation test, stool chymotrypsin activity, abdominal CT
  - ▲ Bacterial overgrowth?: small-bowel quantitative culture (or empiric trial of antibiotics)
- **Inflammatory** diarrhea
  - ▲ SBFT, colonoscopy, abdominal CT
  - ▲ Infection?: stool bacterial culture, O&P × 3, *Clostridium difficile* toxin × 3; serum HIV screen

Management
General Measures
- Hydration if needed
- If specific cause is found, treat it (below).

- Otherwise
  - ▲ Try dietary changes: cut out dairy, caffeine, diet foods (sorbitol), fruit (fructose), ethanol.
  - ▲ Treat symptoms: if noninflammatory, loperamide or diphenoxylate with atropine (Lomotil) can be used, as under "Acute."

Irritable Bowel Syndrome (Diarrhea-Predominant)
- May not meet strict definition for diarrhea (frequent bowel movements, but usually normal stool volume)
- Definition: chronic, recurrent abdominal pain with altered bowel movements; characterized further by the Rome criteria
- Treatment
  - ▲ Education
  - ▲ Food, dairy: triggers?
  - ▲ Fiber helps in some cases
  - ▲ Loperamide or diphenoxylate with atropine
  - ▲ Treat pain
    - Daily cramps: tricyclic antidepressant or selective serotonin-reuptake inhibitor
    - Occasional cramps: as needed, antispasmodic—dicyclomine, hyoscyamine (Levsin)

Laxative Use/Abuse or Carbohydrate Malabsorption
- Stop laxative or modify diet as needed.
- Lactase deficiency: lactase supplement (Lactaid)

Bile Salt Malabsorption
- Try cholestyramine.
- May paradoxically *worsen* diarrhea (if it leads to bile salt *deficiency*)
- If so
  - ▲ Stop cholestyramine.
  - ▲ Diet modification: low fat (<50 g/day), may need supplementation with medium-chain triglycerides

Pancreatic Insufficiency
- Pancreatic enzyme supplementation (various formulations)
  - ▲ Nonencapsulated formulations—may be inactivated in acidic stomach, consider adding proton pump inhibitor.

▲ Encapsulated formulations are protected from acid, but capsule may not dissolve in the duodenum.

Bacterial Overgrowth

- Amoxicillin-clavulanate (Augmentin), ciprofloxacin, or metronidazole: 1- to 2-week course
- If symptoms improve and recur, treat again.
- May need long-term rotating antibiotics

Celiac Sprue

- A response to a gluten-free diet is *part of the diagnosis* as well as the only available treatment.
  - ▲ Lack of effect of diet or recurrent symptoms in a previously compliant patient, consider
    - Noncompliance
    - Alternate diagnosis—small-bowel lymphoma, refractory sprue, microscopic colitis

Inflammatory Bowel Disease

- See chapter on Inflammatory Bowel Disease

DIZZINESS AND VERTIGO

Yoon-Hee K. Cha, M.D.
Scott D. Eggers, M.D.
David A. Froehling, M.D.

IS THE PATIENT'S LIFE AT RISK?

- Dizziness or vertigo can be the presenting symptom of vertebrobasilar ischemia or hemorrhage, particularly in older patients with thromboembolic risk factors (e.g., hypertension, diabetes mellitus, arrhythmia, valvular disease) or a bleeding diathesis.
- Most serious cerebrovascular lesions causing vertigo, such as infarction or hemorrhage of the brainstem or cerebellum, are associated with focal neurologic deficits, including extremity and gait ataxia, dysarthria, diplopia, facial pain or weakness, Horner syndrome, sensory changes, or unilateral weakness.
- Transient ischemic attacks generally resolve in minutes, before the physician has seen the patient, so the history and context are critical to making the diagnosis.

ADDRESSING THE RISK

- The most important step in the evaluation of patients with dizziness is to clarify the nature and temporal course of the symptoms with a detailed history.
  - ▲ Are symptoms precipitated by head movement?
  - ▲ Are there focal neurologic deficits?
  - ▲ What are associated symptoms (e.g., palpitations, headache, paresthesias, tinnitus, hearing loss, angina, nausea, vomiting)?
  - ▲ Has there been head trauma or exposure to ototoxic medications?
  - ▲ What are the patient's other medical problems (e.g., diabetes mellitus, cardiac disease, psychiatric problems)?

Special abbreviation used in this chapter: BPPV, benign paroxysmal positional vertigo.

DIFFERENTIAL DIAGNOSIS

- Dizziness is classified in Table 1.

DIFFERENTIATING THE DIFFERENTIAL

- Features of peripheral and central vertigo are compared in Table 2.

DIAGNOSTIC TEST ORDERING

Bedside Exam—Determine Whether Symptoms Arise From the Vestibular System or Elsewhere

Baseline

- Vital signs—including orthostatic blood pressure
- Cardiac exam—carotid bruits, arrhythmia, aortic stenosis

Table 1. Classification of Dizziness

Vertigo—the illusion of movement (spinning, rocking, tumbling)
    Recurrent positional vertigo
        Benign paroxysmal positional vertigo
        Craniocervical junction abnormalities (uncommon)
        Brain neoplasms (rare)
    Recurrent spontaneous episodes of vertigo
        Vertebrobasilar transient ischemic attacks
        Meniere syndrome
        Vestibular migraine
        Autoimmune/syphilitic
    Prolonged spontaneous episode of vertigo
        Vestibular neuritis
        Infarction or hemorrhage of labyrinth, brainstem, or
          cerebellum
        Multiple sclerosis
Dysequilibrium—a loss of balance or equilibrium
    Visual disturbance, peripheral neuropathy, ataxia, extrapyra-
      midal syndrome, Wernicke's encephalopathy
Presyncope—the feeling of impending loss of consciousness
    Orthostatic hypotension, myocardial infarction, vasovagal
      reaction, cardiac arrhythmia, vascular disease
Psychogenic
    Anxiety, depression, panic attack, hyperventilation, hypo-
      chondriasis

Table 2. Comparison of Peripheral and Central Causes of Vertigo

Feature	Peripheral	Central
Symptoms/signs		
Nausea/vomiting	Severe	Variable
Imbalance	Mild (fall to side of lesion)	Severe (unable to stand)
Hearing loss	May occur	Rare
Neurologic symptoms	Rare	Common
Romberg sign	Present	Variable
Nystagmus	Horizontal ± torsional	Vertical or torsional
	Same direction in all gaze positions	Direction changes with gaze position

- Neurologic exam—focal deficits, especially cranial nerve abnormalities or ataxia
- Medication list—aminoglycosides, anticonvulsants, antihypertensives, diuretics, tranquilizers
- If age >45 years, order ECG and glucose.
- Consider giving thiamine if Wernicke encephalopathy is a possibility

Neuro-otologic Testing

Nystagmus

- Central—clues to central causes of nystagmus include pure vertical, torsional or direction-changing nystagmus, lack of fatigability, or lack of suppression with visual fixation
  - ▲ Note effect with convergence (e.g., downbeat converting to upbeat in Wernicke encephalopathy). Other neurologic signs/symptoms suggest central cause.
- Peripheral
  - ▲ Nystagmus occurs in one direction regardless of eye position and is often suppressible by visual fixation.
  - ▲ Note direction of the nystagmus (named by the fast phase) and effect of eye position on nystagmus.

▲ Peripheral lesions usually produce mixed horizontal/torsional (vestibular neuritis) or vertical/torsional (benign paroxysmal positional vertigo [BPPV]) nystagmus.

Head Thrust (Head Impulse) Testing
- A simple, effective bedside test to determine peripheral vestibular hypofunction but requires practice to interpret (see Arch Neurol. 1988;45:737-9).

Occlusive Ophthalmoscopy
- Observe for movement (spontaneous nystagmus) of the optic disk with the patient visually fixating on a distant target with the other eye.
- Then cover the other eye with your hand and observe whether nystagmus develops or intensifies.
- Nystagmus enhanced by removing visual fixation is generally of peripheral origin.

Positional Testing—Dix-Hallpike Maneuver
- With the head turned 45° to the side, the patient is rapidly taken from a sitting to supine position, with the head hanging 30° over the table (Fig. 1). The test is repeated for each side.
- A positive test for BPPV includes a 3-10–second latency, followed by a mixed upbeat/torsional nystagmus, with the top pole of the eye beating toward the affected (lower) ear. This usually reproduces the patient's vertigo.

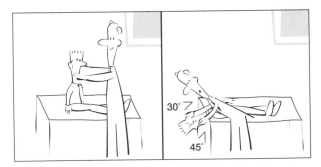

Fig. 1. Dix-Hallpike maneuver.

- Nystagmus usually lasts <30 seconds and fatigues with repeated testing.

Dynamic Visual Acuity
- Patient reads letters on handheld Snellen chart as the examiner rocks patient's head horizontally or vertically twice per second.
- Loss of more than 1 line of visual acuity suggests bilateral vestibular hypofunction.

Vestibulospinal Reflexes
- Romberg sign—elicited by having patient stand with feet together and then closing eyes
  - ▲ If either proprioceptive or vestibular reflexes are diminished, patient loses balance.
  - ▲ If problem is vestibular, patient tends to fall to side of lesion.
- Tandem gait—assessed by having patient walk forward and backward heel to toe

INITIAL MANAGEMENT
Suspected Cerebral Infarction or Hemorrhage
- Emergent non-contrast head CT
- Stroke work-up and treatment (tissue plasminogen activator?) as indicated
- Caveat: large cerebellar infarction or hemorrhage may produce life-threatening edema and brainstem compression requiring neurosurgical decompression

Benign Paroxysmal Positional Vertigo
- The most common cause of vertigo; more frequent with advancing age
- Characterized by vertigo and nystagmus associated with changes in head position
- Vertigo generally lasts <1 minute, frequent episodes
- Cause—dislocation of calcium carbonate crystals from labyrinthine utricle into posterior semicircular canal
- Diagnosis—based on history and appearance of latent, fatigable, torsional/vertical nystagmus on Dix-Hallpike maneuver

- Treatment—canalith repositioning (Epley) maneuver, which attempts to liberate the crystals from posterior semicircular canal (see N Engl J Med. 1999;341:1590-6).

Vestibular Neuritis (Also Called Vestibular Neuronitis, Acute Labyrinthitis)
- Second most common cause of vertigo
- Spontaneous vertigo and nausea lasting days and gradually recovering
- Diagnosis—spontaneous unidirectional horizontal/torsional nystagmus from the acute peripheral unilateral vestibular hypofunction (fast phases away from the affected ear).
- Absence of other signs/symptoms, caloric testing
- If hearing loss, fever, recent otitis media, rule out bacterial labyrinthitis
- Head CT or MRI with gadolinium if any suspicion of central cause
- Treatment—oral prednisone 100 mg daily with 3-week taper improves recovery if started within 2 days after disease onset. Vestibular suppressants (meclizine, promethazine) for 24-72 hours as needed, early vestibular rehabilitation

DYSPNEA

Lin Y. Chen, M.D.
Guilherme H. M. Oliveira, M.D.
Joseph G. Murphy, M.D.

IS THE PATIENT'S LIFE AT RISK?

- Is problem acute, chronic, or acute on chronic?
- If acute or acute on chronic, what is the severity?
- Indications of increased severity
  - ▲ Altered mental status
  - ▲ Hemodynamic instability
  - ▲ Oxyhemoglobin saturation <88%
  - ▲ Altered respiratory pattern
    - Inability to speak normally in full sentences
    - Posture—sitting up and hunching forward
    - Rapid and shallow breathing
    - Accessory muscle use with supraclavicular retractions
    - Thoracoabdominal dyssynchrony (signals impending respiratory failure)
    - Stridor (signals upper airway obstruction)
- Always consider the following life-threatening conditions:
  - ▲ Pulmonary—tension pneumothorax, asthma/COPD exacerbation, pneumonia, pulmonary embolism
  - ▲ Cardiac—acute myocardial infarction, congestive heart failure, cardiac tamponade, valvular disease

ADDRESSING THE RISK

- Determine patient's cardiopulmonary history.
- Establish the following fundamental factors:
  - ▲ Patent airway—exclude upper airway obstruction (in sedated patient, tilt head back and lift mandible while standing at head of bed).
  - ▲ Hemodynamic stability

Special abbreviations used in this chapter: ABG, arterial blood gas; FIO_2, fraction of inspired oxygen.

- ▲ Adequate oxygenation
  - • Target PaO_2 >60 mm Hg and/or oxygen saturation >90% (Table 1)
  - • Call Respiratory Therapy for assistance.
  - • If hypercarbia is not a concern, start with high FIO_2 and titrate oxygen flow by pulse oximeter or arterial blood gas (ABG) results.
  - • If hypercarbia is a concern, slower oxygen titration with serial ABGs is required.
  - • To ICU for high flow oxygen delivery or assisted ventilation (invasive or noninvasive) if satisfactory oxygenation, mental status, and acid-base status (pH ≥7.30) not achieved

DIFFERENTIAL DIAGNOSIS
The differential diagnosis of acute dyspnea is broad and can be organized as shown in Table 2.

DIFFERENTIATING THE DIFFERENTIAL
Constellation of certain history, physical exam, and lab data suggest the diagnosis, as shown in Table 3.

DIAGNOSTIC TEST ORDERING
The order and urgency of tests depends on patient's status (Table 4). All patients should have a pulse oximeter check and most need ABGs, chest X-ray, ECG, and CBC.

INITIAL MANAGEMENT
Asthma Exacerbation
- ▪ Oxygen to correct hypoxemia, goal is saturation >90%
- ▪ Nebulized albuterol (0.5 mL of 0.5% solution [2.5 mg] in 1.25 mL normal saline) ± ipratropium bromide (2.5 mL of 0.02% solution [0.5 mg])
  - ▲ Frequency depends on severity of symptoms and medication side effects.
  - ▲ Range—continuous to every 20-60 minutes to every 2-6 hours
  - ▲ Titrate frequency to patient's exam and peak flows.
- ▪ Methylprednisolone (60-80 mg IV every 6-8 hours)
- ▪ Identify and treat precipitating cause(s); consider antibiotics if purulent sputum.

Table 1. Low Flow Methods for Administration of Acute Oxygen Therapy

Oxygen delivery device	Indications	Oxygen	FIO$_2$	Advantages	Disadvantages
Nasal canula (also applies to nasal masks such as nasal "scoop" or nasal cup)	Less hypoxic patients	0.25-6 L/min	0.24-0.40, depends on patient's minute ventilation	Simple to use Free access to mouth	Imprecise, limited FIO$_2$ Difficult to exceed flow rates >6 L/min
Venturi mask	Controlled oxygen therapy (e.g., acute-on-chronic hypercapnic respiratory failure from COPD)	Flow rate varies with FIO$_2$ setting	0.24, 0.26, 0.28, 0.30, 0.35, 0.40, 0.50	Precise FIO$_2$	Maximum FIO$_2$ 50%
Simple face mask	FIO$_2$ needs >0.40	5-10 L/min	0.30-0.60, depends on patient's minute ventilation & mask fit	Useful in patients with moderate oxygen requirements	Mask may be difficult to tolerate (tight-fitting mask essential)
Partial rebreather mask (no valves in mask, first 1/3 of expired air enters reservoir bag & is rebreathed)	Severely hypoxic patients	10-15 L/min (enough to keep reservoir bag 2/3 full during inspiration)	0.50-0.80	Useful in patients with high oxygen requirements	Mask may be difficult to tolerate
Non-rebreather mask (1-way valves on mask direct exhaled air out of mask, not into reservoir bag)	Severely hypoxic patients	10-15 L/min (same as for partial rebreather mask)	0.60-0.90	Useful in patients with high oxygen requirements	Mask may be difficult to tolerate

- Beware: history of intubation during exacerbations, elderly patient, pregnant, significant comorbidities, history of steroid-induced problems
- Follow with exams and peak expiratory flows at least twice daily.
- To ICU if P_{CO_2} >40 with severe airflow obstruction, no improvement or deterioration in speech, mental status, vital signs despite therapy

Table 2. Causes of Acute Dyspnea

Pulmonary
  Asthma exacerbation
  COPD exacerbation
  Pneumonia
  Pulmonary embolism
  Tension pneumothorax
  Upper airway obstruction (trauma, neoplasm, epiglottitis, laryngeal edema, foreign body)
  Pleural disease
  Interstitial lung disease
  Neoplasm
  Atelectasis
Cardiac
  Acute myocardial infarction
  Congestive heart failure
  Cardiac tamponade
  Arrhythmias
  Valvular disease
  Cardiomyopathy
Neuromuscular
  Myopathy
  Myasthenia gravis
  Spinal cord disorder
  Guillain-Barré syndrome
Others
  Anemia
  Hyperthyroidism
  Acidosis
  Sepsis
  Shock
  Pain
  Intra-abdominal process
  Anxiety

Table 3. Diagnosis of Cause of Dyspnea

History	Exam	Chest X-ray	Diagnosis
Acute dyspnea, chest pain, cough	Trachea deviates away from hyperresonant lung field with ↓ breath sounds	Visceral plural line visible	Pneumothorax
Obstructive lung disease	Wheezing, prolonged expiration, accessory respiratory muscle use, ↓ peak expiratory flow rate, pulsus paradoxus (↓ systolic blood pressure >10 mm Hg in inspiration vs. expiration)	Hyperinflated lung fields	Asthma/COPD exacerbation
Cough, phlegm production, pleuritic chest pain	Fever, bronchial breath sounds, crackles	Infiltrates, effusion	Pneumonia
Acute dyspnea, pleuritic chest pain, risk factors for venous thromboembolism	Tachypnea, crackles, tachycardia	Nonspecific (↑ hemidiaphragm, atelectasis, parenchymal densities, unilateral effusion)	Pulmonary embolism
Chest pain/pressure	↑ or ↓ blood pressure & heart rate, crackles, murmurs, ST-segment changes on ECG, ↑ CK, ↑ CK-MB, ↑ tropon n	May be normal, signs of congestive heart failure	Acute myocardial infarction
More gradual-onset dyspnea, orthopnea, paroxysmal nocturnal dyspnea	Bibasilar crackles, 3rd heart sound, ↑ jugular venous pressure	Kerley B lines, pleural effusion, perihilar congestion, engorged upper lung zone vessels, cardiomegaly, interstitial or alveolar infiltrates	Congestive heart failure
	Ptosis, dysphagia, fatigability, proximal weakness	--	Myasthenia gravis
	Ascending weakness, areflexia	--	Guillain-Barré syndrome

COPD Exacerbation

- Oxygen to correct hypoxemia, administer carefully if hypercapnia is a concern
- Nebulized bronchodilators
- Methylprednisolone (60-125 mg IV every 6-8 hours)
- Identify and treat precipitating cause(s); give antibiotics if new onset of sputum production or change in sputum quality.

Table 4. Tests According to Signs, Symptoms, and Diagnosis

Symptoms/signs	Diagnosis	Tests ordered
Wheezing, prolonged expiration	COPD or asthma exacerbation	CXR, ABG, pre-/post-bronchodilator peak expiratory flow
Fever, productive cough, bronchial breath sounds or crackles	Pneumonia	CXR; ABG; sputum Gram stain/culture; blood cultures ($\times2$); CBC with differential, chemistry panel; thoracocentesis with stains/cultures & pH, LDH, protein, glucose
Pleuritic chest pain, hemoptysis, right parasternal heave, loud P_2, jugular venous distension, tachycardia	Pulmonary embolism	CXR, ABG, ECG, D-dimer, CT angiography vs. V/Q lung scan vs. pulmonary angiography
Chest pain radiating to arm & jaw, diaphoresis, nausea	Acute myocardial infarction	Serial enzymes (CK, CK-MB, troponin T), serial ECG, CXR
Orthopnea, PND, jugular venous distension, displaced PMI, 3rd heart sound	Congestive heart failure	Serial enzymes (CK, CK-MB, troponin T), ECGs to rule out acute myocardial infarction, CXR, echocardiogram
Muffled heart sounds, Kussmaul sign ($\uparrow$ jugular venous pressure during inspiration), pulsus paradoxus	Cardiac tamponade	Emergent bedside echocardiogram

ABG, arterial blood gas; CXR, chest X-ray; P_2, pulmonic 2nd sound; PMI, point of maximal impulse; PND, paroxysmal nocturnal dyspnea; V/Q, ventilation-perfusion.

- Beware: history of intubation during exacerbation, elderly patient, important comorbidities, history of steroid-induced problems, hemodynamic instability
- To ICU for noninvasive or invasive assisted ventilation if pharmacologic therapy fails to reverse respiratory failure (pH <7.30, PaO_2 <55) and/or symptoms

Pneumonia

- Oxygen to correct hypoxemia
- Hydration
- Antibiotics after sputum Gram stain/culture & blood cultures (×2)
  - ▲ Antibiotic choice depends on severity of illness, etiologic factors, exposures, comorbidities, microbiology results, drug resistance concerns, tolerability/side effects of drugs; typical alternatives: fluoroquinolone, macrolide, or third-generation cephalosporin
  - ▲ Likely pathogens for community-acquired pneumonia in hospitalized patients
    - Streptococcus pneumoniae, Haemophilus influenzae, polymicrobial, aerobic gram-negative bacilli, Legionella sp. respiratory viruses
    - Consider Mycobacterium tuberculosis with upper lobe infiltrates and/or high-risk patients
    - Consider aspiration if altered mental status, bulbar weakness, alcohol abuse
- Chest tube if empyema
- Acetaminophen (1 g PO 2-4 times/day as needed—not to exceed 4 g/day)
- Chest physiotherapy

Pulmonary Embolism

- Oxygen to correct hypoxemia
- Heparin (80 U/kg IV bolus, followed by infusion of 18 U/kg per hour)
  - ▲ If clinical suspicion for venous thromboembolism is high, begin heparin before confirmatory testing if no contraindications (e.g., intracranial disease, recent surgery,

history of sensitivity to heparin products, active bleeding, blood dyscrasias).
  - ▲ Recheck aPTT in 4-6 hours, titrate infusion to goal of 60-90 seconds.
- If clinical deterioration, consider bedside transthoracic echocardiogram to evaluate for right ventricular strain and then thrombolysis or surgical thrombectomy.

Pneumothorax
- Tension pneumothorax is a clinical diagnosis and medical emergency.
  - ▲ If suspected, do not wait for chest X-ray, use 14-16–gauge needle to aspirate at 2nd intercostal space in mid-clavicular line.
- Symptomatic or large pneumothoraces without tension require chest-tube drainage.
- Oxygen to correct hypoxemia

Acute Myocardial Infarction
- Transfer patient to ICU or coronary care unit as soon as possible.
- Oxygen
- Aspirin (325 mg PO or rectally)
- Morphine (2-4 mg IV as needed until pain is relieved)
- Angiotensin-converting enzyme inhibitor
- β-Blocker
- Nitrates
- Thrombolysis vs. percutaneous transluminal coronary angioplasty

Congestive Heart Failure
- Oxygen
- Restrict salt and fluid intake, bedrest, prophylaxis for deep venous thrombosis
- Furosemide IV, follow daily weight and input/output
- Angiotensin-converting enzyme inhibitors
- Consider digoxin.
- Determine cause(s) or precipitating factor(s) for heart failure.

ELECTROLYTE DISTURBANCES

Lawrence K. McKnight, M.D.
Robert C. Albright, Jr., D.O.

NORMAL FLUIDS
- Values for fluids are given in Tables 1 and 2.

HYPONATREMIA
Is the Patient's Life at Risk?
- Severity of symptoms and treatment depend on degree of hyponatremia and on rate of onset.
- Rapid correction results in central nervous system swelling and central pontine myelinolysis.
  - ▲ This is worse than the hyponatremia.
  - ▲ Look for mental status changes—lethargy, anorexia, headache, vomiting, agitation, severe weakness, disorientation, coma, seizures.
  - ▲ Check previous lab values, if available, to evaluate progression.
  - ▲ Sodium levels <110-115 mEq/L are generally severe, but this depends on rate of decline.

Addressing the Risk
- If there are mental status changes and hyponatremia is acute, correct more rapidly, up to 1 mEq/hour, and up to half the deficit in the first 24 hours (see Management).
- Find and treat the underlying cause.

Differential Diagnosis
- The differential diagnosis for hyponatremia is listed in Table 3.

Special abbreviations used in this chapter: DI, diabetes insipidus; TTKG, transtubular potassium gradient.

Table 1. Values for Ionic Composition of Normal Fluids*

Fluid	Na$^+$	Cl$^-$	K$^+$	HCO$_3^-$	Quantity/24 hours	Normal replacement, mL/mL
Sweat/burns	50	40	5	0	--	LR
Saliva	60	15	36	50	1.5 L	--
Stomach	80	100	10	0	1.5-2.5 L	D$_5\frac{1}{2}$NS + 20 mEq K$^+$
Duodenum	130	90	5	0-10	0.3-2 L	--
Bile	145	100	5	15	0.1-0.8 L	D$_5$LR + 25 mEq HCO$_3^-$
Pancreas	145	75	5	115	0.1-0.8 L	D$_5$LR + 50 mEq HCO$_3^-$
Ileum	140	100	2-8	30	0.1-9 L	--
Diarrhea	120	90	25	45	--	D$_5$LR + 15 mEq K$^+$

D$_5$LR, 5% dextrose in lactated Ringer solution; LR, lactated Ringer solution; NS, normal saline.
*Ionic values in mEq/L.

Table 2. Contents of IV Fluids

IV fluid	Contents
D$_5$	50 g glucose/L = 170 kcal
D$_{50}$	500 g glucose/L = 1,700 kcal
Normal saline	154 mEq Na$^+$, 154 mEq Cl$^-$
LR	130 mEq Na$^+$, 110 mEq Cl$^-$, 4 mEq K$^+$, 3 mEq Ca$^+$, 27 mEq HCO$_3^-$ per liter

D$_5$, 5% dextrose; D$_{50}$, 50 g/dL dextrose; LR, lactated Ringer solution.

Differentiating the Differential

- Hyponatremia is divided into hyperosmotic, isosmotic, and hypo-osmotic conditions (hypo-osmotic is most common).
- First step in evaluating hypo-osmotic hyponatremia is to assess fluid balance.
  - If the patient is hypovolemic, check spot urine sodium to differentiate renal from nonrenal loss.
  - If the patient is euvolemic, the cause is likely syndrome of inappropriate antidiuretic hormone, but this is a diagnosis of exclusion after thyroid, renal, and adrenal functions have been checked.
  - If hypervolemic, the cause is likely heart, liver, or renal failure.

Table 3. Differential Diagnosis for Hyponatremia

Condition	Suspect when...
Hypovelemic	Orthostatics, skin turgor, ↑BUN:Cr ratio
Renal losses (urine Na >20 mEq/L)	Renal tubular acidosis, polycystic kidney, interstitial nephritis, pyelonephritis, obstruction, diuretics, adrenal insufficiency
	Note: hypokalemia & HCO_3^- loss can potentiate hyponatremia
Nonrenal (urine Na <10 mEq/L)	
GI losses	Vomiting, diarrhea, fistulas
Third space	Pancreatitis, peritonitis, burns
Osmotic diuresis	Mannitol
Euvolemic	
SIADH	↑ADH; low normal serum osmolarity & blood pressure; normal renal, adrenal, thyroid function
	Cancer —lung, duodenum, pancreas, brain, bladder, prostate, lymphoma
	Pulmonary—pneumonia, asthma, TB
	Brain—trauma, infection, hemorrhage, sarcoidosis
	Medications
	Chlorpropamide
	Thiazide diuretics
	TCAs and/or MAOI
	Nicotine
	Cyclophosphamide, vincristine, vinblastine
	Morphine, indomethacin (Indocin), acetaminophen (Tylenol)
	Haloperidol (Haldol), chlorpromazine (Thorazine), barbiturates
	Carbamazepine (Tegretol)
	Vasopressin
	AIDS
Hypothyroid	Decreased deep tendon reflexes, toad face
Primary poly-dipsia	History of excessive water intake

Table 3 (continued)

Condition	Suspect when...
Hypervolemic	Edema, ↑ jugular venous pressure
CHF	Rales, S_3
Cirrhosis	Ascites, jaundice
Renal failure	Nephrosis, increased creatinine
"Pseudo" hyponatremia (osmolality is normal)	
Lipids	Uncontrolled diabetes mellitus, familial
Proteins	Multiple myeloma
Hyperosmolar (osmolality >300 mOsm/kg)	Infusions, diabetes mellitus
	Osmolar gap ($Osm_{measured} - Osm_{est}$) >10
	$Osm_{est} = 2\,[Na] + Glucose/18 + BUN/2.8$
	Diabetes mellitus (1.6 mEq Na per 100 mg/dL glucose)
Lab error	Isolated value, asymptomatic patient

ADH, antidiuretic hormone; CHF, congestive heart failure; Cr, creatinine; GI, gastrointestinal; MAOI, monoamine oxidase inhibitor; S_3, third heart sound; SIADH, syndrome of inappropriate antidiuretic hormone; TCA, tricyclic amine.

Test Ordering

- Check previous sodium value to determine rate of decrease.
- If not explained by history, check serum chemistry panel, serum osmolality, and spot urine electrolytes. Calculate osmolar gap.
- Depending on the history, consider checking sensitive thyrotropin, liver function tests, cortisol, lipids, and arterial blood gases.

Management

- If patient is hypovolemic, replete with normal saline.
- If patient is euvolemic, then fluid restriction
- Demeclocycline 300-600 mg PO twice daily for chronic syndrome of inappropriate antidiuretic hormone
- Hypervolemic, sodium-restricted diet, furosemide
- Severe hyponatremia can be corrected with hypertonic saline, but this is rarely needed (remember, too rapid correction can lead to central pontine myelinolysis).

Replacement Formula
- Total body water (TBW) = weight (kg) $\times$ 0.6 (males) or $\times$ 0.5 (females, elderly)
- Na deficit (mEq) = (desired [Na] – measured [Na]) $\times$ TBW
  - ▲ Note: correct 1/2 deficit over first 24 hours. Desired [Na] is goal for the end of the day.
- Free water excess = TBW $\times$ [1 – (measured [Na]/desired [Na])] (= the amount negative fluid balance you are looking for)
- IV fluid rate (mL/hour) = [Na deficit (mEq)/IV fluid Na concentration (mEq Na/L)] $\times$ 1,000 mL/L $\times$ 1 day/24 hours (3% NaCl = 512 mEq Na/L, normal saline = 0.9% = 154 mEq Na/L)

HYPERNATREMIA

Is the Patient's Life at Risk?
- Hypernatremia, like hyponatremia, presents with neurologic abnormalities related to the acuity of change in sodium concentration.
  - ▲ With acute increase and serum sodium >160 mEq/L, mortality rate is 75%.
  - ▲ Chronic changes are tolerated better and are correlated with plasma osmolality.
- Earliest signs—restlessness, irritability, lethargy
- Later signs (plasma osmolality >375 mOsm)—muscle spasticity, seizures, or death

Addressing the Risk
- Therapy for symptomatic hypernatremia is listed below (see Management).
- Depending on severity of symptoms and rate of change, correct the [Na] rapidly, as addressed in Management section.
- Do not correct >2 mOsm/hour and total correction over 48 hours.
- Find and treat the underlying cause.

Differential Diagnosis
- The differential diagnosis for hypernatremia is listed in Table 4.

Table 4. Differential Diagnosis for Hypernatremia

Condition	Suspect when...
Hypovolemic (H_2O>Na^+ loss)	Orthostatic, skin tenting
Renal (urine Na >20 mEq/L)	Diuretics (loop, thiazide, osmotic), hyperglycemia, uremia, postobstructive diuresis, polyuria, acute tubular necrosis
Nonrenal (urine Na <20 mEq/L)	
GI	Vomiting, nasogastric suction, fistulas, diarrhea
Insensible	Fever (500 mL/day per °C↑), sweating, burns Intubation (may look euvolemic)
Euvolemic	
Central DI (decreased ADH)	CNS insult (postoperative, trauma, infection, granuloma, tumor, metastases) with restricted water access (intubated, comatose) Idiopathic
Nephrogenic DI (ADH ineffective)	Chronic renal disease, medications (lithium, sulfonylurea, analgesics, amphotericin B, colchicine), Sickle cell disease, polycystic kidney disease, hypokalemia, hypercalcemia, congenital
Reset osmolar (maximally concentrated urine)	Hypothalamic brain lesion, hypodipsia, pregnancy
Insensible loss	As above, inability to drink
Hypervolemic	
Mineralocorticoid excess	Cushing syndrome, exogenous steroids, adrenal hyperplasia, ectopic ACTH production, Conn syndrome
Iatrogenic	Salt tablets, dialysate error, postcode ($NaHCO_3$), tube feedings
Lab error	Isolated value, asymptomatic patient

ACTH, corticotropin; ADH, antidiuretic hormone; CNS, central nervous system; DI, diabetes insipidus; GI, gastrointestinal.

Differentiating the Differential
- Begin by evaluating the patient's volume status.
  - ▲ Hypovolemic hypernatremia indicates free water loss in excess of sodium loss
- Check spot urine sodium to distinguish between renal and nonrenal loss.
- Hypervolemic hypernatremia is uncommon and usually iatrogenic.
- Euvolemic hypernatremia is the most common presentation.
- If not accounted for by insensible losses, water deprivation test can be used to differentiate central from nephrogenic diabetes insipidus (DI).
  - ▲ To perform this test, hold all fluids and check urine and plasma osmolality every hour until plasma osmolality is >288 mOsm/kg, weight is down 1-2 kg, and urine osmolality plateaus to within 30 mmol/kg for at least 3 hours
  - ▲ Next, give desmopressin, 1 μg SQ or 10 μg intranasally and check urine and plasma osmolality in 1 hour.
  - ▲ Neither central DI nor nephrogenic DI will be able to concentrate urine with water deprivation.
  - ▲ Central DI will respond to vasopressin with >9% increase in urine osmolality; nephrogenic DI will not.

Test Ordering
- Check previous sodium value to determine rate of increase.
- Urine sodium and osmolality
  - ▲ If hypo-osmolar urine, perform water deprivation test (see above).
- Depending on the history, consider serum chemistry panel, calcium level, dexamethasone suppression test

Management
- If patient is hypovolemic, replenish with half normal saline.
- If patient is euvolemic
  - ▲ If symptomatic, calculate free water deficit.
    - • Free water deficit (L) = weight (kg) × 0.6 × [1 − measured [Na] (mEq/L)/desired [Na] (mEq/L)]
    - • Remember to include patient's normal fluid requirements.

- ▲ Replace half deficit with 5% dextrose or oral free water over first 24 hours
- ▲ Longer term specific therapy:
  - • Central DI—desmopressin 10 µg intranasally once or twice daily
  - • Nephrogenic DI—hydroclorothiazide 12.5-50 mg PO daily, low sodium diet
- ■ If patient is hypervolemic
  - ▲ Furosemide ± 5% dextrose
  - ▲ Dialysis if patient has renal failure

HYPOKALEMIA

Is the Patient's Life at Risk?

- ■ If the patient has symptoms (decreased deep tendon reflexes, paralysis), potassium <2.5 mEq/L, or is receiving digoxin, obtain an ECG.
  - ▲ Look for flat T waves, U waves, increased QT, and arrhythmias.

Addressing the Risk

- ■ If evidence of digitalis intoxication or paralysis, admit patient to ICU for ECG and respiratory monitoring.
- ■ Potassium can be administered IV up to 40 mEq/hour.
- ■ Monitor potassium level every 4 hours.
- ■ Avoid glucose- and alkali-containing solutions because they can precipitate further hypokalemia.

Differential Diagnosis

- ■ The differential diagnosis for hypokalemia is listed in Table 5.

Differentiating the Differential

- ■ After historical exam, including medicine review and patient symptoms, spot urine potassium test can help determine renal cause from extrarenal loss.
- ■ If blood pressure is normal, ensure magnesium level is normal and look for low bicarbonate level to indicate acidosis.
- ■ If there is coexisting hypertension, check renin and aldosterone levels to distinguish between renal artery stenosis and primary hyperaldosteronism.

Table 5. Differential Diagnosis for Hypokalemia

Condition	Suspect when...
Renal loss (urine K >20 mEq/day)	
Hyperaldosteronism	Hypertension (except Bartter syndrome)
Primary hyperaldosteronism	(Low renin)
Increased renin	Renal artery stenosis, renin-secreting tumor, Bartter syndrome
Mineralocorticoid excess	Conn syndrome, congenital adrenal hyperplasia, licorice, Liddle syndrome
RTA (low HCO_3^-)	
RTA 1 (distal)	Hypercalcemia, renal stones, amphotericin B, connective tissue disease, lithium, toluene
	Inability to acidify urine
RTA 2 (proximal)	Multiple myeloma, heavy metals, 6-mercaptopurine, acetazolamide
	Able to acidify urine
Magnesium depletion	Tetany, cardiac arrhythmias
Volume depletion	Vomiting (Na resorbtive state, alkalosis)
Diuretics	High urinary Cl
Antibiotics	High-dose penicillin, carbenicillin (anions)
Extrarenal loss (urine K <25 mEq/day)	
GI	Diarrhea, fistula, nasogastric suction (alkalosis), laxative abuse, villous adenoma, VIPoma, clay ingestion (clay absorbs potassium & iron)
Cutaneous	Fever
Cellular shift	Alkalosis, insulin excess, β-agonists
	Hypokalemic periodic paralysis
	Barium poisoning, digoxin immune FAB (Digibind)
	Leukemia, lymphoma
Inadequate intake (<20 mEq/day)	Rare
Pseudohypokalemia	In whole blood, leukocytosis (>10⁵/mL), check serum potassium

GI, gastrointestinal; RTA, renal tubular acidosis.

Test Ordering

- Check spot urine potassium to sort between renal (>20 mEq/day) and extrarenal causes.
- If renal cause and normotensive, check bicarbonate level (to look for renal tubular acidosis) and magnesium level.
- If renal cause and hypertensive, check simultaneous renin and aldosterone levels.
- Depending on history, consider ECG, repeat serum potassium, arterial blood levels, digoxin level, diuretic screen.

Management

- Route—PO preferred when possible.
- Type
  - ▲ Acidosis—potassium bicarbonate (or gluconate, acetate, citrate)
  - ▲ Diabetic ketoacidosis—potassium phosphate
  - ▲ All the rest—potassium chloride
- Quantity
  - ▲ Serum potassium decreases only when total body stores are decreased by 100-200 mEq. Replace generously (Table 6).
- Rate
  - ▲ PO 40-120 mEq/day
  - ▲ Peripheral vein 10-15 mEq/hour
  - ▲ Central line (femoral) 40 mEq/hour
  - ▲ Alternatives—spironolactone, triamterene
- Note
  - ▲ Replace more cautiously with renal impairment (creatinine >3 mg/dL, BUN >45 mg/dL, creatinine clearance <30 mL/minute).
  - ▲ Avoid potassium-sparing diuretics and angiotensin-converting enzyme inhibitors.

Table 6. Potassium Replacement

Plasma potassium, mEq/dL	Estimated replacement, mEq
3.0-3.5	100
2.5-3.0	200
2.0-2.5	350
1.5-2.0	500
<1.5	800

▲ Oral replacement can be associated with gastrointestinal ulcers.

▲ IV replacement burns and is associated with phlebitis.

■ For refractory hypokalemia, check and replace magnesium.

HYPERKALEMIA

Is the Patient's Life at Risk?

■ If potassium is >6.5 mEq/L, obtain an ECG and place patient on a monitor. Look for peaked T waves, wide QRS, depressed ST segments.

■ Treat immediately based on ECG changes if present. Otherwise repeat serum potassium measurement with arterial blood gases, calcium, magnesium, and electrolyte panel.

Addressing the Risk

■ If potassium is high (ECG changes, potassium >6 5 mEq/L), treat immediately, as indicated in Table 7.

Differential Diagnosis

■ The differential diagnosis for hyperkalemia is listed in Table 8.

Differentiating the Differential

■ Most cases of hyperkalemia are due to decreased excretion.

■ First, ensure that the hyperkalemia is real and severe.

■ Obtain an ECG, and repeat serum potassium measurement.

■ If severe, treat empirically while searching for the cause.

■ Look for oliguria and renal insufficiency.

■ Stop angiotensin-converting enzyme inhibitors and NSAIDs.

■ Calculate the transtubular potassium gradient (TTKG)

▲ TTKG = (urine K/plasma K) × (plasma osmolality/urine osmolality)

▲ TTKG <10 indicates decreased excretion.

▲ Give 0.2 mg fludrocortisone (Florinef), and repeat the TTKG to differentiate hypoaldosteronism from aldosterone-unresponsive states.

■ A simultaneous renin and aldosterone level will help differentiate hyporeninemic hypoaldosteronism from primary adrenal insufficiency.

Table 7. Treatment of Hyperkalemia

Drug	Action	Duration	Mechanism	Comment
Calcium gluconate—10 mL of 10% solution over 2 minutes, repeat every 5 minutes to effect	1-5 minutes	30-60 minutes	Membrane stabilization	First-line therapy
$NaHCO_3$—1 ampule = 44.6 mEq over 5 minutes	30 minutes	2 hours	Redistribution	Give after calcium (can precipitate seizures if hypocalcemic) Do not give in same line as calcium because it will precipitate
Insulin/glucose—15 U regular in 50 mL of 5% dextrose	30-60 minutes	4-6 hours	Redistribution	
Sodium polystyrene sulfonate (Kayexalate)—15-30 mg PO with 20 mL 70% sorbitol, or 30 mg prn in 200 mL H_2O, repeat every 4-6 hours prn	1-2 hours	4-6 hours	Removal	50 mg will lower serum potassium by 0.5-1 mEq/L & will also raise sodium by 1-2 mEq Watch fluid balance Constipating; give oral form with sorbitol, but associated with intestinal necrosis in postoperative patients, especially if given PR*
Furosemide—20-40 mg IV	15 minutes	4 hours	Removal	Watch fluid balance Cautious use with renal insufficiency
Hemodialysis	Immediate	Variable	Removal	Peritoneal dialysis is much less efficient

PR, per rectum; prn, as needed.
*Note that rectal administration of sodium polystyrene sulfonate *is contraindicated* for hemodynamically unstable patients.

Table 8. Differential Diagnosis for Hyperkalemia

Condition	Suspect when...
Decreased excretion	
Oliguric renal failure	TTKG >10, GFR <5 mL/minute
	Dehydration, congestive heart failure, NSAIDs, ACE inhibi-, tors, protein malnutrition
Hypoaldosterone (TTKG >10 with fludrocortisone [Florinef])	
Primary hypoaldos-teronism (increased renin)	Addison disease, congenital adrenal hypoplasia, heparin
Hyporeninemic (suppressed renin)	
Aldosterone unresponsive (TTKG <10 with fludro-cortisone)	
Tubulointerstitial disease	Sickle cell disease, SLE, renal transplant, AIDS, multiple myeloma
Medications	Potassium-sparing diuretics (spironolactone, triamterene, amiloride), trimethoprim, pentamidine, cyclosporine
RTA 4	Diabetic glomerulosclerosis, pyelonephritis, heavy metals
Hereditary	Gordon syndrome
Redistribution	
Acidosis	Potassium 0.4 mEq, pH = 0.1
Tissue breakdown	Tissue necrosis, tumor lysis, hemolysis, hypercatabolism, rhabdomyolysis
Insulin deficiency	
Hyperkalemic periodic paralysis	Autosomal dominant, intermittent attacks last about 1 hour
Medications	Succinylcholine, digoxin toxicity, β blockers, arginine, radiocon-trast dye
Excess intake	TPN, penicillin (1 MU = 1.7 mEq potassium), salt substitutes (14 mEq/g)
Pseudohyperkalemia	Hemolysis, thrombocytosis (>10^6), leukocytosis (>10^5)

ACE, angiotensin-converting enzyme; GFR, glomerular filtration rate; RTA, renal tubular acidosis; SLE, systemic lupus erythematosus; TPN, total parenteral nutrition; TTKG, transtubular potassium gradient.

- Hyporeninemic states also occur in renal tubular acidosis and Gordon syndrome.

Test Ordering
- ECG
- Repeat serum potassium measurements with electrolyte panel and BUN and creatinine.
- TTKG and fludrocortisone trial
- Simultaneous renin and aldosterone measurements
- Depending on history, consider arterial blood gases, glucose, creatinine clearance, digoxin level, CK, aldolase.

Management
- For acute hyperkalemia, treat emergently (as noted above).
- For chronic hyperkalemia, treat underlying cause.
- Hyporeninemic hypoaldosteronism—fludrocortisone, furosemide, or thiazide diuretic.

FEVER OF UNKNOWN ORIGIN

Ramona S. deJesus, M.D.
Randall S. Edson, M.D.

DEFINITIONS

Classic Fever of Unknown Origin (FUO)
- Illness of at least 3 weeks' duration
- Temperature >101°F (38.3°C) on several occasions
- No diagnosis after 1 week in hospital*

Nosocomial FUO*
- Temperature ≥101°F on several occasions in a hospitalized patient receiving acute care

Neutropenic FUO*
- Temperature ≥101°F on several occasions
- Neutrophils in peripheral blood <0.5 × 10⁹/L (<500/mm³) or expected to decrease to <0.5 × 10⁹/L within 1-2 days

HIV-associated FUO*
- Temperature ≥101°F on several occasions in person with serologically confirmed HIV infection

IS THE PATIENT'S LIFE AT RISK?
- Immediate mortality for FUO is low, but some patients have underlying diseases that are ultimately fatal.
- Three most common causes of FUO are the following:
  - ▲ Infection (30%-40%)
  - ▲ Malignancy (20%-30%)
  - ▲ Collagen vascular disease (10%-20%)

---

*Revised defintion is no diagnosis after 3 days of inpatient investigation or 3 outpatient visits.

Special abbreviation used in this chapter: FUO, fever of unknown origin.

- Look for stigmata of bacterial endocarditis.
- Note degree of immunosuppression in patients with HIV infection or neutropenia.
- Consider age—visual disturbances with headache in person >50 years may indicate giant cell arteritis.
- Evaluate for signs of dehydration, especially with persistent fever and decreased oral intake.
- Subtle behavioral changes may indicate central nervous system infection; perform a thorough neurologic exam.

ADDRESSING THE RISK
- Routine and orthostatic vital signs, oxygen saturation
- Hydration
- Thorough physical exam
- Initial testing (see below)
- Discontinue all possible offending medications.
- Look for localizing signs/symptoms.
- Evaluate accordingly if nosocomial, neutropenic, or HIV-related FUO.

DIFFERENTIAL DIAGNOSIS
- The differential diagnosis of FUO is given in Table 1.
- The causes of drug fever are listed in Table 2.

DIFFERENTIATING THE DIFFERENTIAL
- The history, lab, and physical exam findings for various causes of fever are listed in Table 3.

TEST ORDERING
- Be sure that fever is documented before beginning expensive, potentially invasive tests.
- Take a careful history, including travel, immunizations, previous surgical procedures, exposure to animals/TB, alcohol intake, familial disorders, history of any rash, HIV risk factors, tick bites, sexual preference).
- Consider patient's age.
- On physical exam, check the eyes, including ophthalmoscopy, lymph nodes, and entire skin and mucous membranes.
- Unless another diagnosis is probable, consider drug fever early and withdraw all medications the patient was taking when fever began.

Table 1. Differential Diagnosis for Fever of Unknown Origin

Infections	Neoplasia	Rheumatologic disorders	Miscellaneous
Endocarditis,* extrapulmonary/ miliary TB	Lymphomas, metastasis to liver or central nervous system	Still disease (adult)	Drug fever, factitious fever, habitual hyperthermia, Castleman disease, familial Mediterranean fever
Intra-abdominal/GU abscesses	Solid tumors (e.g., hyper-nephromas)	Giant cell arteritis, polymyalgia rheumatica	Granulomatosis (e.g., sarcoidosis)
Osteomyelitis, infected prosthesis, HIV	Lymphoproliferative disease	Systemic lupus erythematosus, rheumatoid arthritis, Sjögren disease, Reiter syndrome	Alcoholic hepatitis, hepatomas
Cytomegalovirus, Epstein-Barr virus, zoonotic fevers, Lyme disease	Myelodysplastic diseases	Cryoglobulinemia, Behçet syndrome, mixed connective tissue disorder	Pulmonary embolism
Malaria, fungal, dental abscess, Kikuchi lymphadenitis, Whipple disease, salmonellosis	Preleukemias, atrial myxomas	Hypersensitivity vasculitis, other vasculitis (polyarteritis nodosa, Takayasu arteritis, Wegener granulomatosis)	Endocrine (thyroiditis, hyperthyroid, ACTH insufficiency), inflammatory bowel disease

ACTH, corticotropin; GU, genitourinary.
*More likely culture-negative or hard-to-isolate organisms (e.g., *Bartonella, Coxiella,* HACKE).

Table 2. Causes of Drug Fever

Antibiotics (sulfonamides, penicillin, nitrofurantoin, antimalarial agents)
Diuretics
Antiarrhythmics (quinidine, procainamide)
Antiepileptic drugs (phenytoin)
Antihistamine (H_1 & H_2 blockers)
Allopurinol
Sedatives (barbiturates)
Antihypertensives (hydralazine, methyldopa)
Bleomycin
Iodides
Antithyroid drugs

- Initial tests (minimum recommended evaluation)
  - Lab tests—CBC with differential; ESR; blood cultures (bacterial, fungal) ×3 off antibiotics; thyroid-stimulating hormone (TSH); BUN/creatinine; routine blood chemistry panel (liver enzymes, LDH, bilirubin, serum calcium, alkaline phosphatase, rheumatoid factor, antinuclear antibodies), urinalysis with microscopy; urine, stool, sputum cultures; guaiac stools; HIV serology
  - Radiology tests—chest X-ray; abdominal CT/MRI; CT/MRI of chest, pelvis, head (if appropriate); echocardiography
  - Tuberculin testing with control(s)
  - Invasive tests—biopsy of any suspicious lymph nodes or skin lesions
- Follow-up tests
  - Bone marrow biopsy if miliary TB or cancer suggested
  - Gallium 67/indium 111–labeled leukocyte whole body scans
  - Repeat CT/MRI with thinner sections to detect small lesions
  - Transesophageal echocardiography (positive in >90% of cases of infective endocarditis presenting as FUO)
  - Prolonged incubation of blood cultures
  - Polymerase chain reaction for *Mycobacterium* TB
  - Liver biopsy if suggested by diagnostic clues
  - Bronchoscopy/colonoscopy if indicated

Table 3. Cause of Fever Correlated With History, Lab, and Physical Exam Findings

Cause	History	Lab & physical findings
Infection		
Subacute bacterial endocarditis	IV drug use	Osler nodes, new regurgitant murmur, Janeway lesions, splinter hemorrhage
Granulomatous meningitis	Subtle behavioral changes	
Malaria	Fever every 2-3 days	Microscopy of stained thin & thick blood films, antigen detection
Intra-abdominal abscess	History of intra-abdominal infections (hepatic, pelvic, pancreatic, subphrenic)	Localized tenderness
CMV	History of blood transfusion, immunosuppression	CMV IgM/viral isolation from blood, rash, hepatomegaly, splenomegaly
Lyme disease	Tick exposure, history of rash, endemic location	Lyme serology +
Kikuchi lymphadenitis	Women <40 years	Enlarged cervical lymph nodes, neutropenia, maybe abnormal LFTs
Whipple disease	Triad of diarrhea (malabsorption); weight loss; transient, migratory, recurring arthralgia	Increased ESR (>30 mm/hour)

Table 3 (continued)

Cause	History	Lab & physical findings
Malignancy		
Lymphoma	Pel-Ebstein fever (increased temperature for several days alternating with normal temperature), weight loss, "B" symptoms	Lymphadenopathy, splenomegaly, increased LDH
Hypernephromas	Hematuria, flank pain	Palpable mass, hypercalcemia, erythrocytosis
Rheumatologic		
Still disease	Young (16-35 years), high fever, myalgias, sore throat, arthralgias	Evanescent, macular rash primarily on trunk during fever, increased ferritin level
Giant cell arteritis	>50 years, headache, visual loss, jaw claudication; associated with polymyalgia rheumatica	Increased ESR, anemia, scalp tenderness, abnormal palpable temporal artery; 25% have increased alkaline phosphatase
Polyarteritis nodosa	Associated with hepatitis C	Mononeuritis multiplex (in 60%), skin lesions (palpable purpura, livedo reticularis), abnormal renal function
Behçet syndrome	Painful, recurrent oral/urogenital ulcerations, arthralgias, myalgias	Minor/major aphthous ulcers, anterior uveitis, erythema nodosum, positive pathergy test/ urate crystal test

Table 3 (continued)

Cause	History	Lab & physical findings
Miscellaneous		
Adrenocortical insufficiency	Nausea/vomiting, weight loss	Hypotension, skin hyperpigmentation
Castleman disease	Mostly <30 years (for localized form), painless mass, "B" symptoms	Peripheral lymphadenopathy with anemia
Factitious fever	Multiple hospitalizations & diagnostic testing	Healthy looking, fever lacks diurnal pattern with rapid defervescence

CMV, cytomegalovirus; LFT, liver function test.

- ▲ Temporal artery biopsy to check for giant cell arteritis or biopsy of infected area to diagnose vasculitic process (e.g., polyarteritis nodosa)
- ▲ Exploratory laparotomy (rarely required with CT or percutaneous biopsy)
- ▪ Despite meticulous investigation, the cause of FUO is not discovered in 5%-15% of cases.

MANAGEMENT
- ▪ Empiric antibiotic trials, except for culture-negative endocarditis, have *no* place in management of FUO.
- ▪ Empiric antibiotic therapy is prudent for seriously ill or deteriorating patients.
- ▪ High-dose corticosteroid treatment should be given only to patients with biopsy-proven vasculitis.
- ▪ Particularly in elderly patients with suspected miliary TB, empiric anti-TB therapy is acceptable, especially if patient has an exposure history or known positive PPD.

FUO IN SUBPOPULATIONS

- Nosocomial FUO
  - ▲ Diverse causes, underlying disease, and complications of hospitalization must be considered.
- Patients with known cancer (neutropenic-associated fever)
  - ▲ Infectious cause in 1/2 of cases reviewed, gram-negative bacilli and gram-positive cocci or fungi the usual causes (typically as complication of neutropenia)
  - ▲ Extension or progression of tumor also causes fever
- Patients infected with HIV
  - ▲ Infectious in 75% of patients, usually with advanced disease (CD4 cell count <100/mm^3 [<0.1 × 10^9/L])
  - ▲ Most common organism—*Mycobacterium* (*M. tuberculosis* or *M. avium-intracellulare*)
  - ▲ Other common organisms—cytomegalovirus, *Toxoplasma gondii* (toxoplasmosis), *Pneumocystis carinii*, *Cryptococcus*
  - ▲ Non-Hodgkin lymphoma or drug fever in 10%

GASTROINTESTINAL TRACT BLEEDING

Marina G. Silveira, M.D.
Amindra S. Arora, M.B., B.Chir.

IMMEDIATE EVALUATION AND MANAGEMENT

Is the Patient's Life at Risk?

- Initial focal point—hemodynamics
- Presence of orthostatic tachycardia and/or hypotension (systolic blood pressure drop >10 mm Hg or heart rate increase >15 beats/minute) or shock
  - ▲ Indicates moderate to massive blood loss—*the patient is at risk*
  - ▲ Baseline hypertensive patients—can be normotensive despite substantial blood loss
- Patients with unstable vital signs—often bleeding from major vascular source
- Unstable patients—poorer prognosis than for those with normal vital signs
- Other important clues—mental status changes, profuse diaphoresis and intense pallor, cyanosis, and low oxymetry levels. *Do not miss!*
- Hemodynamic instability—warrants immediate resuscitation efforts and call for assistance

Addressing the Risk

- Resuscitation—should take precedence over diagnostic or therapeutic procedures that could place patient at higher risk
- Goal—restore and maintain normal vital signs
- Key importance—immediate and constant assessment of vital signs

---

Special abbreviations in this chapter: GI, gastrointestinal; PPI, proton pump inhibitor.

- General management of *all* unstable patients must include the following:
  - ▲ Two large-bore (≥18 gauge) peripheral intravenous catheters
  - ▲ Rapid infusion of colloid (normal saline or lactated Ringer solution) as tolerated per comorbidities
  - ▲ Transfusions—virtually all unstable patients need packed RBCs; if actively bleeding and coagulopathic (INR >1.5 or platelets <50,000 mm^3 [50 × 10^9/L]), transfuse fresh frozen plasma and platelets, respectively
  - ▲ Supplemental oxygen
  - ▲ Monitoring of vital signs and urine output
  - ▲ ICU monitoring—high risk for adverse outcomes include patients who do not respond to initial resuscitation measures and have greater prevalence of significant comorbidities
  - ▲ Surgery consultation if patient refractory to initial resuscitation, requires >4 units RBCs over 24 hours, has massive active bleeding, has recurrent bleeding
- Do not use nasogastric lavage to assess bleeding activity; vital signs are more effective.
- Early diagnostic and therapeutic procedures should be instituted and may alter prognosis, especially with upper gastrointestinal (GI) tract bleeding. Always follow assessment of hemodynamic stability and adequate resuscitation.
- General measures—consider endotracheal intubation for aspiration prevention, especially if patient has altered mental status, massive hematemesis, and variceal hemorrhage.

Differential Diagnosis
The differential diagnosis for GI tract bleeding is listed in Table 1.

Differentiating the Differential
- The presentation typical of upper and lower GI tract bleeding sites is listed in Table 2.
- The risk factors for various conditions producing GI tract bleeding are listed in Table 3.
- History and physical exam (Table 4)
  - ▲ Important in assessing severity of bleeding and making a preliminary assessment of the site and cause of bleeding
  - ▲ Are rarely diagnostic of the source of bleeding

Table 1. Differential Diagnosis for Gastrointestinal (GI) Tract Bleeding

Site	Condition
Nasopharyngeal bleeding	Epistaxis
	Gingival bleeding
Pulmonary hemorrhage	Airway disease
	Pulmonary parenchymal disease
	Pulmonary vascular disorders
	Miscellaneous pulmonary or systemic disorders
GI bleeding	
Upper tract (proximal to ligament of Treitz)	Peptic ulcer disease
	Esophagogastric varices
	Mallory-Weiss tears
	Mucosal erosions
	Arteriovenous malformation
	Neoplastic
	Other: Dieulafoy lesions, portal hypertensive gastropathy, gastric antral vascular ectasia ("watermelon stomach"), perforated/ruptured esophagus (Boerhaave syndrome), hemobilia, hemosuccus pancreaticus, aortoenteric fistula
Lower tract (distal to ligament of Treitz)	Diverticulosis
	Angiodysplasia
	Radiation-induced
	Vasculitis
	Inflammatory bowel disease
	Ischemic colitis
	Infectious colitis
	Neoplastic
	Polyps
	Other: postpolypectomy/biopsy, stercoral ulcers, aortocolonic fistula, anastomotic bleeding, intussusception, Meckel diverticulum, portal colopathy & colonic varices, endometriosis, Dieulafoy lesions
Anorectal bleeding	Hemorrhoids
	Fissure
	Idiopathic rectal ulcers

- Upper GI tract bleeding—approximately 5 times more common than lower GI tract bleeding
- Patients with upper GI tract bleeding are more likely to be hemodynamically unstable at presentation because of severe blood loss and to require blood transfusions than patients with lower GI tract bleeding.
- Patients with unstable vital signs are often bleeding from a major vascular source, such as an ulcer with a visible vessel or gastroesophageal varices.

Ordering Tests
All Patients
- Complete CBC
  - ▲ Initial hemoglobin or hematocrit may not reflect the degree of blood loss
  - ▲ Serial measurements (every 6 hours) are recommended.
- Type and crossmatch
- Electrolytes
  - ▲ BUN/creatinine especially—Watch for disproportionate increase in BUN:creatinine often seen in upper GI tract bleeding.
  - ▲ Poor renal function is an indication of higher risk patient
- Coagulation profile (INR, platelets)

Upper and Lower GI Tract Bleeding
- Initial evaluation with suggestive history and physical exam
- Nasogastric aspirate has *no role* in distinguishing between upper and lower GI tract bleeding.

Table 2. Usual Clinical Presentation of Gastrointestinal (GI) Tract Bleeding

Bleeding site		Presentation
Upper GI tract	Hematemesis	Vomiting of blood—fresh bright red blood or old, "coffee-grounds" appearance
	Melena*	Black, tarry, foul-smelling stools
Lower GI tract	Hematochezia[†]	Bright red blood from rectum

*Melena can result from distal small bowel or even ascending colon bleeding, especially with high colonic transit time.

[†]About 10% of patients with upper GI tract bleeding present with hematochezia.

Table 3. **Risk Factors**

Risk factor	Condition
Advanced age	Diverticula, ischemic colitis, neoplastic
Younger age	PUD, esophagitis, varices, Meckel diverticulum
Known liver disease	Portal hypertension, esophagogastric varices/portal hypertensive gastropathy
Known gastrointestinal disease, previous bleeding	Diverticular disease, ulcer disease, hereditary hemorrhagic telangiectasia, inflammatory bowel disease
Helicobacter pylori	PUD, neoplastic
Acute nonbleeding critical illness	PUD
Increased gastric acid production	PUD
NSAIDs/aspirin	Gastroduodenal ulceration, colitis, diverticular bleeding, pill-induced esophagitis
Ethanol ingestion	Erosive esophagitis, PUD
Abdominal pain	PUD, mesenteric and/or colonic ischemia
Previous surgery	Aortic surgery & aortoenteric/aortocolonic fistula, colon resection & anastomotic bleeding
Radiotherapy	Radiation colitis/proctitis, radiation-induced telangiectasia
Hepatic parenchymal or biliary tract injury	Hemobilia
Retching/vomiting	Mallory-Weiss tears, esophageal rupture
Weight loss/anorexia, change in bowel habits	Neoplastic

PUD, peptic ulcer disease.

Table 4. History and Physical Exam Findings Associated With Various Causes of Gastrointestinal Tract Bleeding*

Etiology	Physical exam	History
Peptic ulcer disease	Epigastric tenderness	History of epigastric pain, GERD, NSAID/aspirin use, alcohol ingestion, tobacco use
Portal hypertension/esophago-gastric varices	Cutaneous signs (spider angiomata, Dupuytren contractures, palmar erythema), splenomegaly, ascites, caput medusae	History of alcohol abuse
Mallory-Weiss tear		Retching/vomiting
Vascular	Telangiectasias of skin & mucous membranes	History of hereditary hemorrhagic telangiectasia
Erosive		Alcohol, NSAID/aspirin use, tobacco use, GERD
Neoplasia (gastric)	Acanthosis nigricans, Virchow node, Sister Mary Joseph nodule, Blumer (rectal) shelf	Weight loss, dysphagia
Neoplasia (colonic)	Pallor	Weight loss, bowel-habit changes, iron deficiency anemia
Ischemic colitis	Normal physical exam + severe abdominal pain	Previous hypotension, shock
Postpolypectomy		History of recent colonoscopy/polypectomy
Aortocolonic/aortoenteric fistulas		History of previous aortic graft surgery
Stercoral ulcers		Chronic constipation
Radiation colitis		Previous radiotherapy (pelvic/prostatic)

GERD, gastroesophageal reflux disease.
*Historical information or physical findings will not be present all the time.

Upper GI Tract Bleeding
- Upper endoscopy
  - ▲ Diagnostic modality of choice for acute upper GI tract bleeding
  - ▲ Highly sensitive and specific for locating and identifying bleeding lesions and is potentially therapeutic
- Barium radiography is *not recommended* in acute upper GI tract bleeding.

Lower GI Tract Bleeding
- Colonoscopy—initial exam of choice for diagnosis and treatment
- Radiographic studies (plain abdominal films)— should precede colonoscopy if perforation or obstruction is suspected
- Anoscopy and sigmoidoscopy
  - ▲ Can be useful for diagnosis of anorectal and left colon bleeding sites but do not rule out synchronous lesions
  - ▲ Role unclear if colonoscopy readily available
- Other possibly useful diagnostic procedures—radionuclide imaging and mesenteric angiography
- Radionuclide imaging
  - ▲ Detects bleeding at a rate of 0.1-0.5 mL/minute
  - ▲ Is more sensitive than angiography but less specific than positive endoscopy or angiography
  - ▲ Disadvantages—poor localization and nontherapeutic procedure
  - ▲ Can be used before angiography to determine which patients are bleeding sufficiently to make a positive angiographic result likely
- Angiography
  - ▲ Requires active bleeding at a rate of 1-1.5 mL/minute to be positive
  - ▲ Potentially therapeutic—vasopressin infusion and embolization can be performed through the catheter
  - ▲ Has a role in patients in whom endoscopy is not feasible and in those with persistent or recurrent bleeding and nondiagnostic colonoscopic findings

- Barium studies have *no role* in evaluation of acute lower GI tract bleeding.

Initial Management of GI Tract Bleeding
- The initial management is outlined in Table 5.

PEPTIC ULCER DISEASE
- Endoscopy with therapeutic procedure in high-risk lesions
- Early use of proton pump inhibitor (PPI)—pantoprazole, 80 mg IV bolus, 8 mg/hour infusion over 24 hours, then pantoprazole, 40 mg/day PO, or omeprazole, 20 mg/day PO, or if IV PPI not available, high-dose oral PPI (e.g., omeprazole, 40 mg PO twice daily)
- Rebleeding after successful endoscopy—second endoscopic treatment
- Surgery
  - ▲ If bleeding is not responsive to standard therapy
  - ▲ For recurrent bleeding after second endoscopic procedure
  - ▲ If poor surgical candidate, angiographic therapy
- If endoscopy is unavailable, contraindicated, or unsuccessful, some evidence for treatment with somatostatin, 250 μg bolus then every hour for 3-7 days, or octreotide, 10-50 μg bolus + 25 μg/hour up to 3 days
- Prevention of recurrence—treat underlying disease (eradicate *H. pylori*, discontinue NSAIDs)

ESOPHAGOGASTRIC VARICES
- Octreotide, 50 μg bolus followed by 50 μg/hour IV infusion for 5 days, or somatostatin, 250 μg bolus followed by 250 μg/hour IV infusion for 5 days; plus

Table 5. Initial Management of GI Tract Bleeding

Always—*assess* hemodynamic stability & *resuscitate* if needed!
Keep in mind—there is evidence that in most patients bleeding stops without any intervention
Preparation for endoscopy
- Nasogastric or orogastric lavage to remove particulate matter, fresh blood, & clots to facilitate procedure & decrease risk of aspiration
- Erythromycin IV 3 mg/kg over 20-30 minutes, 30-90 minutes before endoscopy

- ▲ Endoscopy with band ligation (esophageal varices) or sclerotherapy
- If initial therapy fails, a second endoscopic trial is reasonable; balloon tamponade is also effective for achieving short-term hemostasis (Sengstaken-Blakemore tube, Minnesota tube, or Linton-Nachlas tube).
- Persistent or recurrent bleeding may require more definite therapy—either transjugular intrahepatic portosystemic stent shunt or surgery (shunt-surgery procedures).
- General management for variceal bleeding includes
  - ▲ Aspiration prevention—airway protection and gastric decompression by nasogastric aspiration
  - ▲ Infection prophylaxis
    - Usually quinolone (ofloxacin, 400 mg; norfloxacin, 400-800 mg; ciprofloxacin, 400-1,000 mg) for 7-10 days; initially IV, followed by completion with administration PO
    - Optimal choice of drug and duration of therapy are not clear.
  - ▲ Treatment of hepatic encephalopathy—lactulose
  - ▲ Avoidance of renal failure—appropriate volume replacement, avoidance of nephrotoxic drugs
- Primary prophylaxis—propranolol or nadolol (dosage as tolerated, decrease resting heart rate 25%)
- Secondary prophylaxis—band ligation or sclerotherapy with or without propranolol or nadolol (controversial subject)

MALLORY-WEISS TEARS
- Endoscopic therapy—indicated for actively bleeding lesions or for patients with bleeding stigmata
- No definite evidence for treatment with PPIs

ESOPHAGITIS
- Treatment of underlying cause—high-dose PPI
- Endoscopic therapy—if ulcerations and/or visible vessels

COLONIC DIVERTICULA
- Colonoscopy for recurrent bleeding, with endoscopic therapy for bleeding lesion or bleeding stigmata

- Recurrent bleeding—usually requires combination of colonoscopic treatment, angiographic intervention, and surgical resection of identified site
- Poor outcome after blind subtotal colectomy, especially in elderly

ANGIODYSPLASIAS
- Upper endoscopy/colonoscopy, with endoscopic therapy for bleeding lesion or bleeding stigmata
- Angiography in cases of continuing or recurrent bleeding; therapeutic intervention with intra-arterial vasopressin or embolization
- Surgery—rarely necessary

HEMORRHOIDS
- Nonsurgical management is usually effective—sitz baths, avoidance of straining and stool softeners, dietary modifications.
- Because of high prevalence, rule out other causes of bleeding, especially in patients >50 years.
- Refractory disease—therapeutic options are rubber-band ligation, coagulation therapy, surgical hemorrhoidectomy.

HEADACHE

Douglas J. Creedon, M.D.
Anna M. Georgiopoulos, M.D.
J. D. Bartleson, M.D.

IS THE PATIENT'S LIFE AT RISK?

- Headache
  - ▲ Common reason patients present to emergency department; can be common complaint of hospitalized patients
  - ▲ Initial evaluation should include following life- or neurologic function-threatening secondary causes of headache:
    - • Subarachnoid hemorrhage—typically from ruptured aneurysm or arteriovenous malformation
    - • Intracerebral hemorrhage— usually hypertensive
    - • Ischemic stroke—embolism, thromboembolism, stenosis, dissection
    - • Meningitis
    - • Giant cell arteritis—can cause sudden irreversible blindness
    - • Epidural or subdural hemorrhage—often with trauma history
    - • Enlarging brain mass—tumor, abscess, aneurysm
    - • Pituitary apoplexy
- The history often provides the best clue to headache cause. Warning signs are listed in Table 1.

ADDRESSING THE RISK

- First step in ruling out life-threatening causes of headache— neuroimaging
- If intracranial bleeding (subarachnoid hemorrhage, hemorrhagic stroke, posttraumatic bleeding) is a consideration
  - ▲ Immediate noncontrast CT of head should be performed.
  - ▲ Acute blood will appear bright.
  - ▲ If this is negative, as in approximately 5% of subarachnoid hemorrhages, proceed to lumbar puncture.

- ▲ Lumbar puncture—"gold standard" for evaluating blood in the CSF, look for xanthochromia
  - ▲ To guard against being misled by a bloody tap, the RBCs in both the first and last tubes of CSF should be assayed.
- Do *not* perform lumbar puncture on patient with signs of a mass or increased intracranial pressure (midline shift, blunting of gyri on CT) because sudden release of pressure can cause brainstem herniation and death.
- If pituitary apoplexy is part of the differential diagnosis, examine coronal CT slices.

DIFFERENTIAL DIAGNOSIS
- After potentially life-threatening causes of headache have been addressed, consider a more extensive differential list (Table 2).
- History is key—many migraine patients know they are having a migraine and are able to tell you what has and has not worked in the past.

Table 1. Warning Signs in the Headache History

Think of the following	If you hear—
Subarachnoid hemorrhage	"Worst headache of my life"
	Sudden onset, thunderclap headache (timing is more telling than severity)
	Stiff neck
Mass	Increasing frequency or duration of headaches
	New-onset headache in patients >50 years
	New-onset neurologic signs or symptoms (e.g., weakness, visual disturbances)
Giant cell arteritis, cerebrovascular accident	Headaches in elderly (>60 years)
Intracranial bleeding	History of trauma (may be several weeks past & a mild injury, especially in elderly, alcoholics, & patients taking anticoagulants)
Meningitis	Stiff neck, especially if associated with fever
Mass, cerebrovascular accident	Weakness, numbness, or specific neurologic deficits

Table 2. Differential Diagnosis for Headache

Primary headache disorders
    Migraine headache
    Tension headache
    Cluster headache
Secondary causes of headache
    Systemic illness
    Giant cell (temporal) arteritis
    Meningitis
    Subarachnoid hemorrhage
    Subdural hemorrhage
    Epidural hemorrhage
    Stroke
    Tumors
        Metastases: lung, breast, melanoma
        Primary tumors: gliomas, meningiomas, pituitary adenomas
    Arteriovenous malformation
    Hypertension (usually >200/120 mm Hg)
    Carotid dissection
    Vertebrobasilar insufficiency
    Cerebral venous thrombosis
    Pseudotumor cerebri
    Trauma, including posttraumatic headaches
    Cholesteatomas
    Brain abscess
    Hydrocephalus
    Sinusitis
    Dental abscess
    Acute-angle closure glaucoma
    Temporomandibular joint disorders
    Postherpetic neuralgia
    Trigeminal neuralgia
    Carbon monoxide poisoning
    Prescription drug-induced headache
    Rebound withdrawal headaches

DIFFERENTIATING THE DIFFERENTIAL

- A chief complaint of headache or new development of headache warrants a complete neurologic exam, including ophthalmoscopic exam.
- Often, even life-threatening secondary causes of headaches can present with a paucity of physical signs.
- When evaluating a headache, consider the following: location, quality, radiation, severity (scale of 1-10), temporal profile, exacerbating factors, ameliorating factors, and associated symptoms (Tables 3 and 4).

Table 3. Symptoms That May Be Associated With Certain Causes of Headache

	If yes, consider
Did the headache begin abruptly?	Subarachnoid hemorrhage
Is the headache associated with new neurologic signs or symptoms?	Mass lesion, stroke, or giant cell arteritis
Is the headache associated with fever or myalgias?	Meningitis
Is the headache worsened by coughing or Valsalva maneuver?	Mass, increased intracranial pressure, Arnold-Chiari malformation
Does the headache awaken patient from sleep?	Mass lesion
Is the headache bandlike?	Tension headache
Does patient have a history of cancer?	Metastasis
Is the headache associated with nausea & vomiting?	Mass lesion (especially in posterior fossa), vertebrobasilar cerebrovascular accident
Does patient have scalp tenderness, jaw claudication, malaise, arthralgias, or polymyalgia rheumatica?	Giant cell arteritis
Do any visual or auditory changes precede the headache?	Migraine
Is the headache associated with photophobia or phonophobia?	Migraine, meningitis
Is the pain sharp and lancinating?	Trigeminal neuralgia, cluster headache, postherpetic neuralgia
Do eating, drinking, or tooth brushing trigger the headache?	Trigeminal neuralgia, temporomandibular joint dysfunction

Table 3 (continued)

	If yes, consider
Is there a history of facial grimacing?	Trigeminal neuralgia
Is the headache associated with lacrimation or rhinorrhea (especially one-sided)?	Cluster headache
Do the headaches come in bunches, followed by headache-free periods?	Cluster headache, trigeminal neuralgia
Is the patient immunosuppressed or immunocompromised?	Infection (cryptococcosis, histoplasmosis, toxoplasmosis), primary central nervous system lymphoma

Table 4. Signs That May Be Associated With Certain Causes of Headache

If on exam you find	Consider
Horner syndrome (ptosis, miosis, anhidrosis)	Cluster headache, carotid dissection
Papilledema	Mass lesion, pseudotumor cerebri, cerebral venous thrombosis
Bitemporal field loss	Pituitary mass, suprachiasmatic lesion (e.g., craniopharyngioma)
Focal motor or sensory deficits	Mass lesion, stroke, cerebral venous thrombosis
Disorientation or depressed level of consciousness	Mass lesion, toxic metabolic disease, cerebral venous thrombosis, epidural or subdural hematoma, subarachnoid hemorrhage

TEST ORDERING

- The tests should be dictated by the differential diagnosis.
- Some tests that may prove helpful, and the indications for each, are listed in Table 5.

MANAGEMENT

- Management for some causes of headache is given in Table 6.

Table 5. Tests to Order When Working Up a Headache

If your differential includes	Consider the following test
Subarachnoid hemorrhage	Head CT without contrast (with contrast, if suspicion of mass is high), lumbar puncture
Subarachnoid hemorrhage, meningitis	CSF analysis: glucose, protein, RBCs, WBCs, and cultures or polymerase chain reaction (e.g., for herpes simplex virus) if indicated
Metastasis, infection, drugs or toxins	Blood tests: CBC, electrolytes, glucose, carbon monoxide levels (and other toxins if suggested by history)
Infection, drugs or toxins	Urinalysis, especially in elderly
Mass lesion	CT without and with contrast, MRI if CT is negative & suspicion is high or if CT shows mass lesion that cannot be characterized
Giant cell arteritis	ESR, temporal artery biopsy (do not wait to begin treatment if suspicion for giant cell arteritis is high; steroids will not affect biopsy results if the biopsy is performed within 48 hours after starting therapy)
Cerebral venous thrombosis, encephalitis (e.g., infection)	MRI with gadolinium, magnetic resonance venography

Table 6. Management of Some Causes of Headaches

Subarachnoid hemorrhage	Pain management
	Antiemetics for nausea
	Monitor blood pressure & maintain at or below normal
	Neurovital signs every 2 hours; maintain NPO
	Call neurosurgery to clip/coil
	Control vasospasms (days 4-14 after hemorrhage) with nimodipine
Meningitis	
Bacterial	Head CT without contrast
	Lumbar puncture if CT is negative (do lumbar puncture first if suspicion is high)
	If CSF is positive for bacteria, cefotaxime
Viral	Supportive treatment, antiviral for herpes simplex
Tension headache	Analgesics (e.g., ibuprofen, parenteral ketorolac)
Migraine headache	The key is to use whatever is needed to break the headache. Try the following in descending order:
	Triptan of choice (e.g., sumatriptan)
	NSAID—parenteral ketorolac
	Opioid analgesics (PO or parenteral)
	Dihydroergotamine mesylate (DHE 45)—do NOT mix triptans, DHE 45 & other ergots
	Chlorpromazine
	IV fluids if patient has not been able to eat/drink
	Triptans, dihydroergotamine & other ergots are contraindicated in pregnancy, severe hypertension, & known or suspected coronary artery disease
Migraine headache in pregnancy	Meperidine
	Promethazine

Table 6 (continued)

Cluster headache	Sumatriptan, usually SQ
	100% oxygen through nasal cannula or nonrebreather at 7-10 L/minute for 10-15 minutes
	Dihydroergotamine, usually parenterally
Giant cell arteritis	Prednisone
	Schedule temporal artery biopsy within 48 hours
Trigeminal neuralgia	Carbamazepine
Brain mass	Dexamethasone
	Chest X-ray, CT of chest & abdomen to look for primary tumor
	Neurology & neurosurgery consults
Pseudotumor cerebri	Serial lumbar punctures to decrease intracranial pressure
	Acetazolamide
	Prednisone
	Weight loss

HEMATURIA

Amy S. Oxentenko, M.D.
Fernando C. Fervenza, M.D.

IS THE PATIENT'S LIFE AT RISK?

- Normal urinalysis can include <3 RBCs per high-power field of centrifuged urine.
- Hematuria, either microscopic or macroscopic, is defined as ≥3 RBCs per high-power field.
- In very few circumstances is hematuria deemed life-threatening, but such circumstances do exist and need prompt recognition to prevent morbidity or mortality.

Acute Conditions and Associated Findings

- Renal trauma—posterior rib fractures, flank ecchymosis, hypotension, penetrating injury below the nipple line
- Renal infarction (embolic vs. thrombotic)—irregular heart rhythm, new murmurs, livedo reticularis, blue toes, recent angiography, recent myocardial infarction, multiorgan dysfunction, severe hypertension, flank/abdominal bruits
- Accelerated hypertension—mental status changes, visual impairment, headache
- Severe bleeding diathesis—pallor, ecchymosis, oozing from other sites
- Sickle cell crisis—African American, dehydration, infection, diffuse pain

Subacute Conditions and Associated Findings

- Renal vein thrombosis—history of clotting disorder, history of nephrotic syndrome or paroxysmal nocturnal hemoglobinuria
- Glomerulonephritides—arthralgias or arthritis, skin rashes or

---

Special abbreviations used in this chapter: ANA, antinuclear antibody; ANCA, antineutrophil cytoplasmic antibody; ASO, antistreptolysin O; ENA, extractable nuclear antigen; GBM, glomerular basement membrane; MPO, myeloperoxidase.

lesions, hypertension, edema, oliguria, history of pharyngitis or pyoderma
- Multisystem disorders (systemic lupus erythematosus, microscopic polyangiitis, Wegener granulomatosis, Goodpasture syndrome, scleroderma, Henoch-Schönlein purpura, hemolytic uremic syndrome, thrombotic thrombocytopenic purpura)—rashes, arthralgias or arthritis, neuropathies, rhinosinusitis, hemoptysis, sclerodactyly, abdominal pain, melena, recent diarrheal illness
- Arteriovenous fistulas—abdominal/flank bruits, tachycardia
- Pyelonephritis—fever, costovertebral angle tenderness
- Bladder, ureteral, or urethral trauma—blood at meatus, pelvic trauma or fracture
- Enterovesical fistula—fecaluria, pneumaturia

ADDRESSING THE RISK
- If gross hematuria
  - ▲ Stabilize blood pressure.
  - ▲ IV fluids to hydrate and prevent obstruction from clotting
  - ▲ CBC, type and crossmatch, coagulation studies (PT/INR, PTT), peripheral blood smear
  - ▲ Creatinine to evaluate renal function
  - ▲ Dipstick, then formal urinalysis, with cultures as directed
  - ▲ C3, C4, CH50, antistreptolysin O (ASO), ESR, antinuclear antibody (ANA), extractable nuclear antigen (ENA) panel, antineutrophil cytoplasmic antibody (ANCA), anti–myeloperoxidase (MPO), anti–proteinase 3, anti–glomerular basement membrane (GBM), cryoglobulins.
  - ▲ Reverse coagulopathy if present.
- Trauma
  - ▲ CT kidneys/pelvis
  - ▲ Retrograde urethrography if blood at meatus
- Suspected renal artery or vein thrombosis or embolism
  - ▲ Renal ultrasound with Doppler studies vs. CT, depending on availability
  - ▲ Magnetic resonance angiography
  - ▲ Renal arteriography
- Seek critical care—refractory hypotension, severe hypertension, fulminant hemolysis, acutely compromised renal function, multiorgan dysfunction

DIFFERENTIAL DIAGNOSIS FOR HEMATURIA

- The differential diagnosis is given in Table 1, and the causes of hematuria are listed by age and sex in Table 2. The history, physical exam, and lab findings for various causes of hematuria are listed in Table 3.

Table 1. Differential Diagnosis for Hematuria

Site	Conditions
Renal	
Glomerular	
Proliferative glomerulonephritis	IgA nephropathy, HSP, postinfectious glomerulonephritis (strep), membranoproliferative glomerulonephritis, vasculitides (SLE, Goodpasture syndrome, ANCA-positive vasculitis [microscopic polyangitis, Wegener granulomatosis, Churg-Strauss syndrome], scleroderma, cryoglobulinemia)
Nonproliferative glomerulonephropathies	Minimal change disease, focal segmental glomerulosclerosis, membranous nephropathy, HUS/TTP
Familial	Alport syndrome, Fabry disease, thin basement membrane nephropathy (or benign familial hematuria)
Others	Renal allograft rejection, postradiotherapy
Nonglomerular	
Neoplasms	Renal cell & transitional cell carcinoma, simple renal cysts
Familial	Polycystic kidney disease, medullary sponge kidney
Vascular	Renal infarction (thrombotic, embolic), renal vein thrombosis, aneurysms, arteriovenous malformation, arteriovenous fistula
Infectious	Pyelonephritis, xanthogranulomatous pyelonephritis, TB, *Cryptococcus*
Metabolic	Hypercalciuria, hyperoxaluria

Table 1 (continued)

Site	Conditions
Nonglomerular (continued)	
Trauma	Laceration, contusion, stones
Others	Acute interstitial nephritis, loin pain—hematuria syndrome, malignant hypertension, papillary necrosis
Lower urinary tract	
Ureteral	Stones, trauma, transitional cell carcinoma
Bladder	Cystitis (also interstitial vs. postradiotherapy), transitional cell & papillary carcinoma, rapid emptying of distended bladder, *Schistosoma haematobium*, stones, trigonitis, post-cystoscopy, enterovesical fistula
Urethral	Urethritis, meatal stenosis, caruncle, stricture, prolapse, foreign body, trauma from Foley catheter, urethral neoplasm, stones
Prostatic	BPH, prostatitis, prostatic adenocarcinoma, post-prostatectomy
Others	
Hematologic	Over anticoagulation, anticoagulation unmasking genitourinary lesion, thrombocytopenia, hemophilia, bleeding diathesis, sickle cell
Drug/toxin	Cyclophosphamide (hemorrhagic cystitis), NSAID, phenacetin
Miscellaneous	Vulvovaginitis, menstruation, endometriosis, vaginal foreign body, sexual abuse, anal fissure, vigorous exercise (runners), factitious
False-positives	Myoglobinuria, hemoglobinuria, food coloring, rifampin, beetroot

ANCA, antineutrophil cytoplasmic antibody; BPH, benign prostatic hypertrophy; HSP, Henoch-Schönlein purpura; HUS, hemolytic uremic syndrome; SLE, systemic lupus erythematosus; TTP, thrombotic thrombocytopenic purpura.

DIFFERENTIATING THE DIFFERENTIAL

Characteristics of Hematuria

- Glomerular or renal—brown or cola-colored urine, dysmorphic red cells (>25%), red cell casts
- Extrarenal—gross hematuria with complete clearing between; pink or red urine; more likely to clot
- Urethral source—hematuria at initiation of stream
- Prostatic or bladder neck source—hematuria present in last few drops of urine
- Bladder, ureteral, or renal source—hematuria present throughout stream
- Gynecologic source—cyclical through the month (vaginal bleeding with menses), endometriosis of bladder or urethra

Urinalysis

- Glomerular hematuria—RBC casts, dysmorphic RBCs, proteinuria (gross hematuria alone may be responsible for up to 500 mg protein/24 hours)
- Nonglomerular hematuria—clotting, rounded RBCs

Table 2. Common Causes of Hematuria by Age

Age, y	Causes (in descending order)
<20	UTIs
	Glomerulonephritides
	Congenital tract anomalies
20-40	UTIs
	Stones
	Carcinoma (bladder/kidney)
40-60	UTIs
	Stones
	Carcinoma (bladder/kidney)
>60	UTIs
	Carcinoma (bladder/kidney)
	BPH
	Systemic vasculitis

BPH, benign prostatic hypertrophy; UTI, urinary tract infection.

Table 3. Causes of Hematuria, Clinical Presentation, and Lab Findings

Cause	History	Physical exam	Test
Urinary tract infection, pyelonephritis	Frequency, dysuria	Fever, CVA tenderness	Positive urinalysis Gram stain
Stones	Colicky flank pain radiates to groin, frequent in Asian children (calcium oxalate), family history	Orthostatism, CVA tenderness	80% seen on KUB, may need spiral CT
Poststreptococcal glomerulonephritis	Pharyngitis (latency, 7-10 days), skin infection (latency, 21-30 days), brown or cola-colored urine, oliguria	HTN, edema, fever, residual pharyngitis, healing pyoderma	Low levels of complement, positive ASO titer, dysmorphic RBCs in urine, RBC casts
IgA nephropathy	Most common type of glomerulo-nephritis in children		Renal biopsy
	Hematuria (microscopic or macro-scopic), proteinuria after URI or exercise	Normal, may have HTN/edema	
	Most common cause of hematuria in world (30%)		
Prostatitis	Perineal pain, terminal hematuria in males	Boggy tender prostate	WBCs in urinalysis
Benign prostatic hypertrophy	Hesitancy, weak stream, dribbling	Enlarged, soft, smooth prostate	Mildly elevated prostate-specific antigen

Table 3 (continued)

Cause	History	Physical exam	Test
Papillary necrosis	Diabetes mellitus, sickle cell anemia, analgesics, TB, ethanol, ankylosing spondylosis, obstructive uropathy	May correspond to predisposing cause	Elevated hemoglobin A_{1c}, sickle cell screen, urine acid-fast bacteria
Renal artery embolism/thrombosis	Recent angiogram or myocardial infarction, palpitations or pulse irregularity, subacute bacterial endocarditis	HTN, irregular pulse, new murmurs, flank bruits, livedo reticularis	Doppler study, angiography
Renal vein thrombosis	History of nephrotic syndrome or paroxysmal nocturnal hemoglobinuria	Orthostasis	Doppler study, angiography
Renal laceration or trauma	History of motor vehicle accident, blunt trauma to abdomen, back	Hypotension, flank ecchymosis	CT abdomen
Urethral injury	History of motor vehicle accident, pelvic fracture	High-riding, ballotable prostate; perineal ecchymosis; urethral blood	Pelvic X-rays, retrograde urethrography
Malignant HTN	Headaches, visual changes, TIA-like symptoms	HTN, fundus arteriovenous nicking, exudates/hemorrhage, S_4	ECG, CT head, urinalysis, creatinine
Bleeding dyscrasia	Family history, ethnicity, abnormal coagulation, bleeding, bruising	Pallor, ecchymosis, joint deformities	Special coagulation studies, hemoglobin electrophoresis

Table 3 (continued)

Cause	History	Physical exam	Test
Sickle cell anemia	Males>females, source from left>right kidney, associated with papillary necrosis, glomerulopathy, bacteria, hyperuricemia, incomplete renal tubular acidosis, nephrogenic diabetes insipidus	Orthostatism, pallor, pain	Sickle cell screen
ANCA-positive vasculitis	Paresthesias, arthralgias, skin lesions, abdominal pain, anemia, hematuria, proteinuria, sinusitis, epistaxis	Neuropathies, skin rash, purpura, others	ANCA testing (anti-MPO, anti-PR3) biopsy
HUS/TTP	Prodrome of bloody diarrhea	Pallor, ecchymosis, fever, mental status changes	Peripheral blood smear, stool culture, creatinine
Henoch-Schönlein purpura	Usually boys 2-11 years old, arthralgias, crampy abdominal pain, melena	Non-thrombocytopenic purpura of lower extremities or buttocks, arthritis	Need to exclude other causes of purpura
Alport syndrome	High-frequency sensorineural hearing loss, family history of end-stage renal failure in 2nd-3rd decade, X-linked, ocular abnormality, defect α 5 chain, type IV collagen chain	Deafness, anterior lenticonus, yellow perimacular flecks	Clinical diagnosis, may need renal biopsy

Table 3 (continued)

Cause	History	Physical exam	Test
Goodpasture syndrome	Hemoptysis, hematuria, proteinuria	Coarse breath sounds, rales, pallor	anti-GBM, MPO, PR3, renal biopsy
Scleroderma	Finger changes white to red to blue, arthritis, dyspnea	Sclerodactyly, ulcerated fingers, calcifications, wide split S_2 with loud P_2	Anti-centromere & anti-Scl70
Systemic lupus erythematosus	Females>males, 2nd-3rd decades, fevers, rash, arthritis. As ans>African Americans>whites	Butterfly rash, arthritis, pulmonary rales or rubs	ANA, anti-dsDNA, anti-histone (drug-induced)
Bladder carcinoma	Previous pelvic radiotherapy, chemotherapy with cyclophosphamide, smoking; work in textile, metal, rubber, paint, or printing industry	Suprapubic mass, pelvic lymphadenopathy	Cystoscopy with biopsy
Renal cell carcinoma	Smoking; work in tannery, asbestos, cadmium, lead acetate, or petroleum industry; family history of von Hippel-Lindau disease	Fever, flank mass, left-sided varicocele	CT or MRI

Table 3 (continued)

Cause	History	Physical exam	Test
Prostate adenocarcinoma	High fat diet, family history	Firm, irregular, nodular prostate	Transrectal ultrasonography with biopsy, elevated prostate-specific antigen
Exercise-induced	Transient 24–48 hours after exertion, distance runners, 15%–20% of normal persons	Normal	Urine normalizes
Enterovesicular fistula	History of pelvic surgery or radiotherapy	Fecaluria, pneumaturia	Urinalysis with polyenteric organisms

ANCA, antineutrophil cytoplasmic antibody; ANA, antinuclear antibody; ASO, antistreptolysin O; CVA, costovertebral angle; dsDNA, double-stranded DNA; GBM, glomerular basement membrane; HTN, hypertension; HUS, hemolytic uremic syndrome; KUB, kidney, ureter, bladder; MPO, myeloperoxidase; P_2, 2nd pulmonic sound; PR3, proteinase 3; S_2, 2nd heart sound; S_4, 4th heart sound; TIA, transient ischemic attack; TPP, thrombotic thrombocytopenic purpura; URI, upper respiratory tract infection.

DIAGNOSTIC TEST ORDERING

- An algorithm for evaluating hematuria is provided in Figure 1.

INITIAL MANAGEMENT

- Urinary tract infection or pyelonephritis
  - ▲ Urine culture, blood culture if hypotensive (positive in up to 20%)
  - ▲ Antibiotics
    - IV if unable to take PO, pregnant, or unstable (quinolones, 3rd-generation cephalosporins)
    - Oral antibiotics when stable (trimethoprim-sulfamethoxazole, quinolones)
    - Treat for 3-5 days for cystitis and 10-14 days for pyelonephritis
- Calculi
  - ▲ Aggressive IV hydration, pain control (may need morphine patient-controlled analgesia)
  - ▲ Strain urine for stone analysis.
  - ▲ 24-Hour urine for calcium, phosphorus, urate, cystine, citrate, oxalate, creatinine, sodium, potassium
  - ▲ Urology consult for large stones (>4 mm) in need of extracorporeal shock wave lithotripsy
- Bladder carcinoma
  - ▲ Urology consult
  - ▲ Staging
    - CT of chest, abdomen, and pelvis to evaluate spread and metastasis
    - Liver function tests, bone scan
    - Proctoscopy to rule out rectal involvement if invasive
    - Preoperative medical evaluation
- Renal cell carcinoma
  - ▲ Urology consult
  - ▲ Staging
    - Creatinine clearance, liver function tests, calcium, bone scan
    - CT of chest, abdomen, and pelvis to evaluate spread and metastasis

- MRI to evaluate for renal vein and inferior vena cava tumor thrombus
- Preoperative medical evaluation
- Benign prostatic hypertrophy
  - Bladder scan to rule out retention
  - Lab tests
    - Creatinine
    - Prostate-specific antigen, if baseline available to compare, to rule out malignancy (do not draw blood sample after Foley placement or aggressive digital rectal exam because these cause false-positive results)
  - May begin tamsulosin, 0.4 mg PO daily
  - If obstruction, consult urology to consider transurethral resection of prostate
- Glomerulonephritis
  - Lab tests—C3, C4, CH50, ASO, ESR, ANA, ENA panel, ANCA (anti-MPO, anti-GBM), cryoglobulins, creatinine, serum protein electrophoresis
  - Urine studies—eosinophils, hemosiderin, myoglobin, 24-hour urine creatinine and protein, urinary immunoelectrophoresis
  - Chest X-ray
  - Nephrology consult
- Anticoagulation
  - Discontinue anticoagulation if INR/aPTT supratherapeutic
  - May need vitamin K or fresh frozen plasma to reverse warfarin or protamine sulfate to reverse heparin if bleeding is severe
  - If anticoagulation is essential but limited by bleeding, fully reverse the warfarin and titrate heparin as bleeding allows.
  - Bleeding while therapeutic on anticoagulation, requires same work-up as above given likelihood of disease (80% of the time if therapeutically anticoagulated)

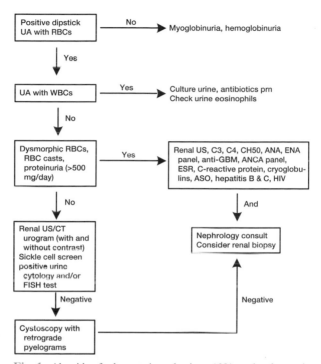

Fig. 1. Algorithm for hematuria evaluation. ANA, antinuclear antibody; ANCA, antineutrophil cytoplasmic antibody; ASO, antistreptolysin O; ENA, extractable nuclear antigen; FISH, fluorescence in situ hybridization; GBM, glomerular basement membrane; IVP, intravenous pyelography; MPO, myeloperoxidase; prn, as needed; UA, urinalysis; US, ultrasonography.

HEMOPTYSIS

Otis B. Rickman, D.O.
Udaya B. S. Prakash, M.D.

IS THE PATIENT'S LIFE AT RISK?

- Hemoptysis
  - ▲ Definition—expectoration of blood from respiratory tract
  - ▲ Common respiratory symptom (patient complains about it before it is seen)
  - ▲ Most commonly due to bronchitis
  - ▲ Frequently portends an ominous diagnosis
  - ▲ Expedient evaluation is required.
- Massive hemoptysis—life-threatening!
  - ▲ Definition (arbitrary)—≥200 mL blood expectorated in 24 hours
  - ▲ Occurs in 1%-4% of patients with hemoptysis
  - ▲ Death—usually caused by asphyxiation, occasionally by exsanguination
- Look for signs of respiratory failure or hemodynamic collapse
- Lung blood supply
  - ▲ Dual supply—low-pressure pulmonary artery and high-pressure bronchial arteries
  - ▲ Bronchial artery—90% of cases of hemoptysis
  - ▲ Can die of hemoptysis of low pressure side (Rasmussen aneurysm)

ADDRESSING THE RISK

- Airway, breathing, circulation, and differential
- Evaluate and manage concurrently.
- If patient is actively bleeding, high operative mortality; thus, stop the bleeding.
- Surgery—only for a good operative candidate with localized bleeding
- High-resolution CT and bronchoscopy are complementary

DIFFERENTIAL DIAGNOSIS

- Hemoptysis is a symptom with a broad differential diagnosis (Table 1).
- Mnemonic device—very fast **docs pitch in** (**v**ascular, **f**actitious, **d**rugs/toxins, **o**ther, **c**avitary, **s**ystemic disease, **p**ulmonary, **i**atrogenic, **t**rauma, **c**ardiac, **h**ematologic, **i**nfection, **n**eoplastic) (Table 1)

DIFFERENTIATING THE DIFFERENTIAL

- Diagnoses suspected on the basis of the history and physical exam findings are listed in Table 2.

DIAGNOSTIC TEST ORDERING

- For every patient with hemoptysis—chest X-ray, CBC, type and screen, and arterial blood gases
- Also, sputum with Gram stain, culture, acid-fast bacteria, and cytology if clinically indicated
- Depending on what is suspected—high-resolution CT, ventilation-perfusion scan, echocardiography, bronchoscopy (Fig. 1)

INITIAL MANAGEMENT

- The algorithm in Figure 1 includes a strategy for managing hemoptysis.

Table 1. Differential Diagnosis for Hemoptysis

Vascular
- Pulmonary embolism (clot, tumor, fat, septic)
- Pulmonary hypertension
- Arteriovenous malformation
- Aneurysm
- Leaking graft

Factitious

Drugs/toxins
- Aspirin
- Warfarin/heparin
- Nitrofurantoin
- Penicillamine
- Solvents

Other
- Catamenial
- Broncholithiasis
- Foreign body
- Lymphangioleiomyomatosis
- Cryptogenic

Cavitary
- TB
- Mycetoma
- Abscess
- Bronchogenic cancer
- Wegener granulomatosis
- Sarcoidosis

Systemic disease/diffuse alveolar hemorrhage
- Goodpasture syndrome
- Wegener granulomatosis
- Microscopic polyangiitis/ polyarteritis nodosa
- Churg-Strauss syndrome
- Rheumatoid arthritis
- Systemic lupus erythematosus
- Behçet syndrome
- Idiopathic pulmonary hemosiderosis

Pulmonary
- Bronchitis
- Bronchiectasis
- Cystic fibrosis

Iatrogenic
- Pulmonary artery catheter
- Transthoracic biopsy
- Bronchoscopy

Trauma
- Puncture
- Laceration
- Contusion
- Bronchial disruption

Cardiac
- Mitral stenosis
- Congestive heart failure
- Congenital heart disease

Hematologic
- Thrombocytopenia
- Platelet dysfunction
- Coagulopathy
- Uremia
- Disseminated intravascular coagulation

Infection
- Bronchitis
- Pneumonia (bacterial, fungal, viral)
- Abscess
- TB
- Parasites

Neoplastic
- Squamous cell
- Adenocarcinoma
- Carcinoid
- Endobronchial adenoma
- Metastases

Table 2. Diagnosis Suggested by History and Physical Exam

History and physical exam clues	Suspected diagnosis	Further testing
Fever, blood-streaked mucopurulent sputum, normal chest X-ray, seasonal	Acute bronchitis	None
Large-volume, purulent sputum; history of severe infection or TB	Bronchiectasis	High-resolution CT
Fever, rigors, adventitious sounds, consolidation, infiltrate on chest X-ray	Pneumonia	Sputum & blood cultures
Chronic aspiration (alcoholic, dysphagia, seizures), poor dentition	Lung abscess	CT chest
Positive PPD, exposure, previous history of/risk factors for TB	TB	Sputum acid-fast bacteria, PPD, chest X-ray
Neutropenic, immunocompromised	Invasive aspergillosis	Biopsy
Past history of cavitary disease, now fever & chills	Mycetoma	Chest X-ray or CT chest
Smoker, weight loss, >40 years old	Bronchogenic cancer	Sputum cytology, flexible fiberoptic bronchoscopy
Pleuritic chest pain, dyspnea, immobility, pleural rub, deep venous thrombosis	Pulmonary embolism	Spiral CT or V/Q scan
Recent bronchoscopy, lung biopsy, pulmonary artery catheter	Trauma	See Figure 1
Status post thoracic aneurysm repair	Fistula	Aortography
Hematuria	Vasculitis	Anti-GBM, ANCA
Pneumothorax, effusion, child-bearing age female	Lymphangioleiomyomatosis	Thoracentesis, high-resolution CT

Table 2 (continued)

History and physical exam clues	Suspected diagnosis	Further testing
Cyclic hemoptysis occurring with menses	Catamenial hemoptysis	Suppress menses
S$_3$, edema, elevated jugular venous pressure	Congestive heart failure	Echocardiography
Opening snap, diastolic murmur	Mitral stenosis	Echocardiography
Telangiectasias, bruit over chest	Osler-Weber-Rendu disease	Family history

ANCA, antineutrophil cytoplasmic antibody; GBM, glomerular basement membrane; S$_3$, 3rd heart sound; V/Q, ventilation-perfusion.

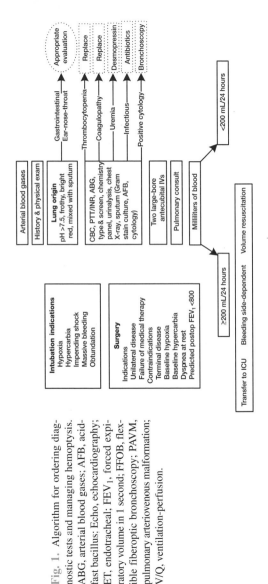

Fig. 1. Algorithm for ordering diagnostic tests and managing hemoptysis. ABG, arterial blood gases; AFB, acid-fast bacillus; Echo, echocardiography; ET, endotracheal; FEV$_1$, forced expiratory volume in 1 second; FFOB, flexible fiberoptic bronchoscopy; PAVM, pulmonary arteriovenous malformation; V/Q, ventilation-perfusion.

Arterial blood gases

History & physical exam

Lung origin
pH >7.5, frothy, bright red, mixed with sputum

CBC, PTT/INR, ABG, type & screen, chemistry panel, urinalysis, chest X-ray, sputum (Gram stain culture, AFB, cytology)

Gastrointestinal ──→ Appropriate evaluation

Ear-nose-throat

── Thrombocytopenia ──→ Replace
── Coagulopathy ──→ Replace
── Uremia ──→ Desmopressin
── Infectious ──→ Antibiotics
── Positive cytology ──→ Bronchoscopy

Two large-bore antecubital IVs

Pulmonary consult

Intubation indications
Hypoxia
Hypercarbia
Impending shock
Massive bleeding
Obtundation

Surgery
Indications
Unilateral disease
Failure of medical therapy
Contraindications
Terminal disease
Baseline hypoxia
Baseline hypercarbia
Dyspnea at rest
Predicted postop FEV$_1$ <800

Milliliters of blood

≥200 mL/24 hours

<200 mL/24 hours

Transfer to ICU   Bleeding side-dependent   Volume resuscitation

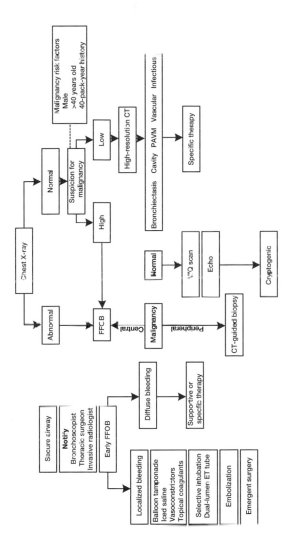

Fig. 1 continued

HEPATOMEGALY

T. Jared Bunch, M.D.
Santhi Swaroop Vege, M.D.

IS THE PATIENT'S LIFE AT RISK?

- The most life-threatening conditions that must be ruled out immediately include
  - ▲ Fulminant hepatic failure (most cases may not have hepatomegaly because of marked hepatic necrosis and shrinkage of the liver)
  - ▲ Closed abdominal trauma with liver or splenic rupture
  - ▲ Acute hepatic vein thrombosis
  - ▲ Sepsis
  - ▲ Hepatic infarction
  - ▲ Severe biliary obstruction
- The following features are suggestive of the above:
  - ▲ Acute onset of symptoms (<10 weeks)
  - ▲ History of toxic ingestion (drugs such as acetaminophen)
  - ▲ Fever
  - ▲ Hypotension
  - ▲ Early signs of encephalopathy (changes in sleep-wake cycle, agitation-anxiety, personality change, altered mental status)
  - ▲ Hypoglycemia
  - ▲ PT >3 seconds
  - ▲ Bilirubin >20 mg/dL
  - ▲ Acute abdominal pain and distension
  - ▲ Signs of peritonitis

ADDRESSING THE RISK

- If any of the above conditions is suspected, proceed as follows:

Special abbreviations used in this chapter: ERCP, endoscopic retrograde cholangiopancreatography; HAV, hepatitis A virus; HBc, hepatitis B core; HBsAg, hepatitis B surface antigen; HBV, hepatitis B virus; HCV, hepatitis C virus.

- ▲ Obtain good intravenous access and start IV fluids.
- ▲ Give nasal oxygen.
- ▲ Start empiric treatment with antibiotics (piperacillin-tazobactam) after blood cultures if sepsis or trauma is suspected.
- ▲ Start acetylcysteine immediately if acetaminophen ingestion is suspected.
- ▲ Call ICU immediately.
- ▲ Contact liver transplant service for fulminant hepatic failure—the sooner the better.
- ▲ Obtain as a priority
  - • Bilirubin, ALT, AST, alkaline phosphatase, PT, albumin, hepatitis viral serologic studies (IgM anti-HAV, IgM anti-HBc, HBsAg, and anti-HCV), blood gases, blood cultures, acetaminophen level
  - • Abdominal ultrasound with Doppler study of venous and/or arterial system

DIFFERENTIAL DIAGNOSIS

- ▫ The causes of hepatomegaly may be subdivided into the following categories: venous congestion, biliary obstruction, infectious/inflammatory, infiltrative, cystic liver disease, and others (Table 1).
- ▫ Note—50% of all cases of hepatomegaly in hospitalized patients are due to congestive heart failure.

DIFFERENTIATING THE DIFFERENTIAL

History of Present Illness
- ▫ Acute vs. chronic disease
  - ▲ The abrupt onset of symptoms suggest an acute liver injury such as infectious or inflammatory (most likely viral), toxic, congestive (acute right-sided heart failure)
- ▫ Characteristics of the symptoms
  - ▲ Confusion, somnolence, agitation, tremulousness: hepatic encephalopathy
  - ▲ Nausea and vomiting: acute liver insult and/or necrosis
  - ▲ Anorexia—common symptom in acute and chronic liver disease
  - ▲ Right upper quadrant pain—infectious or inflammatory
  - ▲ Increase in abdominal girth—suggestive of ascites, spontaneous bacterial peritonitis, hepatic malignancy, venous outflow obstruction

Table 1. **Causes of Hepatomegaly**

Venous
  Congestive heart failure
  Tricuspid regurgitation
  Constrictive pericarditis
  Cor pulmonale
  Budd-Chiari syndrome
  Veno-occlusive disease (chemotherapy, radiation, bone marrow
    transplant, pyrrolizidine alkaloids)
Biliary obstruction
  Common duct gallstones
  Biliary stricture
  Pancreatitis
  Neoplasm (pancreatic, biliary, ampullary)
Inflammatory
  Infectious
        Diffuse—hepatitis (A, B, or C), CMV, infectious
          mononucleosis, herpes simplex, HIV, TB, histoplasmosis,
          actinomycosis, brucellosis, schistosomiasis, falciparum
          malaria
        Localized—pyrogenic abscess, *Entamoeba histolytica*
    Noninfectious—alcohol, toxin- & drug-induced hepatitis,
      autoimmune hepatitis, primary biliary cirrhosis, primary
      sclerosing cholangitis, Wilson disease, Reye syndrome
Infiltrative
  Primary or metastatic cancer
  Lymphoma
  Nonalcoholic steatohepatitis—diabetes mellitus,
    alcohol, hyperalimentation, malnutrition
  Amyloidosis
  Hemochromatosis
  Sarcoidosis
  Glycogen storage disease
  Alpha$_1$-antitrypsin deficiency
Cystic
  Adult polycystic kidney disease
  Pyogenic abscess
  Entamoeba histolytica
  Echinococcus granulosus
Other
  Riedel lobe
  Nonhepatic mass

CMV, cytomegalovirus.

- ▲ Pruritus—cholestasis
- ▲ Jaundice—Painless jaundice suggests a neoplasm obstructing the bile duct (check for a palpable gallbladder on exam, Courvoisier law).
  - • Intermittent jaundice, suggests a stone in the bile duct with cholangitis.
  - • With dark urine and light stools—cholestasis
  - • Without pruritus—acute hepatitis (viral- or drug-induced)
- ▲ Hyperpigmentation—chronic cholestatic liver disease (e.g., primary sclerosing cholangitis, primary biliary cirrhosis), hemochromatosis
- ▲ Ecchymoses—advanced chronic liver disease with/without hypersplenism (may occur with petechiae, gingival bleeding)
- ▲ Urticaria—HBV or HCV infection (with synovitis), immune complex disease (with petechiae)
- ▲ Pharyngitis, rash, and lymphadenopathy—Epstein-Barr virus or cytomegalovirus

Family History
- ▪ Genetically linked chronic liver disease—Wilson disease, hemochromatosis, alpha$_1$-antitrypsin deficiency, polycystic kidney disease, autosomal dominant polycystic liver disease, autoimmune disease
- ▪ Hereditary predisposition—alcoholic liver disease, drug abuse
- ▪ Perinatal exposure to HBV (high prevalence of hepatitis B in Asia and Africa)

Social History
- ▪ Household contact with hepatitis A or food contamination
- ▪ Promiscuous sexual activity, ilicit drug use, history of blood transfusion—viral hepatitis
- ▪ Exposure to a hepatotoxic medication or environmental toxin, including ethanol use
- ▪ Institutional exposure—health care experience, institutionalized or imprisoned (viral hepatitis)
- ▪ Oral contraceptives—hepatic vein thrombosis, cholestasis, hepatic adenoma

Physical Exam
- General
  - Cushingoid features (chronic corticosteroid treatment of liver disease, autoimmune chronic active hepatitis) and signs of chronic liver disease
  - Cachexia—malnutrition (ethanol), malignancy
- Head
  - Scleral icterus—jaundice
  - Kayser-Fleischer rings—Wilson disease
  - Dry eyes/mouth (sicca syndrome/autoimmune disease, primary biliary cirrhosis), buccal icterus (jaundice)
- Neck
  - Adenopathy—lymphoproliferative or metastatic disease, viral hepatitis, granulomatous disease
  - Distended neck veins and hepatojugular reflex—congestive heart failure
  - Kussmaul sign (elevated jugular venous pressure with a paradoxical elevation during inspiration)—constrictive pericarditis or tamponade
- Chest
  - Gynecomastia, spider angiomas—chronic liver disease, usually ethanol
- Chest hyperresonance (emphysema)—alpha$_1$-antitrypsin deficiency
- Cardiac
  - Third heart sound gallop—congestive heart failure
  - Cardiomegaly (displaced apical impulse)—congestive heart failure, alcoholism, hemochromatosis, or amyloidosis
  - Right ventricular heave—right ventricular failure, pulmonary hypertension, cor pulmonale
  - Increased second pulmonic sound—pulmonary hypertension
  - Holosystolic murmur that increases with inspiration—tricuspid regurgitation–pulmonary hypertension, cor pulmonale, advanced congestive heart failure
  - Constrictive pericarditis—diastolic pericardial knock, widening of the split between the aortic and pulmonic

183

components of the second heart sound may occur, a friction rub is best heard using the diaphragm of the stethoscope at the left lower sternal border. The friction rub is easier to hear if respirations are suspended.

- Abdomen
  - ▲ Liver
    - • Displaced liver/benign hepatomegaly—increased height and weight, hyperinflated lungs, Riedel lobe, males
    - • Tenderness—acute, infectious, or inflammatory causes more likely
    - • Nodularity—tumor, polycystic disease, macronodular cirrhosis
    - • Pulsation—*increases* with inspiration (tricuspid regurgitation), *decreases* with inspiration (constrictive pericarditis)
    - • Friction rub—inflammation, recent trauma (liver biopsy), malignancy (surface implants), gonococcal perihepatitis
    - • Bruits—vascular tumor, arteriovenous fistula, acute alcoholic hepatitis
    - • Venous hum—severe tricuspid regurgitation, severe congestion, collateral blood flow from portal hypertension
    - • Splenomegaly—portal hypertension
    - • Caput medusae—collateral blood flow from portal hypertension
- Extremities
  - ▲ Edema—congestive heart failure, cirrhosis
  - ▲ Clubbing of fingers and toes—arteriovenous fistula, congenital cyanotic heart disease, chronic liver disease (hepatitis C)
  - ▲ Dupuytren contractures—ethanol abuse
- Nervous system
  - ▲ Disorientation, tremor, asterixis—encephalopathy
  - ▲ Cerebellar dysfunction, gross tremor (particularly in wing-beating position), slurred speech, hypertonicity—ethanol abuse, Wilson disease

DIAGNOSTIC TEST ORDERING

- An algorithm for examining a patient who has hepatomegaly is presented in Figure 1.

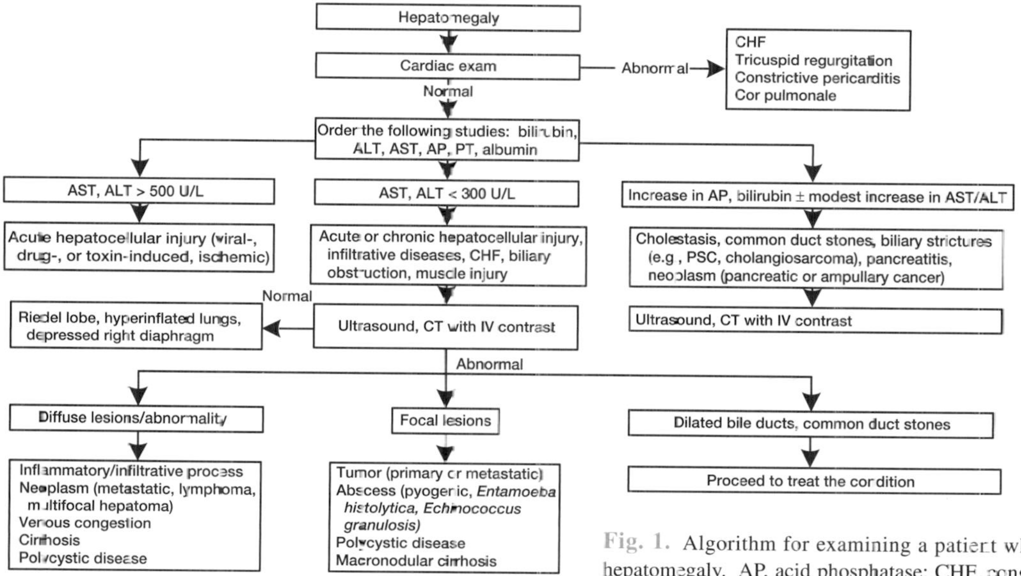

Fig. 1. Algorithm for examining a patient who has hepatomegaly. AP, acid phosphatase; CHF, congestive heart failure; PSC, primary sclerosing cholangitis.

185

- If there is ascites, always obtain a diagnostic sample for
  - Serum-ascitic fluid albumin gradient: >1.1 = cirrhosis-related causes (97% specificity)
  - Cytology
  - CBC and differential: >250 neutrophils = spontaneous bacterial peritonitis
  - Amylase: >1,000 mg/dL = pancreatic ascites
  - Gram stain and cultures

INITIAL MANAGEMENT

Venous Congestion

- Congestive heart failure—low salt diet, diuretics, spironolactone, digoxin, β-blockers, angiotensin-converting enzyme inhibitors
- Suprahepatic vein thrombosis (Budd-Chiari syndrome)—thrombolysis, anticoagulation, surgical shunt, and liver transplant

Biliary Obstruction

- Common bile duct gallstones—endoscopic retrograde cholangiopancreatography (ERCP) and sphincterotomy
- Biliary stricture
  - Cholangitis—blood cultures, CBC, and IV piperacillin-tazobactam
  - ERCP—diagnosis, biopsy, dilation with stent placement
- Neoplasm—surgical resection if resectable, otherwise palliative bypass procedure, chemotherapy, radiotherapy

Inflammatory

- Ethanol hepatitis—abstinence from ethanol, vitamin replacement (folate, thiamine), nutritional support, and corticosteroids if criteria are met: discriminant function (DF) >32 [DF = 4.6 (PT − PT$_{control}$) + bilirubin] or presence of encephalopathy
- Viral hepatitis—Order hepatitis serology tests; give supportive care treatment, with the patient avoiding strenuous exertion, ethanol, and hepatotoxic agents.
  - Hepatitis A—immune globulin is given to all close personal contacts.
  - Hepatitis B—immune globulin is effective if given within 7 days of exposure, followed by the vaccination series for sexual contacts.

- Acetaminophen overdose—Empty the stomach by emesis or gastric lavage; if 1-2 hours after ingestion, administer activated charcoal. Begin acetylcysteine at 140 mg/kg PO, then 70 mg/kg every 4 hours for 17 doses if
  - History of acetaminophen abuse and lab evidence of hepatoxicity
  - Serum acetaminophen concentration is above the "possible hepatic toxicity line" of the Rumack-Mathew nomogram
  - A single ingestion of >7.5 g acetaminophen by history and results of serum concentration are not available
  - Serum concentration is >10 µg and time of ingestion is not known

Infiltrative
- Nonalcoholic steatohepatitis—gradual weight loss, lipid management, diabetes mellitus control, low fat diet
- Ethanol steatohepatitis—reversible with discontinuation of ethanol or treatment of underlying condition
- Neoplasm (metastatic>primary)—Treatment and management depend on the cause of the tumor and associated symptoms.

JOINT PAIN

Peter D. Kent, M.D.
Thomas G. Mason, M.D.

IS THE PATIENT'S LIFE AT RISK?

- First, rule out the possibility of a musculoskeletal emergency.
- The presence of a warm, swollen, tender joint mandates immediate evaluation.
- Red flags include
  - ▲ Fever, chills, weight loss, night sweats
  - ▲ Trauma to a limb or joint area
  - ▲ Neurologic compromise
  - ▲ Acute onset of symptoms
- Septic arthritis is the most important cause of acute joint pain to rule out; it is a medical emergency.

ADDRESSING THE RISK

- If septic arthritis is a possibility, aspirate synovial fluid from the involved joint(s).
- The following studies should be ordered on synovial fluid:
  - ▲ Culture
  - ▲ Gram stain
  - ▲ Cell count and differential
  - ▲ Crystal analysis
- Base the choice of antibiotics for empiric treatment on the Gram stain results.
- X-ray the joint area if trauma is involved or tumor is suspected.

DIFFERENTIAL DIAGNOSIS

- Inflammatory arthritis may be distinguished from noninflammatory by the following:
  - ▲ Warmth over the joint
  - ▲ Synovitis (boggy, swollen synovial tissue)
  - ▲ Pronounced morning stiffness by history

- Joint effusions may be present in both inflammatory and noninflammatory arthritis.
- Arthralgias without arthritis
  - ▲ Viral illness
  - ▲ Subacute bacterial endocarditis
  - ▲ Fibromyalgia
  - ▲ Bursitis
  - ▲ Tendinitis
  - ▲ Fasciitis
  - ▲ Metabolic bone disease (osteomalacia, hyperparathyroidism)
  - ▲ Soft tissue injury
  - ▲ Neuropathy

DIFFERENTIATING THE DIFFERENTIAL

Is There a History of Trauma or Focal Bone Pain?

- If so, obtain an X-ray, with at least two views at 90° angles from each other.
- If film is abnormal, the possibilities include fracture, tumor, or metabolic bone disease.

Is the Joint Pain Articular or Periarticular?

- Articular (joint) pain
  - ▲ Similar with passive and active range of motion
  - ▲ Swelling over the joint
  - ▲ Tenderness along the joint margin
  - ▲ Focuses diagnostic evaluation on the joint(s)
- Periarticular pain
  - ▲ Markedly less severe with passive than active movement
  - ▲ Often maximal at beginning of task and improves with activity
  - ▲ Aggravated with resisted movement or stretch
  - ▲ Site of tenderness may extend perpendicular to joint line
  - ▲ Suggests a diagnosis such as bursitis or tendinitis

Is an Inflammatory Arthritis or Effusion Present?

- Look for boggy synovitis or a bulge sign (knee joint).
- Ask about morning stiffness, which typically lasts for more than 1 hour in inflammatory arthritis.
- Perform arthrocentesis if not contraindicated.
- Inflammatory fluid (>2,000 WBCs/μL with >75% PMNs) suggests crystalline, infectious, or systemic rheumatic disease.

- Fluid from a septic joint usually has >50,000 (50 × 10⁹/L) WBCs/µL.
- Noninflammatory fluid suggests osteoarthritis, soft tissue injury, or viral infection.
- Marrow elements in the fluid suggest intra-articular fracture.
- Bloody effusions occur with coagulopathy, pseudogout, tumor, trauma, or Charcot joints

Is Monoarticular or Polyarticular Arthritis Present?

- The differential diagnostic possibilities are different for the two conditions (Tables 1 and 2)

What Is the Time Course?

- Acute monarthritis, in which symptoms become maximal within 12-24 hours, is likely to result from trauma, an infectious process, or crystal-induced synovitis.
- Polyarthritis that progresses with a subacute course (few weeks) occurs with viral arthritis, spondyloarthropathy, and rheumatoid arthritis.
- More insidious and chronic disorders include osteoarthritis and fibromyalgia.

What Is the Distribution of the Arthritis?

- Symmetric involvement of the metacarpophalangeal joints and proximal interphalangeal joints is characteristic of rheumatoid arthritis.

Table 1. Differential Diagnosis for Inflammatory and Noninflammatory Monarthritis

Inflammatory	Noninflammatory
Infection: viral, bacterial, fungal, mycobacterial	Fracture or internal derangement
Crystalline: gout, pseudogout	Osteoarthritis
Other: psoriatic, reactive, rheumatoid, systemic lupus erythematosus	Other: tumor, hemarthrosis, amyloidosis

Table 2. Differential Diagnosis for Inflammatory and Noninflammatory Polyarthritis

Inflammatory	Noninflammatory
Infection: parvovirus, HIV, rubella, gonococcal, Lyme disease, Whipple disease, endocarditis Systemic inflammatory arthritis: rheumatoid arthritis, systemic lupus erythematosus, Still disease, Behçet syndrome, relapsing polychondritis, familial Mediterranean fever, other Seronegative spondyloarthropathy: Reiter syndrome, psoriatic, ankylosing spondylitis, inflammatory bowel disease Reactive arthritis: enteric or urogenital infection, rheumatic fever Polyarticular crystalline Sarcoidosis Malignancy	Osteoarthritis Hematologic: amyloidosis, leukemia, hemophilia, sickle cell disease Hypertrophic pulmonary osteoarthropathy

- Distal interphalangeal joint involvement occurs in osteoarthritis, Reiter syndrome, and psoriatic arthritis.
- Gout has a predilection for the first metatarsophalangeal joint (podagra) and the ankle.
- Pseudogout usually involves the knees and wrists.
- Migratory polyarthritis occurs in gonococcal arthritis, viral infections, sarcoidosis, rheumatic fever, endocarditis, and systemic lupus erythematosus.
- Oligoarthritis with axial involvement occurs in spondyloarthropathies.

DIAGNOSTIC TEST ORDERING
- The tests ordered according to signs, symptoms, and findings are summarized in Table 3.
- ESR and C-reactive protein
  - ▲ Sensitive but not specific
  - ▲ Can be used as a marker of disease activity

- Rheumatoid factor
  - ▲ Useful in confirming the diagnosis and assessing prognosis for patients with inflammatory polyarthritis
  - ▲ Frequently false-positive result
- Antinuclear antibody
  - ▲ Frequently false-positive result
- Extractable nuclear antigens
  - ▲ These should only be ordered if the clinical suspicion is high for systemic lupus erythematosus, Sjögren syndrome, scleroderma, or mixed connective tissue disease.
- Other tests
  - ▲ Lyme, parvovirus, rubella, and HIV serologic tests are useful only when clinical suspicion is strong.

Table 3. **Summary of Tests Ordered According to Signs, Symptoms, and Findings**

Signs, symptoms, findings	Diagnosis	Tests ordered
Trauma, focal bone pain, ecchymosis	Fracture, dislocation, tumor, metabolic bone disease	X ray of affected joint area
Effusion or synovitis	Trauma, crystalline arthropathy, infection, systemic rheumatic disease, sarcoidosis, spondyloarthropathy, hemarthrosis, tumor	Joint aspiration & synovial fluid analysis for Gram stain, CBC, culture, crystal exam with polarized light microscope
Urethritis, cervicitis, migratory arthritis, tenosynovitis, vesiculopustular lesions	Gonococcal arthritis	Cultures of blood, skin lesions, synovial fluid, cervix, urethra, pharynx, and rectum for *Neisseria gonorrhoeae* inoculated at bedside on Thayer-Martin medium

Table 3 (continued)

Signs, symptoms, findings	Diagnosis	Tests ordered
Podagra	Gout >> pseudogout	Polarized light microscopy of synovial fluid Uric acid crystals are needle-shaped, negatively birefringent
Erythema marginatum, new murmur, chorea, subcutaneous nodules, polyarthritis, recent pharyngitis	Rheumatic fever	Antistreptolysin O titer, throat culture
Axial arthritis	Ankylosing spondylitis, psoriatic arthritis, Reiter syndrome, inflammatory bowel disease	Consider lumbosacral X-ray with sacroiliac views
Risk factors or clinical findings suggestive of HIV/AIDS	HIV arthritis	HIV serology
Enthesitis, keratoderma blennorrhagicum, urethritis, balanitis, oral ulcers, iritis, conjunctivitis, history of STD or gastroenteritis	Reiter syndrome	Consider serology tests for *Campylobacter*, *Chlamydia*, *Salmonella*, *Shigella*, *Ureaplasma*, & *Yersinia*
Chondrocalcinosis & arthritis affecting knees, wrists, elbows, & ankles	Pseudogout	Calcium, phosphate, iron studies, & TSH (to rule out secondary causes) CPPD crystals are rhomboid-shaped, positively birefringent with polarized light microscopy
Arthritis, crythema nodosum, hilar adenopathy	Sarcoidosis or other granulomatous disease	ACE level, biopsy to check for noncaseating granulomas
Fever, heart murmur, arthritis	Endocarditis	Blood cultures

Table 3 (continued)

Signs, symptoms, findings	Diagnosis	Tests ordered
High fever, evanescent pink rash, polyarthritis, sore throat	Still disease	Markedly increased ferritin with absence of autoantibodies Hemoglobin, leukocyte count, erythrocyte count
Polyarthritis, fever, rash	Viral arthritis	Serologic tests (parvovirus, hepatitis, rubella)
Nail pitting	Psoriatic arthritis	Clinical diagnosis
Arthritis, diarrhea, constitutional symptoms, neurologic symptoms, lymphadenopathy, hyperpigmentation	Whipple disease	PCR on joint fluid, for Whipple disease small-bowel biopsy
Oral/nasal ulcers, rash, iritis, photosensitivity, nodules, Raynaud disease, sicca symptoms, morning stiffness, pericarditis, pleuritis, neurologic abnormalities	Systemic rheumatic disease	CBC, ESR, rheumatoid factor, synovial fluid analysis, ANA, ENA, hepatitis, serologic tests
Immunocompromised host	Fungal or mycobacterial arthritis	Fungal & mycobacterial cultures on synovial fluid
Tick bite, history of erythema migrans	Lyme arthritis	Lyme serologic test

ACE, angiotensin-converting enzyme; ANA, antinuclear antibody, CPPD, calcium pyrophosphate dihydrate; ENA, extractable nuclear antigens; PCR, polymerase chain reaction; STD, sexually transmitted disease; TSH, thyroid-stimulating hormone.

INITIAL MANAGEMENT

- Fracture
  - ▲ Assess neurovascular status.
  - ▲ Stabilize
  - ▲ X-ray
- Septic arthritis
  - ▲ Perform blood and urine cultures.
  - ▲ *Staphylococcus aureus* is the most common cause of non-gonococcal bacterial arthritis.
  - ▲ Start empiric antibiotic therapy based on Gram stain and clinical scenario.
    - If Gram stain shows gram-negative organisms, start ceftriaxone or cefotaxime.
    - If Gram stain shows gram-positive cocci, start nafcillin.
    - If Gram stain is negative, both ceftriaxone and nafcillin are reasonable.
  - ▲ For gonococcal infection, start ceftriaxone and treat coexistent sexually transmitted diseases (chlamydia) with doxycycline or azithromycin.
  - ▲ Consult orthopedic surgeon to consider open debridement and irrigation.
  - ▲ Lyme disease and Whipple disease require treatment with special antibiotic regimens.
- Gout
  - ▲ Check serum uric acid level (1/3 of patients with acute gouty attack have normal uric acid level).
  - ▲ NSAIDs are effective in relieving pain and inflammation; indomethacin is commonly given.
  - ▲ If NSAIDs are contraindicated, intra-articular or parenteral corticosteroids are useful.
  - ▲ Colchicine may be used to treat acute gout, and it may be given during the transition to chronic therapy.
  - ▲ In chronic tophaceous gout or multiple attacks, consider a uricosuric agent (probenecid) or allopurinol, starting 2 months *after* the current attack resolves.
    - Uricosurics are not effective if creatinine clearance is <50 mL/minute.
    - Uricosurics should not be given if there is a history of uric acid renal stones or 24-hour urine for uric acid is >1,000 mg.
    - Allopurinol requires adjustment for renal function.

- Pseudogout (calcium pyrophosphate dihydrate crystal arthritis)
  - ▲ X-ray to look for chondrocalcinosis
  - ▲ NSAID if not contraindicated
  - ▲ Intra-articular corticosteroid injections (often effective)
- Rheumatoid arthritis
  - ▲ Synovial fluid analysis to rule out infection
  - ▲ Check acute phase reactants and rheumatoid factor.
  - ▲ NSAID if not contraindicated
  - ▲ Consider a disease-modifying antirheumatic drug, usually in consultation with a rheumatologist.
  - ▲ Physical therapy to prevent deformity
- Seronegative spondyloarthropathies
  - ▲ Sacroiliac X-ray
  - ▲ NSAID if not contraindicated
  - ▲ Physical therapy to prevent deformity
- Postinfectious reactive arthritis
  - ▲ If recent enteric or urogenital infection, antibiotics may be helpful.
  - ▲ Rheumatic fever should be treated with aspirin, penicillin V potassium to eradicate group A streptococci, and sometimes prednisone.
- Hemarthrosis
  - ▲ Evaluate for coagulopathy or thrombocytopenia.
  - ▲ Consider orthopedic evaluation.
- Sterile inflammatory arthritis
  - ▲ CBC, ESR, rheumatoid factor, and synovial fluid analysis
  - ▲ Creatinine level, urinalysis
  - ▲ Antinuclear antibody, extractable nuclear antigens, complement levels, plain X-rays
  - ▲ Consider liver function tests and serologic tests for hepatitis B and C, Lyme disease, and parvovirus.
  - ▲ Treatment is based on the underlying cause but may involve corticosteroids.
- Osteoarthritis
  - ▲ NSAID or acetaminophen if not contraindicated
  - ▲ Physical therapy

- ▲ Injection of affected joint with corticosteroid may provide temporary relief.
- ▲ Surgery for patients not controlled on medical therapy
- ▪ Tendinitis and/or bursitis
  - ▲ NSAID if not contraindicated
  - ▲ Consider anesthetic and corticosteroid injection.
  - ▲ Physical therapy
- ▪ Polymyalgia rheumatica
  - ▲ Evaluate for coexistent giant cell arteritis.
  - ▲ Check ESR.
  - ▲ Start prednisone.
  - ▲ Once symptoms have resolved and ESR has returned to normal, prednisone may be tapered with close monitoring for symptom recurrence or increasing ESR.

LOWER EXTREMITY PAIN

David H. Pfizenmaier II, M.D., D.P.M.
Thom W. Rooke, M.D.

IS THE PATIENT'S LIFE (OR LIMB) AT RISK?

- Lower extremity pain can be a manifestation of a local or systemic process.
- The following conditions must be recognized and treated expeditiously:
  - ▲ Deep venous thrombosis (DVT)
  - ▲ Phlegmasia alba dolens
  - ▲ Phlegmasia cerulea dolens
  - ▲ Acute arterial insufficiency
  - ▲ Compartment syndrome
  - ▲ Vasculitis
  - ▲ Infections
- Most other causes of lower extremity pain are nonemergent and can be diagnosed and treated in due time.

ADDRESSING THE RISK

- Inspect the lower extremities, and examine for symmetry, skin lesions, color changes, edema, and deformity.
- Palpate femoral, popliteal, posterior tibial, and dorsalis pedis arterial pulses. If they are nonpalpable, use portable Doppler ultrasound to determine whether arterial blood flow is present.
- Palpate along muscle groups and joints for tenderness, and note areas of edema, erythema, and warmth.
- Neuromuscular exam
  - ▲ Assess range of motion of all joints, first allowing the patient to move each joint without assistance.
  - ▲ Note loss of function.

Special abbreviations used in this chapter: ANCA, antineutrophil cytoplasmic antibody; DVT, deep venous thrombosis; HIT, heparin-induced thrombocytopenia; LMWH, low-molecular-weight heparin; LR, likelihood ratio.

Table 1 (continued)

Spirochetal
  Syphilis (osteochondritis, periostitis, polyarthritis)
  Lyme disease (angiitis and arthritis, especially the knee)
Viral
  Herpes zoster
  Arthritis (hepatitis, rubella, human parvovirus B19, HIV)
  HIV angiitis
Rickettsial—angiitis
Rheumatologic
  Skin
    Erythema nodosum
    Rheumatoid nodule
    Scleroderma
  Subcutaneous—panniculitis
  Synovial
    Gout
    CPPD/pseudogout
    Rheumatoid synovitis
    Baker cyst (popliteal synovial cyst)
    Bursitis
  Muscle
    Polymyositis
    Dermatomyositis
    Inclusion body myositis
    Fibromyalgia (fibrositis)
  Tendon—tendinitis
  Joint
    Infectious (septic)
    Connective tissue (systemic lupus erythematosus)
    Rheumatoid
    Spondyloarthropathies (psoriatic, Reiter syndrome,
      enteropathic)
    Neuropathic (Charcot joint)
    Hemarthrosis (hemophilia, von Willebrand disease)
    Hypertrophic osteoarthropathy (periostitis of tubular bones)
  Cartilage—osteoarthritis
  Enthesopathy—HLA-B27 spondyloarthropathies (ankylosing
    spondylitis, Reiter syndrome, enteropathic [Crohn disease,
    ulcerative colitis])
  Vasculitic
    Polyarteritis (polyarteritis nodosa, microscopic polyangitis)
    Wegener granulomatosis
    Behçet syndrome
    Thromboangiitis obliterans
    Churg-Strauss syndrome
    Henoch-Schönlein purpura
    Leukocytoclastic
    Hypersensitivity
    Cryoglobulinemia

Table 1 (continued)

Neurologic
    Peripheral (for isolated lower extremity)
        Radiculopathy
        Sciatica
        Mononeuritis
        Tarsal tunnel syndrome
        Neurapraxia
        Neuropathy
        Reflex sympathetic dystrophy
Musculoskeletal
    Muscle
        Myalgia
        Myositis
        Trauma
        Cramp
        Tendon rupture
    Bone
        Osteonecrosis (skeletal infarct—ischemic, aseptic, avascular
          necrosis)
        Chondritis
        Tumor
        Periostitis
Neoplastic
    Muscle—sarcoma
    Bone
        Metastatic lesion (breast, lung, prostate, renal, gastrointesti-
          nal, thyroid)
        Paget disease (osteitis deformans)
        Osteoid osteoma
        Osteosarcoma
        Ewing tumor
    Joint
        Carcinomatous polyarthritis
        Osteochondroma
        Chondrosarcoma
        Pigmented villonodular synovitis
Traumatic
    Fracture
    Frostbite
    Burns
    Compartment syndrome

CPPD, calcium pyrophosphate dihydrate deposition.

- Venous
  - Patients display varicose veins, pitting edema, cyanosis, brawny hyperpigmentation, induration, stasis dermatitis, skin ulceration, and lipodermatosclerosis.
  - In superficial thrombophlebitis, exam may show tenderness, erythema, and a firm cord along an affected vein.
  - Maneuvers can demonstrate an accelerated venous filling time (due to incompetent valves).

Infectious
- Bacterial
  - Local signs include erythema, edema, warmth, pain, loss of function, exudate, subcutaneous crepitus (gas gangrene).
  - Systemic signs include fever, chills, sweats, nausea, vomiting.
- Spirochetal
  - Bull's eye lesion (erythema chronicum migrans of Lyme disease)
  - Maculopapular lesions on palms and soles (syphilis)
- Viral
  - Dermatomal distribution and vesicular lesions (herpes zoster)
  - Digital infarction (human parvovirus B19)

Rheumatologic
- Examine associated areas of skin involvement, morphology of skin lesions, joint involvement (mono- or polyarticular, symmetric vs. asymmetric) to determine if local or systemic process.

Neurologic
- History and neuromuscular exam (see above)

Musculoskeletal or Traumatic
- History and musculoskeletal exam

Neoplastic
- History and physical exam

DIAGNOSTIC TEST ORDERING
Vascular
- For arterial occlusive disease, obtain the ankle-brachial

systolic pressure ratio (ankle-brachial index), which is abnormal if <0.9.

▲ Segmental systolic blood pressures of the lower extremity can help locate a stenotic lesion.

▲ Transition from triphasic to biphasic or monophasic Doppler waveforms in duplex ultrasonography also suggests the location and extent of stenosis.

▲ Segmental measurements of transcutaneous oxygen levels can help with determining healing potential and amputation levels.

▲ Arteriography is the gold standard.

■ For venous disease, history and physical exam are most helpful.

▲ DVT usually is confirmed by Doppler (duplex) compression ultrasonography, with venography considered the gold standard.

▲ D-dimer is a highly sensitive assay that leads to many false-positive results. Thus, D-dimer is most helpful when it is negative (low) because this likely rules out DVT.

▲ A clinical prediction guide (Table 2) can be used to stratify patients with suspected DVT into low, moderate, or high probability groups. A scoring system can be used to improve the pretest probability of DVT being present by combining relevant signs and symptoms, risk factors for DVT, and the presence or absence of an alternative diagnosis (musculoskeletal injury, cellulitis, inguinal lymphadenopathy). With this stratification, the combination of pretest probability and the results of compression ultrasonography markedly enhances the reliability of diagnosing DVT.

▲ DVT is reliably diagnosed in patients with high or moderate pretest scores and abnormal compression ultrasonograms (positive LR = infinity and 72, respectively). Therefore, treatment should be initiated. DVT can be excluded reliably in patients with low pretest scores and normal compression ultrasonograms (negative LR = 0.2). All other or discordant groups likely require further testing (venography or serial compression ultrasonography).

Infectious

- If infection is suspected, begin with the basics: CBC with differential, blood cultures, and ESR.
  - ▲ For joints, perform diagnostic arthrocentesis and obtain a plain X-ray.
  - ▲ For bones, the first step is to obtain plain X-rays.
    - Generally, 3-phase technetium bone scintigraphy is the next diagnostic test if no superimposed condition complicates bone remodeling (recent surgery, trauma, rheumatologic or neoplastic bone disease). In these situations, adjunctive gallium scans or indium-labeled leukocytes may be useful in identifying areas of inflammation or infection, respectively.
    - MRI and CT offer good anatomic resolution and are excellent adjuncts or alternatives to nuclear imaging studies.

Table 2. Clinical Measures for Scoring Suspected DVT*

Major points
    Active cancer (treatment within previous 6 months or palliative)
    Paralysis, paresis, or recent cast immobilization of the lower extremities
    Recently bedridden for >3 days and/or major surgery within 4 weeks
    Localized tenderness along distribution of deep venous system
    Thigh and leg swelling
    Calf swelling that is >3 cm that of asymptomatic leg (measured 10 cm below the tibial tuberosity)
    Strong family history of DVT (>2 first-degree relatives)
Minor points
    Pitting edema in symptomatic leg (or greater than asymptomatic leg)
    Dilated (nonvaricose) collateral superficial veins in symptomatic leg
    Recent trauma (≤60 days in the symptomatic leg)
    Hospitalization within previous 6 months
    Erythema

DVT, deep venous thrombosis.
*Scoring: "High probability" if alternative diagnosis not likely *and* either 1) ≥3 major points or 2) ≥2 major and ≥2 minor points. "Low probability" if alternative diagnosis is likely *and* either 1) 1 major point plus ≤2 minor points or 2) 0 major and ≤3 minor points; also, if an alternative diagnosis is not likely *and* 1) 1 major and ≤1 minor point or 2) 0 major and ≤2 minor points. "Moderate probability" for all other combinations.

Rheumatologic

- ESR, C-reactive protein, antinuclear antibodies, extractable nuclear antigens, rheumatoid factor, complement, X-rays
- Conditions
  - ▲ Polyarteritis (polyarteritis nodosa and microscopic polyangiitis)—90% of cases of microscopic polyangiitis are antineutrophil cytoplasmic antibody (ANCA)-positive.
    - Evaluate polyarteritis nodosa for associated hepatitis B.
    - Angiography and/or biopsy are confirmatory tests.
  - ▲ Churg-Strauss syndrome—This is defined by presence of allergic rhinitis, nasal polyposis, asthma, eosinophilia, and systemic vasculitis of at least 2 extrapulmonary organs.
    - Palpable purpura is present.
  - ▲ Thromboangiitis obliterans (Buerger disease)—Young adult smokers who have claudication in the lower extremities with ischemic digital injury
    - Biopsy shows intraluminal thrombus with microabscesses.
  - ▲ Wegener granulomatosis—Necrotizing granulomatous inflammation of the upper and lower respiratory tract, focal segmental necrotizing glomerulonephritis, skin lesions (palpable purpura is present)
    - Can involve the nervous system (sensory neuropathy, mononeuritis multiplex)
    - Confirmatory diagnosis is biopsy.
    - More than 90% of patients are positive for c-ANCA.
  - ▲ Henoch-Schönlein purpura—Small-vessel vasculitis classically in the setting of abdominal pain with gastrointestinal tract hemorrhage, lower extremity palpable purpura, arthritis, and hematuria
    - Biopsy shows IgA deposition in vessel walls.
    - Complement levels are normal.
  - ▲ Leukocytoclastic vasculitis—Small-vessel vasculitis with immune complex deposition in vessel walls in combination with fibrin and PMNs
    - Often related to rheumatoid arthritis, Sjögren disease, systemic lupus erythematosus, and other connective tissue diseases
    - Palpable purpura is the classic clinical finding.

▲ Cryoglobulinemia—Type II is frequently associated with chronic infection (usually hepatitis C) and immune disorders.
  • Small-vessel vasculitis with palpable purpura, urticaria, cutaneous ulcers, neuropathy, and arthralgias or arthritis are common.
▲ Hypersensitivity vasculitis—Associated with drugs, malignancy, or infection
  • Complement levels (especially C4) may be low.

Neurologic
■ If a neurologic process is suspected, perform nerve conduction studies, EMG, MRI of spine when indicated.

Musculoskeletal/Traumatic
■ To evaluate for a musculoskeletal/trauma-related cause, perform EMG, imaging study (X-ray, CT, MRI), serum CK.

Neoplastic
■ Imaging studies (X-rays, CT, MRI)
■ Biopsy is definitive.

INITIAL MANAGEMENT
Vascular
■ Acute arterial insufficiency
  ▲ Thrombolytic therapy if risk factors for bleeding are low
                         or
  ▲ Vascular surgery with options including
    • Percutaneous transluminal angioplasty
    • Thromboendarterectomy with or without graft replacement
    • Bypass graft
■ Phlegmasia alba dolens and phlegmasia cerulea dolens (venous gangrene)
  ▲ Massive ileofemoral DVT causing secondary arterial insufficiency
  ▲ Phlegmasia alba dolens: swelling, pain, pallor
  ▲ Phlegmasia cerulea dolens: limbs are cyanotic.
  ▲ Requires immediate anticoagulation
    • Consider thrombolytics.
    • Obtain immediate surgical evaluation for possible intervention.

- ▲ If unrecognized and untreated, then excessive morbidity (including limb amputation)
- DVT
  - ▲ Initial treatment is anticoagulation with IV heparin or SQ low-molecular-weight heparin (LMWH).
    - Unfractionated heparin can be given as an initial IV bolus of 60-80 U/kg, followed by continuous infusion of 14-16 U/kg per hour.
    - Monitor the PTT in 6 hours, and adjust the infusion rate accordingly for a goal level that is 1.5-3.0 times higher than baseline value.
    - Monitor the PTT every 6 hours after each adjustment and then every 24 hours once therapeutic levels are achieved.
    - Check platelets daily for potential heparin-induced thrombocytopenia (HIT), with usual onset in 3-4 days.
    - For patients with HIT, alternatives to heparin include hirudin or argatroban.
  - ▲ SQ LMWH is an alternative to IV heparin, especially because it can be used on an outpatient basis.
    - With LMWH, it is not necessary to measure PTT, but platelets should be checked during treatment because HIT can develop.
    - Dosing of LMWH varies with each derivative used (e.g., enoxaparin, dalteparin).
  - ▲ Oral anticoagulation with warfarin should begin with 5 mg on the first or second day following heparinization.
    - Heparin/LMWH therapy should overlap warfarin therapy for 3-5 days after the INR is therapeutic.
    - Warfarin should be administered for 3-6 months in first episodes of DVT and lifelong therapy (and thrombophilia work-up) should be considered if episodes recur.
    - If DVT is untreated, there is risk of pulmonary embolism.

Infection
- Cellulitis, necrotizing fasciitis, gas gangrene, septic arthritis
- Initially, treat with broad-spectrum antibiotics and change on the basis of culture results and sensitivities.

- Surgical consultation and intervention required for
  - Necrotizing fasciitis
  - Gas gangrene (seen with X-rays or appreciated with subcutaneous crepitus)
  - Septic arthritis

Rheumatologic and Vasculitic
- The cornerstone of therapy in most cases of vasculitis is corticosteroids.
  - Cytotoxic and antimetabolite drugs are often used in combination with corticosteroids, especially in rapidly progressive or nonsteroid-responsive conditions.
- For Buerger disease, treatment is to stop smoking.
- For small-vessel vasculitis, treatment of the underlying disease or infection or discontinuation of the offending agent or drug leads to improvement.

Compartment Syndrome
- Increase in closed compartment pressure, with compromise of local vasculature leading to muscular and neural ischemia.
- History and physical exam findings (e.g., pain, pallor, pulselessness, paralysis) are hallmarks for diagnosis.
  - Measurement of compartment pressures is adjunctive.
- Orthopedic surgery evaluation is imperative.
- Treatment begins with placing the patient supine to avoid dependent edema and elevational ischemia.
- Fasciotomy is the mainstay of limb salvage.

NAUSEA AND VOMITING

Luke T. Evans, M.D.
Darrell S. Pardi, M.D.

IS THE PATIENT'S LIFE AT RISK?

- Determine if the patient has
  - ▲ A surgical abdomen
  - ▲ A medical emergency manifesting as nausea and vomiting
  - ▲ A central nervous system (CNS) emergency
  - ▲ A life-threatening electrolyte abnormality caused by prolonged nausea and vomiting
- Surgical emergencies include
  - ▲ Acute appendicitis
  - ▲ Ascending cholangitis
  - ▲ Bowel infarction
  - ▲ Perforated gastric or duodenal ulcer
  - ▲ Perforated bowel
- These emergency conditions are suggested by abdominal pain, fever, tachycardia, poor urine output, and peritoneal signs (absent bowel sounds, abdominal rigidity, rebound tenderness, involuntary guarding).
- Medical emergencies that may manifest with nausea or vomiting include
  - ▲ Diabetic ketoacidosis
  - ▲ Myocardial infarction
  - ▲ Occult drug overdose
  - ▲ Renal failure
  - ▲ Upper gastrointestinal tract bleeding
  - ▲ Sepsis
  - ▲ Alcohol or drug withdrawal
  - ▲ Pregnancy should also be ruled out early to prevent teratogenic exposures.

Special abbreviation used in this chapter: CNS, central nervous system.

- CNS emergencies include
  - CNS hemorrhage or tumor causing increased intracranial pressure
  - Encephalitis
  - Meningitis
- CNS emergency conditions are suggested by headache, mental status changes, meningeal signs, and focal neurologic abnormalities.
- Potentially fatal complications of nausea and vomiting include
  - Severe dehydration
  - Metabolic alkalosis
  - Hypokalemia
  - Hypernatremia
  - Aspiration
  - Esophageal rupture

ADDRESSING THE RISK

- First, assess airway, breathing, and circulation
  - Airway—Determine if patient can protect the airway from aspiration. If patient is unable to protect the airway, intubate the patient.
  - Breathing—The patient should be ventilated mechanically if unable to breathe on own.
  - Circulation—Tachycardia, hypotension, poor urine output, and fever indicate severe dehydration and/or sepsis. Begin IV fluid rehydration with normal saline and blood pressure support with pressors if indicated.
- Next, assess for emergencies noted above.
  - Abdomen—Examine for signs of peritonitis. If present, consult general surgery immediately.
  - Other complaints—Address the presence of anginal symptoms, shortness of breath, headache, and neurologic symptoms. Evaluate and treat accordingly.

DIFFERENTIAL DIAGNOSIS

- The differential diagnosis for nausea and vomiting is listed in Table 1.

DIFFERENTIATING THE DIFFERENTIAL

- Generally, a focused history and physical exam are needed to evaluate new or persistent nausea and/or vomiting.

- Historical clues to the cause of nausea and/or vomiting are listed in Table 2.
- Physical exam findings to narrow the differential diagnosis
  - ▲ Vital signs, including orthostatics, to assess for systemic inflammatory response syndrome and dehydration
  - ▲ Mental status—assess ability to protect airway from aspiration.
    - • Agitation, somnolence, hallucinations, and confusion suggest toxin ingestion.
  - ▲ Intake and output to assess fluid status
  - ▲ Jaundice and/or scleral icterus suggest cirrhosis, hepatitis, or biliary obstruction.
  - ▲ Fruity smell of ketones suggests ketoacidosis.
  - ▲ Neurologic exam to identify focal cranial nerve or cerebellar abnormalities, meningismus suggesting meningitis, or intracranial mass or intracranial bleed
  - ▲ Ophthalmoscopic exam to look for papilledema suggesting increased intracranial pressure
  - ▲ Abdominal exam—Look for the presence and character of the following:
    - • Bowel sounds
    - • Rebound tenderness
    - • Guarding
    - • Peritoneal signs
    - • Murphy sign
    - • Tenderness over McBurney point
    - • Obturator sign
    - • Hernias
    - • Flank pain
  - ▲ Rectal exam, including occult blood testing, to rule out fecal impaction and occult blood loss

DIAGNOSTIC TEST ORDERING

- The work up for serious or persistent nausea and vomiting should include
  - ▲ Flat and upright or left lateral decubitus X-rays
  - ▲ CBC with differential count
  - ▲ Electrolytes (sodium, potassium, chloride, bicarbonate,

Table 1. Differential Diagnosis for Nausea and Vomiting

Surgical emergencies associated with nausea & vomiting	Medical emergencies associated with nausea & vomiting
Bowel obstruction	Diabetic ketoacidosis
Perforated viscus	Acute myocardial infarction
Acute appendicitis	Upper gastrointestinal tract bleeding
Acute cholecystitis	Digoxin toxicity
Intracranial hemorrhage	Renal failure
Incarcerated hernia	Acute pancreatitis
Mesenteric ischemia	Acute cholangitis
Central nervous system hemorrhage	Toxin ingestion
Increased intracranial pressure (tumor, pseudotumor)	Alcohol withdrawal
	Sepsis
	Meningitis
	Peritonitis
	Hypercalcemia

Nonemergency causes of nausea & vomiting

Infectious causes
    Viral
        Rotavirus
        Norwalk agent
    Bacterial enterotoxin-mediated
        Staphylococcus aureus
        Bacillus cereus
        Clostridium perfringens
Iatrogenic causes
    Narcotics
    Digoxin
    Theophylline
    Chemotherapy
    Antibiotics
    NSAIDs
    Radiation enteritis
Metabolic derangements
    Hyperthyroidism
    Addison disease
Motility disorders
    Gastroparesis (diabetic & others)
    Ileus
    Collagen vascular disorders
    Postgastric surgery

Motility disorders (continued)
    Constipation
    Autonomic insufficiency
    Chronic intestinal pseudo-obstruction
    Gastroesophageal reflux disease
Systemic conditions
    Pregnancy
    Hyperemesis gravidarum
    Hypertensive urgency
    Idiopathic cyclic vomiting
    Porphyria
Primary central nervous system cause
    Benign positional vertigo
    Motion sickness
    Labyrinthitis (Meniere disease)
    Migraine headache
Psychiatric conditions
    Anxiety
    Bulimia
    Anorexia nervosa
    Rumination syndrome

BUN, creatinine, glucose, calcium, magnesium, phosphorus)
- ▲ Liver chemistry panel (alkaline phosphatase and ALT)
- ▲ Amylase and lipase
- ▲ If the patient is female, determine β-human chorionic gonadotropin to rule out pregnancy.
- ▲ If abdominal pain is present, consider CT or ultrasound of the abdomen, urinalysis with culture, INR, and serum lactate level
- ▲ If a headache, local neurologic signs, or altered mental status is present, consider CT of the head, lumbar puncture, toxicology screen, and gastric lavage.
- ▲ If fever is present, consider blood cultures, urinalysis with culture, abdominal CT or ultrasound, and chest X-ray.
- ▲ If the patient is diabetic, obtain a stat finger-stick glucose value, serum ketones, and arterial blood gases to rule out diabetic ketoacidosis.
- ▲ If bleeding is from the gastrointestinal tract, type and crossmatch for blood transfusion and obtain INR and PTT.
- ▲ For chronic nausea and vomiting, consider
  - • Esophagogastroduodenoscopy to rule out peptic ulcer disease
  - • Gastric emptying study to rule out gastroparesis
  - • Small-bowel follow-through study to rule out a partial small-bowel obstruction

INITIAL MANAGEMENT
- ■ Management must address the primary cause of nausea and vomiting while treating ongoing symptoms and complications.
- ■ Gastroenteritis
  - ▲ IV fluid resuscitation
  - ▲ Monitoring of electrolytes
  - ▲ Antiemetic therapy with phenothiazines (prochlorperazine [Compazine] or promethazine [Phenergan])
- ■ Small-bowel obstruction
  - ▲ Nasogastric tube to low intermittent suction
  - ▲ NPO
  - ▲ Serial abdominal exams

Table 2. Historical Clues to Cause of Nausea and/or Vomiting

	Historical clues	Suggestive of	Supportive tests
Temporal characteristics	Nausea & vomiting with fever or diarrhea	Gastroenteritis	± Stool studies
	Pain precedes nausea, vomiting, & distension	Mechanical obstruction	Flat & upright abdominal X-ray
	Reproducible postprandial pain with history of vasculopathy	Mesenteric ischemia	Doppler ultrasound of abdomen or mesenteric angiography
	Early morning vomiting with morning headache	Increased intracranial pressure	Head CT
	Early morning nausea & vomiting	Pregnancy	β-HCG Confirm viability of pregnancy
Presence & character of abdominal pain	Colicky pain (intermittent)	Obstructed viscus	Flat & upright abdominal X-ray
	Pain out of proportion to abdominal exam	Mesenteric ischemia	CT or mesenteric angiography
	Well-localized pain with jostling movement	Peritoneal irritation	Abdominal CT
Diabetes mellitus	Polyuria, polydipsia, & weight loss	Untreated/undiagnosed diabetes ± DKA	Serum glucose, serum pH, serum ketones
	Long-term poor glucose control	Diabetic gastroparesis or mesenteric vasculopathy	Gastric emptying study/mesenteric angiogram

Table 2 (continued)

	Historical clues	Suggestive of	Supportive tests
Infectious	Nausea, vomiting, & diarrhea 1-6 hours after a meal (ham, potato or egg salad, cream pastries, & poultry)	S. aureus gastroenteritis	Contaminated food can be cultured
	Nausea, vomiting, & diarrhea 1-6 hours after eating fried rice or refried beans	B. cereus gastroenteritis	Stool culture for organism
Cardiopulmonary	Anginal symptoms, dyspnea	Acute coronary syndrome	ECG & cardiac enzymes
Miscellaneous	Altered mental status ± previous suicide attempts	Intentional overdose	Gastric lavage, drug screen, including acetaminophen level
	Alcohol dependence or history of withdrawal	Alcohol withdrawal	
	New or increased doses of medications (especially narcotics, chemotherapy, & antibiotics)	Medication side-effect	

DKA, diabetic ketoacidosis; HCG, human chorionic gonadotropin.

217

- ▲ IV fluid resuscitation with additional fluid to match nasogastric output
- ▲ Surgical consultation
- Chemotherapy
  - ▲ IV fluid resuscitation
  - ▲ Antiemetic therapy with 5-HT$_3$ receptor antagonists
  - ▲ Dexamethasone and lorazepam may also be helpful.
- Motion sickness or vestibular disturbances
  - ▲ Antiemetic therapy with antihistamines
- Adverse drug reactions
  - ▲ Consider discontinuing drug.
  - ▲ Antiemetic therapy with phenothiazines

MANAGEMENT OF COMPLICATIONS OF NAUSEA AND VOMITING

- Intravascular depletion—Resuscitate with normal saline.
- Hypokalemia—Replace potassium IV or PO, and monitor for cardiac events.
- Hyponatremia—Resuscitate with normal saline. (See chapter on Electrolyte Disturbances.)
- Metabolic alkalosis—Limit nasogastric suctioning if possible and replete intravascular space.
- Esophageal mucosal tear (Mallory-Weiss tear)—Treat the same way as a gastrointestinal tract bleed.
- Esophageal rupture (Boerhaave syndrome) characterized by severe epigastric pain, cyanosis, dyspnea, subcutaneous or mediastinal emphysema, a left-sided pleural effusion, and dyspnea—Obtain an emergency general or thoracic surgery consult for consideration of thoracotomy and esophageal repair.
- Aspiration
  - ▲ Intubate if the patient is unable to protect own airway.
  - ▲ Provide aggressive pulmonary hygiene.
  - ▲ Consider initiating antimicrobial coverage if you are certain of aspiration and the patient is experiencing respiratory distress.

OCULAR AND VISUAL ABNORMALITIES

Sanjay V. Patel, B.M., B.S.
Jonathan M. Holmes, B.M., B.Ch.

IS THE PATIENT'S VISION AT RISK?

- Immediate intervention for the following conditions can save vision:
  - ▲ Acute angle-closure glaucoma
  - ▲ Giant cell arteritis causing either
    - Anterior ischemic optic neuropathy or
    - Central retinal artery occlusion
  - ▲ Nonarteritic central retinal artery occlusion
  - ▲ Endophthalmitis
  - ▲ Corneal ulcer and/or infectious keratitis
  - ▲ Retinal detachment

ADDRESSING THE RISK

- For any ocular or visual complaint
  - ▲ Measure visual acuity in each eye. Use distance or near chart, and test each eye separately, with patient wearing his or her usual glasses if available.
    - Has visual acuity changed from previously? By patient history? By previous and current examination?
    - Check the eye history for previous documented visual acuity.
  - ▲ Is the complaint acute or chronic, unilateral or bilateral?
  - ▲ Does the patient have a systemic disorder that could be related to the visual problem, e.g., hypertension, diabetes mellitus, hypercoagulable state, rheumatoid arthritis, other autoimmune disease?
  - ▲ Does the patient have a history of recent eye trauma, injury, foreign body, or eye surgery?

Special abbreviation used in this chapter: RAPD, relative afferent pupillary defect.

- ▲ Does the patient wear contact lenses? If so, is the patient wearing them now?
- ■ For the red eye
  - ▲ Is the eye painful or painless?
    - • Painless sectoral redness suggests subconjunctival hemorrhage.
    - • Most other causes of red eye are inflammatory and, thus, cause discomfort.
      - – Grittiness, itching, or a foreign body sensation suggests a surface problem (tear film defect, conjunctivitis, or true foreign body).
      - – Deep, severe, boring pain or photophobia suggests a deeper problem (scleritis, keratitis [corneal inflammation], uveitis, endophthalmitis, or acute glaucoma).
  - ▲ How is the redness distributed?
    - • Redness can be localized or diffuse.
    - • Diffuse conjunctival redness, involving the entire conjunctiva, suggests conjunctivitis.
    - • Redness at the corneoscleral junction (or limbus) is termed "ciliary flush," and when more pronounced than the surrounding injection, it suggests a more serious corneal or intraocular process (e.g., keratitis or uveitis). These conditions are often associated with severe pain.
  - ▲ Has vision changed?
    - • More serious conditions are often, but not always, associated with decreased visual acuity. Halos suggest corneal edema, e.g., in acute glaucoma.
  - ▲ Is there a hypopyon (layer of white cells within the anterior chamber)?
    - • It is associated with very severe disease.
    - • It suggests corneal inflammation (e.g., infectious keratitis) or intraocular inflammation (e.g., uveitis or endophthalmitis).
  - ▲ Is the cornea cloudy (caused by corneal edema and may be recognized as obscured iris details)?
    - • It suggests acute glaucoma or keratitis.
    - • A distinct white spot (infiltrate) on the cornea may represent an acute corneal ulcer.
      - – If the defect is dendritic in shape, suspect herpes simplex keratitis.
      - – If the defect is associated with a white infiltrate, a

corneal ulcer or microbial keratitis is likely.

- Any epithelial defect not associated with trauma is cause for concern.

▲ How do the pupils look?

- Anterior uveitis can cause miosis (constriction) or an irregular margin (due to posterior synechiae, i.e., adherence of the pupillary margin to the lens).
- Acute glaucoma often causes a semidilated and fixed pupil.
- Check previous documentation of the pupils in the eye history.
  - Careful documentation of the pupil exam is important.
  - Remember that pupils can remain dilated, fixed, or irregular after previous ocular surgery.

■ For the eye with painless visual loss (quiet white eye)

▲ This suggests a posterior segment process, i.e., retina or optic nerve.

▲ Assess visual fields to confrontation.

- A vertical field cut most likely represents a chiasmal or postchiasmal lesion.
- A horizontal field cut (altitudinal defect) most likely represents optic neuropathy (e.g., optic neuritis).
- A central scotoma suggests optic or retrobulbar neuritis or macular disease.
- A retinal detachment can cause any pattern of field defect in the affected eye.

■ Are the red reflexes present and symmetric?

▲ Absence of a red reflex is due to media opacity (e.g., corneal opacity, cataract, vitreous hemorrhage, or retinal detachment).

■ Is there a relative afferent pupillary defect (RAPD)?

▲ This is detected with the swinging flashlight test.

▲ RAPD suggests an asymmetric large retinal lesion (e.g., large retinal detachment) or an asymmetric optic nerve lesion (e.g., ischemic optic neuropathy).

■ Examine and compare both fundi, looking for symmetry and asymmetry between optic discs, veins, arterioles, maculae, and peripheral retinae.

- ▲ Look for pallor of the macula (edema) surrounding the classic "cherry-red spot" of a central retinal artery occlusion.
- ▲ Look for the swollen optic disc of acute anterior ischemic optic neuropathy or increased intracranial pressure.
- ▲ Look for the cloudy vitreous and poor view of the retina in an inflamed eye with endophthalmitis or in a diabetic person with a vitreous hemorrhage.

DIFFERENTIAL DIAGNOSIS
- ■ The differential diagnoses for painful red eye and loss of vision in a quiet white eye are listed in Table 1.

DIFFERENTIATING THE DIFFERENTIAL
- ■ For painful red eye and for loss of vision in a quiet white eye, see Tables 2 and 3, respectively.

ORDERING TESTS
- ■ Diagnosis of visual abnormalities is made primarily by history and exam, including inspection, red reflex, ophthalmoscopy.

Table 1. Differential Diagnoses for Painful Red Eye and for Sudden Loss of Vision in a Quiet White Eye

Painful red eye	Sudden loss of vision in a quiet white eye
Conjunctivitis (with or without blepharitis)	Vitreous hemorrhage, e.g., diabetes mellitus
Exposure keratopathy	Central or branch retinal artery occlusion
Abrasion or foreign body associated with trauma	Central or branch retinal vein occlusion
Keratitis (infectious or noninfectious)	Anterior ischemic optic neuropathy (arteritic or nonarteritic)
Episcleritis	Optic or retrobulbar neuritis (pain with eye movement)
Scleritis	Exudative age-related macular degeneration
Acute anterior uveitis or iritis	Retinal detachment
Acute angle-closure glaucoma	
Posterior uveitis	
Endophthalmitis	
Hyphema (usually posttraumatic)	
Subconjunctival hemorrhage (not painful)	

- When possible, measure intraocular pressure (unless you suspect severe trauma to the eye, when it should be assessed by the ophthalmologist).
- Ophthalmologist should perform specialized tests, including slit-lamp exam.
- Diagnosis and management of suspected arteritic ischemic optic neuropathy or arteritic central retinal artery occlusion are aided by ESR (>50 mm/hour by Westergren method) and increased C-reactive protein, and diagnosis is confirmed by temporal artery biopsy.

MANAGEMENT

- Management of painful red eye is described in Table 4.
- Management of loss of vision in a quiet white eye is described in Table 5.

Table 2. Painful Red Eye

Features	Diagnosis
Blurriness, cleared with blinking Purulent or watery discharge Eyelids stick together Slight discomfort of foreign body sensation Upper respiratory tract infection May be associated with blepharitis May be itchy if allergic cause Usually viral, may be bacterial Usually bilateral Diffuse conjunctival (*not* ciliary) injection Discharge	Conjunctivitis

Table 2 (continued)

Features	Diagnosis
Localized redness, almost always painless Localized redness concealing conjunctival vessels (may be diffuse or patchy) Visual acuity unchanged Idiopathic or associated with coughing, straining, bleeding dyscrasias, anticoagulant or antiplatelet agents, hypertension, trauma	Subconjunctival hemorrhage
Painless or dull ache Young adult Localized sectorial redness Dilated vessels that blanch with phenylephrine 2.5% drops Visual acuity unchanged Idiopathic or associated with collagen vascular disease, gout, herpes zoster May be recurrent	Episcleritis
Blurred vision Severe deep pain Headaches Photophobia Dilated scleral vessels that do not blanch with phenylephrine, sectorial or diffuse Scleral nodules Decreased visual acuity Violacious hue Associated with connective tissue disease or granulomatous systemic disease (particularly rheumatoid arthritis, Wegener granulomatosis) May be recurrent	Scleritis

Table 2 (continued)

Features	Diagnosis
Pain or deep ache Blurred vision Photophobia Usually unilateral Visual acuity—unchanged or decreased Ciliary flush Miosis or irregular pupil (posterior synechiae) Small deposits on cornea (keratic precipitates) Cloudy anterior chamber & hypopyon if severe Idiopathic or associated with systemic disease, e.g., HLA-B27 related disorder, inflammatory bowel disease, juvenile rheumatoid arthritis, Behçet syndrome, sarcoidosis If history of intraocular surgery, trauma, or sepsis, consider endophthalmitis May be recurrent	Anterior uveitis (iritis)
Pain Photophobia Poor vision Unilateral Decreased visual acuity Ciliary flush Corneal infiltrate (white opacity in corneal stroma) Corneal epithelial defect (stains with fluorescein) May have hypopyon May have purulent discharge If dendritic stain pattern, herpes simplex virus is likely Associated with corneal injury, contact lens wear, immunosuppression In noninfectious keratitis, infiltrate parallel to limbus, with or without ulceration, associated with Wegener granulomatosis, rheumatoid arthritis, severe blepharitis	Keratitis

Table 2 (continued)

Features	Diagnosis
Irritation Foreign body sensation Dryness Poor blinking Redness Corneal infiltrate if superimposed infection Associated with CN VII palsy, sedation (ICU), proptosis Particularly severe if associated with CN V palsy	Exposure keratopathy
Intense pain or ache Poor vision, halos Headache Nausea & vomiting Unilateral Decreased visual acuity Corneal edema (cloudy) Shallow anterior chamber Semidilated & fixed pupil Globe feels "stony-hard" to palpation Associated with hyperopia (farsightedness), elderly age, pupillary dilation	Acute angle-closure glaucoma
Floaters Blurred vision Photophobia Occasionally redness or pain Unilateral Decreased visual acuity Vitreous cells or opacities Retinal exudates Scarring Pigmentation Associated with toxoplasmosis, sarcoidosis, cytomegalovirus, others	Posterior uveitis

Table 3. Loss of Vision in a Quiet White Eye

Features	Diagnosis
Unilateral acute loss of vision Painless Sometimes history of amaurosis fugax Relative afferent pupillary defect Pale retina (sectorial if only a branch is occluded) Cherry-red spot at macula Narrow retinal arterioles ± arteriolar emboli May have other symptoms of giant cell (i.e., temporal) arteritis (jaw claudication, headache, polymyalgia)	Occlusion of central or branch retinal artery (must exclude giant cell arteritis)
Unilateral acute loss of vision Painless Relative afferent pupillary defect Tortuous dilated retinal veins Diffuse flame-shaped retinal hemorrhages Cotton wool spots Disc edema Neovascularization (late) Associated with hypertension, athero-sclerosis of adjacent artery, glaucoma, hypercoagulable state, vasculitis	Occlusion of central or branch retinal vein
Sudden decrease in vision, with appearance of floaters or webs Loss of red reflex Poor retinal view because of blood in vitreous If mild, partial retinal obscurity & evidence of underlying retinopathy Associated with proliferative diabetic retinopathy, sickle cell disease, subarachnoid hemorrhage, retinal or vitreous detachment, vein occlusion, trauma	Vitreous hemorrhage

Table 3 (continued)

Features	Diagnosis
Flashes & floaters Curtain across vision impairing central & peripheral vision Visual field defect May have relative afferent pupillary defect Elevation of retina Retinal tear Myopia	Retinal detachment
Sudden unilateral visual loss Temporal headache Jaw claudication Systemic symptoms associated with polymyalgia rheumatica Scalp tenderness Nonpulsatile temporal arteries Relative afferent pupillary defect Optic disc swelling ± pallor Altitudinal field defect Markedly increased ESR & C-reactive protein	Arteritic anterior ischemic optic neuropathy
Sudden unilateral visual loss Altitudinal visual field loss (classically inferior) Relative afferent pupillary defect Optic disc swelling (may be partial in accordance with field defect ± pallor) Normal ESR Idiopathic or may be associated with arteriosclerosis, diabetes, hypertension	Nonarteritic anterior ischemic optic neuropathy

Table 3 (continued)

Features	Diagnosis
Subacute visual loss (days) Usually unilateral Impaired color vision Pain with eye movement Young adult Decreased visual acuity Color (red) desaturation Optic disc swelling ± pallor Variable field defect Fundus may be normal Idiopathic or may be associated with multiple sclerosis, post-viral infections, granulomatous disease	Optic neuritis If no fundus abnormality, then retrobulbar neuritis
Sudden loss of central vision Central scotoma Distortion of straight lines Objects appear distorted Decreased visual acuity Macular retinal & subretinal hemorrhages (gray-green subretinal membrane) Drusen & pigmentation at macula	Exudative age-related macular degeneration
Gradual loss of central vision (chronic) Usually bilateral Drusen & pigmentation at macula	Dry age-related macular degeneration

Table 4. Management of Painful Red Eye

Diagnosis	Management
Conjunctivitis	Trimethoprim-polymyxin B drops or erythromycin ointment
	But most cases of conjunctivitis are viral or allergic & can be treated symptomatically with artificial tears
	If contact lens wearer, lenses should be removed for at least 7 days
	If purulent, consider culture to rule out gonococcus
	If resistant to antibiotic treatment, consider *Chlamydia* infection
Subconjunctival hemorrhage	No treatment, check for underlying cause if recurrent
Episcleritis	Mild—may resolve spontaneously
	Moderate—try topical NSAID, e.g., ketorolac tromethamine
	Severe—refer to ophthalmologist for topical steroid treatment
Scleritis	Urgent referral to ophthalmologist for systemic steroid treatment and/or oral NSAID
	Refer to rheumatology for systemic work-up
	In severe cases, immunosuppression may be needed
Anterior uveitis (iritis)	Urgent referral to ophthalmology for topical steroids
	Cycloplegic/mydriatic agents help with discomfort & prevent posterior synechiae
	Consider associated systemic disorders
Endophthalmitis	Refer immediately to ophthalmology for vitreous ± aqueous culture and intravitreal antibiotics
Keratitis	Immediate referral to ophthalmologist
	Will require culture of corneal scrapings & aggressive topical antibiotic, antifungal, antiviral treatment
Exposure keratopathy	Keep the cornea moist: frequent artificial teardrops or lubricant ointment
	Refer to ophthalmology if no response to lubrication or secondary infection is suspected
Acute angle-closure glaucoma	Immediate referral to ophthalmology
	Treat with timolol 0.5% drops, acetazolamide 500 mg IV, consider mannitol 1-2 g/kg IV over 60 minutes
	Topical steroids & pilocarpine per ophthalmology
	May need laser iridotomy or surgery
Posterior uveitis	Urgent referral to ophthalmology
	Consider associated systemic disorders

Table 5. Treatment of Loss of Vision in a Quiet White Eye

Central or branch retinal artery occlusion	Best treatment results are with earliest intervention
	Immediate referral to ophthalmology
	Immediate digital massage of globe, acetazolamide 500 mg IV, timolol 0.5% drops to reduce pressure
	Ophthalmologist to consider anterior chamber paracentesis
	Immediate ESR, C-reactive protein, & systemic steroids if giant cell arteritis suspected
Central or branch retinal vein occlusion	Early referral to ophthalmology to determine if "ischemic vein occlusion" for treatment to reduce risk of neovascular glaucoma
	Treat underlying conditions (e.g., diabetes & hypertension)
Vitreous hemorrhage	Bed rest, elevate head of bed
	Stop antiplatelet agents or anticoagulants if possible
	Immediate ophthalmology referral for ultrasound investigation of posterior pole to exclude retinal detachment
	If diabetic, likely to be due to proliferative retinopathy but retinal detachment must be ruled out immediately
Retinal detachment	Strict bed rest with bilateral eye patching if macula is threatened
	Immediate referral to ophthalmology for surgery
Arteritic anterior ischemic optic neuropathy (AION)	High-dose oral prednisone (60-100 mg daily)
	Start steroids before ESR & C-reactive protein results are known
	Refer to ophthalmology; should have temporal artery biopsy within 1 week
Nonarteritic AION	Rule out arteritic AION; if unsure, ESR, C-reactive protein, & biopsy, treat as arteritic with steroids until diagnosis made
	Nonarteritic AION cannot be treated; management of underlying disorder is required
Optic neuritis/ retrobulbar neuritis	Check for focal neurologic signs & refer to neurologist if present
	Order MRI (predictive value for multiple sclerosis)
	Ophthalmology referral is also indicated
	IV steroids may increase rate of recovery (methylprednisolone 1 g/day IV for 3 days, then prednisone 1 mg/kg/day PO × 11 days)

Table 5 (continued)

Exudative age-related macular degeneration	Urgent referral to ophthalmology for potential laser, surgical, or drug treatment
Dry age-related macular degeneration	Is not an emergency Routine ophthalmology referral

PALPITATIONS

Kevin A. Bybee, M.D.
Stephen L. Kopecky, M.D.

IS THE PATIENT'S LIFE AT RISK?

- Palpitations
  - ▲ This refers to conscious sensation of cardiac activity.
  - ▲ Can signify a primary cardiac problem or can be of noncardiac origin
  - ▲ Can be symptom of a benign process, life-threatening arrhythmia, or serious underlying noncardiac disorder
- Patient with palpitations must be evaluated quickly to rule out arrhythmia or other serious disorder
- Because any patient with a tachyarrhythmia and hemodynamic instability needs urgent cardioversion, initial evaluation should focus on indications for emergent electrical cardioversion.

ADDRESSING THE RISK

- Obtain a stat 12-lead ECG.
- On history, assess if the patient has symptoms of a hemodynamically significant arrhythmia such as chest pain, dyspnea, presyncope, or confusion.
- Assess for hemodynamic stability: tachycardia, hypotension, hypoxia, or changes in mental status.
- Focus the physical exam on vital signs and the cardiorespiratory systems.
  - ▲ Determine heart rate and rhythm.
    - • Is the patient tachycardic?
    - • If so, is the rhythm regular or irregular; if irregular, is it regularly irregular or irregularly irregular?
  - ▲ Look for signs of heart failure and depressed cardiac output, e.g., hypoxemia, increased jugular venous pressure,

Special abbreviation used in this chapter: AV, atrioventricular.

presence of third heart sound (S_3) gallop, bibasilar crackles, cyanosis, impaired peripheral perfusion.

- Call for code team response if the patient has signs or symptoms of a hemodynamically significant arrhythmia.
- Place supplemental oxygen at 3-4 L by nasal cannula.
- Establish IV access.
- Efficiently and accurately interpret the 12-lead ECG.
- Tachyarrhythmias >150 beats/minute and bradyarrhythmias <50 beats/minute when associated with hypotension signify a hemodynamically significant arrhythmia.
- Evaluate for and address life-threatening noncardiac causes of palpitations: sepsis, hypoglycemia, severe anemia, acute blood loss (gastrointestinal tract bleed, retroperitoneal bleed), thyrotoxicosis, adrenal insufficiency, pheochromocytoma.

DIFFERENTIAL DIAGNOSIS

- The differential diagnosis for palpitations of arrhythmic origin is listed in Table 1 and that for palpitations of nonarrhythmic origin, in Table 2.

DIFFERENTIATING THE DIFFERENTIAL

ECG Interpretation

Regular Tachycardia With Narrow QRS Complex (<0.10 ms)
- Sinus tachycardia
- Atrioventricular (AV) nodal reentrant tachycardia
- AV reentrant tachycardia with orthodromic conduction (Wolff-Parkinson-White syndrome)
- Atrial flutter with fixed conduction

Regular Tachycardia With Wide QRS Complex (>0.12 ms)
- Sinus tachycardia with delayed or aberrant conduction (sinus tachycardia with a bundle branch block)
- Atrial flutter with fixed conduction and delayed or aberrant conduction
- Supraventricular tachycardia with delayed or aberrant conduction
- Ventricular tachycardia
- AV reentrant tachycardia with antidromic conduction

Irregular Tachycardia With Narrow QRS Complex
- Atrial fibrillation

- Atrial flutter with variable conduction
- Multifocal atrial tachycardia
- Sinus rhythm with frequent atrial premature contractions
- Sinus rhythm with frequent premature ventricular contractions, which will have a wide QRS

Irregular Tachycardia With Wide QRS Complex
- Atrial fibrillation with delayed or aberrant conduction
- Atrial flutter with variable conduction and delayed or aberrant conduction
- Torsades de pointes

Note: If the patient has known coronary artery disease and a wide complex tachycardia, assuming it is ventricular tachycardia will be correct >90% of the time.

Sinus Tachycardia
- Can be a secondary response to many underlying conditions
  - Sepsis
  - Fever
  - Hypovolemia
  - Hypoxia
  - Thyrotoxicosis
  - Anemia

Table 1. Differential Diagnosis for Palpitations of Arrhythmic Origin

Tachyarrhythmia	Bradyarrhythmia
Sinus tachycardia	Sinus bradycardia
Atrial fibrillation	Second degree heart block
Atrial flutter	(Mobitz II)
Paroxysmal supraventricular tachycardia	Third-degree heart block
Multifocal atrial tachycardia	Vagal (cardioinhibitory) bradycardia
Atrioventricular reentrant tachycardia (Wolff-Parkinson-White syndrome)	
Ventricular tachycardia	

Noncardiac	Cardiac
Sepsis	Atrial septal defect
Fever	Ventricular septal defect
Anemia	Aortic regurgitation
Thyrotoxicosis	Aortic stenosis
Hypoglycemia	Pericarditis
Anxiety/postoperative pain	Hyperkinetic heart syndrome
Pheochromocytoma	Acute mitral regurgitation
Medications (theophylline, albuterol, other stimulants)	
Diaphragmatic flutter	

- ▲ Hypoglycemia
- ▲ Adrenal insufficiency (addisonian crisis)
- ▲ Stimulants (albuterol, theophylline, cocaine, amphetamines)
- ▲ Anxiety or pain

ORDERING TESTS
- All patients complaining of palpitations need immediate evaluation, including a stat bedside 12-lead ECG.
- Tests for various suspected diagnoses are listed in Table 3.

INITIAL MANAGEMENT
Arrhythmia Management
- Place patient on continuous bedside monitor with 3 limb leads.
- Obtain IV access if not already available, and place supplemental oxygen.
- Refer to American Heart Association ACLS algorithms for detailed arrhythmia management information.
- The following are suggestions for initial arrhythmia management with first-line treatments.

Tachyarrhythmia—Unstable
- Considered unstable if chest pain, dyspnea, mental status change, hypotension, shock, pulmonary vascular congestion, or acute myocardial infarction
  - ▲ Consider electrical cardioversion.

Table 3. **Suspected Diagnosis and Tests Ordered**

Suspected diagnosis	Tests/lab
Myocardial infarction, arrhythmia	12-lead ECG, CK, CK MB, troponin I or T, CBC, electrolytes (magnesium, creatinine, sTSH)
Thyrotoxicosis	sTSH, free T_4, total T_3
Anemia	CBC, stool hemoccult, ferritin, serum iron, total iron-binding capacity, peripheral blood smear, reticulocyte count
Sepsis	Blood cultures ×2, chest X-ray, urinalysis with Gram stain & culture, CBC
Valvular heart disease	Transthoracic echocardiogram, ECG
Adrenal insufficiency	Serum cortisol, cosyntropin stimulation test, electrolytes

T_3, triiodothyronine; T_4, thyroxine; sTSH, sensitive thyroid-stimulating hormone.

▲ Indications for cardioversion are hypotension, chest pain, congestive heart failure, or depressed cerebral perfusion manifested as change in mental status.
▲ Use unsynchronized cardioversion for all unstable tachyarrhythmias without a pulse.

Tachyarrhythmia—Stable
■ Considered stable if no chest pain, dyspnea, mental status change, hypotension, shock, pulmonary vascular congestion, or acute myocardial infarction
■ Atrial fibrillation/flutter
  ▲ Diltiazem (Cardizem)
    • Bolus IV 0.12-0.25 mg/kg or 10-20 mg IV over 2 minutes
    • Repeat in 15 minutes if needed.
    • Consider diltiazem drip at 5-15 mg/hour.
■ Paroxysmal supraventricular tachycardia
  ▲ Consider vagal maneuvers if not contraindicated.
  ▲ Adenosine, 6 mg IV push and quickly flush with normal saline; repeat with 12 mg IV push if no response.

- ▲ Consider verapamil, 2.5-5.0 mg, if narrow QRS and no response to adenosine.
- ▲ Consider lidocaine, 1.0-1.5 mg/kg IV, if wide QRS and no response to adenosine.
- ■ Wide complex tachycardia of uncertain type
  - ▲ Lidocaine, 1.0-1.5 mg/kg IV; repeat 0.5-0.75 mg/kg if needed.
  - ▲ Start maintenance lidocaine infusion 2-4 mg/minute if initial response to lidocaine.
  - ▲ Consider adenosine, 6-12 mg IV, if no response to lidocaine.
  - ▲ Consider procainamide, 20-30 mg/minute (maximum 17 mg/kg), if no response to adenosine.
- ■ Ventricular tachycardia
  - ▲ Lidocaine, 1.0-1.5 mg/kg IV push; repeat 0.5-0.75 mg/kg if needed.
  - ▲ Start lidocaine infusion, 2-4 mg/minute, if initial response to lidocaine.
  - ▲ Consider procainamide if no response to lidocaine.
- ■ Torsades de pointes
  - ▲ Magnesium sulfate 2 g IV
  - ▲ If no response to magnesium, consider atrial or ventricular pacing.

Bradyarrhythmia—Unstable
- ■ Considered unstable if chest pain, dyspnea, mental status change, hypotension, shock, pulmonary venous congestion, or acute myocardial infarction
  - ▲ Atropine, 0.5-1.0 mg IV
  - ▲ Use transcutaneous pacemaker as a bridge (verify patient tolerance, may need analgesia and sedation).
  - ▲ Prepare for transvenous pacemaker insertion.

Bradyarrhythmia—Stable
- ■ Considered stable if no chest pain, dyspnea, mental status change, hypotension, pulmonary venous congestion, or acute myocardial infarction
  - ▲ Consider atropine, 0.5-1.0 mg IV, or observe.
  - ▲ Monitor and follow vital signs closely.
  - ▲ Ensure availability of transcutaneous pacing if needed.

RASH

Rochelle R. Torgerson, M.D., Ph.D.
Lisa A. Drage, M.D.

IS THE PATIENT'S LIFE AT RISK?
- Although most rashes may be managed in an outpatient setting, there are instances when an acute presentation or flare of a chronic condition requires intensive therapy.

Rashes That Require Inpatient Care—Two General Categories
- Rashes that cause altered metabolism and have a considerable risk of infection
- Rashes that are key diagnostic clues to major underlying illnesses

Presence of the Following Indicate Increased Severity
- Angioedema and tongue swelling
- Mucous membrane involvement
- Skin pain or tenderness
- Generalized erythema
- Extensive blistering, bullae, or desquamation
- Systemic symptoms: fever, hypotension, headache, myalgias, arthralgias
- Systemic involvement: lymphadenopathy, nephritis, hepatitis, agranulocytosis
- Immunosuppression

ADDRESSING THE RISK
- If airway compromise or hypotension
  - ▲ Airway, breathing, circulation (ABCs)
- Severe desquamation or blistering

Special abbreviation used in this chapter: ABCs, airway, breathing, circulation.

- ▲ Fluid resuscitation, aseptic technique, topical or systemic antibiotics
- ▲ ICU if hemodynamically unstable
- If infectious cause
  - ▲ Cultures, broad-spectrum antibiotic coverage
- Blistering or urticaria/angioedema (not infectious)
  - ▲ Systemic corticosteroids (after appropriate diagnostic cultures/studies)

DIFFERENTIAL DIAGNOSIS
- The extensive differential diagnosis can be grouped according to the morphology of individual skin lesions.
  - ▲ Terms used to describe skin lesions are listed in Table 1.
  - ▲ Causes of rash are listed in Table 2.
  - ▲ The differential diagnosis is listed in Table 3.

DIFFERENTIATING THE DIFFERENTIAL
Relevant Information to Obtain From the History
- Rash: onset, location, spread, associated symptoms (e.g., itch, pain)
- Systemic symptoms: fever, headache, myalgia, arthralgia
- Medications: recent changes as well as current oral, topical, over-the-counter, herbal
- Previous skin diseases or reactions
- Allergies: drug or contact
- Exposures: sick contacts, travel, animals, bugs, food
- Family history: atopic or psoriasis
- Immune status

Table 1. Terms Used to Describe Skin Lesions

Term for lesion	Appearance
Macule	Flat, color variation from surrounding skin
Papule	Elevated, diameter = 0.5 cm
Vesicle	Fluid-filled (clear) blister, diameter <0.05 cm
Bulla	Fluid-filled (clear) blister, diameter >0.05 cm
Pustule	Pus-filled blister
Scale	Dry, thickened flakes of stratum corneum
Purpura	Purple, nonblanchable, macular (nonpalpable) or papular (palpable)
Wheal (hive)	Indurated papule, central pallor, evanescent

Table 2. Causes of Rash

Generalized	Patterned/localized erythema	Purpura
Dermatomyositis	Abscess & furuncle	Actinic purpura
Drug eruption	Cellulitis	Disseminated intra-
Lupus erythematosus	Erythema migrans	vascular coagulation
Photosensitive	Erythema multiforme	Steroid-associated
eruptions	Erythema nodosum	purpura
Sézary syndrome	Urticaria	Thrombocytopenic
(cutaneous T-cell		purpura
lymphoma)		Trauma-associated
Stevens-Johnson		purpura
syndrome		Vasculitis (palpable
Toxic epidermal		purpura)
necrolysis		
Viral exanthem		

Vesicles and bullae	Pustules	Inflammatory papules
Bullous impetigo	Infectious	Insect bite reactions
Bullous pemphigoid	Bacterial	Lichen planus
Contact dermatitis	Fungal	Miliaria
(acute)	Noninfectious	Scabies
Coxsackievirus	Pustular psoriasis	
Dermatitis herpeti-	Drugs	
formis		
Herpes simplex		
Herpes zoster		
Pemphigus vulgaris		
Porphyria cutanea		
tarda		
Varicella		

Eczematous rashes	Scales	White spots
Atopic dermatitis	Discoid lupus	Pityriasis alba
Contact dermatitis	erythematosus	Postinflammatory
Lichen simplex	Fungal infections	hypopigmentation
chronicus	Mycosis fungoides	Tinea versicolor
Seborrheic derma-	(cutaneous T-cell	Tuberous sclerosis
titis	lymphoma)	Vitiligo
Stasis dermatitis	Pityriasis rosea	
	Psoriasis	
	Secondary syphilis	

Table 3. Differential Diagnosis of Rash

Rash	History and symptoms	Diagnosis
Target lesions especially on palms or soles	Herpes simplex, *Mycoplasma*, new drug	Erythema multiforme
Lesions ranging from dark red macules with necrotic centers to epidermal detachment with prominent mucosal lesions	Drugs—sulfa, other antibiotics, carbamazepine, barbiturates, allopurinol	Stevens-Johnson syndrome, toxic epidermal necrolysis
Urticaria or swelling of central face, respiratory distress	Insect bite, food exposure, drug	Urticaria, angioedema
Sunburn-like erythroderma, mucosal hyperemia, strawberry tongue, desquamation of hands & feet (late)	Tampon use, nasal packing, wound infection, barrier contraceptive, influenza	Staphylococcal toxic shock syndrome
Diffuse petechial eruption evolving to palpable purpura with gray necrotic centers	Fever, headache, nausea, vomiting, myalgia, close-quartered living conditions, splenectomy	Meningococcal disease
Subtle evidence of soft tissue infection (pain, swelling, warmth), bullae, necrotizing fasciitis	Fever, hypotension, pain out of proportion to exam, rapid progression	Streptococcal toxic shock syndrome
Centripetally spreading macular papular rash evolving to petechial purpuric rash	Travel or residence in endemic area, tick bite, fever, malaise, headache, myalgias, vomiting	Rocky Mountain spotted fever
Palpable purpura	Evidence of systemic involvement: abdominal pain, arthritis, epistaxis, iritis, nephritis, peripheral neuropathy, pulmonary hemorrhage	Vasculitis

Table 3 (continued)

Rash	History and symptoms	Diagnosis
Painful red plaques	Fever, URI, hematologic malignancy	Sweet syndrome (acute febrile neutrophilic dermatosis)
Diffuse sterile pustules	Steroid use or taper, NSAIDs, β-hemolytic streptococcus infection, viral URI, fever, adenopathy	Generalized pustular psoriasis
Grouped vesicles on an erythematous base in a dermatomal distribution	Pain or pruritus in a dermatomal distribution	Herpes zoster

URI, upper respiratory tract infection.

TEST ORDERING

Rash-Specific Testing
- Skin biopsy for hematoxylin-eosin sections, immunofluorescence, and electron microscopy to support or rule out a diagnosis (clinicopathologic correlate often required)
- Cultures of infected lesions to direct antibiotic therapy

Other Tests May Be Dictated by an Underlying Illness
- Cutaneous findings, associated disease, and tests to consider are listed in Table 4.

INITIAL MANAGEMENT

Urticaria or Angioedema (Drug, Food, Insect Bite)
- ABCs
- For severe cases
  ▲ Large-bore IV access with 0.9% normal saline
  ▲ Diphenhydramine
  ▲ Famotidine

- ▲ Methylprednisolone
- ▲ Epinephrine
- ▪ Followed by diphenhydramine or hydroxyzine
- ▪ Short course of prednisone
- ▪ In less severe cases, diphenhydramine or hydroxyzine 50 mg every 4 hours may be enough
- ▪ Discontinue or avoid any identifiable triggers
- ▪ Epinephrine (EpiPen) education

Table 4. Tests Dictated by Cutaneous Finding and Associated Disease

Cutaneous finding	Associated disease	Tests to consider
Aphthous ulcers	Crohn disease, gluten-sensitive enteropathy, Behçet syndrome	Colonoscopy, small-bowel biopsy
Café au lait spots, neurofibromas	Neurofibromatosis	Genetic testing
Dermatitis herpetiformis	Gluten-sensitive enteropathy	Serum IgA endomysial antibody, antigliadin antibodies, small-bowel biopsy
Erythema marginatum	Rheumatic fever	Throat culture, streptococcal antibody titer, ESR, ECG, Echo
Erythema migrans	Lyme disease	ELISA/Western blot 4-6 weeks after infection
Erythema nodosum	Strep pharyngitis, sarcoidosis, inflammatory bowel disease, Behçet syndrome, histoplasmosis, coccidioidomycosis	Throat culture, ACE level, serum calcium, CXR, colonoscopy, fungal stains, cultures, antigen detection, serologic tests for fungal-specific antibodies
Gottron papules, heliotrope rash	Dermatomyositis	Plasma CK, LDH, AST/ALT, aldolase, ANA, anti-Jo-1 antibody, EMG, muscle biopsy

Table 4 (continued)

Cutaneous finding	Associated disease	Tests to consider
Livedo reticularis	Thromboembolic events, vasculitis, connective tissue disorders, pancreatitis, syphilis, TB	Platelet count, D-dimer fibrin degradation products, peripheral smear, PT, aPTT, Echo, amylase, lipase, PPD, AFB smear, CXR (also see tests for dermatomyositis, syphilis, & vasculitis)
Malar rash	Lupus erythematosus	ANA, dsDNA, Sm
Palpable purpura	Churg-Strauss syndrome, cryoglobulinemic vasculitis, Henoch-Schönlein purpura, microscopic polyangiitis, Wegener granulomatosis	CBC, ESR, serum complement levels, serum creatinine, BUN, urinalysis, LFTs, hepatitis serologic tests, ANA, c-ANCA, p-ANCA, & cardiac, respiratory, neurologic, & gastrointestinal tests
Petechial rash	Endocarditis, thromboembolic events, thrombocytopenia, DIC	Blood cultures, Echo, platelet count, D-dimer, fibrin degradation products, peripheral smear, PT, aPTT
Pinch purpura & waxy papules	Amyloidosis	SPEP/UPEP with immunofixation, abdominal wall fat biopsy, skin lesion biopsy
Pretibial myxedema	Graves disease	TSH, T_4
Pyoderma gangrenosum	Inflammatory bowel disease, rheumatoid arthritis, hematologic malignancy, chronic active hepatitis	CBC, colonoscopy, rheumatoid factor, ESR, X-rays, LFTs, hepatitis serologic tests

Table 4 (continued)

Cutaneous finding	Associated disease	Tests to consider
Scaling papules, especially on palms & soles	Secondary syphilis	Rapid plasma reagin, VDRL
Sweet syndrome (acute febrile neutrophilic dermatosis)	Hematologic malignancies, solid tumors	CBC, skin biopsy, preventive cancer screening appropriate for patient age
Telangiectasia, on mucosa & acrally	Rendu-Osler-Weber syndrome	CBC, CXR, colonoscopy, CT of head
Painful ulcerative mucocutaneous lesions, generalized rash (often but not always maculopapular)	Primary HIV infection	HIV RNA test (viral load), HIV antibody test (initially negative but baseline needed for later seroconversion)
Kaposi sarcoma, molluscum contagiosum, severe HSV	HIV	HIV testing (with consent), ELISA/Western blot

ACE, angiotensin-converting enzyme; AFB, acid-fast bacillus; ANA, antinuclear antibody; ANCA, antineutrophil cytoplasmic antibody (c-, cytoplasmic; p-, perinuclear); CXR, chest radiography; DIC, disseminated intravascular coagulation; dsDNA, double-stranded DNA; Echo, echocardiography; HSV, herpes simplex virus; LFT, liver function test; RF, rheumatoid factor; RPR, rapid plasma reagin; SPEP, serum protein electrophoresis; Strep, streptococcal; T_4, thyroxine; TSH, thyroid-stimulating hormone; UPEP, urine protein electrophoresis.

Drug Eruption (Exanthem, Stevens-Johnson Syndrome, Toxic Epidermal Necrolysis)

- ABCs
- Obtain a complete drug history—prescription, nonprescription, topical, ophthalmic.
- Identify and discontinue or find substitutes for likely culprits—antibiotics, anticonvulsants, NSAIDs, angiotensin-converting enzyme inhibitors, thiazide diuretics, dyes.

- Measure drug levels.
- Rash may worsen for several days despite stopping the inciting agent.
- If mild, treat symptomatically (e.g., antihistamines, topical corticosteroids).
- If blistering and exfoliation, administer fluids and use aseptic technique.
- If signs of infection, culture and give broad-spectrum antibiotics.
- If eye is involved, request ophthalmology consult.
- Skin biopsy
- Patient education to avoid recurrence
- After a severe reaction, never rechallenge a patient with drug or skin testing.

Rocky Mountain Spotted Fever

- ABCs
- Diagnosis is made on basis of the clinical and epidemiologic features.
- Doxycycline
- Supportive therapy
- Remain alert for mental status changes, renal dysfunction, myocarditis, and respiratory failure.
- Common but nonspecific changes in lab values: leukopenia, thrombocytopenia, hyponatremia, elevated ALT and AST levels
- Antibody serologic tests will not be positive for 7-10 days after symptom onset.

Staphylococcal Toxic Shock Syndrome

- ABCs
- Vancomycin (until penicillin and oxacillin sensitivities known)
- Removal of tampons, packings, dressings
- Surgical exploration and debridement if indicated
- Clindamycin 900 mg every 8 hours IV may be added to reduce toxin production
- IV immunoglobulin 0.5 g/kg daily IV × 4 days may neutralize circulating toxins

Streptococcal Toxic Shock Syndrome
- ABCs
- Ceftriaxone + clindamycin 900 mg every 8 hours IV
- Aggressive supportive care
- Surgical exploration and debridement are most important.
- Tissue (intraoperative) cultures and sensitivities
- IV immunoglobulin 0.5 g/kg daily × 4 days may neutralize circulating toxins.

Meningococcal Meningitis
- ABCs
- Gram stain, culture, and susceptibilities performed on
  - Blood
  - CSF
  - Skin biopsy (may be positive even after initiation of antibiotic therapy)
- Bacterial antigen testing on CSF
- Ceftriaxone

Bullous Pemphigoid
- Oral corticosteroids to achieve remission
- After remission, reduce prednisone dose to half and then slowly taper
- Steroid-sparing drugs may be tried (e.g., azathioprine, dapsone, methotrexate)
- In mild cases—dapsone may be adequate
- For localized mild cases, topical corticosteroids may suffice.
- Aseptic technique
- Antibiotic coverage as indicated by severity or signs of infection

SPLENOMEGALY

T. Jared Bunch, M.D.
Thomas M. Habermann, M.D.

IS THE PATIENT'S LIFE AT RISK?

- Splenic rupture
  - ▲ An uncommon cause of splenomegaly
  - ▲ Caused by penetrating or nonpenetrating trauma or may be spontaneous
  - ▲ Requires immediate, emergent treatment
  - ▲ Presentation of splenic rupture may be delayed 24-48 hours after trauma.
- Systemic illnesses predisposing to traumatic splenic rupture
  - ▲ Myeloproliferative and lymphoproliferative disorders
  - ▲ Endocarditis
  - ▲ Infection: TB, brucellosis, cytomegalovirus, Epstein-Barr virus, HIV, viral hepatitis, histoplasmosis, toxoplasmosis, malaria

ADDRESSING THE RISK (ACUTE VS. CHRONIC)

- Splenic rupture
  - ▲ History reveals abdominal pain that may be referred to left shoulder (diaphragm irritation).
  - ▲ Physical exam may show orthostasis, peritoneal signs, or hypotension.
  - ▲ If splenic rupture is suspected, rapid assessment with abdominal CT and collaboration with a surgical team are essential.

DIFFERENTIAL DIAGNOSIS

- The differential diagnosis for splenomegaly is listed in Table 1.
- The causes of splenomegaly
  - ▲ Work hypertrophy from immune response or RBC destruction
  - ▲ Congestive
  - ▲ Myeloproliferative
  - ▲ Infiltrative (nonneoplastic and neoplastic)

Table 1. Differential Diagnosis for Splenomegaly

Work hypertrophy
    Immune response
        Bacterial infection—TB, subacute bacterial endocarditis
        Viral infection—cytomegalovirus, Epstein-Barr virus,
          HIV, viral hepatitis
        Fungal infection—histoplasmosis
        Parasitic infection—toxoplasmosis, malaria
        Felty syndrome
        Systemic lupus erythematosus
        Serum sickness
    RBC destruction
        Hereditary spherocytosis
        Thalassemia major
        Pyruvate kinase deficiency
        Hemolytic diseases
Congestive
    Cirrhosis & portal hypertension
    Portal, hepatic, or splenic vein thrombosis
    Congestive heart failure
Myeloproliferative
    Chronic myelogenous leukemia
    Extramedullary hematopoiesis—myeloid metaplasia from
      myelofibrosis, marrow damage by toxins, radiation, infiltra-
      tion by tumor or leukemia
    Polycythemia vera
Lymphoproliferative
    Lymphoma
    Chronic lymphocytic leukemia
    Acute lymphocytic leukemia
    Hairy cell leukemia
Infiltrative
    Nonneoplastic—sarcoidosis, amyloidosis, Gaucher disease
    Neoplastic—acute nonlymphocytic leukemia, metastatic tumor
Other
    Trauma
    Splenic cyst(s)
    Pyogenic abscess
    Hemangioma
    Idiopathic splenomegaly

DIFFERENTIATING THE DIFFERENTIAL

History of Present Illness

- Acute vs. chronic disease
  - ▲ Abrupt onset of symptoms suggests a traumatic, infectious, or inflammatory cause.
  - ▲ Chronic history of constitutional complaints suggests a neoplastic cause.
- Characteristics of the symptoms
  - ▲ Fatigue and malaise—common symptoms in acute and chronic liver disease, hematologic malignancy, and chronic systemic infection
  - ▲ Anorexia—common symptom in acute and chronic liver disease, weight loss, hematologic malignancy
  - ▲ Persistent dull ache or fullness in left upper quadrant—moderate-massive splenomegaly (may be accompanied with early satiety)
    - • Differential diagnosis is of massive splenomegaly: myeloproliferative disorders, non-Hodgkin lymphoma, hairy cell leukemia, splenic cyst, Gaucher disease.
  - ▲ Increase in abdominal girth—suggestive of ascites and advanced chronic liver disease, hepatic malignancy, venous outflow obstruction
  - ▲ Pruritus—lymphoma, cholestasis
  - ▲ Urticaria—hepatitis B infection (with synovitis), immune complex disease (with petechiae), lymphoma
  - ▲ Pharyngitis, rash, and lymphadenopathy—Epstein-Barr virus or cytomegalovirus
  - ▲ History of congestive heart failure or cirrhosis—congestive disease

Family History

- Genetic anemic diseases—sickle cell anemia (SS, SC), thalassemia major or minor, hereditary spherocytosis
- Genetic association—alcoholic liver disease

Social History

- Promiscuous sexual activity, illicit drug use (endocarditis if IV drugs), or history of blood transfusion—viral hepatitis, HIV

- Exposure to a marrow-toxic medication or environmental toxin, including heavy use of ethanol.

Physical Exam
- Evaluate for lymphadenopathy.
- Perform a thorough cardiac and liver exam to look for signs of dysfunction, infection or inflammation, and portal hypertension
- Exam of the spleen should involve percussion and palpation.
  - ▲ Normal spleen is not palpable in adults.
  - ▲ Tenderness suggests peritoneal inflammation from infection, infarction, or rapid enlargement.

ORDERING TESTS
Lab Tests
- Initial laboratory evaluation of splenomegaly includes a CBC, with differential and platelet count, and peripheral blood smear (Tables 2 and 3).
- Perform liver tests to evaluate for hepatic abnormality and measure bilirubin as an index of cholestasis or hemolysis.

Radiographic Evaluation
- CT with IV contrast/MRI
  - ▲ Useful for evaluating parenchymal splenic disease
  - ▲ CT can accurately assess size.
  - ▲ CT may demonstrate lymphadenopathy in deeper nodal groups and is especially useful for suspected lymphoma.
  - ▲ CT can identify tumors and small lacerations not detected by other imaging methods.
  - ▲ MRI allows visualization of vessels without IV contrast, but is occasionally used for this purpose.

Tissue Biopsy
- Bone marrow aspiration is indicated for evaluation of hematologic disorders and infectious disease.
  - ▲ Allows cytologic and histologic exam of bone marrow cells
  - ▲ Specimen may provide information about infection through culture and staining (acid-fast bacilli, yeast, fungus).

Table 2.   Initial Evaluation of Splenomegaly: CBC With Differential and Platelet Count

Anemia
  Microcytic: thalassemia, hereditary sideroblastic anemia
  Macrocytic: polychromasia (check reticulocyte count), myeloid metaplasia, target cells (thalassemia; hemoglobins C, D, E, S; liver disease), spherocytosis
  Normocytic: acute blood loss, splenic rupture, bone marrow infiltration (lymphoma, myeloproliferative diseases)
Erythrocytosis
  Polycythemia vera
  Secondary polycythemia
  Hypoxic erythrocytosis: pulmonary disease, chronic cor pulmonale
  Hemoglobinopathies
Leukopenia
  Myelodysplastic disease
  Hypersplenism: congestive disease, malaria, sarcoidosis
  Infection: mononucleosis, HIV, overwhelming bacterial infection
  Systemic lupus erythematosus
  Felty syndrome
Leukocytosis
  Neutrophilic
    Acute bacterial infections
    Lymphocytosis
      High ($\geq 15 \times 10^9$/L cells): infectious mononucleosis (atypical lymphocytes), acute & chronic lymphocytic leukemia
      Moderate (<15×10^9/L cells): viral infections (infectious mononucleosis, hepatitis, cytomegalovirus, HIV), toxoplasmosis, neoplasm (carcinoma, Hodgkin disease)
  Eosinophilic
    Hypersensitivity reaction
    Neoplasm: Hodgkin and non-Hodgkin lymphoma
    Collagen vascular disease
  Basophilic
    Myeloproliferative disorder
  Monocytosis
    Subacute bacterial endocarditis
    Chronic infection: TB, malaria
    Collagen vascular disease

Table 2 (continued)

Thrombocytopenia
  Lymphoma
  Aplastic anemia
  Marrow damage—chemicals, ionizing radiation, alcohol,
    infection, leukemias, metastatic disease, myelofibrosis
  Increased destruction of platelets—chronic lymphocytic
    leukemia, lymphoma, systemic lupus erythematosus
  Infection—infectious mononucleosis, cytomegalovirus, HIV,
    malaria, sepsis
  Thrombotic thrombocytopenic purpura
  Thrombocytopenia—idioipathic or secondary
  Hemolytic uremic syndrome
Thrombocytosis
  Primary
      Polycythemia vera
      Chronic myelocytic leukemia
      Myelofibrosis
  Secondary
      Infection
      Inflammatory disease
      Neoplasm
      Asplenia
      Postsurgical procedure

- Lymph node biopsy is indicated for patients with persistent,
  unexplained, localized or generalized lymphadenopathy >1
  cm and persisting more than 1 month.
- Diagnostic laparotomy with splenectomy may be indicated
  after complete diagnostic evaluation does not disclose a cause
  of splenomegaly and primary splenic lymphoma is suspected.

MANAGEMENT
Work Hypertrophy
- Immune response
    ▲ Bacterial endocarditis—blood cultures, echocardiogram,
      empiric antibiotic treatment to cover *Staphylococcus*,
      Streptococcus, and *Enterococcus* while culture results are
      pending
    ▲ Infectious mononucleosis
      • Primarily Epstein-Barr virus but may be cytomegalovirus

Table 3. Initial Evaluation of Splenomegaly: Peripheral Blood Smear

Feature	Condition
Target cells	Thalassemia
	Hemoglobins C, E, SC
	Liver disease
	Splenectomy
Basophilic stripping	Hemolysis
	Lead poisoning
	Thalassemia
Schistocytes (fragmented RBCs)	Thrombotic thrombocytopenic purpura
	Disseminated intravascular coagulation
	Vasculitis
Teardrop cells	Myelofibrosis
	Myelophthisis
Spherocytes	Autoimmune hemolytic anemia
	Hereditary spherocytosis
	Burns
	Clostridium infections
Sickle cells	Sickle cell anemia (hemoglobin SS, SC)
	Hemoglobin S β-thalassemia
Acanthocytes	Chronic or severe liver disease
"Bite" cells	Unstable hemoglobinopathy
Howell-Jolly bodies	Postsplenectomy
	Acquired hyposplenism
Intraerythrocytic parasite	Malaria

- No treatment available other than symptomatic treatment with acetaminophen or NSAIDs.
- For thrombocytopenia, autoimmune hemolytic anemia, or airway obstructive lymphoid tissue, a course of corticosteroids may be beneficial.
- Vigorous activity is avoided for 1 month or until splenomegaly regresses.

RBC Destruction
- Sickle cell anemia
  - Hydration and oxygen treatment if patient is hypoxic
  - Folic acid supplementation and transfusion for hemolytic and aplastic crises
  - Patient may be functionally asplenic and require vaccination against encapsulated organisms.
- Hemolytic anemia
  - CBC with peripheral smear and reticulocyte count
  - For hereditary membrane defect, hemoglobin <8.0 g/dL, and reticulocyte count >11%, splenectomy may be indicated.
  - Autoimmune hemolytic anemia is confirmed with a direct Coombs test and immunosuppressive therapy instituted dependent on the disease.
  - Intravascular hemolysis treatment is directed at the underlying disorder.
  - Folate supplementation and iron replacement may be necessary for patients with valve hemolysis.
  - Acute intravascular hemolysis, disseminated intravascular coagulation, or acute renal failure may require transfusion support or hemodialysis.

Congestive
- Cirrhosis and portal hypertension
  - Doppler ultrasonography to assess patency of blood vessels and direction of flow
  - Treat underlying disease.
  - Consider shunt surgery or percutaneous placement of a shunt.
  - Watch for signs of hepatic encephalopathy or intestinal ischemia if thrombus involves the portal or hepatic veins.
- Congestive heart failure—low salt diet, diuretics (spironolactone), angiotensin-converting enzyme inhibitor, β-blocker, digitalis

Infiltrative
- Nonneoplastic
  - Sarcoidosis—diagnosed with chest X-ray for staging and biopsy of easily accessible sites; treatment with corticosteroid if clinically indicated

- ▲ Amyloidosis—diagnosed with clinical suspicion, fat aspiration, and protein electrophoresis
- ▲ Gaucher disease—treatment with synthetic glucocerebrosidase and symptomatic treatment, including blood transfusions for anemia and partial splenectomy for severe cardiopulmonary compromise or hypersplenism
- ■ Neoplastic
  - ▲ Lymphoma, acute and chronic lymphocytic leukemia, hairy cell leukemia, metastatic tumor
  - ▲ Treat underlying disease

THROMBOCYTOPENIA

Tait D. Shanafelt, M.D.
Rafael Fonseca, M.D.

IS THE PATIENT'S LIFE AT RISK?

- Active bleeding (i.e., gastrointestinal tract bleed) in patient with thrombocytopenia can lead to life-threatening hemorrhage.
- Platelet counts $<10 \times 10^9$/L are associated with spontaneous intracerebral hemorrhage and require immediate evaluation.
- Heparin-induced thrombocytopenia (HIT) activates platelets and is associated with potentially life-threatening thrombosis (myocardial infarction, cerebrovascular accident, deep venous thrombosis or pulmonary embolism, arterial thrombosis)
- Hemolytic uremic syndrome (HUS) and thrombotic thrombocytopenic purpura (TTP) are life-threatening conditions that cause thrombocytopenia and hemolytic anemia requiring immediate hospitalization and plasma exchange.
- Disseminated intravascular coagulation can be a life-threatening complication of tissue injury that leads to thrombosis or hemorrhage.

ADDRESSING THE RISK

In Hemorrhaging Patient

- Obtain IV access, and prepare for immediate platelet transfusion
- Immediate hematology consult
- Check PT and PTT to identify any coexisting coagulopathy
- Be mindful of possible coexistent qualitative platelet defect due to NSAID use, uremia, alcoholism, cirrhosis, myeloma,

---

Special abbreviations used in this chapter: HIT, heparin-induced thrombocytopenia; HUS, hemolytic uremic syndrome; ITP, idiopathic thrombocytopenic purpura; TTP, thrombotic thrombocytopenic purpura.

Waldenström macroglobulinemia or myeloproliferative disorders.

- Avoid invasive procedures (central catheter at noncompressible site, lumbar puncture, nasogastric tube, or surgery) in patients with platelet counts <50 × 10^9/L until platelet deficit is corrected.

In Patient With Possible HUS or TTP

- Request immediate hematology consult.
- Prepare for possible plasma exchange.

In Patient With Possible HIT

- Stop all heparin (including line flushes).
- Consider alternative anticoagulant (lepirudin, danaparoid, argatroban).
- Consult hematology.

DIFFERENTIAL DIAGNOSIS

- Rule out spurious thrombocytopenia due to platelet clumping. This can be done by reviewing the smear and drawing a repeat platelet count in a citrated tube.
- The two main causes of thrombocytopenia are production failure or destruction (Tables 1 and 2). Other causes are sequestration (Table 3) and dilution. Platelets are diluted by massive RBC transfusions.

Table 1. Decreased Platelet Production

Nutritional deficiencies:* vitamin B$_{12}$, folate
Aplastic marrow, usually pancytopenic
Myelodysplastic syndromes or leukemia
Toxin-mediated marrow suppression: alcohol, drugs
Cirrhosis
Sepsis
Medications: H$_2$-blockers, proton pump inhibitors, thiazide diuretics, many others
Viral infection: Epstein-Barr virus, HIV, hepatitis C, mumps
Myelophthisis
Congenital platelet deficiencies

*The decrease usually is moderate but can be severe.

Table 2. Destruction or Consumption of Platelets

Immune-mediated	Mechanical, consumption
Idiopathic thrombocytopenic purpura	Disseminated intravascular coagulation
Heparin-induced thrombocytopenia	Hemolytic uremic syndrome, thrombotic thrombocytopenic purpura
Treatment-induced: quinine, quinidine, valproic acid	HELLP (hemolysis, elevated liver enzymes, low platelet count) syndrome, seen in pregnancy
Evans syndrome	Endocarditis
	Prosthetic cardiac valves
	Infection: *Rickettsia* or ehrlichiosis
	Anti–phospholipid antibody syndrome
	Vasculitis

Table 3. Sequestration of Platelets

Splenomegaly—common causes include the following:
chronic myelogenous leukemia, polycythemia vera,
agnogenic myeloid metaplasia, lymphoma, Hodgkin disease,
Mycobacterium avium complex, cirrhosis with portal
hypertension, TB, malaria, histoplasmosis, endocarditis,
autoimmune hemolysis

DIFFERENTIATING THE DIFFERENTIAL

General Principles

- If thrombocytopenia began *after admission* to hospital, focus evaluation on new medications, HIT, or disseminated intravascular coagulation as cause of thrombocytopenia.
- If patient *presents* to hospital with thrombocytopenia, consider idiopathic thrombocytopenic purpura (ITP), HUS or TTP, acute leukemia, or HIV.
- An algorithm for thrombocytopenia is shown in Figure 1.

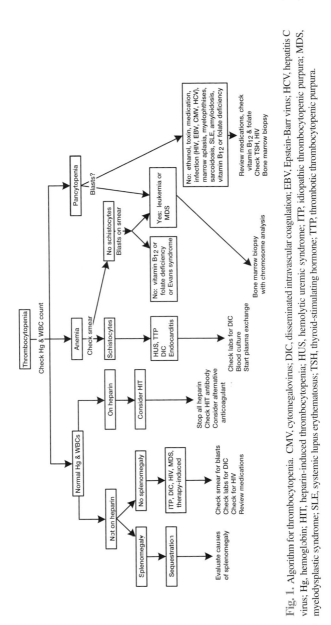

Fig. 1. Algorithm for thrombocytopenia. CMV, cytomegalovirus; DIC, disseminated intravascular coagulation; EBV, Epstein-Barr virus; HCV, hepatitis C virus; Hg, hemoglobin; HIT, heparin-induced thrombocytopenia; HUS, hemolytic uremic syndrome; ITP, idiopathic thrombocytopenic purpura; MDS, myelodysplastic syndrome; SLE, systemic lupus erythematosus; TSH, thyroid-stimulating hormone; TTP, thrombotic thrombocytopenic purpura.

History

- Personal history or family history of bleeding disorder (i.e., uncontrolled bleeding with dental procedures or previous surgical procedures)
- Menorrhagia?
- New medications: thiazide, H_2-blocker, quinidine, proton pump inhibitor, valproic acid, quinine, sulfa, gold?
- Recent viral illness (associated with ITP, aplastic anemia)?
- Diarrhea or gastrointestinal symptoms (associated with HUS)?
- Headache, confusion, somnolence? Consider intracranial bleed if platelets $<10 \times 10^9/L$.
- Identify the neurologic symptoms of TTP.
- NSAID use? Identify coexistent qualitative platelet defect.
- Is patient on heparin? Consider HIT.
- Pregnant or recent delivery? Consider HELLP syndrome.

Physical Exam

- Petechiae
- Purpura (mucous membrane purpura = "wet purpura")
- Bruising, ecchymosis
- Neurologic exam with focal deficit
- Ophthalmoscopic exam
- Stool guaiac
- Lymphadenopathy or splenomegaly

SPECIFIC THROMBOCYTOPENIC CONDITIONS

Disseminated Intravascular Coagulation

- A systemic thrombotic state triggered by tissue injury and leading to intravascular thrombosis and consumption of clotting factors
- Patients become coagulopathic secondary to consumption of coagulation factors and may subsequently bleed.
- Diagnosis is suggested clinically by diffuse oozing or overt hemorrhage at surgical sites and line sites.
- Patient may have simultaneous evidence of thrombosis (skin necrosis, digital ischemia, deep venous thrombosis, myocardial infarction) and bleeding.

- *Presence of soluble fibrin monomers is the most specific lab finding.*
- Lab findings of increased INR, increased PTT, and positive D-dimer support the diagnosis.
- Peripheral blood smear may or may not show schistocytes.
- Four principle underlying causes of disseminated intravascular coagulation
  - ▲ Sepsis, infection
  - ▲ Tissue injury: ischemia, trauma, pancreatitis
  - ▲ Malignancy
  - ▲ Obstetric complications

HUS or TTP
- HUS or TTP is an inflammatory state characterized by endothelial injury leading to formation of microthrombi and fibrin strands in small blood vessels.
  - ▲ Pathophysiology—thought to be a deficiency or absence of metalloprotease enzymes that cleave von Willebrand factor. Without these cleaving enzymes, large von Willebrand multimers accumulate, leading to endothelial injury that initiates thrombosis.
  - ▲ HUS or TTP causes thrombocytopenia secondary to platelet consumption and anemia secondary to fragmentation of erythrocytes by fibrin strands in microvasculature.
  - ▲ Majority of patients with TTP *do not* have the full clinical pentad: fever, thrombocytopenia, microangiopathic hemolytic anemia, renal disease (ranging from microscopic hematuria to acute renal failure), and neurologic symptoms (headache, confusion, seizure).
  - ▲ Only requirements for the diagnosis and the only requirements to initiate empiric treatment (plasma exchange) while work-up is pursued: microangiopathic hemolytic anemia and thrombocytopenia
  - ▲ Without plasma exchange, mortality approaches 90%, but with treatment it is reduced to 20%-25%.
  - ▲ HUS is associated with *E. coli* O157:H7 infection.
  - ▲ TTP can be idiopathic, medication-induced (clopidogrel, ticlopidine, mitomycin C), or hereditary.

HIT
- Two types of HIT

- ▲ Type I
  - Benign
  - Characterized by mild decrease (20%-30%) in platelet count caused by platelet agglutination that typically occurs within first 48 hours after heparin exposure
  - Occurs in 20% of patients exposed to heparin
  - No important clinical sequellae of type I HIT
  - Does not require cessation of heparin therapy
- ▲ Type II
  - Caused by immune-mediated platelet destruction due to heparin exposure
  - Pathophysiology—thought to be secondary to immune-mediated consumption of platelets due to IgG antibody that reacts to heparin bound to platelet factor 4 antigen.
  - *In addition to causing platelet destruction, antibodies activate platelets, leading to major thrombotic (80% venous, 20% arterial) complications.* This immune-mediated reaction occurs in 1% of persons exposed to heparin.
  - Type II HIT typically occurs after 4-5 days of heparin exposure but can occur in <12 hours if person was exposed to heparin in the last 100 days.
- ■ HIT is a clinical diagnosis based on thrombocytopenia developing after exposure to heparin.
  - ▲ Characterized by a 50% decrease or $>100 \times 10^9$/L decrease in platelets
  - ▲ Lab testing (presence of anti-platelet factor 4 antibody) has good specificity and can support diagnosis of type II HIT, but low sensitivity and long processing time make HIT a clinical diagnosis.

ITP

- ■ Diagnosis of exclusion and can be made only after other causes of thrombocytopenia (problems with production, destruction, or sequestration) have been excluded.
- ■ Cause—anti-platelet antibodies leading to immune-mediated platelet destruction.
- ■ Anti-platelet antibody testing has poor sensitivity and specificity and is not indicated in the work-up or diagnosis of ITP.

- Rule out HIV in patients with risk factors.
- Bone marrow biopsy should be performed before ITP is diagnosed in patients older than 60 and in younger patients if the diagnosis is unclear.

TESTS AND WORK-UP

Everyone

- CBC with differential count (note: automated platelet count is inaccurate if count is $<10 \times 10^9/L$)
- Blood smear—critical component of work-up of thrombocytopenia
  - ▲ Rule out platelet clumping.
  - ▲ Schistocytes indicate TTP or HUS, disseminated intravascular coagulation, or endocarditis
  - ▲ Blasts indicate acute leukemia or myelodysplastic syndrome; next step is order bone marrow biopsy
- Creatinine—may be increased in HUS or TTP
- Urinalysis—microscopic hematuria in HUS or TTP

Febrile?

- Consider HUS/TTP, subacute bacterial endocarditis, disseminated intravascular coagulation
- Blood culture to identify possible endocarditis
- PT, PTT, D-dimer, soluble fibrin monomers to identify disseminated intravascular coagulation
- Consider echocardiography if new murmur or risk factors for endocarditis.
- Stool culture for *E. coli* O157:H7

Other

- Possible ITP
  - ▲ Check HIV test.
  - ▲ Bone marrow biopsy in patients older than 60
- Neurologic symptoms
  - ▲ CT of head to rule out intracranial bleed
  - ▲ Consider TTP.
- Blasts on peripheral smear—bone marrow biopsy
- On heparin—test for HIT antibody.
- Other considerations—vitamin B_{12}, folate, thyroid-stimulating hormone (rarely cause platelets <50,000 by themselves)
- Unclear cause—bone marrow biopsy

MANAGEMENT

General

- Risk of bleeding or hemorrhage with surgery or trauma increases with platelets $<50\text{-}100 \times 10^9/L$.
- Avoid invasive procedures until platelet count is corrected.
- Transfusion thresholds
    - Platelets $<10 \times 10^9/L$—Transfuse platelets in all patients, with possible exception of ITP (see ITP below).
    - Bleeding patient—Transfuse platelet count to $>50 \times 10^9/L$.
    - Preoperative
        - General surgery—Transfuse platelet count to $>50 \times 10^9/L$.
        - Neurosurgery or ophthalmologic surgery—Transfuse platelet count to $>100 \times 10^9/L$.

Disseminated Intravascular Coagulation

- Supportive care
- Identify and treat underlying cause.
- Most authorities believe transfusing platelets and fresh frozen plasma "fuels the fire" by enhancing cytokine cascade: *avoid transfusion unless active hemorrhage.*
- In refractory disseminated intravascular coagulation with thrombotic or hemorrhagic complications, some hematologists begin heparin therapy while simultaneously giving fresh frozen plasma. The intent of this counterintuitive approach is to use heparin to arrest the prothrombotic state while simultaneously replacing depleted coagulation factors to prevent hemorrhage. This approach requires technical expertise and experience in treating disseminated intravascular coagulation and should be initiated under the direction of a hematologist.

HUS or TTP

- Stop clopidogrel and ticlopidine.
- Stop nephrotoxic medications.
- Hydrate
- *Prepare for immediate plasma exchange* (consult hematology and nephrology).

- If no plasma exchange at your center, give 4 units fresh frozen plasma, and arrange for immediate transfer.
- Microangiopathic hemolytic anemia (i.e., schistocytes on peripheral blood smear) and thrombocytopenia are only requirements to initiate plasma exchange while work-up is pursued.
- Value of adding corticosteroids to plasma exchange is debated but usually recommended initially (IV methylprednisolone).
- Follow daily LDH and platelet counts while patient has plasma exchange.
- Generally, patients receive daily plasma exchange until platelets $>150 \times 10^9$/L and LDH is normal and then can be considered for tapering of frequency of plasma exchange.

HIT
- Stop *all* heparin (including line flushes).
- Do *not* convert to low-molecular-weight heparin (20%-30% cross-reactivity of antibodies).
- Evaluate for symptoms or physical exam findings of arterial (myocardial infarction, cerebrovascular accident) or venous (deep venous thrombosis, pulmonary embolism) thrombosis.
- Test for HIT antibody (ELISA-based anti-platelet factor 4 antibody).
- Studies suggest discontinuation of heparin alone may not be adequate to decrease risk of thrombosis and recommend alternative anticoagulation for *all* patients with HIT—even those without thrombosis at time of diagnosis.
- Consult hematology for other options for anticoagulation (i.e., lepirudin, argatroban, danaparoid).

ITP
- Start prednisone, 1 mg/kg
- Patients with ITP generally respond poorly to platelet transfusions, and their remaining platelets are large and hyperfunctional.
- General principle—Avoid platelet transfusions in ITP patients.
- Splenectomy for refractory ITP
- IV immunoglobulin or anti-D immunoglobulin (Whinrho) can be used to temporarily maintain platelet count before splenectomy.
- Consult hematology.

Splenomegaly
- Identify the cause.
  - ▲ Most common cause varies by population studied.
  - ▲ For patients at risk for HIV, *Mycobacterium avium* complex, TB, or other infection is most likely cause.
  - ▲ In general population, chronic myelogenous leukemia, lymphoma, polycythemia vera/myeloproliferative disorder, or cirrhosis with portal hypertension is most likely cause.
  - ▲ In immigrants, consider malaria, TB, leishmaniasis.
- Role of splenectomy for treatment depends on underlying process and severity of thrombocytopenia.
- Consult hematology if splenectomy is considered.

TREMOR AND MOVEMENT DISORDERS

Matthew L. Flaherty, M.D.
Andrea C. Adams, M.D.

IS THE PATIENT'S LIFE AT RISK?

- The most common causes of tremor and movement disorder (including ataxia in this chapter) usually are not acutely life threatening. However, several less common conditions may be rapidly fatal or debilitating and should be considered.

Three Disorders of Neuromuscular Rigidity

Neuroleptic Malignant Syndrome

- Idiosyncratically induced by dopamine blockers, including neuroleptics (antipsychotics) and antiemetics (e.g., promethazine)
- Characteristics—muscular rigidity, involuntary movement, unstable blood pressure, decreased mental status, fever
- Mortality up to 30%

Malignant Hyperthermia

- Disorder of excessive muscle contraction leading to hyperthermia, most often associated with succinylcholine and halothane anesthesia
- Responsible gene defect is often familial

Tetanus

- Caused by wound contamination with *Clostridium tetani*, which produces the neurotoxin tetanospasmin
- Occurs in unimmunized or underimmunized person
- Typical incubation period: 7-21 days (range, 5 days-15 weeks)
- Often begins with stiff jaw (trismus), stiff neck, dysphagia, and irritability
- Progresses to generalized rigidity and muscle spasms triggered by minor stimuli

Three Causes of Ataxia
Cerebellar Hemorrhage
- Acute onset of ataxia (particularly gait), often with headache, vertigo, vomiting, decreased mental status, variable ocular signs (including ipsilateral cranial nerve VI palsy), nuchal rigidity
- Excessive intracranial pressure may cause brainstem compression and death.

Wernicke Encephalopathy
- Classic triad: gait ataxia, ophthalmoplegia, confusion
- Nystagmus is often present
- Associated with alcoholism, caused by thiamine deficiency
- If inadequately treated, may progress to chronic amnestic state, Korsakoff psychosis
- Death is usually due to associated illnesses (e.g., hepatic failure, infection)

Drug Toxicity
- Phenytoin, carbamazepine, valproic acid, lithium, alcohol, benzodiazepines, other sedatives
- Overdose may lead to hemodynamic instability, pulmonary insufficiency, seizures, or dangerous falls

Two Causes of Tremor
Drug Toxicity
- Lithium, valproic acid, stimulants (including cocaine and amphetamine)
- Classically produces "action tremor," which increases as outstretched hand approaches a target

Drug Withdrawal
- Remember the "3 Bs" of fatal withdrawal: booze (ethanol), benzodiazepines, barbiturates.
- Consider hepatic encephalopathy as cause of decreased mental status and movement disorder (especially asterixis) because benzodiazepines make the condition of these patients worse.

ADDRESSING THE RISK
- Pay attention to airway, breathing, and circulation and general medical management. Patients with above conditions often require monitoring in ICU.

Specific Management Points

Neuroleptic Malignant Syndrome

- Withdraw dopamine blockers, lithium, anticholinergics.
- Use antipyretics and cooling as necessary.
- Monitor serum electrolytes (potassium, calcium, phosphorus), renal function, urine output, CK levels, acid-base balance (remember to correct arterial blood gas values for temperature), and CBC.
- Causes of death—renal failure, electrolyte imbalance with arrhythmia, coagulopathy, others
- Pharmacologic treatment with bromocriptine or dantrolene

Malignant Hyperthermia

- Monitor as for neuroleptic malignant syndrome.
- Treat with dantrolene.
- Anesthesiologists are usually familiar with diagnosis and treatment.

Tetanus

- Tetanus immune globulin, 500 units IM, followed by tetanus toxoid immunization at a different site
- Consider surgical debridement of causative wounds.
- Use penicillin, metronidazole, or other antibiotic appropriate for *Clostridium* infection.
- Mild sedation with benzodiazepines to reduce spasms
- Assess respiratory status frequently; mechanical ventilation may be needed.

Cerebellar Hemorrhage

- If concerned about cerebellar hemorrhage, CT of head
- If hemorrhage is confirmed, urgent neurosurgical consultation (decompression can be life saving)

Wernicke Encephalopathy

- Immediate treatment—thiamine, 50-100 mg IV immediately + 50 mg PO/IM per day for 3 days
- Provide balanced diet and multivitamin.
- Always administer thiamine when giving glucose to

alcoholics or poorly nourished persons because glucose alone may precipitate Wernicke encephalopathy.

Drug Toxicity
- Check drug levels if available—ethanol, phenytoin, carbamazepine, valproic acid, lithium.
- Consult poison control or emergency department physician for overdose management.

Drug Withdrawal
- Monitor vital signs, agitation level, mental status.
- Standardized rating scales (often performed by nursing at frequent intervals) are useful.
- Treatment
  - ▲ Benzodiazepine taper (usually lorazepam or chlordiazepoxide) for ethanol and benzodiazepine withdrawal
  - ▲ Barbiturates (usually pentobarbital or phenobarbital) for barbiturate withdrawal

DIFFERENTIAL DIAGNOSIS
Definitions
- Akathisia—subjective feeling of motor restlessness, classically produced by dopamine blockers (e.g., antipsychotic and antiemetic medications), sometimes confused with psychotic agitation
- Ataxia—muscular incoordination, variously manifested in limbs, head, trunk, or gait
- Athetosis—ceaseless, slow, involuntary writhing movements, especially the hands
- Ballismus—violent, flinging movements of limbs caused by contraction of proximal muscles
- Chorea—continual, complex, rapid movements that appear coordinated but are involuntary
- Clonus—movement marked by contractions and relaxations of a muscle occurring in rapid succession; typically associated with spasticity and upper motor neuron damage
- Dyskinesia—general (nonspecific) term for abnormal, involuntary, hyperkinetic movements
- Dystonia—dyskinetic movements or abnormal postures caused by disordered muscle tone

- Myoclonus—sudden, shocklike contractions of a muscle or muscle group causing a focal or generalized jerk
- Tics—rapid, stereotyped, patterned movements under partial voluntary control
- Tremor—involuntary, rhythmic trembling caused by alternating contraction and relaxation of opposing muscle groups
  - ▲ Action tremor—tremor most prominent when a limb is being used (sometimes applied to "postural tremor")
  - ▲ Intention tremor—usually a description of ataxic limb movements, thus not a true tremor; as the patient's hand approaches a target, it wavers erratically (failed motor compensation for inaccuracy)
  - ▲ Postural tremor—tremor noticeable when a limb is held in a stationary, usually outstretched, posture
  - ▲ Resting tremor—tremor most prominent with limb at rest, often dampens with voluntary limb movement

DIFFERENTIATING THE DIFFERENTIAL
- Conditions associated with tremor, chorea, myoclonus, and dystonia are listed in Table 1.

Tremor
Parkinson Disease
- Classic triad: resting tremor, bradykinesia, rigidity
- Often an unsteady, stooped gait with small steps (festinating gait)
- Masked facies, micrographia
- Generally responsive to levodopa

"Parkinson Plus" Syndromes (Progressive Supranuclear Palsy, Multiple System Atrophy, Others)
- Involve parkinsonism and other neurologic deficits
- Levodopa is less efficacious than in Parkinson disease
- Progressive supranuclear palsy—impaired vertical gaze, dysarthria, dysphagia
- Multiple system atrophy may include autonomic failure, lower motor neuron signs, ataxia

Table 1. Conditions Associated With Tremor, Chorea, Myoclonus, and Dystonia

Tremor
- Parkinson disease
- Parkinsonism
    - Drugs: dopamine antagonists
    - Progressive supra-nuclear palsy
    - Multiple system atrophy
    - Stroke or other disease of basal ganglia
- Physiologic tremor
    - Drug-enhanced
        - Caffeine
        - Theophylline
        - Prednisone
        - Amphetamine
        - Lithium
        - Tricyclics
    - Other enhancers
        - Drug withdrawal
        - Thyrotoxicosis
        - Hypoglycemia
        - Pheochromocytoma
        - Emotion
- Essential tremor

Myoclonus
- Myoclonic epilepsy
- Anoxic brain injury
- Hepatic failure (asterixis is sometimes described as "negative" myoclonus)
- Uremia
- Meningitis
- Encephalitis
- Cephalosporin/penicillin

Tics
- Tourette syndrome
- "Benign" habit spasms

Chorea
- Huntington chorea
- Sydenham chorea
- Chorea gravidarum
- Senile chorea
- Creutzfeldt-Jakob disease
- Wilson disease
- Stroke
- Systemic lupus erythematosus
- Cerebral palsy
- Thyrotoxicosis
- Polycythemia vera
- Hyperosmolar, nonketotic hyperglycemia
- Carbon monoxide poisoning
- Drugs
    - Birth control pills
    - Anticonvulsants
    - Stimulants
    - Anticholinergics
    - Antidepressants
    - Dopamine agonists
    - Dopamine antagonists

Rigidity
- Neuroleptic malignant syndrome
- Malignant hyperthermia
- Tetanus
- Strychnine poisoning
- Severe parkinsonism
- Stiff-person syndrome
- Psychiatric illness

Ballismus
- Subthalamic nucleus infarction or injury

Table 1 (continued)

Dystonia	**Ataxia** (acute or subacute onset)
Drugs (often an acute dystonic reaction)	Cerebellar infarction or hemorrhage
Dopamine antagonists	Brainstem infarction or hemorrhage
Dopamine agonists	Hydrocephalus (including normal-pressure hydrocephalus)
Antidepressants (tricyclics, lithium)	Tumor
Certain antihistamines	Progressive multifocal leukoencephalopathy
Cocaine	Multiple sclerosis
Idiopathic (primary dystonias)	Abscess
Focal dystonias (e.g., torticollis, writer's cramp)	Viral cerebellitis (in children)
Head trauma	Nutritional deficiency (vitamin B_{12}, thiamine)
Anoxia	Paraneoplastic syndromes
Meningitis	Drug toxicity (ethanol, lithium, phenytoin, barbiturates, carbamazepine, valproic acid, mercury, toluene)
AIDS (toxoplasmosis, progressive multifocal leukoencephalopathy)	
Hereditary/degenerative disease (Wilson disease, Parkinson disease, Huntington disease, progressive supranuclear palsy)	

Essential Tremor

- Familial form is autosomal dominant
- May involve arms, head, or voice
- Action tremor without other neurologic impairment
- Suppressed temporarily by ethanol

Physiologic Tremor

- Usually a fine postural tremor
- Often improves with β_2-blockade

Chorea
Wilson Disease

- Can present as chorea or various other movement disorders

- Mental status change, psychiatric disturbance, hepatitis, cirrhosis, dysarthria may accompany or precede the movement disorder
- If young patient, a high level of suspicion is required.

Huntington Disease
- Autosomal dominant inheritance
- Psychiatric disturbance may occur before chorea.

Dystonia
Acute Dystonic Reaction
- Produces variable abnormal and uncomfortable postures, sometimes including oculogyric crisis
- Typically follows new administration of a dopamine blocker
- Most common in young adults

Ataxia
Normal-Pressure Hydrocephalus
- Classic triad: dementia, gait ataxia, urinary incontinence
- Head imaging shows dilated ventricles, but CSF pressure is normal.
- May improve after lumbar puncture

Multiple Sclerosis
- History may suggest previous (sometimes transient) neurologic impairment.
- Involvement of two separate neural systems of central nervous system at two separate times is required for diagnosis.
- MRI often shows white matter lesions but findings are nonspecific

TEST ORDERING
CT of Head
- Useful in acute situations such as ischemic or hemorrhagic stroke
- Can define mass lesions and hydrocephalus
- Usually available on urgent or emergent basis
- Currently the first choice for initial stroke imaging (because of its speed and sensitivity for hemorrhage)
- Low yield for most movement disorders

MRI of Head

- More useful than CT for evaluating nonhemorrhagic ischemia, demyelinating disease, disease of posterior fossa (brainstem and cerebellum)
- Emergent availability of MRI is less than for CT
- Requires prolonged patient immobolization

Drug Levels

- Should be determined as applicable

Serum Creatinine and BUN

- An increase points to uremia as the cause.

CSF

- Should be examined if meningitis or encephalitis is suspected (usually after CT to rule out mass effect)

EEG

- Useful when epileptic movements are a consideration

Thyroid-Stimulating Hormone and Glucose

- Check levels when evaluating enhanced physiologic tremor.

Wilson Screen

- All children and young adults with hyperkinetic movement disorders should have screening test for Wilson disease.
- Initial tests—liver enzymes, serum ceruloplasmin, 24-hour urine for copper, ophthalmologic exam for Kayser-Fleischer rings

MANAGEMENT

Parkinson Disease

- Often managed by neurologists
- Many dopamine agonists and anticholinergic agents are available for treatment.
- Excessive dopamine may cause dystonia, chorea, hallucinations, or sleep disturbance.
- Treatment of psychosis in Parkinson patients should *not* include

traditional neuroleptics; low-dose atypical neuroleptics such as quetiapine (Seroquel) are less likely to worsen rigidity or tremor.

Drug-Induced Parkinsonism
- Withdraw the offending drug.
- If withdrawal is not possible, addition of anticholinergic (benztropine, trihexyphenidyl) may reduce symptoms.
- Anticholinergics may cause cardiac dysfunction, urinary retention, and confusion, especially in elderly patients.

Acute Dystonic Reactions
- Withdraw the offending drug.
- IV diphenhydramine or benztropine is often promptly effective.

Essential Tremor
- β-Blocker therapy (propranolol), be careful if patient has respiratory disease, congestive heart failure, or hypotension
- Second-line agent—primidone

Restless Legs Syndrome
- Treatment—nighttime dopamine agonists (levodopa/carbidopa [Sinemet], pramipexole [Mirapex], ropinirole [Requip]), clonazepam, or opiates (propoxyphene, codeine)

Wilson Disease
- If diagnosis is confirmed, treatment involves copper chelation, usually with penicillamine, which has many side effects.

Tourette Syndrome
- Clonidine is sometimes used but is seldom effective.
- In severe cases, treatment with small oral doses of haloperidol or pimozide is often helpful.
- Pimozide may prolong QT interval dangerously.
- Tardive dyskinesia is serious potential side effect of neuroleptic use.

ARTERIAL BLOOD GASES

Grace K. Dy, M.D.
Kaiser G. Lim, M.D.

BLOOD GAS VALUES

- Arterial pH — 7.35-7.45
- Arterial oxygen pressure (PaO_2) — 75-100 mm Hg
- Arterial carbon dioxide pressure ($PaCO_2$) — 35-45 mm Hg
- Arterial oxygen saturation (SaO_2) — 95%-100%
- Mixed venous oxygen pressure (PvO_2) — 38-42 mm Hg
- Mixed venous oxygen saturation ($S\bar{v}O_2$) — 70%-75%

INDICATIONS

- To assess adequacy of oxygenation for diagnostic and therapeutic purposes
- To determine adequacy of ventilation or carbon dioxide clearance
- To assess acid-base status

OXYGENATION VARIABLES

- Arterial oxygen saturation (SaO_2)
- Arterial oxygen content (CaO_2)
- Arterial oxygen pressure (PaO_2)
- Arterial carbon dioxide pressure ($PaCO_2$)
- Alveolar-arterial oxygen gradient [$P(A-a)O_2$]
- Arterial-alveolar oxygen ratio (PaO_2/PAO_2)
- PaO_2/FIO_2 ratio (FIO_2 = fraction of inspired oxygen)

Arterial Oxygen Saturation (SaO_2)

- Oxygen saturation of hemoglobin varies with PaO_2.
- With the sigmoid characteristic of oxygen saturation curve,

---

Special abbreviations used in this chapter: ABG, arterial blood gas; V/Q, ventilation-perfusion.

the plateau phase is reached at a partial pressure of oxygen (pO_2) of 60 mm Hg (SaO_2 of 90%).
- Practical and most important measurement in titrating oxygen therapy: component in determining oxygen content
- Inability to maintain SaO_2 >90% is considered an indication for oxygen supplementation and, in the acute setting, mechanical ventilation.
- Except in methemoglobinemia, sulfhemoglobinemia, certain hemoglobinopathies, and carbon monoxide poisoning, measured oxygen saturation mirrors measured PaO_2.
- Hemoglobin levels do not affect SaO_2.
    - ▲ Anemia causes dyspnea by decreased oxygen carrying capacity and delivery to peripheral tissues.
- SaO_2 can be measured with carbon monoxide oximeters and modern arterial blood gas (ABG) machines

Arterial Oxygen Content (CaO_2)
- Minimal information needed to assess adequacy of oxygenation and to guide oxygen therapy
- A vital component in determining what we can control for tissue perfusion
- Oxygen delivery depends on both CaO_2 and cardiac output
- $CaO_2 = 1.39 \times SaO_2 \times$ hemoglobin $+ 0.0031$ (PaO_2)
- Normal value, 18-21 mL O_2/dL
- Hemoglobin is equally important because most of the oxygen is transported bound to hemoglobin.
- CaO_2 does not measure peripheral tissue oxygenation, which is the ultimate goal. It is not sufficient for assessing patients with critical illnesses, e.g., shock, sepsis, or compromised cardiac function.

Arterial Oxygen Pressure (PaO_2)
- *Reflects* alveolar oxygen pressure (PAO_2) and the alveolar air-pulmonary capillary interface
- *Not* affected by hemoglobin levels
- PaO_2 does not have a linear relation with SaO_2.
- Decreases by 1.2 mm Hg for every 1 mm Hg increase in $PaCO_2$
- Reduced pulmonary diffusing capacity does not always result in clinically important *resting* hypoxemia. However, it can contribute to hypoxemia during exercise.

- Decreases with age as a result of shifts in ventilation-perfusion ($\dot{V}/\dot{Q}$) ratios in the aging lung
- Simple way to estimate age-dependent norm at room air:

$$Pao_2 = 100 - (age/3)$$

Alveolar Oxygen (Pao_2) Equation
- $Pao_2 = Fio_2 (PB - 47) - (Paco_2 \times 1.2)$ (for $Fio_2 <0.60$)
- $Pao_2 = Fio_2 (PB - 47) - Paco_2$ (for $Fio_2 \geq 0.60$)
  where PB is barometric pressure (760 mm Hg at sea level) and water vapor pressure is 47 mm Hg when fully saturated at 37°C

Significance
- Low barometric pressure results in a low Pao_2 if Fio_2 remains constant.
- Low Fio_2 (e.g., mouth-to-mouth ventilation) results in a low Pao_2
- Increasing $Paco_2$ decreases Pao_2 (and vice versa).

Alveolar-Arterial O_2 Gradient [$P(A-a)O_2$]
- $P(A-a)O_2 = Pao_2 - Pao_2$
- Used to evaluate adequacy of oxygen transfer
- Varies with age, increasing after age 40
- Predicted A-a O_2 gradient at room air with adjustment for age:

$$Age/4 + 4$$

- $P(A-a)O_2$ determination is most useful when Fio_2 is 0.21.
- Thus, normal $P(A-a)O_2$ value is both age- and Fio_2-dependent.

  For Fio_2 of 21%, 5-25 mm Hg
  For Fio_2 of 100%, <150 mm Hg

- A large A-a gradient with patient receiving 100% supplemental oxygen reflects either a physiologic or anatomical shunt (e.g., left-to-right heart shunt)
- A normal A-a gradient (5-25 mm Hg on room air) indicates that hypoxemia is due to hypoventilation or low Fio_2.
  However, prolonged hypoventilation can lead to areas of atelectasis and thus an increase in the A-a gradient.

Arterial-Alveolar O_2 Ratio

- An alternative to $P(A-a)O_2$ for evaluating adequacy of oxygen transfer
- With increasing FIO_2, PaO_2/PAO_2 varies much less than $P(A-a)O_2$.
- This is a more stable variable, remaining fairly constant with increasing FIO_2 as long as the underlying lung condition does not vary; hence, it is useful in the short term (hourly) and in assessment of oxygenation.
- Normal PaO_2/PAO_2 ranges from 0.74 in elderly people to about 0.9 in young subjects (usual range, 0.77-0.82)
- Most reliable when FIO_2 is <0.55

PaO_2/FIO_2 Ratio

- Another alternative to $P(A-a)O_2$ for evaluating adequacy of oxygen transfer
- Obviates need to calculate PAO_2
- Is used as part of the diagnostic criteria for acute lung injury (<300) and acute respiratory distress syndrome (<200 regardless of positive end-expiratory pressure level)
- Most reliably assessed at an FIO_2 of ≥0.5
- Limitation—does not account for $PaCO_2$, but this is not important at high FIO_2.
- Normal PaO_2/FIO_2 by age
  - ▲ ≤60 years: 400-500
  - ▲ >60 years: $400 - [5 (age - 60)]$

VENTILATORY VARIABLE
Arterial Pressure of Carbon Dioxide ($PaCO_2$)

- Necessary for evaluating oxygenation (alveolar oxygen equation)
- Reflects adequacy of alveolar ventilation relative to carbon dioxide production
- An important component of acid-base balance (Henderson-Hasselbalch equation)
- Never diffusion-limited
- Increased physiologic dead space, resulting from V/Q mismatch or severe restrictive disease, is a more common cause of increased $PaCO_2$ than hypoventilation.

In a Nutshell

- In the acute setting, if the saturation is ≤90% on room air, order an ABG.
    - ▲ Confirm hypoxia and rule out possible causes (Fig. 1).
    - ▲ First, rule out acute hypercapnia (i.e., respiratory failure)
    - ▲ Second, observe response to supplemental oxygen (V/Q mismatch vs. shunt)
    - ▲ If hypercapnia is not a problem, oxygen titration can be done while monitoring saturation.
    - ▲ If hypercapnia is a problem (e.g., COPD), monitor oxygen supplementation with another ABG 10-15 minutes after change in therapy.

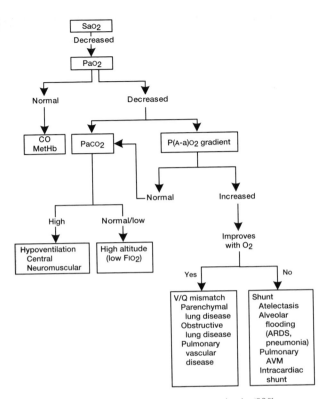

Fig. 1. Algorithm for work-up if oxygen saturation is ≤90% on room air. ARDS, acute respiratory distress syndrome; AVM, arteriovenous malformation; CO, carbon monoxide toxicity; FIO_2, fraction of inspired oxygen; MetHb, methemoglobinemia; SaO_2, arterial oxygen saturation; V/Q, ventilation/perfusion.

CARDIAC BIOMARKERS

R. Scott Wright, M.D.
Dariush S. Takhtehchian, M.D.
Joseph G. Murphy, M.D.

PATHOPHYSIOLOGY OF INCREASED CARDIAC ENZYME LEVELS

- Acute coronary occlusion interrupts blood flow to the myocardium and causes necrosis of myocytes, which leads to loss of cell membrane integrity and release of cellular macromolecules. Myocyte necrosis results in the appearance of biomarkers in the plasma.

CLINICAL IMPORTANCE

- Allows for early diagnosis of acute myocardial infarction (MI)
- Cardiac enzymes differentiate between
  - ▲ Non–ST-segment elevation MI—increased serum markers
  - ▲ Unstable angina—no serum markers released
- Cardiac enzymes provide risk stratification and prognostic information in acute coronary syndromes (e.g., high early levels predict more complications).

TYPES OF CARDIAC BIOMARKERS

- Troponin (Table 1)
  - ▲ Cardiac-specific subtypes (I, T) are measured by current assays.
  - ▲ Accuracy depends partly on assay coefficient of variation (<10% ideal).
  - ▲ Most accurate and specific measure of myocyte necrosis
  - ▲ Appears in plasma 2-4 hours after onset of necrosis
  - ▲ May remain elevated for days
  - ▲ Very sensitive bioassay; may be elevated in conditions other than acute MI, such as congestive heart failure, pul-

Special abbreviation used in this chapter: MI, myocardial infarction.

Table 1. Differential Diagnosis of Elevated Cardiac Troponins

Acute myocardial infarction; there is a rapid rise and fall in levels in patients with cardiac ischemia

Congestive heart failure or circulatory volume overload

Pulmonary embolism

Hypertensive crisis

Infiltrative cardiomyopathies

Myocarditis or myopericarditis

Cardiac injury secondary to chemotherapy or other toxins

Hypotensive spell with "watershed territory"-associated myocyte necrosis

Anemia with "watershed territory"-associated myocyte necrosis

Septic or hypovolemic shock with associated myocyte necrosis

Valvular heart disease-associated myocyte necrosis from pressure and/or volume overload

Pressor agent-associated myocyte necrosis

Apical ballooning syndrome

monary embolism, hypertensive crisis, myocarditis, myopericarditis, traumatic injury, and drug toxicity
  ▲ Troponin I and troponin T are both useful and equal in diagnostic utility.
  ▲ Not elevated in renal failure per se, but is a high-risk marker when elevated in patients with renal failure
- CK, CK-MB
  ▲ Muscle enzyme expressed in skeletal, cardiac, and smooth muscle types
  ▲ CK-MB is highly expressed in cardiac myocytes.
  ▲ Appears in plasma 4-6 hours after onset of myocyte necrosis
  ▲ Equal sensitivity to cardiac troponins but less specific
  ▲ Can be elevated from skeletal muscle injury and after operations on organs that express CK-MB
- Myoglobin
  ▲ A heme protein found in many tissues
  ▲ Elevated very early after onset of myocyte necrosis, appearing as early as 90 minutes after symptom onset in one study
  ▲ Not specific for the heart and may be elevated for other

reasons

- ▲ Release and metabolism may follow an undulating pattern and so may be at a nadir when measured, masking diagnosis of acute MI.
- ▲ Should be used in combination with troponin for diagnosis of acute MI

- ■ C-reactive protein
  - ▲ Inflammatory marker protein, elevated in many conditions
  - ▲ Excellent marker for future cardiovascular risk when elevated (≥3 mg/L) in patients with no underlying inflammatory or malignant conditions
  - ▲ Treatment options—aspirin, statin, lipid-lowering therapy, weight loss, regular exercise, more aggressive control of diabetes

- ■ B-type natriuretic peptide
  - ▲ Released from cardiac myocytes (ventricular >> atrial) secondary to increased filling pressures and in congestive heart failure and restrictive cardiomyopathies
  - ▲ Very sensitive diagnostic marker for acute heart failure
  - ▲ Confers prognostic information in acute coronary syndromes

CHEST X-RAY

Sean M. Caples, D.O.
Edward C. Rosenow III, M.D.

BASIC APPROACH

- The importance of a thorough review of a chest X-ray—Up to 19% of lung cancers of any size and 90% of early (<1 cm) peripheral solitary lung cancers are missed on chest X-rays.
- Primary care providers should develop a comfort level for viewing chest X-rays of all their patients.
- The key to interpreting a chest X-ray is to read hundreds of normal ones. With experience, you will recognize abnormalities more readily, even without knowing what the abnormality is.
- Read the chest X-ray before you read the radiologist's report. It has been estimated that radiologists miss 10%-15% of abnormalities on chest X-rays.
- Describe what you see without necessarily making a diagnosis immediately.
- Do not concentrate on a single abnormality; there may be others.
- Make every attempt to compare a new film with old films.
- Begin by looking at the X-ray from 6-8 feet away.
- Never accept the reading of a chest X-ray as "normal."
- Assess the technical adequacy of the study.
  - ▲ Be sure the entire thorax is seen.
  - ▲ Check the symmetry of the clavicle to assess patient rotation.
  - ▲ With proper X-ray penetration, the lower thoracic vertebrae behind the heart should be faintly visible.
- A bright or "hot" light may be helpful for faint or underpenetrated exams.
- Develop your own systematic review of chest X-rays and be consistent. Use whatever system you are comfortable with,

but be sure to include
- ▲ Chest wall
- ▲ Lung parenchyma and large airways
- ▲ Mediastinum

Chest Wall
- Look for pleural thickening or calcification.
- Costophrenic angles are normally sharp (200-400 mL of pleural fluid is required to blunt the angles).
- Diaphragm
  - ▲ Right hemidiaphragm is normally higher than the left
  - ▲ Subpulmonic effusion may resemble an elevated diaphragm without blunting of the costophrenic angles (decubitus film may be required to demonstrate effusion).
- Bony abnormalities (metastases), rib notching (coarctation), extrathoracic soft tissues (neck, tracheal masses), shoulder joints

Lung Parenchyma and Airways
- Comparing left and right symmetry is most helpful.
- About 15% of the lung parenchyma is hidden by cardiovascular structures and the left diaphragm on front view X-rays; lateral films are helpful in identifying lesions hidden in this area.
- Look carefully behind the heart, diaphragm, and mediastinal structures.
- Carefully scan the apices under the clavicles and first rib.
- Try not to overinterpret interstitial markings, which may be accentuated by a submaximal inspiration. (If inspiration was adequate, it should be possible to count 10 ribs above the right costophrenic sulcus.)
- Normal lung markings (which are predominantly vascular structures) should disappear within about 1 cm of the pleural surface; visible markings extending to the pleura suggests an abnormality (e.g., Kerley B lines); compare the new film with old films.

Mediastinum
- Familiarize yourself with the normal silhouette.
- The left hilus is up to 3 cm superior to the right hilus in 95% of normal persons. An elevated right hilus may suggest volume loss on that side.

- Know the mediastinal compartments and common abnormalities of each.
  - ▲ Superior—thyroid, aortic arch aneurysm
  - ▲ Anterior—neoplasms of various origins
  - ▲ Middle—lymph nodes, heart, great vessels, esophagus
  - ▲ Posterior—neurogenic tumors
- Anteroposterior (portable) films magnify heart size and mediastinum
- CT usually is needed to further characterize mediastinal abnormalities.

SOME PATTERNS OF ABNORMALITIES

Airspace-Filling Disorders

- These typically have ill-defined borders and may be referred to as "consolidation."
- Focal (involving segment or lobe)
  - ▲ Pneumonia (bacterial, viral)
  - ▲ Pulmonary embolus with infarction
  - ▲ Neoplasm (bronchoalveolar cell carcinoma, lymphoma)
  - ▲ Contusion
- Diffuse or patchy/multifocal
  - ▲ Pulmonary edema
  - ▲ Infection (TB, *Pneumocystis jiroveci* [formerly *carinii*] pneumonia, other)
  - ▲ Hemorrhage
  - ▲ Neoplasm (lymphoma)

Two Typical Radiographic Findings

Air Bronchogram

- Visible air-filled bronchus is surrounded by fluid filled lung.
- This occurs when fluid accumulates in the alveoli but not in the conducting airways.

Silhouette Sign

- The loss of the normal air-fluid interface caused by accumulation of fluid within the air spaces. For example, the border of the right side of the heart normally is visualized in sharp contrast against the air-filled right middle lobe. With pneumonia in this lobe, the border of the right side of the heart is lost or "silhouetted out."

Interstitial Patterns
- The accumulation of fluid or cells in the interstitial tissue
- May coexist with air-space filling radiographically

Fine Reticular Pattern
- May be acute (Kerley B lines of cardiogenic pulmonary edema, viral pneumonia)
- May be chronic (interstitial lung disease/idiopathic pulmonary fibrosis or hypersensitivity pneumonitis)

Nodular Pattern
- Miliary TB, fungal disease, sarcoidosis, metastases, alveolar cell carcinoma

Coarse Reticular Pattern
- Honeycombing of advanced idiopathic pulmonary fibrosis
- May also be seen with pulmonary edema superimposed on emphysema

Nodule
- A well-defined opacity <3 cm in diameter
- Is completely surrounded by aerated lung space in the absence of an effusion

Solitary Pulmonary Nodule
- Neoplastic (malignant 30% vs. benign 70%) or infectious granuloma

Multiple Nodules
- Metastases, inflammatory (rheumatoid, Wegener granulomatosis), septic emboli

Mass
- Similar to a nodule but is >3 cm in diameter
- More than 90% are malignant

Increased Lung Radiolucency (Decreased Opacity)
- Air trapping in acute, severe asthma (diffuse) or foreign body

aspiration (regional)
- Emphysema with or without bullae
- Pulmonary embolism with regional oligemia

SELECTED CLINICAL APPLICATIONS

Pneumothorax

- Spontaneous or secondary (COPD, ruptured bullae, trauma, *Pneumocystis jiroveci* pneumonia)
- Most often identified as a white line (visceral pleura) abutted by a paucity of lung markings peripheral to it
- The collapsed lung is *not* always denser than the contralateral lung.
  - ▲ Radiodensity depends on vascular markings, and the pneumothorax causes regional oligemia.
- Importance of patient position
  - ▲ Upright (preferred)—small collections of air usually seen in the apex (often lateral apex)
  - ▲ Recumbent—requires larger volumes of air to appreciate
    - • May see subpulmonic air, a collection along the anterolateral mediastinum *or*
    - • Deep sulcus sign—a deep and wide costophrenic sulcus (between the lateral chest wall and diaphragm)
  - ▲ If the patient cannot sit upright, obtain a lateral decubitus film; air will rise to the upper edge of the lateral chest wall.
- Expiratory films *may* be helpful if the diagnosis is in question, because lung tissue becomes denser and the visceral pleura may be identified more readily. However, the study of first choice is plain inspiratory films.
- Pitfalls
  - ▲ Skin folds or bed sheets, particularly with portable films
    - • These lines often extend out of the thorax or may have lung markings peripheral to them.
  - ▲ Large bullae may mimic a pneumothorax.
- Tension pneumothorax is a clinical diagnosis (hypotension, unilaterally absent breath sounds, and tracheal deviation) and decompression must be performed without waiting for the chest X-ray. It is possible for a stable, nonventilated

patient to demonstrate radiographic signs of a tension pneumothorax, which include ipsilateral hemidiaphragmatic depression and shift of the trachea and mediastinum away from the collapsed lung.

- Any size pneumothorax is important in a mechanically ventilated patient where there is always a risk of a tension pneumothorax.

Cardiovascular Findings
Normal Contours of the Mediastinum
- Right paratracheal stripe (air-lung interface) is normally up to 5 mm in diameter.
  - ▲ Widening here may be due to lymphadenopathy or fat.
  - ▲ The inferior portion is continuous with the azygous vein.
- Aorticopulmonary window
  - ▲ The space below the aortic arch and above the left pulmonary artery
  - ▲ Obliteration of this space suggests adenopathy or tumor.

Heart Size and Chambers
- Loss of the normal heart contour may represent chamber enlargement or pericardial effusion.
- Horizontal width of the heart normally should be no more than half the width of the thorax (cardiothoracic ratio).

Hila
- The normal branching, vascular appearance is lost with lymphadenopathy or tumor.
  - ▲ Pulmonary arterial hypertension is suggested by engorged pulmonary arteries that rapidly taper ("pruned tree").
  - ▲ Pulmonary venous hypertension causes prominence of the superior veins in the upper zones of the hila.

Congestive Heart Failure
- Generalized or focal chamber enlargement
- Pulmonary edema
  - ▲ Cephalization early (increased upper zone markings)
  - ▲ Later, you see evidence of interstitial edema—Kerley B lines (thickening of interlobular septae), peribronchial cuffing (thickening), pleural effusions, prominent superior pulmonary veins.

▲ Alveolar filling, often with a perihilar or "bat-wing" distribution

■ Note: Kerley B lines are also seen in lymphangitic carcinoma and, less often, in interstitial disease.

Thoracic Aortic Aneurysm or Dissection

■ May affect any part of the thoracic aorta

■ Associated with poorly controlled hypertension and Marfan syndrome

■ Dissection usually presents with acute, typical symptoms but may be found incidentally on chest X-ray weeks after the event.

■ The film should be compared with previous ones to assess for enlargement.

■ Up to 20% of chest X-rays that show dissection are interpreted as "normal."

■ Some radiographic features

▲ Widening, blurring, or irregularity of the aortic silhouette

▲ Calcium sign— More than a 6-mm separation of the calcified intima from the outer aortic wall of the ascending or descending aorta may suggest dissection.

▲ Displacement of other thoracic structures
  • Rightward shift of trachea or esophagus
  • Inferior displacement of left mainstem bronchus

▲ Widened mediastinum or pleural effusion (usually left-sided) may suggest hemorrhage or leakage.

■ Further imaging is mandatory, such as CT, transesophageal echocardiography, or MRI.

Coarctation of the Aorta

■ Congenital band-like narrowing of aorta that most often occurs just distal to the origin of the left subclavian artery, although site of origin may vary

■ Milder degrees of narrowing may present in adulthood with hypertension of the upper extremities.

■ Classic chest X-ray findings in adults

▲ Rib notching—This results from prominent tortuous intercostal collateral vessels along the posterior inferior portion

of ribs 3 through 8, which bypass the aortic narrowing to supply the descending aorta.
  - ▲ Irregular contour of the upper descending aorta—Prestenotic and poststenotic dilatation may form the "3 sign" just superior to the left main pulmonary artery
- ■ Associated with bicuspid aortic valve and intracerebral aneurysms.

Pulmonary Embolism
- ■ Chest X-ray has very low sensitivity and specificity.
- ■ Some radiographic features
  - ▲ Normal chest X-ray in ~1/3 of patients
  - ▲ Atelectasis, hemidiaphragm elevation
  - ▲ Westermark sign—localized parenchymal oligemia
  - ▲ Hampton hump—pleural-based, wedge-shaped opacity suggestive of pulmonary infarction (rare)
  - ▲ Pleural effusion
  - ▲ Enlarged pulmonary artery or arteries
- ■ Consider CT angiography, ventilation-perfusion scan, deep venous duplex ultrasonography

Volume Loss With or Without Atelectasis
Causes
- ■ Endobronchial obstruction
  - ▲ May be due to foreign body or mucus plugging
  - ▲ Bronchogenic carcinoma *must* be ruled out.
- ■ Compressive atelectasis—from effusions or pleural-based mass
- ■ Hypoventilation can cause discoid (linear) atelectasis (seen in bedridden or splinting patients)

Radiographic Findings
- ■ About 25% of cases lack chest X-ray findings.
- ■ Findings may include
  - ▲ Displacement of the interlobar septa bounding the affected lobe—This is the most direct and reliable sign.
  - ▲ Hemidiaphragmatic elevation
  - ▲ Mediastinal shift on the obstructed side
  - ▲ Narrowing of rib margins
  - ▲ Hyperinflation or oligemic changes of the remaining lobe(s) or contralateral lung
  - ▲ "Reverse S sign" with collapse of the right upper lobe

Pleural Effusion
- Layering of effusion confirmed by lateral decubitus film, also confirms a subpulmonic effusion that may not blunt the costophrenic angle
- If in doubt, perform thoracentesis with ultrasound guidance.
- During or after a thoracentesis, if the patient develops cough, shortness of breath, or chest pain or becomes hypotensive, obtain a chest X-ray to rule out pneumothorax.

CHEST X-RAY AND DIFFERENTIAL DIAGNOSES
- Common differential diagnoses based on the chest X-ray pattern are listed in Table 1.

ATLAS OF CHEST X-RAYS
- Figures 1-10.

Table 1. Common Differential Diagnoses Based on Chest X-ray Pattern

Consolidation in a nonsegmental distribution with air bronchograms
        Infection—bacterial (most commonly pneumococcus), fungal
        Neoplasia—lymphoma, bronchoalveolar cell carcinoma
        Inflammatory—pulmonary infiltrates with eosinophilia syndrome, bronchiolitis obliterans-organizing pneumonia
        Trauma—contusion, irradiation pneumonitis

Segmental consolidation with mild atelectasis (usually without air bronchogram)
        Infection—bronchopneumonia (bacterial [including mycoplasma], fungal, viral)
        Inflammatory—allergic bronchopulmonary aspergillosis, Wegener granulomatosis
        Neoplasia—benign, primary, or metastatic malignancy
        Other—aspiration, postoperative atelectasis, pulmonary infarction

Cystic and cavitary disease
        Congenital—bronchopulmonary sequestration (almost always in lower lobes)
        Infection—bacterial (rule out TB), fungal, parasitic, septic emboli
        Inflammatory—Wegener granulomatosis, rheumatoid nodules, sarcoidosis
        Neoplasia—squamous cell carcinoma (more commonly), metastatic disease
        Inhalational—pneumoconiosis (silicosis)

Solitary or multiple pulmonary nodules
        Congenital—bronchial cyst, arteriovenous malformation
        Infection—TB, fungal, parasitic (if multiple, think of septic emboli)
        Inflammatory—Wegener granulomatosis, rheumatoid nodule
        Neoplasia—carcinoid, hamartoma, primary & metastatic carcinoma
        Other—amyloidosis, hematoma

Diffuse (bilateral) alveolar infiltrates (airspace disease)
        Infection—viral, airway spread of TB, histoplasmosis
        Inflammatory—alveolar hemorrhage syndrome, vasculitis
        Neoplasia—metastatic disease, bronchoalveolar cell carcinoma
        Pulmonary edema—cardiogenic, noncardiogenic
        Embolic—fat or amniotic fluid
        Drug or inhalation injury
        Alveolar proteinosis

Table 1 (continued)

Diffuse disease with predominant reticular or reticulonodular
pattern

       Infection—rule out miliary TB

       Inflammatory—connective tissue diseases

       Neoplasia—lymphangitic carcinomatosis

       Inhalational—silicosis

       Drug effects

       Idiopathic pulmonary fibrosis, histiocytosis X,
         lymphangioleiomyomatosis

Isolated pleural effusion (without other abnormalities on chest X-ray)

       Infection—TB, subphrenic abscess

       Inflammatory—connective tissue disease

       Neoplasia—lymphoma, metastatic disease

       Embolic—pulmonary embolism

       Congestive heart failure

       Trauma

       Metabolic—renal, thyroid, liver disease

Mediastinal abnormalities by compartment

       Superior (above aortic arch)

            Thyroid (>90%)

            Neurogenic neoplasia

            Vascular structures (aneurysms)

       Anterior (bordered by sternum anteriorly and heart, great
         vessels posteriorly)

            Lymphoma, most commonly Hodgkin disease
               (particularly if <30 years old)

            Thymoma (most common if >30 years old)

            Germ cell tumors

            Castleman disease (angiofollicular giant lymph node
               hyperplasia)

       Middle (contains heart & great vessels, large airways,
         esophagus, vagus & phrenic nerves)

            Lymph node enlargement (lymphoma, metastases,
               granulomatous disease)

            Fibrosing mediastinitis (most often due to histo-
               plasmosis)

            Bronchogenic, enterogenous, and pleuropericardial cysts

            Esophageal lesions

            Mediastinal vessel enlargement (coarctation, aneurysm)

       Posterior (between the anterior aspect of vertebral column
         & posterior chest wall)

            Neurogenic tumors—may arise from peripheral nerves
               (neurofibromas or schwannomas), sympathetic ganglia
               (ganglioneuromas), or paraganglion cells (pheo-
               chromocytomas)

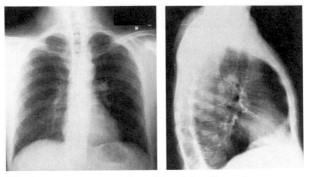

Fig. 1. Normal posteroanterior and lateral chest X-ray of a young man.

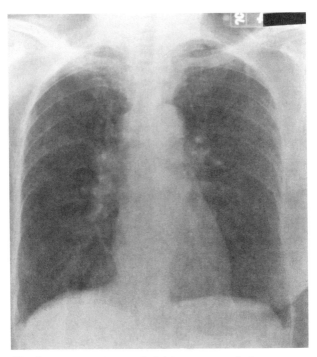

Fig. 2. A 50-year-old woman had right mastectomy for breast cancer. One year later, the follow-up film showed a right paratracheal fullness, which was found to be metastatic adenopathy.

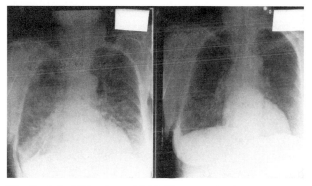

Fig. 3. *Left*, Diffuse interstitial infiltrates and pulmonary venous hypertension from congestive heart failure. *Right*, 12 hours later following diuresis. Note cardiac enlargement.

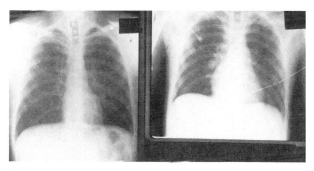

Fig. 4. *Left*, Baseline chest X-ray of middle-aged man. *Right*, Portable film after acute pulmonary embolism. Note enlarged right pulmonary artery, right hemidiaphragm elevation, and right basilar oligemia (Westermark sign).

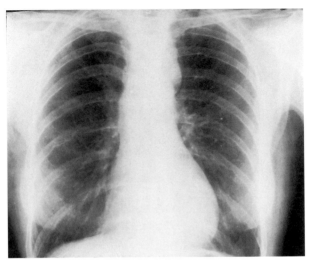

Fig. 5. Coarctation of aorta. Note notching of inferior surface of ribs and irregular contour of upper aorta (the "3" sign).

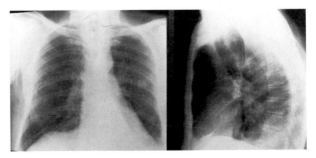

Fig. 6. Posteroanterior and lateral views of collapsed left lower lobe. Note displaced hilum, volume loss, and relative parenchymal lucency (compensatory hyperinflation) on the left. Also note nodular density of left midlung.

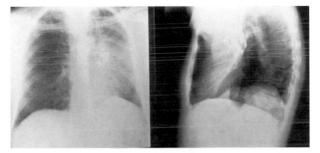

Fig. 7. Posteroanterior and lateral films showing left upper lobe collapse resulting from a broncholith (calcified hilar node that has eroded through bronchus). Lobar boundary is easily seen on lateral film, but also note the elevated hemidiaphragm and relative ground-glass density of upper lung field on the left in the posteroanterior film.

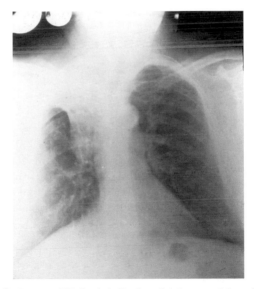

Fig. 8. Reverse "S" sign is indicative of right upper lobe collapse caused by an obstructing airway mass. The lower half of the "S" is a bronchogenic carcinoma.

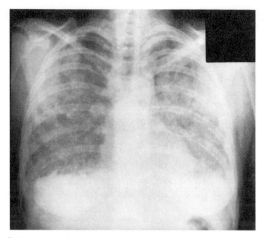

Fig. 9. Lymphangitic metastases in a 25-year-old woman with breast cancer. Diffuse reticulonodular infiltrates with Kerley B lines are seen in the right base. Also note the right paratracheal and hilar adenopathy and small bilateral pleural effusions.

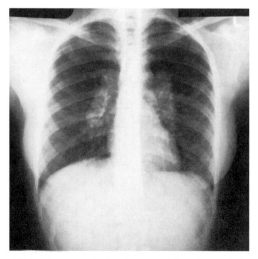

Fig. 10. Right paratracheal and bilateral hilar adenopathy in a young woman with stage I sarcoidosis who presented with arthralgias and erythema nodosum. Histoplasmosis may present in a similar fashion and must be considered in the differential diagnosis.

COAGULATION PANEL

Karin F. Giordano, M.D.
Rajiv K. Pruthi, M.B.B.S.

DECISION TO PERFORM HEMOSTATIC TESTING

- The key to deciding to perform hemostatic testing and choosing the appropriate coagulation tests lies within the patient's history.
- The first step is to determine if the patient's problem is hemostasis (i.e., excessive bleeding) or thrombosis (i.e., hypercoagulability).
- After this has been determined, testing can be appropriately ordered and interpreted.

EVALUATION OF BLEEDING DISORDERS

Bleeding History

- The history continues to be important to guide testing.
- The aims of obtaining a detailed hemostatic history are to determine if there is a bleeding disorder and to differentiate a congenital from an acquired bleeding disorder.
- Questions to ask
  - ▲ Is the bleeding problem lifelong or new? Bleeding during previous surgical procedures is a useful historical factor (remember to ask about wisdom tooth extraction).
  - ▲ Is there a family history of bleeding? It may be useful to ask for presence of specific bleeding disorders (e.g., hemophilia, von Willebrand disease).
  - ▲ Is the patient taking drugs that predispose to bleeding? Consider heparin, warfarin, NSAIDs, and aspirin as potential causes.
  - ▲ Ask about the nature of bleeding. Some clinical clues include

Special abbreviations used in this chapter: DRVVT, dilute Russell viper venom time; RT, reptilase time; TT, thrombin time.

- Mucous membrane bleeding, petechiae—platelet dysfunction, von Willebrand disease
- Hemarthrosis—hemophilia
- Soft tissue hematomas—defect in coagulation cascade (e.g., hemophilia or other factor deficiency)
- Immediate bleeding at time of surgery—defect in primary hemostasis
- Bleeding after initial adequate hemostasis—factor deficiency
- Marked delay in bleeding—factor XIII deficiency

Screening Tests

- The history may allow the physician to focus on particular testing. For example, a history of petechiae or spontaneous bruising may lead the clinician to focus on platelet studies, whereas a family history of hemophilia would lead to detailed testing for factor deficiencies.
- For patients with a history suggestive of a bleeding disorder, the following screening tests are recommended:

Tests of Coagulation

- The extrinsic, intrinsic, and common coagulation pathways are shown in Figure 1.
- The differential diagnosis for abnormal screening test results is listed in Table 1.
- aPTT
  - Measures the integrity of the intrinsic and final common pathway, i.e., prekallikrein, high-molecular-weight kininogen, and factors I (fibrinogen), II, V, VIII, IX, X, XI, XII
  - Most sensitive to deficiencies of factors higher up in the intrinsic pathway
    - Depending on the sensitivity of the aPTT reagents, aPTT may be normal or only slightly prolonged in mild hemophilia (factor VIII or IX deficiency)
- PT
  - Measures integrity of extrinsic and final common pathway, i.e., factors I (fibrinogen), II, V, VII, X
  - PT is not prolonged by heparin, because of a heparin neutralizer in the reagent.

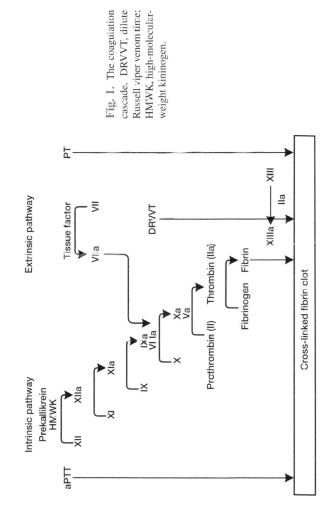

Fig. 1. The coagulation cascade. DRVVT, dilute Russell viper venom time; HMWK, high-molecular-weight kininogen.

Table 1. Differential Diagnosis for Prolonged Screening Test Result

Screening test	Drugs	Inhibitors	Factor deficiency
aPTT	Heparin, warfarin, DTIs*	Factor VIII inhibitors are relatively common Other factor inhibitors are rare Lupus anticoagulant	XII, XI, IX, VIII X, V, fibrinogen, liver disease, vitamin K deficiency, DIC
PT	Warfarin, DTIs*	Factor V inhibitors	VII, X, V, fibrinogen, liver disease, DIC, vitamin K deficiency
DRVVT	Heparin, warfarin, DTIs*	Lupus anticoagulant Factor V inhibitors	X, V, fibrinogen, vitamin K deficiency, DIC
TT	Heparin, DTIs*	Bovine thrombin inhibitor	Dysfibrinogenemia, hypofibrinogenemia, afibrinogenemia, DIC
RT	*Not* heparin	*Not* heparin	Dysfibrinogenemia, hypofibrinogenemia, afibrinogenemia, DIC

DIC, disseminated intravascular coagulation; DRVVT, dilute Russell viper venom time; DTI, direct thrombin inhibitor; RT, reptilase time; TT, thrombin time.

*Examples, lepirudan, argatroban, bivalirudin.

- Generally, abnormalities of PT or aPTT reflect either coagulation factor deficiency or presence of an inhibitor to one or more of the coagulation factors listed. The differentiation is made by performing mixing studies (see below).
- INR
  - Standardized formula to reflect changes in PT secondary to oral anticoagulation
  - INR = (patient PT/mean normal PT)^{ISI}
  - ISI (international sensitivity index) represents sensitivity of thromboplastin to decrease of vitamin K-dependent factors (II, VII, IX, X). This information is supplied by the manufacturer of the PT reagents.

▲ INR is meant only for monitoring oral anticoagulation.
- Dilute Russell viper venom time (DRVVT)
  - ▲ Snake venom used to measure "common" pathway
  - ▲ Directly activates factors V and X
  - ▲ Part of screening for lupus anticoagulant (see below)
- Thrombin time (TT)
  - ▲ Measures conversion of fibrinogen to fibrin; bypasses thrombin
  - ▲ TT is *not* a measure of thrombin activity.
- Reptilase time (RT)
  - ▲ Snake venom that converts fibrinogen to fibrin
  - ▲ Used to determine if prolonged TT is caused by heparin or a fibrinogen dysfunction or deficiency
    - • If both TT and RT are prolonged, consider either a quantitative or qualitative deficiency of fibrinogen, which may be acquired or congenital.
    - • If TT is prolonged but RT is normal, think of heparin.
- Mixing studies
  - ▲ Used to evaluate prolonged aPTT, PT, or DRVVT.
  - ▲ The patient's plasma is mixed with normal plasma in a 1:1 ratio to determine if abnormal aPTT, PT, or DRVVT corrects.
    - • If it corrects to a normal value, think of factor *deficiency*, which could be congenital or acquired (e.g., liver disease, warfarin).
    - • If it does not correct completely, think of an *inhibitor* (specific factor inhibitor, lupus anticoagulant, or heparin).
- Factor assays
  - ▲ Factor results are reported as percentage of normal *activity*.
  - ▲ Factor activity levels are decreased in deficiency or the presence of inhibitor.
  - ▲ Indications for checking specific factor activity levels include clinical suspicion of a factor deficiency or abnormal aPTT, PT, or DRVVT.
  - ▲ Abnormal screening test findings and the differential diagnosis for factor deficiencies are listed in Table 2.
- Factor inhibitors
  - ▲ Antibodies targeted against a specific factor

Table 2. Coagulation Factors

Factor	Abnormal tests	Acquired deficiencies	Congenital deficiencies	Increased levels	Clinical hints
I (fibrinogen)	TT RT (DRVVT, aPTT, PT in some cases)	Dysfibrinogenemia Hypofibrinogenemia Liver disease DIC	Congenital Afibrinogenemia (autosomal dominant)	Inflammation (acute phase reactant)	Chronic hyperfibrinogenemia may predispose to thrombosis
II (prothrombin)	aPTT PT DRVVT	Warfarin Vitamin K deficiency Liver disease Factor inhibitor	Autosomal recessive	NA	TT is *not* a test of prothrombin activity
V	aPTT PT	Liver disease Factor inhibitor DIC Acute leukemia	Autosomal recessive	NA	Factor V level is a sensitive indicator of factor deficiency due to liver failure
VII	PT	Warfarin Vitamin K deficiency Liver disease	Autosomal recessive	NA	Short half-life of factor VII causes rapid increase in PT with warfarin, but other factors are not yet decreased enough for true anticoagulation

Table 2 (continued)

Factor	Abnormal tests	Acquired deficiencies	Congenital deficiencies	Increased levels	Clinical hints
VIII	aPTT (may be normal in mild cases)	Factor inhibitor	Hemophilia A (X-linked) von Willebrand disease	Stress Liver disease Pregnancy Estrogen	Mild deficiency can be missed—stress/ exercise may transiently increase level to normal (e.g., walking up several flights of stairs before blood is drawn)
IX	aPTT (may be normal in mild cases)	Warfarin Vitamin K deficiency Liver disease Factor inhibitor	Hemophilia B (X-linked)	NA	
X	aPTT PT DRVVT	Warfarin Vitamin K deficiency Liver disease Factor inhibitor Amyloidosis	Autosomal recessive	NA	

DIC, disseminated intravascular coagulation; DRVVT, dilute Russell viper venom time; TT, thrombin time.

- ▲ Presence of a factor inhibitor is suggested by lack of complete correction of an abnormal aPPT, PT, or DRVVT in mixing studies.
  - • A decrease in activity level of a specific factor in this setting suggests an inhibitor of that factor.
- ▲ Most common factor inhibitor is factor VIII inhibitor.
  - • Inhibitors of factors V, IX, X and XI are much less common.
- ▲ Factor VIII inhibitors
  - • Alloimmune—inhibiting antibodies that develop in some hemophilia patients, resulting in poor response to factor VIII treatments
  - • Autoimmune—usually idiopathic in the elderly; may be associated with autoimmune disease, malignancy, lymphoproliferative disease, drugs (penicillin, phenytoin, ampicillin, sulfa).
- ▲ Bethesda assay
  - • A measure of the amount of factor inhibitor activity, expressed as Bethesda units (BU).
  - • <1 BU is negative; 1-10 is low.

Platelet Tests
- ▪ Platelet count
  - ▲ Look for thrombocytopenia.
    - • Confirm low platelet count with a peripheral blood smear.
    - • If in vitro clumping (pseudothrombocytopenia) is suspected, draw blood in a citrate tube.
- ▪ Bleeding time
  - ▲ A crude test of the primary hemostatic response (i.e., vasoconstriction, platelet plug formation)
  - ▲ Sensitivity and specificity are low because of variations in test interpretation.
- ▪ Platelet aggregation studies—observation of platelet aggregation in vitro in response to different stimuli
  - ▲ Aggregation with adenosine diphosphate, collagen epinephrine—shows abnormalities of fibrinogen binding (Glanzmann thrombasthenia), arachidonic acid metabolism (COX inhibition), storage pool disease
  - ▲ Aggregation with ristocetin—abnormalities suggest von Willebrand disease, Bernard-Soulier syndrome

▲ Platelet aggregation studies are sensitive to any antiplatelet agents the patient may be taking. Remember to ask about over-the-counter analgesics!

EVALUATION OF HYPERCOAGULABLE STATES

Thrombotic History

- A thorough history is essential in guiding hypercoagulability testing.
- Historical events to consider
  - ▲ Personal or family history of deep venous thrombosis
  - ▲ Oral contraceptives
  - ▲ Recent trauma or surgery
  - ▲ Immobility
  - ▲ Smoking
  - ▲ Malignancy
  - ▲ Fetal loss
  - ▲ Previous arterial events (myocardial infarction, stroke)
- A history of arterial or venous thrombosis may guide testing differently.

Hypercoagulability Testing

- Clinical hint: To avoid ambiguity of test results, try to have blood drawn before starting treatment with heparin and warfarin.
- Acute events (e.g., deep venous thrombosis, stroke) may affect some test results. Ideally, abnormalities should be reconfirmed about 4 weeks after the patient stops taking warfarin.
- Details of hypercoagulability testing are outlined in Table 3.

Activated Protein C Resistance/Factor V Leiden

- In activated protein C resistance, factor V is resistant to inactivation by activated protein C.

Protein C

- Activated by thrombin-thrombomodulin complex to degrade factors Va and VIII

Table 3. Hypercoagulability Testing

	Frequency	Assay	Thrombosis type	Thrombosis risk	Acquired abnormalities	Clinical hints
Activated protein C resistance/ factor V Leiden	Most common genetic risk factor for DVT 20% of patients with idiopathic venous thrombosis	Suboptimal increase in aPTT in response to protein C Confirm with PCR for factor V Leiden mutation	Venous	Heterozygotes (3-7× increase) Homozygotes (80× increase)	NA	Activated protein C resistance assay is not reliable if baseline aPTT is increased 5% of patients with activated protein C resistance (as measured by the first-generation assay) do not have factor V Leiden
Protein C deficiency	3% of patients with idiopathic venous thrombosis	Protein C antigen & activity	Venous	Heterozygotes (7× increase) Homozygotes (purpura fulminans)	Warfarin Vitamin K deficiency Liver disease	In vitamin K deficiency, protein C & factor VII should be decreased proportionally
Protein S deficiency	2% of patients with idiopathic venous thrombosis	Protein S antigen & activity	Venous	Heterozygotes (unknown) Homozygotes (purpura fulminans)	Warfarin Vitamin K deficiency Liver disease	In vitamin K deficiency, protein S & factor II should be decreased proportionally

Table 3 (continued)

	Frequency	Assay	Thrombosis type	Thrombosis risk	Acquired abnormalities	Clinical hints
Antithrombin III deficiency	3%–6% of patients with idiopathic thromboembolic event	Antithrombin III antigen & activity	Venous ? Arterial	Heterozygotes (5× increase) Homozygotes (incompatible with life)	Heparin Liver disease DIC L-asparaginase Nephrotic syndrome Oral contraceptives	Warfarin can cause increased level
Prothrombin 20210G-A	6% of patients with idiopathic venous thrombosis	PCR-based assay	Venous ? Arterial	Heterozygotes (2.8× increase) Homozygotes	NA	

Table 3 (continued)

	Frequency	Assay	Thrombosis type	Thrombosis risk	Acquired abnormalities	Clinical hints
Hyperhomo-cysteinemia	10%–25% of patients with venous thrombosis	Homocysteine level	Venous Arterial Atherosclerotic disease	Heterozygotes (unknown) Homozygotes, (homocystinuria in childhood)	Vitamin B_{12}, B_6, or folate deficiency Renal failure Hypothyroidism Phenytoin Methotrexate	Treat with folate, vitamin B_{12}, B_6 Could check *MTHFR* gene—1 mutation found in some people with increased homocysteine

DIC, disseminated intravascular coagulation; DVT, deep venous thrombosis; PCR, polymerase chain reaction.

Protein S
- Acts as a cofactor with protein C to inactivate factors Va and VIIIa

Antithrombin III Deficiency
- Antithrombin III inhibits thrombin and factors Xa, XIa, XIIa and kallikrein.
- Absence of antithrombin III leads to lack of inhibition, resulting in a hypercoagulable state.

Prothrombin 20210G-A
- This mutation leads to increased plasma levels of prothrombin, predisposing to venous and possibly arterial thromboses.

Hyperhomocysteinemia
- Increased serum level of homocysteine predisposes to venous and arterial thrombosis and to cardiovascular disease.

Antiphospholipid Antibodies
- A heterozygous group of antibodies (IgM and IgG) directed against protein-phospholipid complexes on which coagulation interactions occur, thereby interfering with normal coagulation cascade.
- Two classes of antiphospholipid antibodies that currently can be tested for:
  - Lupus anticoagulant
  - Anticardiolipin antibodies
- Patients with these antibodies are at risk for venous and arterial thrombosis, recurrent spontaneous abortions, and neurologic complications.
- Antiphospholipid antibodies may be idiopathic or associated with autoimmune diseases (e.g., systemic lupus erythematosus), drugs (e.g., hydralazine), or antiphospholipid syndrome.
- They are often associated with immune-mediated thrombocytopenia. Remember to check the platelets!
- Symptomatic patients should be treated with warfarin, with a goal INR of 2.5-3.5.

Lupus Anticoagulant

- Initial tests to suggest lupus anticoagulant—aPTT and DRVVT, which do *not* correct with mixing.
- Further testing (Fig. 2)
  - ▲ DRVVT corrects with addition of phospholipid.
  - ▲ Platelet neutralization procedure—aPTT decreases by at least 4 seconds with addition of platelets (source of phospholipid membranes).
- Other tests (not routinely performed at Mayo Clinic)—dilute PT, kaolin clotting time, dilute tissue thromboplastin inhibition tests, factor Xa-activated aPTT, Taipan venom time
- The patient should have at least two different tests (e.g., aPTT and DRVVT) to appropriately screen for lupus anticoagulant.

Anticardiolipin Antibodies

- These are a different type of antiphospholipid antibody and must be tested for even if lupus anticoagulant screen is negative.
- The presence of anticardiolipin IgM or IgG is tested.
  - ▲ The significance of IgM antibodies is unclear.
  - ▲ The presence of IgM may be related to the acute process.
  - ▲ A positive test should be rechecked after the active disease has resolved.

Deep Venous Thrombosis and Malignancy

- Malignancy itself is an important risk factor for venous thrombosis.
- Hypercoagulability panel is not always indicated.
  - ▲ Does the history suggest another underlying hypercoagulable state?
  - ▲ Would it change your management and the length of anticoagulation?

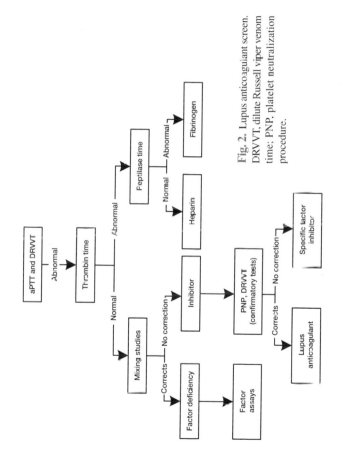

Fig. 2. Lupus anticoagulant screen. DRVVT, dilute Russell viper venom time; PNP, platelet neutralization procedure.

HEPATITIS SEROLOGY

William Sanchez, M.D.
J. Eileen Hay, M.B.Ch.B.

EVALUATION

- Evaluation with viral hepatitis serologic tests is reserved for patients with known exposure or, more commonly, increased serum levels of transaminases.
- Definitions—hepatitis A virus (HAV), hepatitis B virus (HBV), hepatitis C virus (HCV), hepatitis D virus (HDV)

INDICATIONS

- Evaluation of asymptomatic patients with increased serum levels of transaminases
- Evaluation of patients with symptoms suggestive of infectious hepatitis—fevers, jaundice, malaise, right upper quadrant pain
- Evaluation of the cause of chronic liver disease
- Evaluation of patients with recent exposure to possible infectious source—parenteral exposure, needlestick, high-risk sexual contacts
- Evaluation of immunity in patients vaccinated against viral hepatitis
- Evaluation of patients for transplant candidacy

INTERPRETATION

- For interpretation of hepatitis serologic tests, see Table 1.
- Hepatitis A—markers include anti-HAV total and IgM fraction
- Hepatitis B

Special abbreviations used in this chapter: HAV, hepatitis A virus; HBcAg, hepatitis B core antigen; HBeAg, hepatitis B e antigen; HBsAg, hepatitis B surface antigen; HBV, hepatitis B virus; HCV, hepatitis C virus; HDV, hepatitis D virus.

Table 1. Interpretation of Hepatitis Serologic Tests

Disease state	Test results	Comments
Acute hepatitis A	(+) Anti-HAV IgM	
Past exposure to hepatitis A	(+) Anti-HAV IgG	Anti-HAV IgG confers immunity
Acute hepatitis B	(+) HBsAg (+) Anti-HBcAg (IgM)	(+) HBeAg or (+) HBV-DNA indicates high infectivity
Chronic hepatitis B (high infectivity)	(+) HBsAg (+) Anti-HBcAg (IgG) (+) HBeAg	
Chronic hepatitis B (low infectivity)	(+) HBsAg (+) Anti-HBcAg (IgG) (+) Anti-HBeAg	
Recovery from acute hepatitis B	(+) Anti-HBsAg (+) Anti-HBcAg (IgG) (±) Anti-HBeAg	Anti-HBsAg IgG confers immunity
Vaccinated against hepatitis B	(+) Anti-HBsAg	
Exposure to hepatitis C	(+) Anti-HCV	If (+) by ELISA and (−) by RIBA, consider false positive Anti-HCV is not protective against disease
Chronic hepatitis C	(+) Anti-HCV (+) HCV-RNA	
Active hepatitis D	(+) Anti-HDV	Hepatitis D occurs only as coinfection with acute hepatitis B or as superinfection on chronic hepatitis B

HAV, hepatitis A virus; HBcAg, hepatitis B core antigen; HBeAg, hepatitis B e antigen; HBsAg, hepatitis B surface antigen; HBV, hepatitis B virus; HCV, hepatitis C virus; HDV, hepatitis D virus.

- ▲ Markers include HBsAg (surface antigen), anti-HBsAg
- ▲ HBcAg (core antigen), anti-HBcAg (total and IgM fraction)
- ▲ HBeAg ("e" antigen, which indicates active viral replication), anti-HBeAg
- ▲ HBV-DNA (also correlates with active viral replication)
- ■ Hepatitis C
  - ▲ Markers include anti-HCV by ELISA and RIBA
  - ▲ HCV-RNA by polymerase chain reaction
- ■ Hepatitis D—Markers include anti-HDV

ADDITIONAL TESTING

- ■ Evaluation of patients with high-risk exposure (high-risk sexual contact, injection drug use, occupational needlesticks) should include evaluation for HIV.
- ■ When evaluating chronic liver disease of unknown cause, consider important differential diagnoses: occult alcohol abuse, hemochromatosis (ferritin and iron studies), Wilson disease (ceruloplasmin in patients <40 years), alpha$_1$-antitrypsin deficiency (liver involvement can occur without prominent pulmonary symptoms), autoimmune hepatitis (antinuclear antibodies and other autoimmune markers).
- ■ Liver biopsy is indicated in chronic viral hepatitis for diagnosing cirrhosis.
- ■ Patients with chronic viral hepatitis are at increased risk for hepatocellular carcinoma and should be screened with ultrasonography and serum alpha fetoprotein.

INTERPRETATION OF THE ELECTROCARDIOGRAM

Nina Wokhlu, M.D.
Clarence Shub, M.D.

NORMAL ECG

- Rapid and accurate ECG interpretation considered within clinical context can result in appropriate lifesaving treatment.
- ECG interpretation involves first and foremost determining if a patient is clinically stable or unstable.
  - ▲ Unstable signs and symptoms are defined as shock, hypotension (systolic blood pressure <90 mm Hg), decreased consciousness or unresponsiveness, shallow or absent respiration, thready or absent pulse, dyspnea, acute pulmonary edema, chest discomfort, or myocardial ischemia.
- A normal ECG is labeled in Figure 1.

Normal Intervals

- RR interval—time between successive R waves on the ECG
- PP interval—time between successive P waves on the ECG (this is the same as the RR interval on a normal ECG)
- P wave—initial deflection, usually <0.11 second in duration and <2.5 mm tall
- PR interval—time between onset of the P wave and onset of the QRS complex
  - ▲ Duration between 0.12 and 0.2 second
  - ▲ Duration inversely related to heart rate
- QRS complex—time from onset of the Q wave (or R wave if no Q wave is present) to termination of the S wave
  - ▲ Normal duration, 0.06-0.1 second

Special abbreviations used in this chapter: APC, atrial premature contraction; AV, atrioventricular; LAFB, left anterior-superior fascicular block; LBBB, left bundle branch block; LPFB, left posterior fascicular block; PVC, premature ventricular contraction; RBBB, right bundle branch block; SA, sinoatrial.

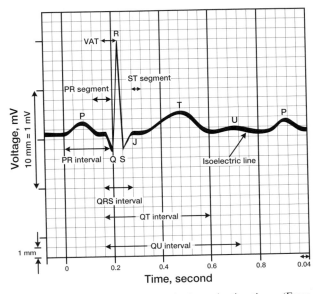

Fig. 1. Normal ECG. VAT, ventricular activation time. (From Goldschlager N, Goldman MJ. Principles of clinical electrocardiography. 13th ed. Norwalk [CT]: Appleton & Lange; 1989. Used with permission.)

- QT interval—time from onset of the Q wave to termination of the T wave
  - Duration should be less than half the preceding RR interval.
  - Corrected QT interval—QT interval (seconds)/square root RR interval (seconds)
    - Usually 0.3-0.46 second
    - Inverse relation to heart rate
- J point—point where the QRS complex ends and the ST segment begins
- PR interval—time from the end of the P wave to onset of the QRS complex
- ST segment—begins after the J point and ends at the onset of the T wave
- Ventricular activation time (VAT)—begins after onset of the Q wave and ends at the R wave

- U wave—positive deflection occasionally present after the T wave and before the P wave
  - ▲ May be indicative of hypokalemia

ECG Determinations
- Three main tasks

Determine if the Rhythm Is Regular or Irregular
- If the distance between successive QRS complexes is constant, the rhythm is regular.

Determine if the QRS Complex Is Wide (>0.1 Second) or Narrow
- If the rhythm is regular, determine the origin: SA (sinoatrial) node, atrioventricular (AV) node (junctional), or ventricular (wide QRS complex).

Search for the P Wave
- If the rhythm is irregular, determine the pattern of the irregularity.
  - ▲ Atrial fibrillation—varying RR intervals, nonexistent P waves, or if P waves are present, they are abnormal with varying P wave contours and variable PR intervals
  - ▲ Multifocal atrial tachycardia—three or more different P wave morphologies with 1:1 conduction and a ventricular rate ≥100 beats/minute
  - ▲ Wandering atrial pacemaker—three or more different P wave morphologies with 1:1 conduction and a ventricular rate <100 beats/minute
  - ▲ Atrial flutter with variable conduction (block)

Narrow Complex, Irregular Tachycardia
- Common causes include atrial fibrillation, multifocal atrial tachycardia, atrial flutter with variable conduction, and sinus tachycardia with atrial premature contractions (APCs)

Ectopic Beats
- Premature beats that occur out of synchrony with the baseline rhythm (extrasystoles)

APC

- Ectopic atrial contraction with a typical P-QRS-T morphology which occurs *before* the next anticipated sinus beat
- There is often a compensatory pause after the APC before the next normal beat.
- An APC may also be nonconducted (isolated premature P wave without a subsequent QRS).

Junctional Premature Contraction

- Ectopic contraction originating in AV node with a narrow QRS complex and no P wave or an inverted P wave (denoting retrograde conduction) preceding or following the QRS complex
- Best seen in leads II, III, and aVF

Premature Ventricular Contraction (PVC)

- Ectopic ventricular contraction that occurs *before* the next anticipated beat.
- Characterized by a wide QRS morphology and no antecedent P wave, or if a P wave is present, the PR interval will usually be abnormal.
- Ventricular bigeminy—a sinus beat alternates with a PVC every other contraction
- Ventricular trigeminy—every third beat is a PVC (ventricular quadrigeminy, every fourth beat is a PVC, and so on)

Intrinsic Rates

- SA node, 60-100 beats/minute
- AV node, 40-60 beats/minute
- Ventricular, 30-40 beats/minute
- Rule of thumb—distance between QRS complexes incrementing by 1 large box = heart rate/minute: $300 \rightarrow 150 \rightarrow 100 \rightarrow 75 \rightarrow 60 \rightarrow 50 \rightarrow 43 \rightarrow 37$ beats/minute
- When there is a regular, narrow QRS complex tachycardia at a rate of 150 beats/minute, consider atrial flutter with 2:1 conduction.
- A wide QRS complex tachycardia at a rate of 150 beats/minute is often ventricular tachycardia, but it could reflect atrial flutter with 2:1 conduction and preexisting or rate-related bundle branch block.

Association (or Dissociation) Between the P wave and QRS Complex

- Determine if the P wave is before or after or bears no relation to the QRS complex.
- If every P wave is not followed by a QRS complex, second- or third-degree heart block (or atrial flutter) may be present.

QRS MORPHOLOGY AND QRS AXIS

- Electrical axis is shown in Figure 2.
- To calculate electrical axis in the frontal plane (net QRS vector)
  - ▲ Measure the net positive or negative deflection (vector sum the positive and negative components in relation to the isoelectric line) of the QRS in lead I—±180° (negative QRS) to 0° (positive QRS), then the same for aVF, –90° (negative QRS) to +90° (positive QRS)
  - ▲ Draw perpendicular lines to each axis at the appropriate vector point.
  - ▲ A diagonal line from the center of the reference system to the point where the two perpendicular lines intersect is the axis in degrees.
- Normal findings
  - ▲ The P wave, QRS complex, and T wave are all inverted in lead aVR.
  - ▲ The P wave is upright in leads I, II, aVF, and most left sided precordial leads.
  - ▲ Note: An isolated Q wave in lead III may be a normal variant, but Q waves should not be seen in limb leads II and aVF; in this case, an inferior infarct pattern should be considered.
  - ▲ Note: The QRS axis shifts leftward with increasing age. Thus, a rightward or even vertical QRS axis in the elderly may be a clue to cardiac disease, e.g., pulmonary hypertension or conduction abnormality.

QRS Morphology
Bundle Branch Block

- Reflects impairment in the left and/or right ventricular conduction system

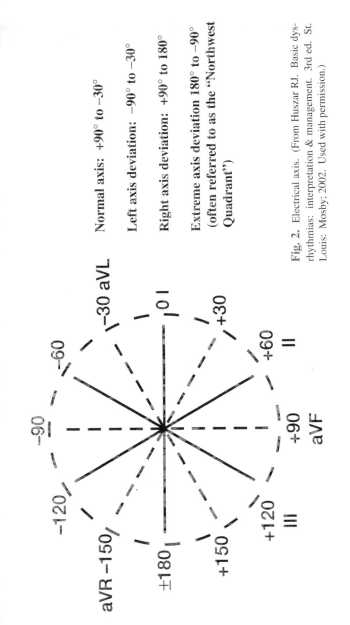

Normal axis: +90° to −30°

Left axis deviation: −90° to −30°

Right axis deviation: +90° to 180°

Extreme axis deviation 180° to −90° (often referred to as the 'Northwest Quadrant')

Fig. 2. Electrical axis. (From Huszar RJ. Basic dysrhythmias: interpretation & management. 3rd ed. St. Louis: Mosby; 2002. Used with permission.)

- ▲ Complete bundle branch block results in a QRS complex ≥0.12 second in duration.
- ▲ Incomplete bundle branch block pattern (or intraventricular conduction delay) results in an intermediate QRS duration of 0.1-0.12 second.
- ■ Bundle branch block morphology in various leads is outlined in Table 1.
- ■ ECG features of left bundle branch block (LBBB) and right bundle branch block (RBBB) are shown in Figures 3 and 4, respectively.
- ■ The ECG in a patient with a pacemaker located in the right ventricle (typical location) exhibits a pseudo-LBBB pattern.
  - ▲ Vertical pacemaker spikes immediately precede the atrial and ventricular impulses or just precede ventricular impulses, depending on the type of pacemaker.
- ■ If a patient with a right ventricular pacemaker has an RBBB (instead of the expected LBBB), consider ventricular septal perforation, with the tip of the pacing apparatus displaced into the left ventricle.
- ■ Causes of bundle branch block include anteroseptal myocardial infarction, Lev disease, Lenègre disease (idiopathic degeneration of the cardiac conduction system), cardiomyopathy, pulmonary embolism, pericarditis, and myocarditis.

Table 1. Bundle Branch Block Morphology in Various Leads

| Lead | Bundle branch block | |
	Left	Right
I, aVL, V_{5-6}	Monophasic wide positive R wave	Small q wave
		Tall R wave
	ST-segment depression	Wide, slurred S wave
	T-wave inversion	
V_{1-2}	Deep, wide negative QS or rS	rSR' pattern
		Possible ST-segment depression
	Small r followed by deep, wide S	T-wave inversion

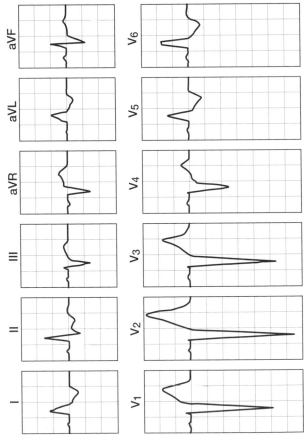

Fig. 3. ECG features of left bundle branch block. (From Huszar RJ. Basic dysrhythmias: interpretation & management. 3rd ed. St. Louis: Mosby; 2002. Used with permission.)

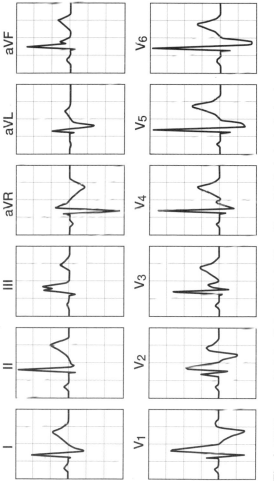

Fig. 4. ECG features of right bundle branch block. (From Huszar RJ. Basic dysrhythmias: interpretation & management. 3rd ed. St. Louis: Mosby; 2002. Used with permission.)

- LBBB
  - ▲ May be persistent or rate-related
  - ▲ May be present only at faster heart rates (e.g., with exercise)
  - ▲ May resolve as the heart rate returns to normal
- "Hemiblock" denotes a fascicular conduction delay usually with a near-normal QRS duration.

Left Anterior-Superior Fascicular Block (LAFB) Criteria
- ECG features (Fig. 5)
  - ▲ Left axis deviation, −30° to −90°
  - ▲ QRS duration <0.10 second, unless accompanied by other blocks
  - ▲ Dominant R wave in leads I and aVL, with/without small preceding q waves
  - ▲ Small R wave followed by a larger, deep S wave in leads II, III, and aVF

Left Posterior Fascicular Block (LPFB)
- ECG features (Fig. 6)
  - ▲ Right axis deviation, +90° to +180°
  - ▲ QRS duration <0.10 second
  - ▲ Small R wave followed by deep S wave in leads I and aVL
  - ▲ Small q wave followed by tall R wave in leads II, III, and aVF
  - ▲ No evidence of right ventricular hypertrophy

Bifascicular Blocks
- RBBB + LAFB—QRS axis often between −60° and −120°
- RBBB + LPFB—QRS axis often greater than +120°
- ECG findings are compared in Table 2.

Trifascicular Blocks
- RBBB + LAFB + first-degree atrioventricular block (AVB)
- RBBB + LPFB + first-degree AVB
- Alternating RBBB and LBBB

Ventricular Hypertrophy
- Left ventricular hypertrophy and right ventricular hypertrophy are compared in Figure 7.

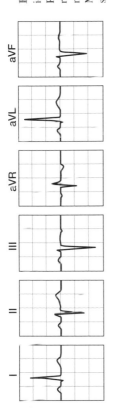

Fig. 5. ECG features of left anterior fascicular block. (From Huszar RJ. Pocket guide to basic dysrhythmias: interpretation and management. 3rd ed. St. Louis: Mosby; 2002. Used with permission.)

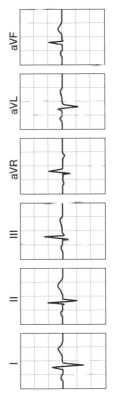

Fig. 6. ECG features of left posterior fascicular block. (From Huszar RJ. Pocket guide to basic dysrhythmias: interpretation and management. 3rd ed. St. Louis: Mosby; 2002. Used with permission.)

Table 2. ECG Findings in Bifascicular Block

ECG finding	RBBB + LAFB	RBBB + LPFB
QRS axis	$-60°$ to $-120°$	$\geq +120°$
Leads I, aVL	QR	RS
Leads II, III, aVF	RS	QR
Leads V_1, V_2	rSR'	rSR'

LAFB, left anterior-superior fascicular block; LPFB, left posterior fascicular block; RBBB, right bundle branch block.
Modified from Hoekstra JW. Handbook of cardiovascular emergencies. 2nd ed. Philadelphia: Lippincott Williams & Wilkins; 2001. Used with permission.

Left Ventricular Hypertrophy Criteria
- Precordial leads (Sokolow, Lyon criteria)
  - ▲ S wave in V_1 + R wave in V_5 (or V_6) >35 mm
  - ▲ R wave in V_5 or R wave in V_6 >26 mm
  - ▲ R wave + S wave in any precordial lead >45 mm
- Limb leads (Gubner, Ungerleider criteria)
  - ▲ R wave in lead I and S wave in lead III >26 mm
  - ▲ R wave in aVL >11 mm
  - ▲ S wave in aVR >15 mm
  - ▲ R wave in aVF >20 mm
- Associated ST-segment depression and T-wave inversion in leads with increased QRS voltage indicates left ventricular hypertrophy with "strain."
- Note: There are multiple sets of criteria for diagnosing left ventricular hypertrophy, such as the Sokolow, McPhie, Cornell, and Estes criteria. No set has gained universal acceptance. Sensitivity and specificity vary. QRS voltage criteria alone have reduced specificity. However, combining QRS voltage criteria and repolarization criteria ("left ventricular hypertrophy with strain") enhances specificity.

Right Ventricular Hypertrophy Criteria
- Right axis deviation
- R wave > S wave in V_1
- qR pattern in V_1 or V_{3R}

Pericardial Effusion/Tamponade
Electrical Alternans
- A specific but not sensitive marker of a large pericardial effusion with or without tamponade (Fig. 8)

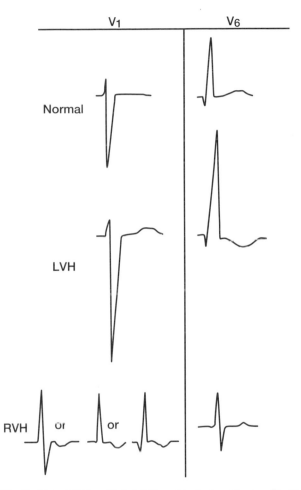

Fig. 7. Right (RVH) and left (LVH) ventricular hypertrophy. The T wave can be upright, flat, or inverted in lead V$_1$ on a normal ECG. (From Goldberger AL. Electrocardiography. In: Kasper DL, Braunwald E, Fauci AS, Hauser SL, Longo DL, Jameson JL, editors. Harrison's principles of internal medicine. Vol. II. 16th ed. New York: McGraw-Hill; 2002. p. 1315. Used with permission.)

- It is related to excess motion of the heart within the pericardial sac, sometimes referred to as "swinging heart."
- The height of every other QRS complex alternately increases then decreases, often accompanied by low-voltage QRS complexes.
  - ▲ Low QRS voltage is defined as <5 mm in the limb leads and <10 mm in the precordial leads.

CARDIAC INJURY

Ischemia
- ST-segment depression in contiguous leads, >1-2 mm with downsloping or horizontal pattern (upsloping less diagnostic)
- Measure ST-segment deviation 0.08 second after the J point.
- Note: Although persistent ST-segment depression can be due to ischemia, it has other causes, including left ventricular hypertrophy with strain, electrolyte disturbance, and digitalis effect.

Infarct
- Terms "ST elevation myocardial infarction" and "non-ST elevation myocardial infarction" are preferred (because it is difficult to differentiate transmural from subendocardial infarction by ECG criteria). The presence of Q waves implies a greater degree of myocardial necrosis than the absence of Q waves.

ST-Segment Configuration
- Marked ST-segment elevation in two or more contiguous ECG leads represents acute myocardial infarction.

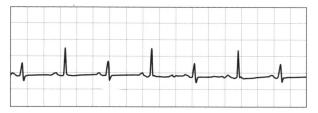

Fig. 8. Electrical alternans. (From Goldberger AL. Electrocardiography. In: Isselbacher KJ, Braunwald E, Wilson JD, Martin JB, Fauci AS, Kasper DL, editors. Harrison's principles of internal medicine. Vol. I. 13th ed. New York: McGraw-Hill; 1994. p. 954-66. Used with permission.)

- Dynamic, transient ST-segment depression generally represents acute cardiac ischemia.
- Always request a previous ECG for comparison.

Acute ST Elevation Myocardial Infarction

- ECG criterion—ST-segment elevation ≥1-2 mm in two contiguous leads
- During an acute ST elevation infarct, the ECG goes through the following sequential changes (Fig. 9):
  - ▲ Early (seconds to minutes)—T waves peak as large upright hyperacute T waves (especially in anterior myocardial infarction); T-wave inversions occur early as well.
  - ▲ This is followed within a short time (<30 minutes) by concave downward ST-segment elevation.
  - ▲ From 2 hours to days later, Q waves appear; T-wave inversions may persist or resolve completely months or years later.
  - ▲ ST segment returns to baseline after a few days.
- Note: Acute ST elevation may also be caused by transient coronary artery spasm with transmural ischemia, which may return to normal as the spasm is relieved and not necessarily cause infarction.
  - ▲ Other inciting causes of myocardial ischemia and acute ST elevation include coronary artery dissection and cocaine-induced coronary spasm.

Where Is the Infarct?

- A scheme for determining the location of an acute myocardial infarction is given in Figure 10.
- Septal
  - ▲ Location: left anterior descending artery and its septal perforators
- Anterior
  - ▲ V_3-V_4 ST-segment elevation may be associated with poor R-wave progression (decreasing or poorly increasing R wave amplitude) in leads V_2-V_5
  - ▲ Location: left anterior descending artery and its diagonal branches

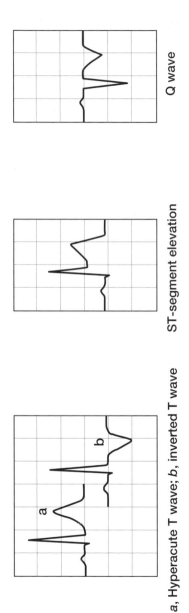

a, Hyperacute T wave; *b*, inverted T wave   ST-segment elevation   Q wave

Fig. 9. Progression of myocardial infarction on ECG. (From Huszar RJ. Basic dysrhythmias: interpretation & management. 3rd ed. St. Louis: Mosby; 2002. Used with permission.)

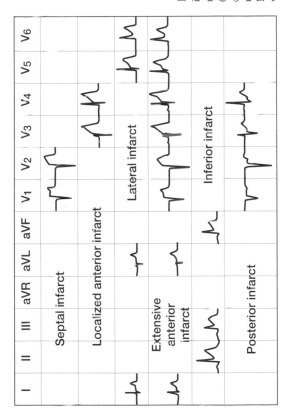

Fig. 10. Scheme for determining the location of an acute myocardial infarction on ECG. (Modified from Huszar RJ. Basic dysrhythmias: interpretation & management. 2nd ed. St. Louis: Mosby-Year Book; 1994. Used with permission.)

- Inferior
  - ▲ ST-segment elevation in leads II, III, and aVF, with reciprocal ST-segment depression in leads I and aVL
  - ▲ Location: right coronary artery and its posterior left ventricular branches or the left circumflex artery
- Lateral
  - ▲ Leads I, aVL, and/or V_5-V_6 ST-segment elevation; reciprocal ST-segment depression in leads II, III, and aVF
  - ▲ V_5-V_6 ST-segment elevation may be combined with an inferior infarct on ECG and is referred to as an "inferolateral myocardial infarction."
  - ▲ Location: left circumflex artery and its obtuse marginal branch or left anterior descending artery and its diagonal branches
- Posterior
  - ▲ Leads V_1-V_2 ST-segment depression, tall R waves in late phase, not deep Q waves
  - ▲ Location: left circumflex artery and/or its posterolateral branch
- Right ventricle
  - ▲ V_{2R}-V_{4R} ST-segment elevation, occasionally V_1-V_3
  - ▲ Location: right coronary artery

Diagnosis of Myocardial Infarction in the Presence of LBBB
- Can be challenging
- ECG features are shown in Figure 11.
- Scoring system to aid in diagnosis of acute myocardial infarction confounded by LBBB on ECG
  - ▲ Score >3 suggests acute infarction.
  - ▲ ST-segment elevation ≥1 mm concordant (the same direction) with the QRS complex is highly suggestive of infarction (score of 5).
  - ▲ ST-segment depression ≥1 mm in leads V_1, V_2, or V_3 is highly suggestive of infarction (score of 3).
  - ▲ ST-segment elevation ≥5 mm discordant (opposite direction) with the QRS complex is suggestive of infarction (score of 2).

ST-Segment Elevation
- Can be associated with coronary artery vasospasm, myocarditis, pericarditis, ventricular aneurysm, and, less frequently, with Brugada syndrome

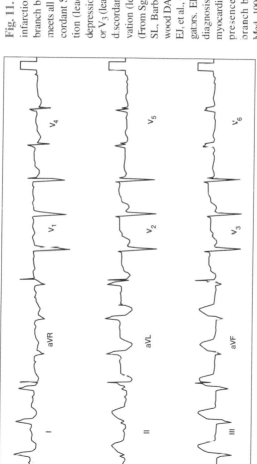

Fig. 11. Acute myocardial infarction with left bundle branch block. This patient meets all three criteria: concordant ST-segment elevation (lead II), ST-segment depression in leads V_1, V_2, or V_3 (leads V_2 and V_3), and discordant ST-segment elevation (leads III and aVF). (From Sgarbossa EB, Pinski SL, Barbagelata A, Underwood DA, Gates KB, Topol EJ, et al., GUSTO-I Investigators. Electrocardiographic diagnosis of evolving acute myocardial infarction in the presence of left bundle-branch block. N Engl J Med 1996;334:481-7. Used with permission.)

- Brugada syndrome—a pattern of ST-segment elevation in leads V_1, V_2, and V_3 with coexisting RBBB
  - ▲ This pattern can be a marker for sudden death (Fig. 12).
- ST-segment elevation is transient with coronary spasm, myocarditis, and pericarditis.
- Persistent ST-segment elevation >1 month after infarction may signal the possibility of ventricular aneurysm.
- Pericarditis
  - ▲ Diffuse concave upward ST-segment elevation associated with PR segment depression (Fig. 13)
  - ▲ Reciprocal depression of ST segment in aVR

T-Wave Abnormalities
- T-wave inversions (similar to ST-segment depression) can indicate cardiac ischemia if they are in two or more contiguous leads, especially if they are symmetric, new, and correspond clinically to time of occurrence of chest pain.
- Tall, peaked T waves, particularly in the precordial leads, can also indicate hyperkalemia.

Q Waves
- Pathologic Q waves in contiguous leads indicate completed transmural infarct, referred to as a "Q-wave infarct."
- Pathologic Q waves are at least 1/4 the height of the succeeding QRS complex and are at least 0.04 second in duration.
- The distribution of the Q waves on the ECG leads indicates the location of the transmural infarct (e.g., anterior, anterolateral, inferior, inferolateral). Multiple Q-wave infarcts may be present.

Abnormal P Wave Morphology
- May indicate right or left atrial enlargement (Fig. 14)
- Left atrial enlargement
  - ▲ Broad, notched P waves ("P mitrale") often seen in lead II
  - ▲ Biphasic P waves in V_1 (positive then negative deflection)
- Right atrial enlargement
  - ▲ Tall, peaked P waves >2.5 mm in leads II, III, and aVF (P pulmonale)

Cardiac Conduction Disturbances
- SA node exit block

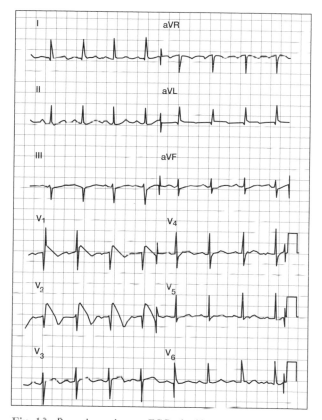

Fig. 12. Brugada syndrome. ECG of a 32-year-old man who had cardiac arrest without evidence of structural heart disease. (From Brugada J, Brugada R, Brugada P. Right bundle-branch block and ST-segment elevation in leads V_1 through V_3: a marker for sudden death in patients without demonstrable structural heart disease. Circulation. 1998;97:457-60. Used with permission.)

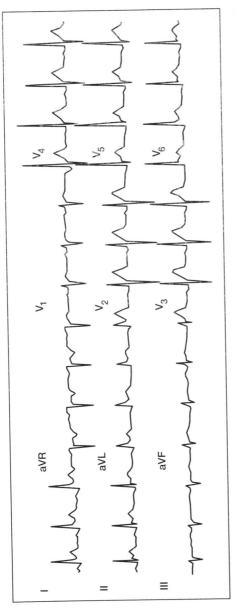

Fig. 13. Pericarditis. Note the classic signs of diffuse concave upward ST-segment elevation with concomitant PR depression. (From Oh JK. Pericardial diseases. In: Murphy JG, editor. Mayo Clinic cardiology board review. 2nd ed. Philadelphia: Lippincott Williams & Wilkins; 2000. p. 509-32. By permission of Mayo Foundation for Medical Education and Research.)

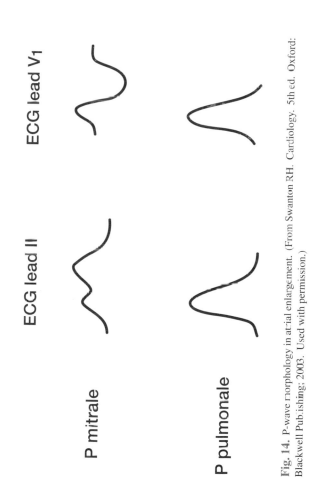

ECG lead II   ECG lead V₁

P mitrale

P pulmonale

Fig. 14. P-wave morphology in atrial enlargement. (From Swanton RH. Cardiology. 5th ed. Oxford: Blackwell Publishing; 2003. Used with permission.)

- ▲ Caused by a block in conduction between the SA node and the atria, resulting in the omission of a complete P-QRS-T complex (Fig. 15)
- ▲ A long pause occurs that is a multiple of the PP interval of the predominant rhythm.
- ■ SA node (Wenckebach)
    - ▲ A cyclical decrease in the PP interval until a P wave is omitted
    - ▲ PR interval is constant.
- ■ Sinus arrest
    - ▲ Caused by failure of the SA node
    - ▲ Standstill of the heart for ≥1.6-2.0 seconds (Fig. 16)
    - ▲ No P wave is generated.
    - ▲ A long pause occurs that is not a multiple of the PP cycle.
- ■ First-degree AV block
    - ▲ Sinus rhythm (Fig. 17)
    - ▲ PR interval ≥0.2 second constant from contraction to contraction.
- ■ Second-degree AV block
    - ▲ Mobitz I (Wenckebach)
        - • Progressive prolongation of the PR interval with eventual omission of the QRS complex with repetition of the same cycle (Fig. 18)
        - • Shortened PR interval succeeding the nonconducted QRS complex
        - • Characterized by progressive decrease in the RR interval
    - ▲ Mobitz II
        - • Fixed PR interval with eventual omission of the QRS complex in a cyclical pattern: often 2:1 (i.e., two cycles of conducted QRS to 1 omitted QRS), 3:1, 3:2, or 4:1, etc. (Fig. 19)
- ■ Third-degree, or complete, heart block
    - ▲ Atrial impulses are completely blocked with two independent rates: an atrial rate and an autonomous slow ventricular rate (Fig. 20).
    - ▲ QRS complexes may be narrow at a rate of about 50-60 beats/minute if the AV junction is the source of ventricular impulses or wide if the origin is below the AV junction, i.e., idioventricular, at a rate of usually <45 beats/minute.
    - ▲ Causes of complete heart block include myocardial infarction, conduction disease of the elderly, Lyme disease,

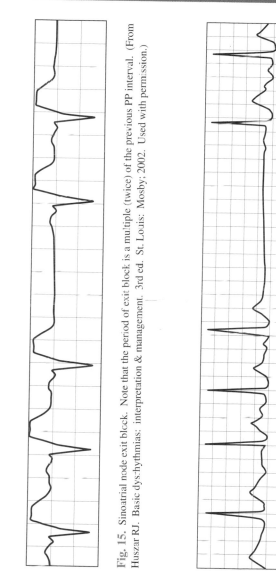

Fig. 15. Sinoatrial node exit block. Note that the period of exit block is a multiple (twice) of the previous PP interval. (From Huszar RJ. Basic dysrhythmias: interpretation & management. 3rd ed. St. Louis: Mosby: 2002. Used with permission.)

Fig. 16. Sinus arrest. (From Swanton RH. Cardiology. 5th ed. Oxford: Blackwell Publishing; 2003. Used with permission.)

Chagas disease, digitalis toxicity, infiltrative disease (e.g., amyloidosis), infective endocarditis, and other, miscellaneous rare diseases.

DISTURBANCES OF RATE

- Tachy-brady syndrome
  - ▲ A form of "sick sinus syndrome" or sinus node dysfunction (Fig. 21)
  - ▲ Definition—periods of alternating tachycardia and bradycardia.

Bradyarrhythmias

- Sinus bradycardia
  - ▲ Sinus rhythm (normal P-QRS-T configuration) with a heart rate <60 beats/minute (Fig. 22)
- AV junctional rhythm
  - ▲ Regular narrow complex QRS rhythm at a rate of 40-60 beats/minute with no P waves or visible retrograde P waves in leads II, III, and aVF (Fig. 23)
- Accelerated junctional rhythm
  - ▲ Regular narrow complex QRS rhythm at a rate of 60-100 beats/minute with no P waves (Fig. 24)
  - ▲ Retrograde P waves preceding or succeeding the QRS in leads II, III, and aVF may occur.
- Idioventricular rhythm
  - ▲ Wide QRS complex, regular (or rarely irregular) ventricular-based rhythm (Fig. 25)
  - ▲ Rate, 30-40 beats/minute
- Accelerated idioventricular rhythm
  - ▲ Ventricular-based rate at 60-120 beats/minute
  - ▲ Note broad QRS complexes without P waves in Figure 26.
  - ▲ Also referred to as "slow ventricular tachycardia"

Tachyarrhythmias

- Sinus tachycardia
  - ▲ Sinus rhythm (normal P-QRS-T configuration) at a heart rate >100 beats/minute
- Atrial flutter
  - ▲ Rapid atrial rate of 250-350 beats/minute with various degrees of AV conduction delay

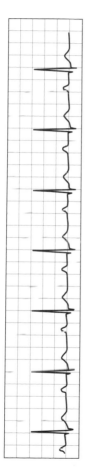

Fig. 17. First-degree atrioventricular block. (From Nolan J, Greenwood J, Mackintosh A. Cardiac emergencies: a pocket guide. Oxford: Butterworth-Heinemann; 1998. Used with permission.)

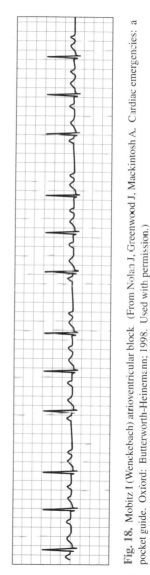

Fig. 18. Mobitz I (Wenckebach) atrioventricular block. (From Nolan J, Greenwood J, Mackintosh A. Cardiac emergencies: a pocket guide. Oxford: Butterworth-Heinemann; 1998. Used with permission.)

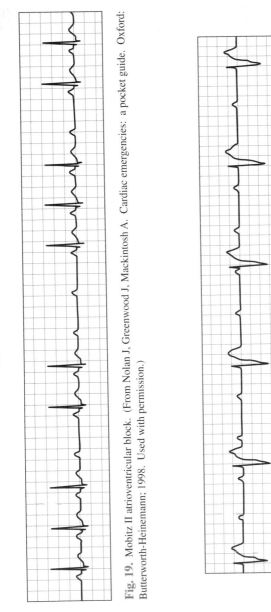

Fig. 19. Mobitz II atrioventricular block. (From Nolan J, Greenwood J, Mackintosh A. Cardiac emergencies: a pocket guide. Oxford: Butterworth-Heinemann; 1998. Used with permission.)

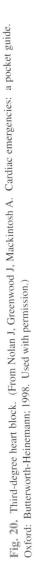

Fig. 20. Third-degree heart block. (From Nolan J, Greenwood J, Mackintosh A. Cardiac emergencies: a pocket guide. Oxford: Butterworth-Heinemann; 1998. Used with permission.)

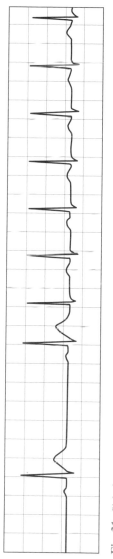

Fig. 21. Sick sinus syndrome. (From Scheinman M. Arrhythmias. In: Braunwald E, editor. Essential atlas of heart diseases. Philadelphia: Current Medicine, Inc.; 1997. p. 6.1-6.36. Used with permission.)

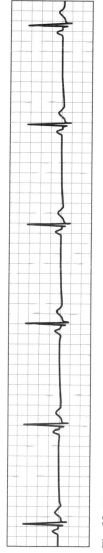

Fig. 22. Sinus bradycardia at a rate of 30 beats/minute. (From Nolan J, Greenwood J, Mackintosh A. Cardiac emergencies: a pocket guide. Oxford: Butterworth-Heinemann; 1998. Used with permission.)

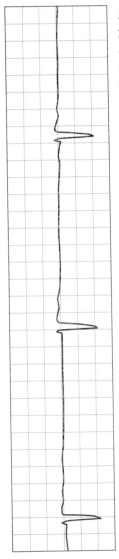

Fig. 23. Junctional rhythm. (From Huszar RJ. Basic dysrhythmias: interpretation & management. 3rd ed. St. Louis: Mosby; 2002. Used with permission.)

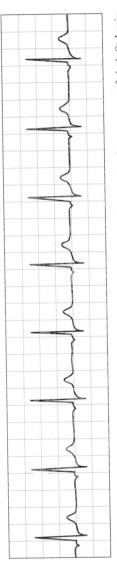
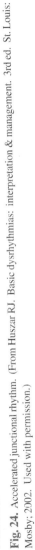

Fig. 24. Accelerated junctional rhythm. (From Huszar RJ. Basic dysrhythmias: interpretaion & management. 3rd ed. St. Louis: Mosby; 2002. Used with permission.)

356

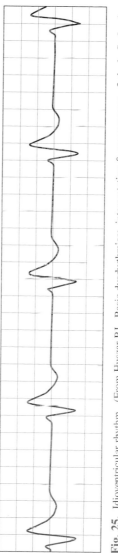

Fig. 25. Idioventricular rhythm. (From Huszar RJ. Basic dysrhythmias: interpretation & management. 3rd ed. St. Louis: Mosby; 2002. Used with permission.)

- ▲ The sawtooth pattern of P waves in classic atrial flutter is seen best in leads II, III, and aVF.
- ▲ AV conduction delays often 2:1, 3:1, 4:1, or variable conduction delay (Fig. 27)
- ▪ Atrial fibrillation
  - ▲ Completely irregular atrial activity resulting in no discernable or consistent P waves, with resultant irregular ventricular activity (Fig. 28)
  - ▲ If the ventricular rate is ≥100 beats/minute, it is said to be "atrial fibrillation with rapid ventricular response."
- ▪ Paroxysmal supraventricular tachycardia
  - ▲ Atrial rate of 150-250 beats/minute (Fig. 29)
  - ▲ Narrow QRS complexes
- ▪ Multifocal atrial tachycardia
  - ▲ Atrial P waves vary with at least three different P wave morphologies (and origins) at a rate ≥110/minute, thus resulting in an irregular ventricular rate (Fig. 30).
  - ▲ Ectopic P waves are seen best in leads II, III, and aVF.
  - ▲ It often coincides with severe pulmonary disease.
- ▪ Junctional tachycardia
  - ▲ Morphologic features similar to those of a junctional rhythm, with a faster ventricular rate, usually >100/minute (Fig. 31)
- ▪ Ventricular tachycardia
  - ▲ Three or more ventricular depolarizations at a rate of 100-200 beats/minute, with QRS >0.12 second
  - ▲ QRS may be uniform ("unifocal") or multiform ("multifocal").
  - ▲ AV dissociation may be found.
  - ▲ Left axis deviation is common but not universal.
  - ▲ Sustained ventricular tachycardia is present when the duration is at least 30 seconds (Fig. 32).
- ▪ Note: The presence of AV dissociation suggests that a wide complex tachycardia is ventricular in origin.
- ▪ Note: Ventricular tachycardia should be regular or nearly so. If it is irregular, then suspect atrial fibrillation or atrial flutter with (rate-related) aberrancy or underlying bundle branch block.
- ▪ Torsades de pointes
  - ▲ A form of polymorphic ventricular tachycardia in which the axis of the QRS complex changes direction in a cyclic fashion (Fig. 33).
  - ▲ Often preceded by a rhythm with a prolonged QT interval

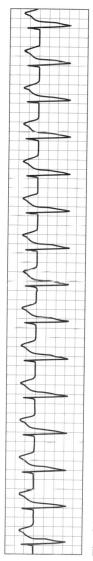

Fig. 26. Accelerated idioventricular rhythm. (From Nolan J, Greenwood J, Mackintosh A. Cardiac emergencies: a pocket guide. Oxford: Butterworth-Heinemann; 1998. Used with permission.)

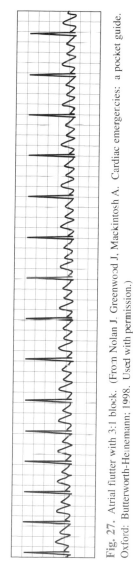

Fig. 27. Atrial flutter with 3:1 block. (From Nolan J, Greenwood J, Mackintosh A. Cardiac emergencies: a pocket guide. Oxford: Butterworth-Heinemann; 1998. Used with permission.)

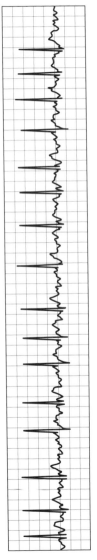

Fig. 28. Atrial fibrillation. (From Nolan J, Greenwood J, Mackintosh A. Cardiac emergencies: a pocket guide. Oxford: Butterworth-Heinemann; 1998. Used with permission.)

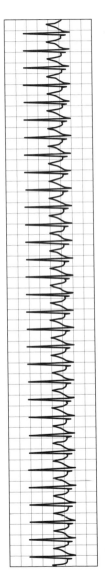

Fig. 29. Paroxysmal supraventricular tachycardia. (From Nolan J, Greenwood J, Mackintosh A. Cardiac emergencies: a pocket guide. Oxford: Butterworth-Heinemann; 1998. Used with permission.)

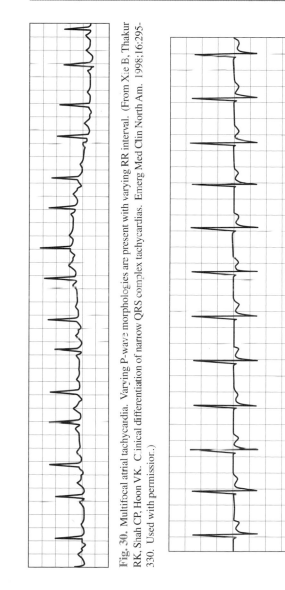

Fig. 30. Multifocal atrial tachycardia. Varying P-wave morphologies are present with varying RR interval. (From Xie B, Thakur RK, Shah CP, Hoon VK. Clinical differentiation of narrow QRS complex tachycardias. Emerg Med Clin North Am. 1998;16:295-330. Used with permission.)

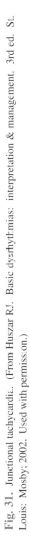

Fig. 31. Junctional tachycardia. (From Huszar RJ. Basic dysrhythmias: interpretation & management. 3rd ed. St. Louis: Mosby; 2002. Used with permission.)

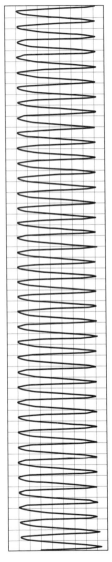

Fig. 32. Sustained monomorphic ventricular tachycardia. (From Nolan J, Greenwood J, Mackintosh A. Cardiac emergencies: a pocket guide. Oxford: Butterworth-Heinemann; 1998. Used with permission.)

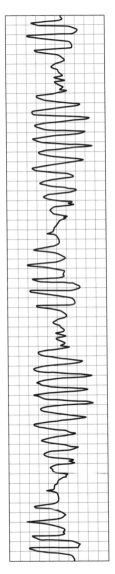

Fig. 33. Torsades des pointes. Note how the QRS axis appears to rotate about an isoelectric line. (From Nolan J, Greenwood J, Mackintosh A. Cardiac emergencies: a pocket guide. Oxford: Butterworth-Heinemann; 1998. Used with permission.)

- Tachyarrhythmias with a wide QRS represent ventricular tachycardia or supraventricular tachycardia with aberrancy or previous bundle branch block (Table 3)
- Factors favoring ventricular tachycardia include
  - ▲ QRS duration >0.12 millisecond
  - ▲ The likelihood improves further if the QRS duration >0.14 millisecond and RBBB morphology or QRS >0.16 millisecond and LBBB morphology

Table 3. **Comparison of Ventricular Tachycardia and Supraventricular Tachycardia**

Factor	Ventricular tachycardia	Supraventricular tachycardia
Rate/minute	Usually 100-200 beats/minute	Usually 150-250 beats/minute
100-130	13% of patients	1% of patients
130-170	47% of patients	27% of patients
170-200	21% of patients	60% of patients
>200	19% of patients	12% of patients
Relation of P waves to QRS complex	AV dissociation Only 33% of patients show a 1:1 P:QRS ratio	1:1 P:QRS ratio (if P waves are visible) 100% of patients
QRS duration, milliseconds	Wide complex	Wide or narrow
<120	14% of patients	76% of patients
120-140	19% of patients	24% of patients
>140	67% of patients	0% of patients
Relation of QRS to previous premature contractions	Similar morphology	Usually different morphology unless bundle branch block was previously present
Capture or fusion beats	Yes (may be observed)	No (not observed)

AV, atrioventricular.
Modified from Shen W-K, Hammill SC. Cardiac arrhythmias. C. Ventricular arrhythmias. In: Giuliani ER, Gersh BJ, McGoon MD, Hayes DL, Schaff HV, editors. Mayo Clinic practice of cardiology. 3rd ed. St. Louis: Mosby; 1996. p. 780-820. By permission of Mayo Foundation.

▲ Left axis deviation, QRS morphology similar to previous PVCs, capture and fusion beats.
- Ventricular tachycardia characteristically may demonstrate fusion or capture beats, especially at relatively slow rates (Fig. 34).
  - ▲ A fusion beat results from merging simultaneous supraventricular and ventricular impulses, producing a QRS complex of intermediate morphology compared with the supraventricular and ventricular impulses.
  - ▲ A capture beat occurs when an atrial impulse passes through the AV node, with a resultant narrow QRS complex that is clearly different from the predominant QRS morphology in a wide complex tachycardia.
- Ventricular fibrillation
  - ▲ Unstable, disorganized ventricular electrical activity (Fig. 35)
  - ▲ Rate >300 beats/minute with QRS waveforms of variable width and regularity.
- Ventricular asystole
  - ▲ Flatline, absence of ventricular activity (Fig. 36)

Preexcitation Syndromes
- Wolff-Parkinson-White syndrome
  - ▲ A triad of short PR interval ≤0.11 second, widening of the QRS complex (≥0.11 second), and slurring of the first portion (upstroke) of the QRS complex (known as the "delta wave," which is referred to as "preexcitation") (Fig. 37)
  - ▲ Complicated by episodes of supraventricular tachycardia that can be either wide or narrow complex, depending on the conduction pathway.
- Lown-Ganong-Levine syndrome
  - ▲ PR interval <0.12 second, with a QRS complex of normal duration associated with paroxysmal supraventricular tachycardia

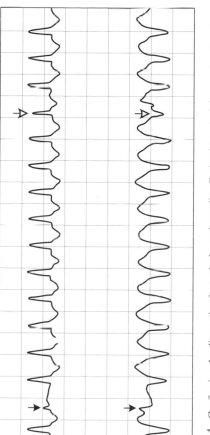

Fig. 34. Confirming the diagnosis of ventricular tachycardia. Fusion beats (*solid arrows*) and capture beats (*open arrows*) are shown. (From Brady WJ, Skiles J. Wide QRS complex tachycardia: ECG differential diagnosis. Am J Emerg Med. 1999;17:376-81. Used with permission.)

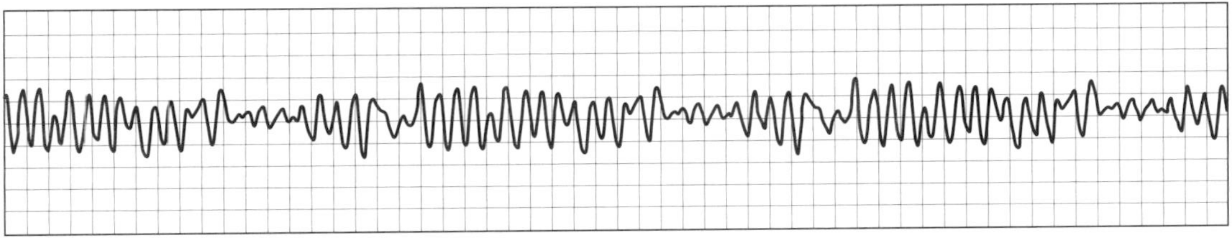

Fig. 35. Ventricular fibrillation. Note the chaotic ventricular activity. (From Nolan J, Greenwood J, Mackintosh A. Cardiac emergencies: a pocket guide. Oxford: Butterworth-Heinemann; 1998. Used with permission.)

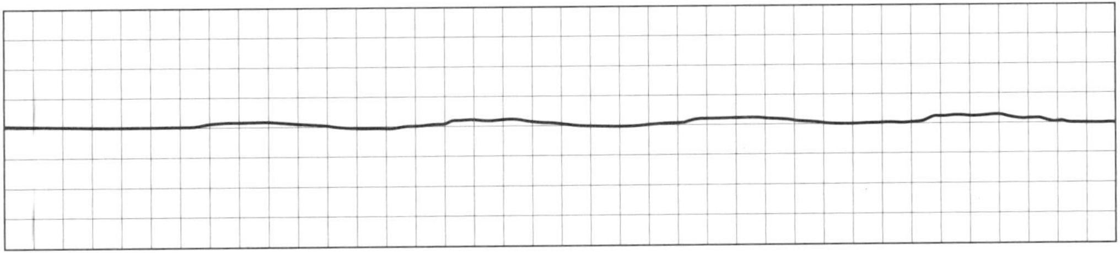

Fig. 36. Asystole. (From Nolan J, Greenwood J, Mackintosh A. Cardiac emergencies: a pocket guide. Oxford: Butterworth-Heinemann; 1998. Used with permission.)

Electrolyte- and Medication-Induced Arrhythmias

- Hyperkalemia
  - ▲ Tall, narrow peaked T waves particularly prominent in the precordial leads→P waves disappear→QRS complexes widen resembling a sine wave (→progressive increase in serum potassium) (Fig. 38)
- Hypokalemia
  - ▲ Prominent U wave, amplitude >1.5 mm (may be larger than the T wave) (Fig. 39)
- Prolonged QT interval
  - ▲ May be caused by hypocalcemia, hypomagnesemia, bradyarrhythmias, amiodarone, sotalol, tricyclic antidepressants, type IA antiarrhythmic agents, phenothiazines, liquid-protein diets, and congenital prolonged QT syndromes (Romano-Ward syndrome [associated with normal hearing] and Jervell and Lange-Nielsen syndrome [associated with deafness]) (Fig. 40)
- Note: Prolonged QT interval predisposes toward ventricular tachycardia, particularly torsades des pointes. The treatment of choice is often to discontinue any offending medication.
- Digitalis toxicity
  - ▲ Characteristic concave upward scooped ST segment, lengthened PR interval or higher degrees of AV block, SA block, paroxysmal atrial tachycardia, sinus bradycardia, PVCs, ventricular tachycardia, ventricular fibrillation, junctional rhythm, or junctional tachycardia (Fig. 41)

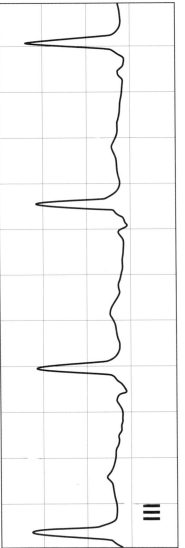
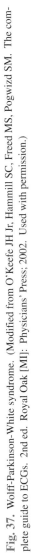

Fig. 37. Wolff-Parkinson-White syndrome. (Modified from O'Keefe JH Jr, Hammill SC, Freed MS, Pogwizd SM. The complete guide to ECGs. 2nd ed. Royal Oak [MI]: Physicians' Press; 2002. Used with permission.)

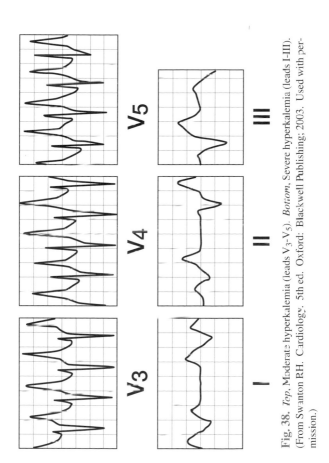

Fig. 38. *Top*, Moderate hyperkalemia (leads V_3–V_5). *Bottom*, Severe hyperkalemia (leads I–III). (From Swanton RH. Cardiology. 5th ed. Oxford: Blackwell Publishing; 2003. Used with permission.)

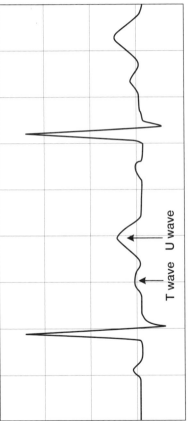

T wave U wave

Fig. 39. Hypokalemia. Note the prominent U wave. (From Thaler MS. The only EKG book you'll ever need. 4th ed. Philadelphia: Lippincott Williams & Wilkins; 2003. Used with permission.)

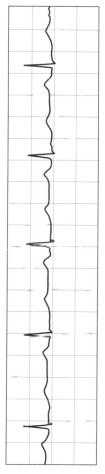

Fig. 40. Prolonged QT interval. Corrected QT interval was 0.5 second. (Modified from O'Keefe JH Jr, Hammill SC, Freed MS, Pogwizd SM. The complete guide to ECGs. 2nd ed. Royal Oak [MI]: Physicians' Press; 2002. Used with permission.)

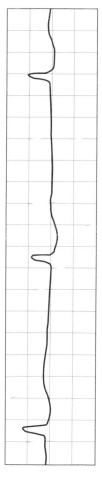

Fig. 41. Digitalis effect. Note upward concavity of the ST segments. (Modified from O'Keefe JH Jr, Hammill SC, Freed MS, Pogwizd SM. The complete guide to ECGs. 2nd ed. Royal Oak [MI]: Physicians' Press; 2002. Used with permission.)

LIVER FUNCTION TESTS

Augustine S. Lee, M.D.
Jason Persoff, M.D.
Stephen M. Lange, M.D.

EVALUATION OF LIVER FUNCTION

- Several lab tests evaluate the presence of liver damage or impairment of liver function. These tests are loosely termed "liver function tests."
- It can be helpful to subcategorize liver function tests to reflect specific patterns of liver injury:
  - ▲ Markers of cholestasis
  - ▲ Markers of hepatocellular injury
  - ▲ Markers of biosynthetic function
- Commonly used liver function tests and their normal values are listed in Table 1.
  - ▲ Normal values can vary with age, sex, ethnicity, and body mass index and are determined by the lab of each institution.

INDICATIONS

- Liver function tests generally are ordered for the following reasons:
  - ▲ To detect hepatobiliary disease
  - ▲ To estimate the degree of injury to the liver
  - ▲ As an indirect or direct measure of abnormality in other organ systems, as in pancreatitis, metastatic cancer, acute myocardial infarction, myopathy, right heart failure, encephalopathy, hemolysis, and shock states
  - ▲ To monitor for adverse drug effects
  - ▲ As a general screen for critically ill patients
- Some indications for which liver function tests may be helpful are listed in Table 2.

Special abbreviation used in this chapter: ALP, alkaline phosphatase.

Table 1. Normal Values for Liver Function Tests

Test	Normal value
Marker of hepatocellular injury	
AST*	12-31 U/L
ALT†	Male, 10-45 U/L Female, 9-29 U/L
Markers of cholestasis	
Bilirubin	
Total	0.1-1.1 mg/dL
Direct (conjugated)	0-0.3 mg/dL (20%-50% of total bilirubin)
ALP	Male, 98-251 U/L Female, 81-312 U/L
Liver isoenzyme	24-158 U/L
Bone isoenzyme	24-146 U/L
Intestine isoenzyme	0-22 U/L
GGT	8-48 U/L
5NT	4.0-11.5 U/L
Markers of biosynthetic function	
Albumin	3.5-5 g/dL
PT	8.4-12 seconds

ALP, alkaline phosphatase; GGT, γ-glutamyltransferase; 5NT, 5'-nucleotidase.
*Also called SGOT (serum glutamic-oxaloacetic transaminase).
†Also called SGPT (serum glutamic-pyruvic transaminase).

- Operating characteristics for identifying specific disease states are described in Table 3.

INTERPRETATION

- The approach to the interpretation of abnormal liver function tests should be guided by the following three important principles:
  - ▲ Liver function tests are sensitive markers of hepatobiliary disease.
  - ▲ Not all liver function test abnormalities reflect abnormalities of the hepatobiliary system.
  - ▲ Additional testing is often required to confirm a specific diagnosis.
- Liver function test abnormalities and the corresponding conditions are given in Table 4.
- Cholestasis of any cause is best suggested by abnormalities

Table 2. Indications for Liver Function Tests

Clinical indications	Nonhepatobiliary indications	Drug effects & monitoring for toxicity*
Jaundice (total bilirubin >2.5 mg/dL)	Pancreatitis	Examples
	Heart failure	HMG-CoA
Ascites	Constrictive	reductase
Tender hepatomegaly	pericarditis	inhibitors
Abdominal pain	Myocardial infarction	Thiazolidine-
(Murphy sign)	Premature	diones
Risk for viral	emphysema	Methotrexate
hepatitis	Metastatic disease	Isoniazid
Risk for primary	Myopathies	Amiodarone
liver neoplasm	Autoimmune	Anticonvul-
Suggestive family	disorders	sants
medical history	Inflammatory bowel	Others
(e.g., hemo-	disease	NSAIDs
chromatosis)	Sepsis	ACE-inhibitors
Suspected cholangitis	Bone disorders	Nicotinic acid
Dark urine	Diabetes mellitus	Sulfonamides
Known toxic	Skin pigmentation	Erythromycin
ingestions	Kayser-Fleischer	Griseofulvin
Suicide attempts	ring	Fluconazole
Encephalopathy,	Chondrocalcinosis	
seizures, coma	(pseudogout)	
Nonspecific malaise	Hemolysis	

ACE, angiotensin-converting enzyme.
*Regular toxicity monitoring is recommended for few select drugs.

in alkaline phosphatase (ALP) and bilirubin (primarily direct bilirubin) out of proportion to the aminotransferases.

- A marked increase in bilirubin (>25-30 mg/dL) is more suggestive of hepatocellular injury than extrahepatic cholestasis. An increase >15 mg/dL itself usually requires a concomitant hemolytic process or renal insufficiency in addition to hepatocellular injury.
- In Gilbert syndrome and hemolysis, total bilirubin is usually <6 mg/dL.

Table 3. Operating Characteristics for Identifying Specific Disease States

Disease	Test	Characteristics			
		Sensitivity, %	+LHR	Specificity, %	–LHR
Obstructive jaundice	Direct bilirubin >50% of total bilirubin	95	1.4	32	0.16
	ALP >3 × normal	85	2.4	65	0.23
		Sensitivity, %		Specificity, %	LHR
Acute viral hepatitis	AST, U/L				
	≤200	99		81	0.4
	201-400	73		98	1.0
	401-600	57		99	7.0
	601-1,000	50		>99	20.0
	>1,000	28		100	∞
	ALP <2 × normal	90		77	
	AST:ALT <1	90			
		Positive predictive value, %			
Alcohol-induced injury	AST:ALT				
	>2	90			
	>3	96			

ALP, alkaline phosphatase; LHR, likelihood ratio.

Table 4. Abnormal Liver Function Tests

Test	Values	
	Increased	**Decreased**
AST	Hepatocellular necrosis (very high levels)	Azotemia
	Acute viral hepatitis	Chronic renal dialysis
	Microsteatosis	Pyridoxal phosphate deficiency states
	Reye syndrome	Less so than with ALT
	Acute fatty liver of pregnancy	(See ALT for associated conditions)
	Liver disease of any cause	
	Cirrhosis	
	Hepatic ischemia	
	Nonalcoholic steatohepatitis	
	Biliary disease	
	Heart failure	
	Neoplasms	
	Granulomas	
	Musculoskeletal injury	
	IM injections	
	Myoglobinuria	
	Myopathies	
	Acute myocardial infarction	
	Pancreatitis	
	Intestinal injury	
	Radiation injury	
	Pulmonary infarction	
	Cerebral infarction	
	Renal infarction	
	Drugs & herbal preparations	
	Burns	
	Mushroom poisoning	
	Lead poisoning	
	Hemolytic anemia	
	Myopathies	
	Trichinosis	
	Macroenzyme AST	

Table 4 (continued)

	Values	
Test	**Increased**	**Decreased**

ALT	Tends to parallel AST, but *lower* in alcoholic liver disease
	Obesity
	Severe preeclampsia
	Rapid progressive acute lymphoblastic leukemia
		Genitourinary tract infections
		Malnutrition
		Pyridoxal phosphate deficiency states
		    Alcoholic liver disease
		    Pregnancy
		    Malnutrition

Bilirubin	Hepatic & posthepatic jaundice
	Prolonged fasting
	Direct bilirubin
	    Biliary obstruction (especially post-hepatic)
	    Dubin-Johnson syndrome
	    Rotor syndrome
	Indirect bilirubin
	    Hemolysis
	    Gilbert disease
	    Crigler-Najjar syndrome
	    Drugs
	        Novobiocin
	    Thyrotoxicosis
	    Large hematomas
		Certain drug ingestions
		    Barbiturates

ALP	Bone
	    Hyperparathyroidism
	    Paget disease
	    Tumors & bony metastasis
	    Osteomalacia, rickets
	    Hyperthyroidism
	    Extensive fractures (healing phase)
	        Osteogenesis imperfecta
		Excess vitamin D
		Milk-alkalai syndrome
		Hypothyroidism, cretinism
		Pernicious anemia
		Celiac disease
		Malnutrition
		Scurvy
		Zinc deficiency
		Magnesium deficiency
		Congenital hypophospha-tasia

Table 4 (continued)

	Values	
Test	**Increased**	**Decreased**

ALP (continued)

    Liver

        Biliary obstruction of
          any cause

        Hyperthyroidism

        Diabetes mellitus

        Neoplasms

        Hepatic venous
          congestion

        Adverse drug toxicity

        Infiltrative (amyloidosis,
          leukemia)

        Liver disease

          Acute hepatitis

          Cirrhosis

          Primary biliary
            cirrhosis

          Hepatosteatosis

    Intestine

        Inflammatory bowel
          disease

        Severe malabsorption

        Intestinal infarction

        Chronic hemodialysis

    Others

        Hyperphosphatasia

        Ectopic production
          from tumors

          Ovarian, cervical
            cancer

        Vascular endothelial
          origin

        Children

        Pregnancy (placental
          isoenzyme)

        Type O & B blood
          after fatty meal

Table 4 (continued)

Test	Values	
	Increased	**Decreased**
GGT*	Alcohol	Hypothyroidism
	Alcoholic hepatitis	
	Biliary obstruction	
	Acute pancreatitis	
	Liver metastasis	
	Nonhepatic neoplasms	
	Hypernephroma,	
	melanoma, lung,	
	breast	
	Acute hepatitis	
	Chronic active hepatitis	
	Cirrhosis	
	Primary biliary cirrhosis	
	Fatty liver	
	Acute myocardial	
	infarction	
	Drug effects	
	Hyperthyroidism	
5NT†	Biliary obstruction of	
	any cause	
	Liver metastasis (often	
	preceding jaundice)	
	Hepatoma	
Albumin	Dehydration	Malnutrition
	IV albumin infusions	Malabsorption syndromes
		Hyperthyroidism
		Pregnancy
		Liver disease (decreased
		synthesis)
		Chronic infection
		Hereditary analbuminemia
		Neoplasms
		Nephrotic syndrome
		Protein-losing enteropathy
		Dilutional
		Iatrogenic, SIADH,
		polydipsia
		Congenital deficiency
		Hemorrhage
		Burns
		Crohn disease

Table 4 (continued)

Test	Values	
	Increased	**Decreased**
PT	Factor deficiency or defect I (fibrinogen), II (prothrombin), V, VII, X	Ovarian hyperfunction Regional enteritis or ileitis
	Inadequate vitamin K	
	Fat malabsorption	
	Severe liver damage (decreased factor synthesis)	
	Drugs Warfarin	
	Idiopathic familial hypoprothrombinemia	
	Circulating anticoagulants Systemic lupus erythematosus	
	Hypofibrinogenemia (factor I) Acquired or inherited	
	Disseminated intravascular coagulation	
	Zollinger-Ellison syndrome	
	Hypervitaminosis	

ALP, alkaline phosphatase; GGT, γ-glutamyltransferase; SIADH, syndrome of inappropriate antidiuretic hormone.

*Normal in pregnancy and postpartum states as well as in bone diseases, unlike ALP.

†Normal in pregnancy and postpartum states, unlike ALP.

Data from Wallach J. Interpretation of diagnostic tests. 7th ed. Philadelphia: Lippincott Williams & Wilkins; 2000.

- The hepatobiliary origin of ALP can be confirmed by an increase in the liver isoenzyme of ALP, 5'-nucleotidase, or γ-glutamyltransferase.
- ALT is more specific to the liver than AST, and an increase in AST alone should prompt evaluation for a nonhepatobiliary cause of the AST abnormality (e.g., in a patient with a history of chest pain, consider acute myocardial infarction).

- An increased AST:ALT ratio >2 is more suggestive of alcohol-induced liver disease (this stems from an alcohol-induced pyridoxal phosphate deficiency). AST does not usually exceed 250 U/L when related to alcoholic hepatitis.
- However, the AST:ALT ratio also increases (i.e., >1) with increasing degrees of hepatic fibrosis and cirrhosis.
- An AST:ALT ratio <1 is more suggestive of viral hepatitis in an acutely jaundiced patient, whereas in an asymptomatic patient, it likely is a reflection of nonalcoholic steatohepatitis.
- Extreme increases in aminotransferase levels (Table 3) are most specific for, and thus suggestive of, the diagnosis of acute viral hepatitis, but they also can occur with acute drug toxicity or shock. (However, sensitivity at these levels diminish, and lower levels should not preclude the physician from considering these diagnoses.)
- The accumulated damage to the liver cannot be gauged by AST, ALT, ALP, or bilirubins alone. PT or albumin reflects the biosynthetic capacity of the liver and is a better marker of the degree of liver function in acute liver failure or chronic liver disease. Factor levels, such as factor V, can test for this more directly.

ADDITIONAL TESTING

- Depending on the specific clinical scenario, additional testing may be indicated to define the specific hepatobiliary or even possibly extrahepatobiliary cause of abnormal liver function tests. Other tests that are often used to follow up an initially abnormal liver test profile are listed in Table 5.
- An initial algorithmic approach to abnormal liver function tests is more appropriate for outpatients than hospitalized patients. For patients who are primarily asymptomatic but have increased AST or ALP, Figures 1 and 2 give two algorithms for the appropriate work-up.

Table 5. Additional Tests to Consider

Tests	Possible clinical features	Suggested diagnosis
Viral hepatitis serologies	Acute febrile illness, predisposing risk factors (IV drug abuse, travel), asymptomatic, vasculitis	Viral hepatitis
Transferrin saturation Iron saturation/TIBC HFE gene mutation	Family history, diabetes, skin pigmentation, cardiomyopathy, hypogonadism, pseudogout & chondrocalcinosis, hypothyroidism, liver disease	Hemochromatosis
Serum ceruloplasmin 24-hour urine copper Serum copper	Kayser-Fleischer rings, family history, <30 years old, risus sardonicus, cognitive impairment, bradykinesia, rigidity, ataxia, tremor, liver disease (can present as acute liver failure)	Wilson disease
Serum protein electrophoresis	α_1-Antitrypsin deficiency Panacinar emphysema, panniculitis, liver disease, family history Autoimmune hepatitis Asymptomatic to fulminant liver disease, other autoimmune disorders	α_1-Antitrypsin deficiency Decrease in α_1-globulin band Autoimmune hepatitis Increase in polyclonal immunoglobulin

Table 5 (continued)

Tests	Possible clinical features	Suggested diagnosis
α_1-Antitrypsin Phenotype Serum levels	(As above)	α_1-Antitrypsin deficiency
Antiendomysial & artigliadin antibodies	Diarrhea, weight loss, anemia, osteomalacia, ataxia, depression, epilepsy, arthritis, dermatitis herpetiformis, autoimmune disorders	Celiac sprue
Antimitochondrial antibodies	Asymptomatic to advanced cholestatic liver disease, fatigue, pruritis, younger woman, hyperpigmentation (not due to jaundice)	Primary biliary cirrhosis
CK/aldolase	Weakness, Gottron papules, dermatoheliosis, significant muscle trauma, drug-induced myositis, underlying malignancy	Muscle injury & inflammation
Troponin	Chest pain, history of atherosclerotic disease	Myocardial infarction
Echocardiography	Congestive heart failure, right-sided heart failure, pericardial calcifications, Kussmaul sign, prominent liver pulsations, murmur of tricuspid regurgitation, elevated ascitic total protein with portal hypertension	Causes of cardiac cirrhosis

Table 5 (continued)

Tests	Possible clinical features	Suggested diagnosis
Antinuclear antibodies & anti-smooth muscle antibodies	(As above)	Autoimmune hepatitis
Toxicology screen	Critically ill patients, history of depression, history of drug or alcohol abuse	Important in acute liver failure Acetaminophen, alcohol, coingestions
Imaging Ultrasound, CT, MRI ERCP	(As per specific diagnoses)	Steatosis, masses, hepatic/portal vein thrombosis, cholelithiasis & related diseases, granulomas, abscesses, infiltrative processes, primary sclerosing cholangitis
Liver biopsy	(As per specific diagnoses)	Often definitive at determining cause of liver lesion & at staging the extent of liver damage Not indicated in acute liver failure (fulminant hepatitis)

ERCP, endoscopic retrograde cholangiopancreatography; TIBC, total iron-binding capacity.

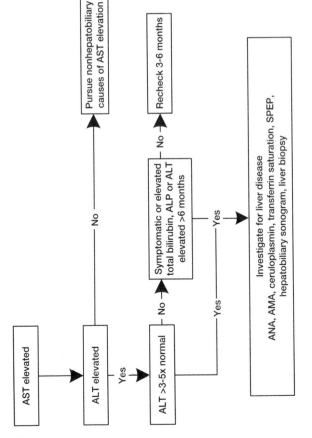

Fig. 1. Increased AST level in a well patient. ALP, alkaline phosphatase; AMA, antimitochondrial antibody; ANA, antinuclear antibodies; SPEP, serum protein electrophoresis. (Modified from Kamath PS. Clinical approach to the patient with abnormal liver tests. Mayo Clin Proc. 1996;71:1089-95. By permission of Mayo Foundation for Medical Education and Research.)

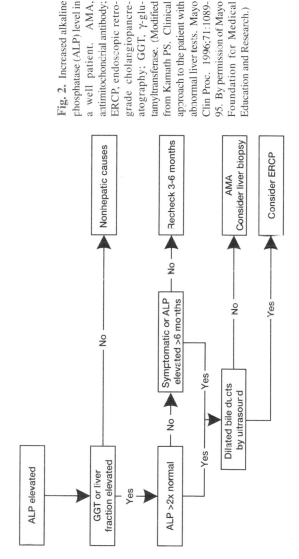

Fig. 2. Increased alkaline phosphatase (ALP) level in a well patient. AMA, antimitochondrial antibody; ERCP, endoscopic retrograde cholangiopancreatography; GGT, γ-glutamyltransferase. (Modified from Kamath PS. Clinical approach to the patient with abnormal liver tests. Mayo Clin Proc. 1996;71:1089-95. By permission of Mayo Foundation for Medical Education and Research.)

PULMONARY ARTERY CATHETER

Kirby D. Slifer, D.O.
William F. Dunn, M.D.

DESCRIPTION

- Pulmonary artery catheter (PAC) is a 110-cm, 7F, heparin-bonded, polyvinylchloride, balloon-tipped, flow-directed catheter inserted through the central venous system into the pulmonary circulation (Fig. 1).
- The balloon is 1-2 cm from the tip and inflated by 0.8-1.5 mL of air, allowing for flotation during insertion.
- The catheter shaft is marked with black bands at 10-cm increments, which aid in determining location of the catheter tip within the central circulation.
- A thermistor wire that ends 4-6 cm proximal to the catheter tip provides for
  - ▲ Cardiac output calculations (via thermodilution technique)
  - ▲ Intermittent measurements of pulmonary artery occlusion pressure (PAOP)
  - ▲ Continuous measurements of central venous pressure and pulmonary artery pressures

Features That Differ By Model and Manufacturer

- Number of lumens (2-5)—The fifth lumen allows administration of fluids or medications.
- Temporary cardiac pacing—atrial, ventricular, or atrioventricular sequential
- Measurements of oxygen saturation
- Continuous determination of right ventricular ejection fraction
- A proximal port 10 cm from the catheter tip measures pressure changes from the right ventricle to the pulmonary artery, helping detect distal migration of the catheter tip (Fig. 2).

Special abbreviations used in this chapter: PAC, pulmonary artery catheter; PAD, pulmonary artery diastolic [pressure]; PAOP, pulmonary artery occlusion pressure.

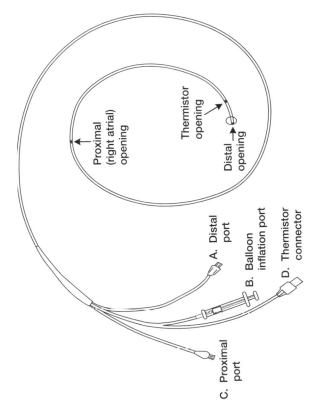

Fig. 1. The quadruple-lumen pulmonary artery catheter. (From Darovic GO. Pulmonary artery pressure monitoring. In: Darovic GO, Franklin CM, editors. Handbook of hemodynamic monitoring. Philadelphia: WB Saunders Company; 1999. p. 121-57. Used with permission.)

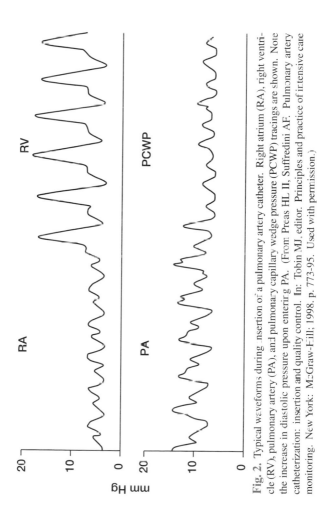

Fig. 2. Typical waveforms during insertion of a pulmonary artery catheter. Right atrium (RA), right ventricle (RV), pulmonary artery (PA), and pulmonary capillary wedge pressure (PCWP) tracings are shown. Note the increase in diastolic pressure upon entering PA. (From Preas HL II, Suffredini AF. Pulmonary artery catheterization: insertion and quality control. In: Tobin MJ, editor. Principles and practice of intensive care monitoring. New York: McGraw-Hill; 1998. p. 773–95. Used with permission.)

INDICATIONS

- Insert PAC only if the answer to both questions below is "yes."
  - ▲ Will the information obtained *likely change* current management?
  - ▲ Is expertise available for optimal placement, data collection, and maintenance of the catheter?

Accepted Diagnostic and Therapeutic Indications

- Shock
  - ▲ Diagnosis
    - Differentiate between different types of shock
  - ▲ Treatment
    - Assess intravascular volume status
    - Guide fluid and pressor therapy
    - Optimize oxygen delivery (controversial)
- Pulmonary edema (cardiogenic and noncardiogenic)
  - ▲ Diagnosis
    - Confirm cause
  - ▲ Treatment
    - Titrate left ventricular preload (cardiac failure)
    - Assess and titrate intravascular volume (renal failure)
- Diagnosis of pulmonary lymphangitic carcinomatosis (wedged catheter cytology)
- Acute myocardial infarction
  - ▲ Diagnosis
    - Assessment of severity of left-to-right shunting in setting of ventricular septal defect
  - ▲ Treatment
    - Right ventricular infarction with hypotension
- Intraoperative monitoring (high-risk surgery)

CATHETER INSERTION

- Complete, sterile barrier precautions should be used when inserting a PAC—sterile mask, gown, gloves, towels, and a full-length sheet covering the patient.
- Internal jugular and subclavian veins are the sites of choice.
- Femoral vein is the least desirable site because of increased incidence of intravascular catheter infections.
- Common insertion sites and their distances to the right atrium, right ventricle, pulmonary artery, and wedge position are listed in Table 1.

General "Dos" and "Don'ts"
"Dos"
- Always have at least one more person in the room.
- Continuously assess the patient for signs of distress.
- Inflate the balloon to the manufacturer's recommended volume (know this ahead of time!).
- Advance the catheter with the balloon inflated.
- Check for distal migration of the catheter tip (balloon inflation volume is suddenly much less than recommended by manufacturer).
- Inflate the balloon slowly and stop at any point a sudden increase in resistance is felt (overwedged) or if *no* resistance is felt (balloon rupture).
- Insert under continuous ECG monitoring with a defibrillator at the bedside.
- Minimize balloon inflation time/cycles.
- Check a chest X-ray after positioning the PAC.

"Don'ts"
- Never withdraw the catheter with the balloon inflated (increases risk for intracardiac trauma, e.g., valve rupture).

Table 1. Insertion Sites and Distances*

Vein	Right atrium	Right ventricle	Pulmonary artery	Wedge position
Right internal jugular	10-15	25	40	45
Left internal jugular	15-20	30	45	50
Subclavian	10	20	35	40
Femoral	40-50	65	80	85
Right ante-cubital	30-40	60	75	80
Left antecubital	35-45	65	80	85

*All distances are in centimeters.
Modified from Darovic GO. Pulmonary artery pressure monitoring. In: Darovic GO, Franklin CM, editors. Handbook of hemodynamic monitoring. Philadelphia: WB Saunders Company; 1999. p. 121-57. Used with permission.

- Do not forcefully pull on a catheter that does not withdraw easily.
- Do not use fluids to inflate the balloon.
- Do not manipulate the catheter frequently (increases risk of infection).
- Do not exceed the recommended inflation volume.
- Do not keep the catheter in place for prolonged periods.

Waveforms
- The typical waveforms obtained during passage of the PAC through the right atrium (central venous pressure), right ventricle, and pulmonary artery are shown in Figure 2.
- Entrance into the pulmonary artery is marked by the appearance of a dicrotic notch.
- A typical PAOP tracing is illustrated in Figure 3. Note the rise and fall in baseline pressure associated with respiratory variation.
  - Depending on whether the patient is breathing spontaneously or is given positive pressure ventilation, PAOP is determined by appropriate measurement of the pressure in relation to the baseline.
    - With positive pressure ventilation, measure PAOP at end-expiration (arrows in Fig. 3).
    - With spontaneously breathing patients, PAOP is also measured at end-expiration (arrowhead), but the inflection point differs from that measured with positive-pressure ventilation because of the generation of negative intrathoracic pressure.

LIMITATIONS
- Controversy surrounds pulmonary artery catheterization.
- No study has shown an increase in survival in catheterized patients; in fact, the observational study of Connors et al. (JAMA. 1996;276:889-97) demonstrated an increased mortality rate. This result is believed to be due to catheter complications, data misinterpretation, and aggressive care.
- Accurate interpretation of data from a PAC is based on the assumption that a continuous, unbroken column of fluid (blood) extends from the left ventricle to the catheter tip.
- Any perturbation that interferes with this column of fluid will affect data accuracy.

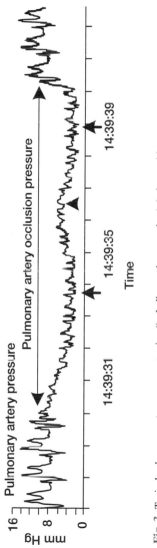
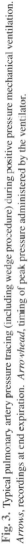

Fig. 3. Typical pulmonary artery pressure tracing (including wedge procedure) during positive pressure mechanical ventilation. *Arrows*, recordings at end expiration. *Arrowhead*, timing of peak pressure administered by the ventilator.

- Various anatomic, physiologic, and extrinsic conditions can affect the accuracy of data:
  - ▲ Severe mitral regurgitation
  - ▲ Severe tricuspid regurgitation
  - ▲ Mitral stenosis/left atrial myxoma
  - ▲ Left ventricular dysfunction (PAOP is a reflection of left ventricular end-diastolic volume [preload]). A noncompliant ventricle will affect the accuracy of data obtained (e.g., ventricular hypertrophy, myocardial ischemia).
  - ▲ Catheter "whip" (e.g., hyperdynamic circulation, excessive catheter length in the right ventricle, catheter tip located near the pulmonic valve)
  - ▲ Miscellaneous (positive pressure ventilation, location of catheter tip in lung zones 1 or 2)

CONTRAINDICATIONS

Relative
- Coagulopathy
- Permanent pacemaker recently implanted
- Left bundle branch block
- Bioprosthetic tricuspid (or pulmonic) valve

Absolute
- Right-sided endocarditis
- Mechanical tricuspid (or pulmonic) valve
- Presence of thrombus or tumor in a right chamber of the heart

TROUBLESHOOTING

Despite proper insertion technique, it may not be possible to obtain a good waveform. Here are some of the possible causes and solutions.

Absence of Pulmonary Artery Waveform Pattern
- Thrombus formation on catheter tip, inability to aspirate blood from the distal port: Replace the catheter.
- Leak in the system: Tighten loose connections.
- Defective transducer: Replace the transducer. If air is suspected in the transducer, purge air.
- Loose cable or electrical connections: Tighten loose connections.

Unable to Obtain PAOP Measurement
- Retrograde movement of the catheter tip into the pulmonary artery: Inflate the balloon and reposition the catheter tip into the wedge position.
- Balloon rupture (see COMPLICATIONS)

Pulmonary Artery Waveform is Damped
- Catheter tip is lodged against vessel wall: Ask patient to cough or move side-to-side. Also, try gentle aspiration, followed by flushing.
- Thrombus formation on catheter tip (see above, Absence of Pulmonary Artery Waveform Pattern)
- Air trapped in tubing: Aspirate air from the system.
- Distal migration of catheter tip into wedged position resulting in a PAOP waveform: Withdraw the catheter until a PAOP tracing is obtained with the recommended inflation volume.

Sudden Changes in Pressure Measurements or Pressure Measurements Inappropriate to the Patient's Condition
- Change in the patient's position: Transducer must be leveled to the patient's right atrium.
- Inaccurate zero referencing: Reset transducer to zero atmosphere.

HEMODYNAMIC VARIABLES
- Normal values for hemodynamic variables used in critical care medicine are given in Table 2.

CLINICAL SCENARIOS
- Examples of common hemodynamic variables are given in Table 3.
- Four principles should guide PAC use and therapy at all times:
  - ▲ Adequate placement and maintenance
  - ▲ Proper data collection
  - ▲ Proper interpretation of hemodynamic data
  - ▲ Appropriate alteration of therapy based on acquired data
- When data obtained by the PAC are no longer being used to actively guide or alter therapy, the catheter should be removed.

Table 2. Normal Hemodynamic Variables

Variable	Unit	Range
Right atrium (CVP)	mm Hg	0-8
Right ventricle	mm Hg	25/0-6
Pulmonary artery	mm Hg	15-30/6-12*
Mean pulmonary artery pressure	mm Hg	9-16
MAP	mm Hg	70-105
PAOP	mm Hg	6-12
CI	L/min per m^2	2.8-4.2
SVRI	dyne·sec·cm^{-5}	1,600-2,400
PVRI	dyne·sec·cm^{-5}	69-177
SVI	mL/beat per m^2	30-65
RVEF		0.40-0.60

CI, cardiac index; CVP, central venous pressure; MAP, mean arterial pressure; PAOP, pulmonary artery occlusion pressure; PVRI, pulmonary vascular resistance index; RVEF, right ventricular ejection fraction; SVI, stroke volume index; SVRI, systemic vascular resistance index.
*Systolic/diastolic.

COMPLICATIONS
- Before, during, and after insertion, beware of complications!

Immediate Complications
- Pneumothorax
  - ▲ Suspected when
    - Air is withdrawn into the venous access needle during initial puncture
    - Patient experiences increased dyspnea or hemodynamic compromise after central access
  - ▲ Chest tube should be placed depending on extent of pneumothorax and patient's clinical picture.
  - ▲ This is why bilateral attempts at central venous access should never be performed unless a chest X-ray shows the absence of pneumothorax.
- Atrial or ventricular dysrhythmias—generally benign
  - ▲ Most likely to occur during passage of the PAC through the right ventricle during flotation or catheter pullback
  - ▲ Further advancement of the PAC terminates dysrhythmias.
- Air embolism—usually occurs during insertion of the catheter
  - ▲ Trendelenberg position reduces the risk.

Table 3. Hemodynamic Variables of Common Clinical Scenarios*

	R atrium, mm Hg	R ventricle, mm Hg	Pulmonary artery, mm Hg	PAOP, mm Hg	Cardiac index, L/min/m²	SVR dynes/s/cm⁻⁵	PVR dynes/s/cm⁻⁵
Hypovolemic shock	0-2	15-20/0-2	15-20/0-6	2-6	**<2.0**	**>1,500**	≤250
Cardiogenic shock	6	45-0/6-8	45-50/30-35	30-35	**<2.0**	**>1,500**	≤250
Distributive shock							
Early	0-2	20-25/0-2	20-25/0-6	**0-6**	**≥2.5**	**<1,500**	<250
Late	0-4	25/4-10	25/4-10	**4-10**	**<2.0**	**>1,500**	>250
Acute pulmonary embolism	8-12	50/12	**50/12-15**	≤12	<2.0	>1,500	**>350**
Cardiac tamponade	**12-18**	**25/12-18**	**25/12-18**	12-18	<2.0	>1,500	≤250
Cor pulmonale	**>6**	**80/>6**	**80/35**	<12	~2.0	>1,500	>350
Pulmonary hypertension	C-6	80-100/0-6	80-100/40	30	<2.0	>1,500	**>350**
Ventricular septal rupture	6	60/6-8	60/35	<12	<2.0	>1,500	>250
Acute R ventricle infarction with failure	**12-20**	30/12-20	30/12	<12	<2.0	>1,500	>250
Acute L ventricle infarction with failure	0-6	**30-40/0-6**	**30-40/18-25**	**>18**	>2.0	>1,500	>250
Acute L ventricle infarction without failure	0-6	25/0-6	25/12-18	**≤18**	**≤2.5**	1,500	≤250

L, left; PAOP, pulmonary artery occlusion pressure; PVR, pulmonary vascular resistance; R, right; SVR, systemic vascular resistance.
*The three most critical data points for each scenario are in bold.

- ▲ Increased risk—hypovolemia with low filling pressures or development of highly negative intrathoracic pressures during inspiration.
- ▲ If suspected, place patient left side down. Small amounts of air are tolerated if confined to the pulmonary circulation, but severe respiratory distress can occur.
- ■ Catheter knotting—more apt to occur in the presence of a dilated right ventricle.
  - ▲ Interventional radiology and surgery are options for deknotting.
  - ▲ Do not attempt to pull PAC back if there is resistance!

Delayed Complications
- ■ Balloon rupture—can be immediate
  - ▲ Risks include multiple inflations, prolonged indwelling time, exceeding recommended inflation volume.
  - ▲ Possibility of fragment or air emboli
  - ▲ If the PAC is needed, you may still keep it in, and if pulmonary artery diastolic (PAD) pressure correlates with PAOP, PAD pressure may be used to monitor filling of left side of the heart.
- ■ Pulmonary artery perforation—caused by overinflation of the catheter with or without distal migration
  - ▲ Risk factors include multiple manipulations, exceeding recommended inflation volume, distal migration of the stiff catheter tip, pulmonary hypertension, severe mitral regurgitation, advanced age, female, anticoagulation.
  - ▲ Usually presents as hemoptysis, often massive
  - ▲ Call surgery immediately!
  - ▲ Intubate the mainstem bronchus of the uninvolved lung if massive bleeding occurs.
  - ▲ Place the affected side in the dependent position.
  - ▲ Positive end-expiratory pressure and proximal positioning of the catheter can be attempted as temporizing measures while waiting for surgery.
- ■ Thromboembolic phenomenon
  - ▲ Often clinically silent, but can present as damped waveforms, poor IV fluid infusion or increased pulmonary artery systolic/diastolic pressure with a widened PAD pressure-to-PAOP gradient (suggestive of pulmonary embolism)
  - ▲ Remove and, if indicated, replace the catheter.

- Infection
  - ▲ Risk increases after 72-96 hours.
  - ▲ There is poor correlation between blood cultures and catheter infection.
  - ▲ If suspected, remove the catheter.
  - ▲ If another catheter is needed, obtain a new site (do *not* exchange the catheter over a guidewire).

STEPWISE APPROACH TO PLACEMENT OF A PAC

- Position the patient supine, and position yourself comfortably.
- Clean the skin with an iodine solution, and drape the area and patient with sterile towels and full-length sheet (the more the better).
- Anesthetize the skin with 1% lidocaine.
- Locate the internal jugular vein with a 21-gauge, 1.5-inch needle attached to a 5-mL syringe. Once the free flowing blood is aspirated, detach the syringe, leaving the locator needle in place. (This step is not needed for the subclavian or femoral vein.)
- Insert an 18-gauge guidewire introducer needle attached to a 5-mL syringe next to the locator needle, aspirating until the free flow of blood is noted. Then, remove the locator needle.
- Detach the syringe from the 18-gauge guidewire introducer needle. Generally, blood will flow freely from the needle hub (a tip that you are still in the right place).
- Thread the guidewire (soft, "J"-end first) through the guidewire introducer needle.
- Holding the guidewire in place, withdraw the guidewire introducer needle.
- With a scalpel blade, make a small incision to enlarge the puncture site.
- Insert the vessel dilator through the introducer (they become a unit).
- Advance, twisting the vessel dilator-introducer unit over the guidewire.
- Remove the guidewire and vessel dilator, leaving the introducer in place.

- Aspirate the introducer and the attached sideport to confirm intravascular placement, then flush.
- Secure in place with sutures.
- Prepare the PAC.
- Wipe the external surface with gauze soaked in sterile saline, and flush the proximal and distal catheter lumens to remove air that may gain access to the circulation.
- Check balloon integrity by submerging the catheter tip in sterile water, inflating the balloon, and checking for air leaks.
- Deflate the balloon and insert the PAC through the sterile sleeve, and pull the sleeve toward you to keep it out of the way.
- With the help of a nonsterile assistant, connect flush-line catheters to the appropriate ports of the PAC (via transducers, providing PAC distal port pressure tracing monitoring during subsequent advancing of the catheter, while preventing air intravasation via any open ports).
- Advance the distal tip of the PAC approximately 10-15 cm. At this point, the waveform typical of the central venous circulation-right atrium will be noted. Further advancement is guided by the observed waveforms (see Fig. 2 while doing this). Attach the sterile sleeve to the introducer hub.

PULMONARY FUNCTION TESTS

David Allan Cook, M.D.
Paul D. Scanlon, M.D.

DEFINITIONS AND NORMAL VALUES

- Most results of pulmonary function tests are reported as a percentage of predicted (the most important exception is FEV_1:FVC ratio).
- Normal ranges for many tests vary with age and/or size.
- "Rule of thumb" normal values (for quick checks before a final report) are given below.
    - ▲ FVC (forced vital capacity): measure of "usable" lung capacity (volume)
        - Normal is >80% of predicted.
    - ▲ FEV_1 (forced expiratory volume in 1 second): rate of expiration = degree of obstruction
        - Normal is >80% of predicted but varies with age and size.
    - ▲ FEV_1/FVC ratio: the presence or absence of obstruction.
        - 0.7 is an acceptable "rule of thumb" (>0.7 = normal); it varies with age.
    - ▲ Provocation (methacholine) challenge
        - Inhalation of a substance such as methacholine induces bronchospasm in susceptible patients (asthma).
        - Decrease in FEV_1 by >20% is "positive" (but is found in 10% of "normals").
    - ▲ Bronchodilator response
        - FVC and FEV_1 measured before and after a bronchodilator

Special abbreviations used in this chapter: ABG, arterial blood gas; DLCO, diffusing capacity of carbon monoxide; FEV_1, forced expiratory volume in 1 second; FVC, forced vital capacity; MEP, maximal expiratory pressure; MIP, maximal inspiratory pressure; MVV, maximal voluntary ventilation; TLC, total lung capacity.

- Improvement of 12% and 200 mL indicate significant reversibility.
▲ DLCO (diffusing capacity of carbon monoxide)
  - It measures how much carbon monoxide is absorbed in a single breath.
  - Result depends on alveolar membrane, blood flow, and hemoglobin.
  - Lower limit for adults (>20 years old): male = predicted − 8; female = predicted − 6.5 (about 75%-80%)
▲ Lung volumes
  - TLC (total lung capacity): measure of total lung volume (FVC + residual volume)
  - Residual volume: volume of gas remaining in lung after complete exhalation
▲ Flow loops
  - Inspiratory flow loops are used to evaluate *extra*thoracic (above thoracic inlet) obstruction.
  - Expiratory flow loops are used to evaluate *intra*thoracic obstruction (asthma, COPD, trachea below thoracic inlet).
▲ MIP (maximal inspiratory pressure) and MEP (maximal expiratory pressure)
  - Measure peak pressure that can be generated with inspiratory and expiratory effort
▲ MVV (maximal voluntary ventilation)
  - Tests both airflow and muscle strength
  - Normal is $\approx FEV_1 \times 40$ (lower limit is $FEV_1 \times 30$).
▲ ABGs (arterial blood gases) can be ordered in conjunction with pulmonary function tests.
  - Can be obtained before and during exercise if desired (requires arterial catheter or multiple arterial punctures)

INDICATIONS
Spirometry
- Includes FVC, FEV_1, and sometimes MVV or bronchodilator testing
- Can be done at bedside
- Most cost-effective pulmonary function test.
- Indications
  ▲ Straightforward diagnostic problem (asthma, uncomplicated COPD)

- ▲ Screening asymptomatic smoker (15%-25% will have abnormal results)
- ▲ Initial evaluation of most pulmonary symptoms (along with chest X-ray)
- ▲ Logistic issues (patient unable to travel for complete exam)
- ▲ Often adequate for monitoring disease
- ▲ Annual certification for use of respiratory protection equipment

"Complete" Pulmonary Function Testing
- ▪ Usually includes spirometry before and after bronchodilator, lung volumes, and D$_{LCO}$.
- ▪ Indications
  - ▲ Complex respiratory symptoms or disease
  - ▲ Distinguish between asthma and COPD
    - • D$_{LCO}$ is decreased in emphysema.
  - ▲ Distinguish between obstructive and restrictive diseases
  - ▲ Distinguish between parenchymal and extraparenchymal restriction
  - ▲ Note: even when complete pulmonary function testing is performed initially, limited studies are often adequate for follow-up.

D$_{LCO}$
- ▪ Indications
  - ▲ Restrictive lung disease (very sensitive to progression)
  - ▲ Obstructive lung disease (abnormal in emphysema)
  - ▲ Vascular disease (chronic pulmonary embolism, pulmonary hypertension [not sensitive])
  - ▲ Before and during treatment with a medication toxic to lung (amiodarone, bleomycin)

Methacholine Challenge
- ▪ Indications
  - ▲ Confirm suspicion of reactive airway disease
  - ▲ Chronic unexplained cough (cough variant asthma)
  - ▲ Evaluate response of asthma to treatment

Lung Volumes
- Indications
  - ▲ Low FVC
  - ▲ Interstitial/restrictive lung disease
  - ▲ Neuromuscular weakness
  - ▲ Obesity

Inspiratory Loops
- Indication
  - ▲ Suspicion of upper airway obstruction

MIP/MEP
- Indication
  - ▲ Suspicion of neuromuscular disease

ABGs
- Indications
  - ▲ Before and during exercise may detect subtle abnormalities
  - ▲ Severe COPD (staging, need for or response to oxygen therapy, surgical risk)
  - ▲ Severe chest wall or neuromuscular restriction (e.g., severe scoliosis, amyotrophic lateral sclerosis, Guillain-Barré syndrome)

INTERPRETATION

General Approach to Pulmonary Function Tests
- Examine FEV_1/FVC ratio and shape of the curve.
  - ▲ Low FEV_1/FVC or "scooped out" (concave) curve = obstruction
  - ▲ Next step, examine FEV_1 to quantitate degree of obstruction.
    - • 60%-80% = mild obstruction
    - • 40%-60% = moderate obstruction
    - • <40% = severe obstruction
  - ▲ Next, check bronchodilator response.
    - • "Significant" reversibility if FEV_1 or FVC improve by *both* ≥200 mL and ≥12%
  - ▲ Check D_{LCO}.
    - • Low = emphysema, otherwise asthma or chronic bronchitis

- Examine TLC (or FVC if TLC is not available).
  - ▲ Low = restrictive disease (parenchyma, chest wall, or neuromuscular)
    - Curve = small; "witch's hat"
    - Next step, check TLC if not already done.
    - If TLC is low, check DLCO.
      - Low DLCO = parenchymal lung disease (e.g., interstitial lung disease)
      - Disproportionately high residual volume (high residual volume/TLC) and normal DLCO, consider neuromuscular disease.
      - Normal DLCO and residual volume = chest wall deformity/limitation (e.g., kyphosis, obesity, weakness)
    - FVC used for quantitation
      - 60%-80% = mild restriction
      - 50%-60% = moderate restriction
      - <50% = severe restriction
- Check DLCO
  - ▲ Normal, with abnormal spirometry
    - Asthma
    - Chronic bronchitis
    - Neuromuscular weakness
    - Chest wall deformity
  - ▲ Low
    - Normal spirometry
      - Anemia (7% decrease in DLCO for each 1 g/dL decrease in hemoglobin)
      - Pulmonary hypertension
      - Pulmonary embolism
      - Obliterative vascular disease (e.g., scleroderma, systemic lupus erythematosus)
    - Abnormal spirometry
      - Emphysema
      - Parenchymal restrictive disease
      - Pulmonary edema

- Decreased lung volume (pneumonectomy)
  - Quantitation
    - 65%-normal = mild (recall that "normal" range varies)
    - 50%-65% = moderate
    - <50% = severe
  - ▲ High (spirometry usually normal)
    - Obesity
    - Asthma
    - Exercise (nonresting state)
    - Polycythemia
    - Left-to-right shunt
    - Pulmonary hemorrhage
- ■ Check MVV
  - ▲ Low MVV with otherwise normal spirometry suggests
    - Inspiratory (extrathoracic) obstruction
    - Neuromuscular weakness
    - Poor performance
- ■ Other tests
  - ▲ Methacholine challenge—if considering asthma
    - "Positive" if >20% decrease in FEV_1
  - ▲ MIP/MEP—if considering neuromuscular weakness
    - Low MIP and normal MEP suggest diaphragmatic weakness.
    - Low MEP and normal MIP suggest spinal cord injury below C4.
    - Both low MEP and MIP suggest muscle weakness or poor performance

ADDITIONAL TESTING
- ■ Chest X-ray—if not already done, get one.

Restrictive Parenchymal Lung Disease
- ■ CBC, rheumatoid factor, antinuclear antibodies, cryoglobulins, ABGs
- ■ Usually proceed with high-resolution CT of chest
- ■ Consider lung biopsy in appropriate setting.

Isolated Low D$_{LCO}$
- ■ CBC (calculate "correction" as above if anemic), rheumatoid factor, antinuclear antibodies, ABGs

- Consider ventilation-perfusion scan or contrast chest CT (acute or chronic pulmonary embolism)
- Echocardiography (evaluate for pulmonary hypertension)

Neuromuscular Weakness
- Careful physical exam
- CBC, electrolytes (potassium, calcium, magnesium, phosphate), ABGs, CK, serum protein electrophoresis
- EMG is crucial.
- Consider acetylcholine receptor-binding antibodies (myasthenia gravis?).

THYROID FUNCTION TESTS

Lisa S. Chow, M.D.
Rebecca S. Bahn, M.D.

PRINCIPLES

- Need to correlate thyroid function test results with clinical suspicion and physical exam findings
- Symptoms and signs suggestive of hyperthyroidism
  - ▲ Symptoms—heat intolerance, increased sweating, weight loss, increased appetite, anxiety, palpitations, fatigue
  - ▲ Signs—tachycardia (especially new-onset atrial fibrillation), hyperkinetic movements, tremor, abnormal thyroid exam, exophthalmos
- Symptoms and signs suggestive of hypothyroidism
  - ▲ Symptoms—cold intolerance, decreased sweating, slow movements, weight gain, constipation, hoarseness, paresthesias
  - ▲ Signs—bradycardia; delayed relaxation of reflexes; dry, coarse, cool skin; periorbital puffiness
- Prevalence of thyroid disease—~0.6% in the population (hypothyroidism/hyperthyroidism ratio is 1:1)
- Comorbid acute illness often leads to inaccurate values. If thyroid dysfunction is suspected, repeat tests after acute illness resolves.
- Thyroid-stimulating hormone (TSH) level is the initial test for evaluating thyroid function.
- If TSH is abnormal, the next test should be a free thyroxine (T_4) level. Free T_4 index is another option.
- In inpatient setting, drugs (especially iodine in contrast dye) frequently cause abnormal thyroid function tests.
- Normal values for thyroid function tests are listed in Table 1.

Special abbreviations used in this chapter: T_4, thyroxine; TSH, thyroid-stimulating hormone.

Table 1. Normal Values (Mayo Clinic Laboratory) for Thyroid Function Tests

Test	Comment	Normal value
TSH	Test of choice	0.3-5.0 mIU/L
Total T_4	Direct measurement of bound & free T_4	5.0-12.5 µg/dL
Free T_4	Measurement of functional (free) T_4	0.7-2.0 ng/dL
Total T_3	Used only in hyperthyroidism evaluation	80-180 ng/dL
Free T_3	Rarely used	2.3-4.2 pg/mL
Thyroid autoantibodies	Positive in Hashimoto disease	Thyroglobulin antibody titer, <1:100
		Microsomal antibody titer, <1:100
TSI	Positive in Graves disease	≤1.3 (index value, no unit used)
Thyroglobulin	Used to follow-up thyroid cancer	Depends on circumstances

T_3, triiodothyronine; T_4, thyroxine; TSH, thyroid-stimulating hormone; TSI, thyroid-stimulating immunoglobulin.

INDICATIONS

- Indications for thyroid function tests are listed in Table 2.
- An algorithm for evaluating high or low levels of TSH is given in Figure 1.

FURTHER EVALUATION

- Hyperthyroidism
  - ▲ Radioiodine uptake with or without scan
- Thyroid nodule
  - ▲ Fine-needle aspiration biopsy of palpated nodule
- Hypothyroidism
  - ▲ Antithyroid antibodies
    - • If positive, consider Hashimoto thyroiditis.
    - • If negative, consider a non-Hashimoto cause.
- Subclinical hypothyroidism
  - ▲ Repeat thyroid function tests in 6 months.
- Sick euthyroid
  - ▲ Repeat thyroid function tests after acute illness resolves.

Table 2. Indications for Thyroid Function Tests and the Corresponding Sensitivity and Specificity

Indication	Test	Sensitivity, %		Specificity, %	
		Hyperthyroid	Hypothyroid	Hyperthyroid	Hypothyroid
Evaluation of a "healthy" patient	TSH	>99	99	>99	99
(i.e., seen in clinic)	Free T$_4$	95	90	95	90
Evaluation of a "sick" patient	TSH	99	99	95	95
(i.e., seen in hospital)	Free T$_4$	95	60	97	80

T$_4$, thyroxine; TSH, thyroid-stimulating hormone.

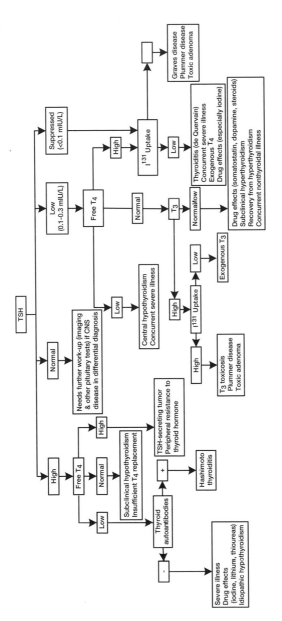

Fig. 1. Algorithm for evaluating high or low levels of thyroid-stimulating hormone (TSH). CNS, central nervous system; T₃, triiodothyronine; T₄, thyroxine.

CAVEAT

- Because of their many comorbid conditions, hospitalized patients often have thyroid function test abnormalities for reasons other than thyroid disease.
- If the diagnosis of thyroid disease is unclear, it is critical to repeat thyroid function tests after hospital discharge.

ACID-BASE DISORDERS

Javier D. Finkielman, M.D.
Robert C. Albright, Jr., D.O.

DEFINITION
- Normal arterial blood pH is 7.40 or $[H^+] - 40$ ($[HCO_3^-] = 24$).
- Under normal conditions, the net amount of acid secreted and the consequent renal production of bicarbonate equals the rate of proton generation, preserving the $[H^+]$ balance.
- Failure to maintain the proton or bicarbonate concentration leads to acidosis or alkalosis.
- When the disorder involves only one process, the result is a simple acid-base disorder; when more than one process, it is a mixed acid-base disorder.

CLASSIFICATION
Simple Acid-Base Disturbances
Metabolic Acidosis
- pH <7.37 → acidosis
- Low $[HCO_3^-]$ → metabolic
- Normal compensation → low P_{CO_2}

Expected Range of Compensation
- $P_{CO_2} = 1.5 \times [HCO_3^-] + 8 \pm 2$
- P_{CO_2} = last 2 digits of the pH

Anion Gap
- Normal anion gap = 12 ± 2
- Anion gap = $[Na^+] - ([Cl^-] + [HCO_3^-])$
- High anion gap → metabolic acidosis with increased anion gap

Metabolic Alkalosis
- pH >7.43 → alkalosis

Special abbreviation used in this chapter: RTA, renal tubular acidosis.

- High $[HCO_3^-] \rightarrow$ metabolic
- Normal compensation $\rightarrow$ high P_{CO_2}

Expected Range of Compensation
- $P_{CO_2} = 40 + 0.6 \times \Delta\,[HCO_3^-]$
- $P_{CO_2} = 0.9 \times [HCO_3^-] + 9$

Respiratory Acidosis
- pH <7.37 $\rightarrow$ acidosis
- High $P_{CO_2} \rightarrow$ respiratory
- Normal compensation $\rightarrow$ high $[HCO_3^-]$

Expected Range of Compensation
- Acute
  - $\uparrow \Delta\,[HCO_3^-] = 0.1 \times \Delta\,(P_{CO_2})$
- Chronic
  - $\uparrow \Delta\,[HCO_3^-] = 0.4 \times \Delta\,(P_{CO_2})$

Respiratory Alkalosis
- pH >7.43 $\rightarrow$ alkalosis
- Low $P_{CO_2} \rightarrow$ respiratory
- Normal compensation $\rightarrow$ low $[HCO_3^-]$

Expected Range of Compensation
- Acute
  - $\downarrow \Delta\,[HCO_3^-] = 0.2 \times \Delta\,(P_{CO_2})$
- Chronic
  - $\downarrow \Delta\,[HCO_3^-] = 0.5 \times \Delta\,(P_{CO_2})$

Mixed Acid-Base Disturbances
- When two or more acid-base conditions are present simultaneously, the patient has a mixed disorder.
- Any combination may occur except for respiratory alkalosis and acidosis, because one can never concurrently overexcrete and underexcrete carbon dioxide.
- To diagnose mixed disorders
  - Know how the simple disorders affect pH, P_{CO_2}, and bicarbonate
  - Know the extent of the compensatory mechanism that ought to occur for any given degree of primary disorder
- If the compensatory change does not fit one of the formulas

or the yellow areas in Figure 1, a mixed acid-base disorder is present.

- For example, in metabolic acidosis the primary disturbance is bicarbonate lost and the compensatory response is increased ventilation, which reduces the P_{CO_2}. If the P_{CO_2} is *lower than expected* based on the compensatory mechanism, respiratory alkalosis is present. If the P_{CO_2} is *higher than expected*, respiratory acidosis is present (Table 1).
- In addition, if the anion gap is high, regardless of the pH and the primary acid-base disorder, a component of metabolic acidosis with high anion gap is present.

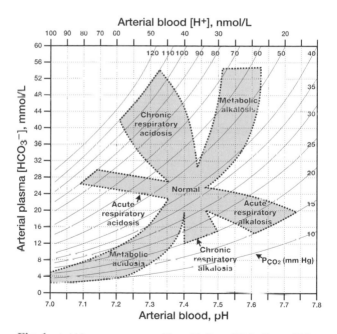

Fig. 1. Acid-base nomogram. (From DuBose TD Jr, Cogan MG, Rector FC Jr. Acid-base disorders. In: Brenner BM, editor. The kidney. 5th ed. Philadelphia: WB Saunders Company; 1996. p. 929-98. Used with permission.)

Table 1. Summary of Simple and Mixed Acid-Base Disorders

Disorder	Initial change	Compensation	Degree of compensation	Second disorder
Metabolic acidosis	HCO_3^- decrease	PCO_2 decrease	Lower	Respiratory alkalosis
			Higher	Respiratory acidosis
Metabolic alkalosis	HCO_3^- increase	PCO_2 increase	Lower	Respiratory alkalosis
			Higher	Respiratory acidosis
Respiratory acidosis	PCO_2 increase	HCO_3^- increase	Lower	Metabolic acidosis
			Higher	Metabolic alkalosis
Respiratory alkalosis	PCO_2 decrease	HCO_3^- decrease	Lower	Metabolic acidosis
			Higher	Metabolic alkalosis

Modified from Narins RG, Emmett M. Simple and mixed acid-base disorders: a practical approach. Medicine (Baltimore). 1980;59:161-87. Used with permission,

- In anion gap metabolic acidosis, it is helpful to compare the "Δ [HCO_3^-]" with the "Δ anion gap." The illustrated concept of the Δ anion gap reflects any increase in the anion gap above normal should lead to ~1:1 titration of 1 mEq of bicarbonate.
  - ▲ For example, an anion gap of 20 reflects an "excess anion gap" of 8 ($20 - 12 = 8$). Therefore, the expected decrease in serum bicarbonate should be 8, or a serum bicarbonate level of 16 ($24 - 8 = 16$).
    - • If the Δ [HCO_3^-] > Δ anion gap, a combination of anion gap and nonanion gap metabolic acidosis is present.
    - • If the Δ [HCO_3^-] < Δ anion gap, a combination of anion gap metabolic acidosis and metabolic alkalosis is present.

METABOLIC ACIDOSIS

- In metabolic acidosis, bicarbonate is lost or nonvolatile acid is gained. Metabolic acidosis does not necessarily mean an abnormal pH because respiratory compensation or the combination with a second acid-base disorder could result in near-normal or normal pH, respectively.

Metabolic Acidosis With Increased Anion Gap
Causes
- Causes are listed in Table 2.

Management
Diabetic Ketoacidosis
- Volume replacement (not in end-stage renal disease) and insulin form the cornerstone of treatment.
- IV insulin bolus (0.1 U/kg) is followed by a continuous infusion of insulin (starting dose 0.1 U/kg per hour).
- 1L of isotonic saline or Ringer lactate should be given rapidly IV on arrival in the first hour, then 0.5-1 L of half normal saline in the second and third hours.
- From the fourth hour, the amount of fluid should be estimated based on urine output and clinical assessment.
- Glucose level should be determined hourly, and when it falls around 200-300 mg/dL, 5% glucose solutions should be added.

Table 2. Causes of Metabolic Acidosis With Increased Anion Gap

Endogenous
Ketoacidosis
Diabetes mellitus
Starvation
Alcohol-induced
Lactic acidosis
Hypoxic (type A)
Nonhypoxic (type B)
Uremia
Exogenous
Methanol
Ethylene glycol
Salicylate
Paraldehyde

From Laski ME, Kurtzman NA. Acid-base disorders in medicine. Dis Mon. 1996;42:90-125. Used with permission.

- Henceforth, insulin infusion and glucose infusion should be adjusted so glucose level remains around 250 mg/dL.
- Potassium replacement is usually needed; if the admission value is normal or low, potassium should be given early.
- Electrolytes should be checked every 3-4 hours.
- Bicarbonate should be considered if pH <7.00, and phosphate should be considered if <1 mg/dL.
- Insulin infusion should be switched to SQ dosage after ketoacidosis has resolved (anion gap and bicarbonate have normalized).

Lactic Acidosis
- Lactic acidosis occurs when oxygen delivery to the cells is inadequate (type A) or the cell is unable to use oxygen.
- Type A results from systemic (shock, carbon monoxide poisoning) or localized (interruption of regional vasculature, mesenteric ischemia, acute arterial thrombosis) tissue hypoxia.
- Type B is the consequence of drugs, toxins, and organ failure (phenformin, metformin, cyanide intoxication, zidovudine, didanosine, zalcitabine, methanol, some hematologic malignancies, liver failure, severe acute pancreatitis).
- The diagnosis is usually one of exclusion and lactate can be measured.

- Treatment consists of restoration of tissue perfusion and oxygenation.

Intoxications

- Methanol and ethylene glycol are metabolized to glycolate or formate.
- An indication of increased alcohol levels is an increase in the osmolar gap: the difference between measured and calculated serum osmolality.
- The calculated (calc) serum osmolality is calculated as follows:
$$\text{Osmolality}_{(calc)} = 2\,[Na^+] + [glucose]/18 + [BUN]/2.8 + [ethanol]/4.6$$
  - ▲ Na is in mEq/L and BUN, glucose, and ethanol in mg/dL (ethanol could be excluded).
  - ▲ If this difference is >15-20, the presence of toxic alcohol is likely.
- Treatment requires infusion of ethanol to produce a serum level of 100-200 mg/dL, followed by hemodialysis, or the use of fomepizole, an alcohol dehydrogenase inhibitor.
- Aspirin can produce respiratory alkalosis, mixed respiratory alkalosis and metabolic acidosis, or (less commonly) pure metabolic acidosis.
  - ▲ Treatment consists of limiting further drug absorption with activated charcoal, urine alkalization, and establishing a high urinary flow rate. Hemodialysis should be considered for patients with renal failure or for severe cases.

Metabolic Acidosis With Normal Anion Gap
Causes
- Causes are listed in Table 3.

Diagnosis
- Urinary anion gap may help to distinguish gastrointestinal from renal loss of bicarbonate as the cause of hyperchloremic metabolic acidosis.
  - ▲ Urinary anion gap = $[Na_u^+ + K_u^+] - [Cl_u^-]$
  - ▲ A negative urinary anion gap results from a nonrenal cause of hyperchloremic acidosis (e.g., diarrhea).

▲ Urinary anion gap is positive in renal tubular acidosis (RTA).

Management
Nonrenal

- Diarrhea is the most common cause of hyperchloremic metabolic acidosis. If renal function is normal, therapy should focus on resolving excessive enteric bicarbonate loss and administering physiologic saline.
- Urinary diversion–related disorders may require thiazide therapy or alkali supplements.
- The most common clinical form of acid ingestion occurs in patients receiving hyperalimentation. Treatment is to adjust composition of the parenteral nutrition.

Table 3. Causes of Metabolic Acidosis With Normal Anion Gap

Nonrenal
    Diarrhea
    Pancreatic fistula
    Urinary diversion
    Acid ingestion
    Arginine infusion
Renal
    Uremia
    Proximal RTA
    Hypokalemic distal RTA
        Classic
        Amphotericin-induced
    Hyperkalemic distal RTA
        Short-circuit distal RTA
            Urinary tract obstruction
            Sickle cell disease
            Drug-induced
        Mineralocorticoid deficiency
            Addison disease
            Selective aldosterone deficiency
            Hyporeninemic hypoaldosteronism

RTA, renal tubular acidosis.

From Laski ME, Kurtzman NA. Acid-base disorders in medicine. Dis Mon. 1996;42:90-125. Used with permission.

Renal

- Proximal RTA (type 2) occurs because the proximal tubule fails to reclaim bicarbonate appropriately.
  - ▲ It occurs in isolation or as part of Fanconi syndrome (aminoaciduria, phosphaturia, uricosuria, glycosuria, and bicarbonaturia).
  - ▲ Proximal RTA is unusual and occurs most commonly as part of Fanconi syndrome that may be caused by Wilson disease, heavy metals, autoimmune diseases, amyloidosis, multiple myeloma, transplant rejection, nephropathy, paroxysmal nocturnal hemoglobinuria, gentamicin, ifosfamide, and other conditions.
  - ▲ Often, treatment is not required, but if acidosis is severe, bicarbonate or a thiazide plus bicarbonate is recommended.
- In classic distal RTA (type 1), hyperchloremic, hypokalemic metabolic acidosis, H^+ secretion in the collecting ducts or the ability to lower urinary pH is impaired.
  - ▲ Several subtypes have been identified.
  - ▲ Causes of distal RTA include autoimmune disorders, cirrhosis, medullary sponge kidney, systemic lupus erythematosus, sickle cell anemia, obstructive uropathy, renal transplantation, amphotericin, lithium, analgesic nephropathy, and drug toxins.
- Hyperkalemic distal RTA (type 4) is caused by defective ammonia production.
  - ▲ Most patients with RTA type 4 have hyporeninemic hypoaldosteronism.
  - ▲ Usual causes include diabetic nephropathy, nephrosclerosis, tubulointerstitial nephropathies, and NSAIDs.
- Without a clear or reversible cause, the treatment of distal RTA relies on providing alkali.
  - ▲ In patients with hyperkalemic distal RTA, potassium restriction is necessary; if aldosterone is absent, fludrocortisone can be used.

METABOLIC ALKALOSIS

- Metabolic alkalosis occurs when bicarbonate accumulates or acid is lost from the body.

- Three major causes of metabolic alkalosis: volume contraction, mineralocorticoid excess, and alkali administration (Table 4)

Management
- For patients with metabolic alkalosis, the history and physical exam should focus on eating habits, drug use, and volume status.
- A low urinary chloride (<20 mEq/L) suggests volume contraction.
  - For volume contraction, therapy focuses on repairing any volume losses and potassium deficiency with the use of physiologic saline and potassium supplementation.
- For non–volume-depleted patients, treatment aims at correcting steroid excess if possible. Spironolactone, up to 400 mg daily, with large amounts of potassium may be considered for some patients.
- For alkali load syndrome, alkalemia should resolve after the exogenous source of alkali is stopped.

RESPIRATORY ACIDOSIS
- Respiratory acidosis is characterized by a decrease in alveolar ventilation relative to carbon dioxide production.

Table 4. Causes of Metabolic Alkalosis

Volume contraction (urinary [Cl$^-$] <20 mEq/L)
Emesis
Gastric suction
Diuretics
Posthypercapnia
Without volume contraction (urinary [Cl$^-$] >20 mEq/L)
Primary & secondary mineralocorticoid excess
Cushing syndrome
Errors of steroid metabolism
Liddle syndrome
Bartter syndrome
Iatrogenic hypermineralocorticoidism
Alkali loads (no volume contraction)
Milk-alkali syndrome
Bicarbonate administration
Lactate or citrate administration

Modified from Laski ME, Kurtzman NA. Acid-base disorders in medicine. Dis Mon. 1996;42:90-125. Used with permission.

- Respiratory acidosis appears to be caused by a primary increase in blood P_{CO_2}.
- Causes are listed in Table 5.

Management

- The problem for most patients with respiratory acidosis is not acidosis but hypoxia of respiratory failure.
- Hypercapnia can result from an acute or chronic process.
  - ▲ Acute hypercapnia develops as a consequence of pneumonia, status asthmaticus, central nervous system depression, and neuromuscular impairment.
    - Treatment should focus on correcting the hypoxia, by mechanical ventilation if necessary, and removing or improving the underlying cause.
  - ▲ Chronic hypercapnia results from many conditions, including COPD, neuromuscular disorders, and chest wall problems.
    - The acidosis is usually well buffered, the decrease in pH is of no consequence, and no treatment is needed regarding pH. However, sometimes, an acute respiratory decompensation (most commonly from pneumonia,

Table 5. Causes of Respiratory Acidosis

Abnormal respiratory drive—excessive sedation, central alveolar hypoventilation, sleep apnea

Neuromuscular—myasthenia gravis, paralytic agents, multiple sclerosis, amyotrophic lateral sclerosis, Guillain-Barré syndrome, botulism, myopathies, myositis

Thoracic cage problems—scoliosis, ankylosing spondylitis, flail chest

Obstructive disease—tracheal, laryngeal, or bronchial obstruction; obstructive sleep apnea

Pulmonary disease—severe interstitial fibrosis, COPD

Pleural disease—fibrothorax, hydrothorax, pneumothorax

Ventilator-management errors—excessive dead space, insufficient tidal volume and/or ventilator rate

Data from Laski ME, Kurtzman NA. Acid-base disorders in medicine. Dis Mon. 1996;42:90-125; Narins RG, Emmett M. Simple and mixed acid-base disorders: a practical approach. Medicine (Baltimore). 1980;59:161-87.

sedation, or uncontrolled oxygen therapy) superimposes the chronic hypercapnia, producing more retention of carbon dioxide and more acidosis.

- Management depends on severity of the acute process and baseline situation of the patient.
- Management usually includes antibiotics, bronchodilators, aspiration of secretions, and, if due to excessive sedation, naloxone or flumazenil could be helpful.
- The minimum amount of oxygen to keep the P_{O_2} about 60 mm Hg should be applied and mechanical ventilation should be used with a conservative approach because of the great difficulty in weaning such patients from ventilators.
- If the patient is encephalopathic from hypercapnia, mechanical ventilation should be instituted.
- ▲ Note: when a patient with chronic hypercapnia is on mechanical ventilation, the goal P_{CO_2} is needed to keep a normal pH (not a normal P_{CO_2}), because, rapid P_{CO_2} reduction produces posthypercapnic alkalosis, with potentially serious consequences.

RESPIRATORY ALKALOSIS

- Respiratory alkalosis is characterized by an increase in alveolar ventilation relative to carbon dioxide production.
- Respiratory alkalosis appears to be caused by a primary decrease in blood P_{CO_2}.
- Causes are listed in Table 6.

Management

- Respiratory alkalosis is the most common acid-base disorder.
- Respiratory alkalosis of <24 hours is considered acute.
- Treatment should be directed toward decreasing hyperventilation and correcting the underlying cause.
- Most cases of respiratory alkalosis, especially chronic cases, pose little risk to health and are not treated.
- In psychogenic respiratory alkalosis, such as panic attacks, management includes reassurance, psychologic therapy, rebreathing into a bag, and sometimes sedation.

Table 6. Causes of Respiratory Alkalosis

Hypoxia
Pulmonary receptor stimulation—pneumonia, pulmonary embolism,
  asthma, pulmonary edema, restrictive disorders
Psychogenic
Drugs—theophylline, salicylates, progesterone
Central nervous system—Cheyne-Stokes breathing, stroke,
  infection
Cirrhosis
Pregnancy
Fever
Sepsis
Hyperthyroidism
Errors in ventilator settings—excessive tidal volume, excessive
  ventilation rate

Modified from Laski ME, Kurtzman NA. Acid-base disorders in medicine.
  Dis Mon. 1996;42:90-125. Used with permission.

ACUTE CORONARY SYNDROMES

Guilherme H. M. Oliveira, M.D.
Arjun Deb, M.D.
R. Scott Wright, M.D.
Joseph G. Murphy, M.D.

DEFINITIONS

- Acute coronary syndromes include
  - ▲ Unstable angina
  - ▲ Non–ST-segment elevation myocardial infarction (NSTEMI)
  - ▲ ST-segment elevation myocardial infarction (STEMI)

Unstable Angina

- Clinical syndrome resulting from rupture of an unstable plaque or from a critically stenotic stable plaque
- It is defined by any of the following:
  - ▲ Rest angina—angina occurring at rest and usually lasting >20 minutes within a week before presentation
  - ▲ New-onset angina—angina of at least Canadian Cardiovascular Society class III severity within 2 months before initial presentation
  - ▲ Worsening angina—previously diagnosed angina that is more frequent, longer in duration or lower in threshold, and has worsened by at least one class within 2 months after initial presentation to at least Canadian Cardiovascular Society class III severity

Myocardial Infarction

- Diagnosed by the presence of at least two of the following three criteria:
  - ▲ Prolonged chest pain (>30 minutes) or anginal equivalent

Special abbreviations used in this chapter: LBBB, left bundle branch block; LMWH, low-molecular-weight heparin; NSTEMI, non–ST-segment elevation myocardial infarction; PCI, percutaneous coronary intervention; PTCA, percutaneous transluminal coronary angioplasty; STEMI, ST-segment elevation myocardial infarction; tPA, tissue plasminogen activator.

- ▲ ECG changes consistent with injury or necrosis
- ▲ Increased levels of cardiac enzymes
- ■ Subdivisions
  - ▲ NSTEMI—characterized by an increase in troponin I or T in the clinical setting of acute coronary syndrome and/or ST-segment depression >1 mm in two or more contiguous leads
  - ▲ STEMI—characterized by ST-segment elevation >1 mm in two or more contiguous leads or left bundle branch block (LBBB) not known to be old
- ■ Unstable angina cannot be distinguished from NSTEMI at presentation.

CLINICAL PRESENTATION

- ■ Chest pain is the most common presenting symptom of acute coronary syndromes.
- ■ Chest pain is more likely due to an acute coronary syndrome if
  - ▲ It is more severe than previous typical episodes of angina.
  - ▲ It lasts >20 minutes but <4 hours.
  - ▲ It started at rest.
  - ▲ It radiates and is accompanied by dyspnea, diaphoresis, nausea, or vomiting.
- ■ Chest pain is more likely to be noncardiac related if:
  - ▲ Sharp pain worsened by coughing or deep breathing
  - ▲ Brief episodes of pain lasting a few seconds
  - ▲ Constant pain lasting >8 hours to days
  - ▲ Pain located solely in the middle or lower abdominal region
  - ▲ Pain reproduced by palpation or movement of chest wall or localized with a finger
- ■ Other less common presenting symptoms of acute coronary syndrome
  - ▲ Loss of consciousness
  - ▲ Sudden onset of dyspnea
  - ▲ Altered mental status
  - ▲ Appearance of an arrhythmia (atrioventricular block, atrial fibrillation, ventricular tachyarrhythmias)
  - ▲ Unexplained hypotension
- ■ Physical findings indicating a high likelihood of an acute coronary syndrome and high cardiovascular risk include
  - ▲ Hypotension
  - ▲ Third heart sound
  - ▲ Increased jugular venous pressure

- ▲ Apical systolic murmur of transient mitral regurgitation
- ▲ Pulmonary rales indicative of pulmonary edema
- The likelihood of coronary artery disease in patients with symptoms suggesting unstable angina is outlined in Table 1 and the short-term risk of death or nonfatal myocardial infarction in Table 2.
- Aim of the initial history and physical examination should be
  - ▲ Assess the likelihood of coronary ischemia as the cause of chest pain
  - ▲ Exclude other life-threatening disorders such as pulmonary embolism and aortic dissection, which may have a similar presentation
  - ▲ Assess the severity of the acute coronary syndrome and provide appropriate triage

ECG AND LABORATORY DIAGNOSIS OF ACUTE CORONARY SYNDROME
ECG Findings
Unstable Angina
- Nonspecific findings are the most common.
- ECG may be normal in up to 40% of cases.
- Transient T-wave inversion is the most sensitive sign for ischemia.
- Transient flat or downsloping ST-segment depression is the most specific sign for ischemia and may represent subepicardial injury.

NSTEMI
- Absence of ST-segment elevation
- Nonspecific changes are most common.
- Persistent ST-segment depression with T-wave inversion is the most specific sign.

STEMI
- ST-segment elevation >1 mm (defined as elevation of the ST segment >1 mm 0.6 millisecond after the J point) in two or more contiguous leads (i.e., leads that represent a myocardial wall, I, aVL-lateral wall; II, III, aVF-inferior wall)
- LBBB not known to be old

Table 1. Likelihood of Coronary Artery Disease (CAD) in Patients With Symptoms Suggestive of Unstable Angina

High likelihood (0.85-0.99)	Intermediate likelihood (0.15-0.84)	Low likelihood (0.01-0.14)
Any of the following features: History of previous MI, sudden death, CABG, or known CAD Definite angina in men >60 or women >70 years Transient hemodynamic or ECG changes with pain Variant angina ST-segment elevation/depression >1 mm Marked symmetrical T-wave inversion in multiple precordial leads	Absence of high-likelihood features & any of the following: Definite angina in men <60 or women <70 years Probable angina in men >60 or women >70 years Chest pain probably not angina in diabetics Chest pain probably not angina with 2 or more risk factors other than diabetes ST-segment depression 0.05-1.0 mm T-wave inversion ≥1 mm in leads with dominant R waves Extracardiac vascular disease	Absence of high- & intermediate-likelihood features & any of the following: Probably not angina One risk factor other than diabetes T-wave inversion or flattening <1 mm in leads with dominant R waves Normal ECG

CABG, coronary artery bypass graft; MI, myocardial infarction.
Modified from ACC/AHA Practice Guidelines [cited 2005 Nov 3]. Available from http://www.acc.org/clinical/guidelines/unstable/incorporated/index.htm. Used with permission.

Table 2. Short-Term Risk of Death or Nonfatal Myocardial Infarction in Patients With Unstable Angina

High risk	Intermediate risk	Low risk
At least 1 of the following has to be present: Prolonged (>20 minute) ongoing chest pain Pulmonary edema Angina with S₃ or new/worsening rales Angina with hypotension Angina with new/worsening mitral regurgitation murmur Angina at rest with dynamic ST changes >1 mm	Absence of any high-risk features & any of the following: Prolonged angina at rest >20 minutes, now resolved in a person with moderate/high likelihood of CAD Rest angina >20 minutes or resolved with rest or nitroglycerin Nocturnal angina Angina with dynamic T-wave changes New-onset CCSC III/IV angina in past 2 weeks with moderate/high likelihood of CAD Pathologic Q waves or resting ST-segment depression <1 mm in multiple leads	Absence of any high- or intermediate-risk feature Increased angina, frequency, severity, duration Angina provoked at lower threshold New-onset angina with onset 2 weeks to 2 months before presentation Normal or unchanged ECG

CAD, coronary artery disease; CCSC, Canadian Cardiovascular Society Class; S₃, third heart sound.
Modified from ACC/AHA Practice Guidelines [cited 2005 Nov 3]. Available from http://www.acc.org/clinical/guidelines/unstable/incorporated/index.htm. Used with permission.

Laboratory Findings

- Elevation of CK, CK-MB, and troponin
  - ▲ Myocardial necrosis—Whether this is acute coronary syndrome will depend on clinical setting.
  - ▲ Other possibilities include
    - Myocarditis—septic, viral, inflammatory, paraneoplastic
    - Trauma
    - Systemic inflammatory response syndrome
    - Catastrophic pulmonary embolism
- Increase in CK and CK-MB with normal levels of troponins
  - ▲ Early myocardial injury if this only happens initially when there was not enough time for troponins to increase, but troponin levels should be increased on further testing.
  - ▲ Persistent increase in CK with normal troponin is found in rhabdomyolysis and severe skeletal muscle injury or necrosis.
- Increased troponins with normal CK and CK-MB
  - ▲ Uncertain pathophysiologic situation, which clinically indicates increased risk for death
  - ▲ If chest pain is present and patient is at obvious risk for coronary artery disease, manage as acute coronary syndrome.
  - ▲ Other possibilities include
    - Pulmonary embolism
    - Severe systemic illness
    - Renal failure (troponin T rather than I is more commonly affected by renal function)

EARLY RECOGNITION OF MYOCARDIAL INFARCTION

- Advise patients prescribed nitroglycerin to call 911 after **1** nitroglycerin if no improvement in chest pain after 5 minutes.
- Family members should be trained in cardiopulmonary resuscitation and use of automatic external defibrillators.

PERIHOSPITAL ISSUES

- After onset of chest pain, patient chews 162 or 325 mg aspirin.
- Advance cardiac life support providers or paramedics perform, interpret, relay 12-lead ECG to hospital.
- Prehospital thrombolysis—physician in ambulance or full-time paramedics who are able to transmit ECGs and are in contact with trained medical personnel

- Patients <75 years with STEMI and shock should be transported to hospital with percutaneous coronary intervention (PCI) capability, with door-to-door transfer time <30 minutes (same for patients with congestive heart failure).

MANAGEMENT OF ACUTE CORONARY SYNDROMES

Immediate Assessment and Treatment

- The following assessment should be completed within the first 10 minutes:
  - ▲ Vital signs, including oxygen saturation
  - ▲ IV access
  - ▲ 12-lead ECG
  - ▲ Brief targeted history and physical as discussed above, including contraindications to thrombolytic therapy
  - ▲ Initial cardiac marker levels
  - ▲ Initial coagulation and electrolyte levels
  - ▲ Possible chest X-ray (<30 minutes)
- The patient should also receive the following during the initial assessment:
  - ▲ Oxygen at 4 L/minute
  - ▲ Aspirin 325 mg chewable
  - ▲ Nitroglycerin sublingual or spray
  - ▲ Morphine IV if pain not relieved by nitroglycerin

Specific Management

Unstable Angina and NSTEMI

- Rapid initiation of antithrombotic and antianginal therapy is the goal of management of acute coronary syndromes.

Aspirin

- All patients with suspected unstable angina should receive 325 mg of crushed aspirin initially, followed by 160-325 mg daily.
- For patients with unstable angina, aspirin has been found to decrease the incidence of death and nonfatal myocardial infarction by 50%.
- Clopidogrel is recommended for patients who have hypersensitivity to aspirin.

β-Blockers

- All patients with an acute coronary syndrome should receive β-blockers.
  - ▲ Metoprolol, 5 mg IV at 5- to 10-minute intervals, followed by oral metoprolol 25-50 mg every 6-12 hours. Titrate the dose to desired heart rate and blood pressure.
- If there is absolute contraindication, use diltiazem or verapamil.
- The goal is to relieve cardiac ischemia and decrease the resting heart rate to 50-60 beats/minute and a mean arterial pressure of 60-70 mm Hg.

Heparin

- The combination of unfractionated IV heparin and aspirin is superior to aspirin alone (reducing the risk of death and myocardial infarction by 33%).
- Low-molecular-weight heparin (LMWH) is as effective as unfractionated heparin, without causing excess bleeding complications.
- Heparin should be continued for a minimum of 3-7 days because its beneficial effects are lost if infusion is discontinued after 2 days.
- If the patient is triaged to early invasive therapy, unfractionated heparin is preferred because it can be reversed quickly.
- For patients with a history of heparin-induced thrombocytopenia, give lepirudin, a direct thrombin inhibitor.
- Heparin, IV bolus 80 U/kg, followed by 18 U/kg per hour
  - ▲ Adjust infusion rate to keep aPTT at 2-2.5 × the upper limit of normal.
  - ▲ Check aPTT 6 hours after starting heparin infusion and 6 hours thereafter until the goal aPTT is reached, then check every 12-24 hours.
  - ▲ Heparin normograms are helpful in adjusting infusion rates.
- Enoxaparin, 1 mg/kg every 12 hours. Dalteparin, 120 U/kg every 12 hours, is as effective without having to monitor serial aPTT.
- Lepirudin, 0.4 mg/kg bolus, followed by 0.15 mg/kg per hour infusions with a goal aPTT of 1.5-2.5 × the upper limits of normal

Glycoprotein IIb/IIIa Receptor Inhibitors

- They inhibit cross linking of platelets and prevent platelet aggregation and thrombus formation.
- In patients with unstable angina and NSTEMI, eptifibatide added to heparin and aspirin reduced the absolute risk of death and nonfatal myocardial infarction at 30 days by 5%, when compared with heparin and aspirin.
- Compared with heparin alone, tirofiban and heparin reduced the relative risk of death, nonfatal myocardial infarction, and refractory ischemia at 7 days by 32%.
- Abciximab should only be given to patients undergoing early revascularization.
- Currently, eptifibatide and trofiban are recommended in addition to heparin and aspirin for patients with unstable angina or NSTEMI who have high-risk characteristics as defined by the TIMI Risk Score or in whom PCI is planned.
- Eptifibatide, 180 µg/kg bolus, followed by 2 µg/kg per minute for 24-48 hours
- Tirofiban, 0.4 µg/kg per minute over 30 minutes, followed by 0.1 µg/kg per minute for 24-48 hours
- Abciximab, 0.25 mg/kg IV bolus, followed by 10 µg/minute for 12 hours for unstable angina and planned PCI

Clopidogrel

- It is a thienopyridine that inhibits the adenosine diphosphate mediated activation of platelets.
- Clopidogrel decreased the rate of major adverse cardiovascular events by 20% in patients admitted with an acute coronary syndrome in the CURE study. In that study, however, patients were not offered early revascularization strategy and not treated with glycoprotein IIb/IIIa inhibitors.
- Currently, the use of clopidogrel in NSTEMI acute coronary syndrome should be limited to patients not undergoing early revascularization in whom glycoprotein IIb/IIIa inhibitors are not used.

Statins
- HMG-CoA reductase inhibitors have benefits other than lipid-lowering effects in patients with an acute coronary syndrome.
- PROVE-IT trial showed that lowering low-density lipoprotein cholesterol to mean of 65 mg/dL in hospitalized patients with high-risk coronary syndromes produced a 16% relative risk reduction in combined end point of death from any cause, myocardial infarction, recurrent unstable angina, or revascularization at 2 years. Therefore, we recommend treating patients with acute coronary syndrome to low-density lipoprotein cholesterol of <80.
- The MIRACLE study showed evidence that statins diminish the rate of recurrent ischemia after an acute coronary syndrome.

Aldosterone Blockers
- Eplerenone 50 mg/day, when started within 3-14 days after myocardial infarction in patients with a left ventricular ejection fraction <40%, reduced morbidity and mortality at 3 months and 2 years compared with placebo.

Nitrates
- They decrease cardiac ischemia and anginal pain by reducing preload and dilating coronary arteries.
- Sublingual nitroglycerin should be administered immediately to patients with an acute coronary syndrome.
- IV infusion can be used for refractory pain or initially for patients who are hypertensive on presentation.
- Tachyphylaxis may develop within 24 hours after a continuous infusion.
- Nitroglycerin, 0.4 mg sublingually, can be given at presentation, and IV nitroglycerin can be started at 10-20 µg/minute and rapidly titrated to decrease pain.

Morphine
- Pain relief is an important therapeutic goal, and patients should receive morphine frequently for pain relief.
- Morphine, 1-3 mg IV every 5-10 minutes until pain is relieved

Oxygen
- All patients with a suspected acute coronary syndrome should receive oxygen, especially if they have respiratory distress or hypoxemia.
- Oxygen saturation should be kept >90%.
- Oxygen, 2-4 L, to keep arterial oxygen saturation >90%

Early Percutaneous Revascularization
- Patients with high and intermediate TIMI risk scores benefit from early revascularization with PCI (<48 hours after admission), according to the FRISC II and TIMI 18 trial results (Table 3).

STEMI
- Emergency department
  - ▲ Door-to-ECG *review* <10 minutes
  - ▲ Right-sided ECG leads for all inferior STEMI patients

Table 3. TIMI Risk Factor Score*

Risk factor score
1. Age >65 years
2. Three or more risk factors for coronary artery disease
3. Previous coronary stenosis >50% or previous percutaneous coronary intervention
4. Two or more anginal events over the past 24 hours
5. ASA use in the past 7 days
6. ST-segment changes
7. Cardiac markers elevation

Risk of adverse cardiac event[†]

No. of risk factors	Risk, %
0-1	4.7
2	8.3
3	13.2
4	19.9
5	26.2
6-7	41.0

*Low risk = score 0-2; intermediate risk = score 3-4; high risk = score 5-7. Patients with elevated cardiac enzymes and/or ST changes should be included in the high-risk category independent of their overall score.
[†]Myocardial infarction, cardiac death, or recurrent ischemia.

- ▲ Door-to-percutaneous transluminal coronary angioplasty (PTCA) time <90 minutes for primary PCI
- Goal of management—immediate reperfusion of the infarct-related artery with reestablishment of TIMI grade 3 flow
- TIMI flow grades—TIMI 0 = complete occlusion of infarct-related artery, TIMI 1 = flow into but not through the obstructive thrombus, TIMI 2 = reperfusion of infarct-related artery with slow flow, TIMI 3 = normal brisk flow.
- Initial emergency department management
  - ▲ Aspirin: patient chews 162 or 325 mg
  - ▲ β-Blocker
    - PO
    - IV, especially if hypertension or tachycardia

Reperfusion Therapy
- Reperfusion therapy can be accomplished with either thrombolytics or percutaneous coronary intervention (which includes the use of stents).
- The choice of reperfusion therapy depends on availability of treatment modalities; ACC/AHA guidelines recommend that thrombolytics be given within 30 minutes after diagnosis or PCI be performed within 90 minutes after diagnosis.
- The GUSTO IIb trial showed that PTCA reduced the combined end point of death, nonfatal myocardial infarction, or nonfatal disabling stroke (13.7% for tissue plasminogen activator [tPA] vs. 9.6% for PTCA) at 30 days, but these differences were nonsignificant after 6 months of follow-up.
- PTCA with stenting decreases the rates of restenosis and reocclusion more than angioplasty alone and may prevent the loss of benefit over time seen in earlier trials.

Thrombolysis
- All patients with new LBBB or ST-segment elevation >1 mm in two contiguous leads are potential candidates for thrombolytic therapy if they present within 12 hours after onset of symptoms.
- ISIS-2 showed a mortality benefit with thrombolytics compared with placebo of about 20% at 30 days that persisted for up to 10 years.
- The maximal benefit was in people with anterior wall infarction.

- Reperfusion therapy
  - ▲ Fibrinolysis if no PCI within 90 minutes available, door-to-needle <30 minutes
  - ▲ Fibrinolysis if true posterior myocardial infarction
  - ▲ Absolute contraindications to fibrinolysis
    - Any previous intracranial hemorrhage
    - Any cerebral aneurysm, arteriovenous malformation, or malignant neoplasm
    - Stroke within last 3 months (except last 3 hours)
    - Active bleeding
    - Suspected aortic dissection
    - Notable head or facial trauma within last 3 months
  - ▲ History of stroke more than 3 months ago is now a relative contraindication.
- The presence of any one of these contraindications also contraindicates PCI, which requires full anticoagulation with heparin, glycoprotein IIb/IIIa inhibitors, clopidogrel, and aspirin.
- GUSTO I showed that tPA decreased 30-day mortality by 15% compared with streptokinase.
- Currently, tenecteplase-tPA is the thrombolytic agent of choice, as it can be given as a one-time bolus with heparin and aspirin.
- Determining whether reperfusion therapy is successful is difficult clinically. The combination of chest pain relief, at least a 50% decrease in ST-segment elevation, and the appearance of accelerated idioventricular rhythm predicts successful reperfusion with high specificity.
- Complete resolution of ST-segment elevation at 90 minutes indicates a 93% likelihood of reperfusion of the infarct-related artery and an 80% likelihood of TIMI grade 3 flow.
- Patients who receive thrombolytic therapy and do not have complete resolution of chest pain or a 50% decrease in ST-segment elevation at 60 minutes should be referred for rescue PCI.
- Combination $\frac{1}{2}$-dose tenecteplase or reteplase with abciximab for those <75 years
- Combination $\frac{1}{2}$-dose lysis and glycoprotein IIb/IIIa inhibitors is *contraindicated* for those >75 years

- Alteplase (recombinant tPA), IV bolus of 15 mg, followed by 0.75-mg/kg (up to 50 mg) IV infusion over 30 minutes, then 0.25-mg/kg (up to 35 mg) IV infusion over 60 minutes, with a total maximal dose of 100 mg over 90 minutes.
- The risk of serious intracranial bleeding is about 0.7% for patients receiving tPA, with a mortality rate >50% if bleeding occurs and higher among patients >75 years.

PCI
- Addressing nonculprit lesions in primary PCI is a class III indication and should not be done routinely.
- Randomized controlled clinical trials show that PCI offers better TIMI grade 3 flow, more sustained patency of the infarct-related artery, and fewer bleeding complications than thrombolytic therapy.
- Thirty-day and long-term mortality also favor PCI in comparison with thrombolytic therapy, and PCI is the reperfusion modality of choice at our and most major institutions in the U.S.
- The "door-to-PTCA" time should be <60-90 minutes.
- If symptoms are <3 hours, primary PCI is preferred if expected door-to-PTCA time minus expected door-to-needle time is <60 minutes.
- Primary PCI is preferred
  - ▲ Congestive heart failure or shock
  - ▲ Symptom duration >3 hours
- Nonculprit vessels should not be treated at time of primary PCI
- Rescue PCI if hemodynamically or electrically unstable or if persistent ischemia
- Routine coronary angiography and PCI if indicated by flow-limiting lesion post-lysis in stable patients
- Glycoprotein IIb/IIIa inhibitors such as abciximab or integrilin should be administered routinely during PCI to decrease the rate of death and recurrent myocardial infarction, as shown in the CADILLAC and ADMIRAL trials.
- Primary PCI is also the treatment of choice for STEMI complicated by cardiogenic shock.
- The SHOCK trial showed a 1-year survival of 47% in the early revascularization group and 33% in the medical stabilization group.

Coronary Artery Bypass Surgery
- Emergency bypass surgery is indicated for left main coronary artery disease or severe three-vessel disease not amenable to percutaneous revascularization.
- Diabetic patients with three-vessel disease appear to have better survival if they undergo surgical bypass.
- For those in whom the left coronary anterior artery is not bypassed, survival benefits are unproven.
- Timing of coronary artery bypass graft
  - ▲ Critical anatomy with preserved left ventricular function— perform coronary artery bypass graft before dismissal
  - ▲ If significant left ventricular dysfunction—delay performing coronary artery bypass graft

Anti-ischemic Therapy
- Aspirin, nitrates, β-blockers, statins, oxygen, and morphine should be administered as for treatment of unstable angina and NSTEMI (see above).
- Unlike their role in unstable angina, β-blockers have been conclusively proven to decrease the mortality rate and occurrence of major cardiovascular events after acute myocardial infarction.

Antithrombotic Therapy
- Heparin should be given as adjunctive therapy after thrombolytic therapy.
- Enoxaparin is *contraindicated* with lysis in patients
  - ▲ >75 years
  - ▲ With increased creatinine (2.0 mg/dL in women, 2.5 mg/dL in men)
- Preferably, a weight-based nomogram should be used.
- For patients undergoing direct angioplasty, heparin should be given in combination with glycoprotein IIb/IIIa inhibitors.

Angiotensin-Converting Enzyme Inhibitors
- Analysis of pooled data shows that angiotensin-converting enzyme inhibitors started within 36 hours after myocardial

infarction significantly decreased 30-day mortality (RRR = 7%).

- Most of this benefit was observed in the first 7 days after myocardial infarction and in high-risk groups such as Killip classes II and III and anterior wall myocardial infarction.
- Angiotensin-converting enzyme inhibitors should be started at the lowest possible dose and titrated up as tolerated.
- Angiotensin-converting enzyme inhibitor in first 24 hours for
  - ▲ Anterior myocardial infarction
  - ▲ Left ventricular ejection fraction <0.40
  - ▲ Heart failure
- Angiotensin receptor blocker (valsartan or candesartan) if patient cannot tolerate angiotensin-converting enzyme inhibitor

Other Adjunctive Measures
- There is no role for the routine use of antiarrhythmic agents or magnesium or calcium channel blockers unless specifically indicated.
- Aggressive blood sugar control has a beneficial effect on the outcome of patients with myocardial infarction.
- Measure left ventricular function in all infarct patients

Implantable Cardioverter-Defibrillator
- Ventricular fibrillation or significant sustained ventricular tachycardia >48 hours after STEMI, not due to recurrent ischemia or reinfarction
- One month after STEMI if left ventricular ejection fraction is 0.31-0.40 with nonsustained ventricular tachycardia and with inducible ventricular tachycardia or ventricular fibrillation at electrophysiologic study
- One month after STEMI with left ventricular ejection fraction <0.31

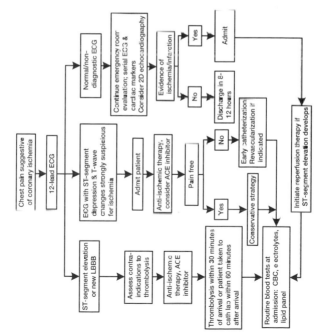

Fig. 1. Algorithm for management, in the emergency department, of patients with suspected myocardial infarction. ACE, angiotensin-converting enzyme; LBBB, left bundle branch block.

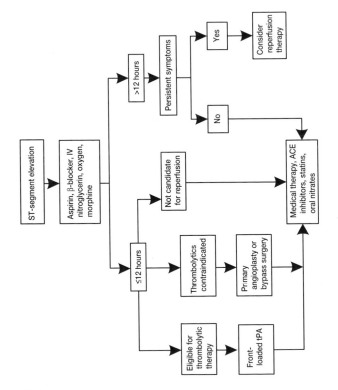

Fig. 2. Algorithm for the management of Q-wave myocardial infarction. ACE, angiotensin-converting enzyme; tPA, tissue plasminogen activator. (Modified from Antman EM. Medical therapy for acute coronary syndromes: an overview. In Braunwald E, editor. Atlas of heart diseases. Vol VIII. St. Louis: Mosby; 1996. p. 10.1-10.25. Used with permission.)

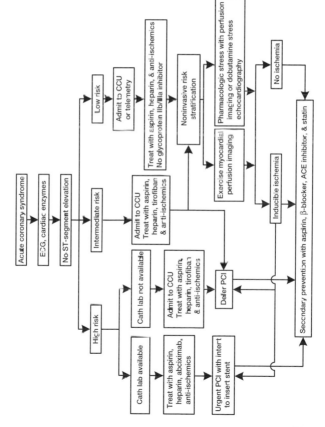

Fig. 3. Algorithm for the management of unstable angina/ NSTEMI. ACE, angiotensin-converting enzyme; CCU, coronary care unit; PCI, percutaneous coronary intervention.

ACUTE RENAL FAILURE

Andrew D. Rule, M.D.
Robert C. Albright, Jr., D.O.

DEFINITION

- Acute renal failure (ARF) is an increase in the serum level of creatinine of 0.5 mg/dL daily or BUN of 10 mg/dL daily over several days, with a decrease in glomerular filtration rate.
- Pseudoacute renal failure can occur when there is an increase in creatinine or BUN without a decrease in the glomerular filtration rate.
  - ▲ Increased creatinine—increase in protein intake, part of rhabdomyolysis, trimethoprim, cefoxitin, flucytosine.
  - ▲ Increased BUN—gastrointestinal tract bleeding, tissue trauma, glucocorticoids, tetracycline.

CLASSIFICATION

Acute vs. Chronic

- Chronic renal failure is suggested by
  - ▲ Electrolyte abnormalities—hypocalcemia and hyperphosphatemia with high level of parathyroid hormone.
  - ▲ High levels of creatinine and BUN without symptoms of uremia
  - ▲ Anemia with low erythropoietin levels
  - ▲ Osteodystrophy and neuropathy
  - ▲ Abnormal renal ultrasound with
    - Small kidneys (<10 cm)
    - Decreased or absent renal cortex
    - Increased echogenicity of renal cortex

Urine Output

- Anuric (<50 mL/day)

Special abbreviation used in this chapter: ARF, acute renal failure.

- ▲ Limited differential diagnosis—complete obstruction, rapidly progressive glomerulonephritis, cortical necrosis, bilateral renal artery occlusion
  - ▲ Not typically seen in acute tubular necrosis
- Oliguric (<400 mL/day)
  - ▲ Poor prognosis compared with nonoliguric
- Nonoliguric (>800 mL/day)
- ARF is also categorized by cause—prerenal, intrinsic, and postrenal

ETIOLOGY
- The causes of ARF are listed in Table 1.

EPIDEMIOLOGY
Prevalence
- ARF occurs in 1% of hospitalized patients and in 20% of ICU patients.
- In the community, ARF occurs in approximately 209 per 1 million population.

Risk Factors
- Radiocontrast dye, especially patients with
  - ▲ Creatinine >2.0 mg/dL
  - ▲ Diabetes mellitus
- Elderly
- Hyperbilirubinemia

Mortality Rate
- 7% for ARF that is prerenal and leads to hospital admission
- 45% for ARF acquired in the hospital
- 70% for ARF acquired in the ICU
- 80% for postoperative ARF

CLINICAL PRESENTATION
- ARF may present without any obvious signs or symptoms.
- Typically, the precipitating condition (e.g., dehydration) suggests the need for a laboratory evaluation for ARF.
- When ARF is severe and prolonged, a patient may present clinically with volume overload (pulmonary edema, hypertension) and/or uremia, as in chronic renal failure.
- Uremia symptoms include fatigue, lethargy, myoclonus,

Table 1. Causes of Acute Renal Failure

Prerenal
    Hypotension—any cause, e.g., sepsis
    Hypovolemia—common in elderly with baseline chronic renal
       failure
    Decrease in effective arterial blood volume—congestive heart
       failure, nephrotic syndrome, cirrhosis, third spacing
    Renal vasoconstriction —hypercalcemia, norepinephrine, epi-
       nephrine, cyclosporine, tacrolimus, amphotericin B, radiocon-
       trast dye, cocaine
    Drugs that impair renal vascular autoregulation (e.g., NSAIDs &
       angiotensin-converting enzyme inhibitors)
    Atheroembolic
    Renal vein thrombosis
    Hepatorenal (diagnosis of exclusion)
Intrinsic
    Glomerular or renal microvasculature—disseminated intravascu-
       lar coagulation, thrombotic thrombocytopenic purpura, hemolyt-
       ic uremic syndrome, toxemia of pregnancy, glomerulonephritis
    Acute tubular necrosis
       Ischemic (from any prolonged prerenal process)
       Medication- or toxin-induced—aminoglycoside antibiotics,
         cisplatin, heavy metals, IV immune globulin, methotrexate,
         foscarnet, pentamidine, organic solvents, cocaine, mannitol,
         cyclosporine, tacrolimus, amphotericin B, radiocontrast dye
       Intrinsic toxins—myeloma light chain, uric acid, hemolysis,
         rhabdomyolysis, oxalate
    Allergic interstitial nephritis—β-lactams, sulfonamides,
       trimethoprim, NSAIDs, ciprofloxacin, thiazide diuretics,
       furosemide, rifampin, phenytoin, allopurinol
    Chinese herb nephropathy ("slimming teas")
    Pyelonephritis
    Infiltrates—lymphoma, sarcoidosis
    Renal allograft rejection
Postrenal
    Ureteral—papillary necrosis, bilateral calculi, retroperitoneal
       fibrosis, compression by tumor
    Bladder—calculi, blood clot, neurogenic, transitional cell cancer
    Medication-induced crystalluria—acyclovir, sulfonamides,
       methotrexate, indinavir
    Urethra—prostate cancer, benign prostatic hypertrophy, stricture,
       phimosis

Modified from Brady HR, Brenner BM. Acute renal failure. In: Braunwald
E, Fauci AS, Kasper DL, Hauser SL, Longo DL, Jameson JL, editors.
Harrison's principles of internal medicine. 15th ed. New York: McGraw-
Hill; 2001. p. 1541-51. Used with permission.

muscle cramps, uremic frost, seizures, pericarditis, arrhythmias, pruritus, ecchymoses, anorexia, nausea, bleeding, hypothermia.

DIAGNOSTIC STRATEGIES

- All patients with acute renal failure need the following diagnostic studies:
  - ▲ History and physical exam (Table 2)
  - ▲ CBC, creatinine, BUN, sodium, potassium, calcium, phosphorus (Table 3)
  - ▲ Urinalysis and fractional excretion of sodium (Table 4)
  - ▲ 24-Hour creatinine clearance and proteinuria
- For selected patients, antinuclear antibodies, antineutrophilic cytoplasmic antibodies, anti-glomerular basement membrane antibodies, cryoglobulins, others

Radiology

- Renal ultrasound to evaluate for hydronephrosis (only 80%-85% sensitive and serial studies may be necessary if suspicion for postrenal ARF is high)
- Renal Doppler ultrasound to evaluate for renal artery stenosis and renal vein thrombosis
- Bladder scan to evaluate for urethral obstruction
- CT of retroperitoneum to evaluate for obstructing masses
- In acute anuria, renal angiography should be considered to rule out acute renal embolization.

Indications for Renal Biopsy

- Generally not necessary in ARF except for following indications:
  - ▲ Suspicion of glomerulonephritis or vasculitis based on serologic markers and/or urinalysis findings (RBC casts)
    - • Example—perinuclear antineutrophilic cytoplasmic antibodies suggest microscopic polyangiitis, and biopsy confirms this with pauciimmune necrotizing glomerulonephritis.
  - ▲ Inconclusive clinical, lab, and radiology studies
  - ▲ Prerenal, postrenal, and toxin/ischemic acute tubular necrosis ruled out
  - ▲ Rule out allograft rejection vs. drug toxicity in renal transplant patients

Table 2. History and Physical Exam Clues

Clue	Suggested cause
Recent angiography	Atheroemboli
Ischemia of extremity	Rhabdomyolysis
Anuria	Postrenal
Rash, fever, arthralgias	Allergic interstitial nephritis
Bone pain	Multiple myeloma
Livedo reticularis, digit ischemia	Atheroemboli
Palpable purpura	Vasculitis
Hemoptysis	Vasculitis
Flank pain	Renal artery occlusion, severe glomerulonephritis, or pyelonephritis, nephrolithiasis
Papilledema	Malignant hypertension
Enlarged prostate	Benign prostatic hypertrophy
Anticholinergic medications	Neurogenic bladder
Alcoholic	Rhabdomyolysis
Prosthetic heart valve	Postinfectious glomerulonephritis
Chronic lymphocytic leukemia or lymphoma or chemotherapy	Uric acid nephropathy
Polyuria	Postrenal, hypokalemia nephropathy
Abdominal pain, flank pain, palpable bladder	Postrenal

Data from Brady HR, Brenner BM. Acute renal failure. In: Braunwald E, Fauci AS, Kasper DL, Hauser SL, Longo DL, Jameson JL, editors. Harrison's principles of internal medicine. 15th ed. New York: McGraw-Hill; 2001. p. 1541-51.

- Biopsy has <1% risk of serious complications (arteriovenous fistula, hematoma, infection, surgery, or death).
- Biopsy alters management of patients in approximately three of four cases.

MANAGEMENT
- Treatment generally varies depending on the underlying cause.
  - Prerenal—Increase renal perfusion (IV fluids, blood transfusions, dopamine).

Table 3. Blood Tests

Suspected cause	Confirmatory marker
Prerenal	BUN:creatinine ratio >20:1
Malignancy	Hypercalcemia & hyperuricemia
Rhabdomyolysis	Increased CK level
Multiple myeloma	Monoclonal gammopathy on SPEP
Acute interstitial nephritis	Eosinophilia
Exogenous nephrotoxin (e.g., ethylene glycol)	Osmolar gap
Renal transplant rejection	Immunosuppressive agent trough level
Glomeruloncphritis	ANA, ANCA, cryoglobulins, anti-GBM antibodies, ASO titer

ANA, antinuclear antibodies; ANCA, antineutrophilic cytoplasmic antibodies; ASO, antistreptolysin O; GBM, glomerular basement membrane; SPEP, serum protein electrophoresis.

▲ Postrenal—Relieve obstruction (place Foley catheter, consult urology).

▲ Intrinsic—Look out for uremic complications and take supportive measures.

GENERAL MEASURES

- Check urinalysis, urine sodium, and urine creatinine—important to check before IV fluids or diuretics.
- Exclude postrenal and prerenal causes.
  ▲ Consider a volume challenge if indicated.
- Stop all nephrotoxic agents.
- Consider furosemide.
  ▲ Diuretics have not been shown to be advantageous in the outcome of ARF but should be considered if patient is volume overloaded or if toxins need to be excreted (e.g., heme pigments in rhabdomyolysis).
- Treat with high dose of furosemide (100-200 mg IV 2 or 3 times daily).
- Furosemide and/or mannitol drip may be helpful in obtaining diuresis.
- Avoid doses of furosemide >600 mg/day because of ototoxicity.
- Indications for dialysis in ARF are listed in Table 5.

Table 4. Urinalysis

Condition	Dipstick	Sediment	Urine osmolality, mOsm/kg	FENa*
Prerenal	Trace/no protein	Hyaline casts	>500	<1
Intrinsic				
Acute GN	Moderate-severe protein	RBCs, RBC casts	>500	<1
	Hemoglobin	Dysmorphic RBCs		
ATN	Mild-moderate protein	Granular casts	<350	>1
AIN	Mild-moderate protein	WBCs, WBC casts	<350	>1
	Leukocytes	RBCs, eosinophils		
	Hemoglobin			
Postrenal	Trace/no protein	Crystals, RBCs	<350	>1
	Leukocytes, mercury possible	WBCs		

AIN, acute interstitial nephritis; ATN, acute tubular necrosis; FENa, fractional excretion of sodium; GN, glomerulonephritis.

$$*FENa = \frac{Urine\ Na \times plasma\ creatinine}{Plasma\ Na \times urine\ creatinine} \times 100$$

Modified from Thadhani R, Pascual M, Bonventri JV. Acute renal failure. N Engl J Med. 1996;334:1448-60. Used with permission.

SUPPORTIVE MEASURES

- Nutritional management emphasizes sufficient calories without nitrogenous waste.
  - ▲ Calories between 126 and 147 kJ/kg daily
  - ▲ Protein between 0.6 g/kg and 1.4 g/kg daily
- Restrict intake of fluid (1 L/day), sodium (90 mEq/day), potassium (60 mEq/day), and phosphorus (800 mg/day).
- Hyperkalemia
  - ▲ Check for ECG changes (peaked T waves or sinusoidal pattern).
  - ▲ Treat with calcium gluconate, bicarbonate, insulin and glucose, furosemide, sodium polystyrene sulfonate, and dialysis.
- Metabolic acidosis
  - ▲ Do not treat with sodium bicarbonate unless bicarbonate decreases to <15 mmol/L or arterial pH is <7.2.
  - ▲ Indication for dialysis
- Hypocalcemia
  - ▲ Does not require replacement unless severe
- Hyperphosphatemia
  - ▲ Calcium acetate or sevelamer HCl (Renagel)
- Stress ulcer prophylaxis
  - ▲ H_2-Blockers
- Adjust drug doses, especially digoxin, antibiotics, antihypertensives, and benzodiazepines.
- Avoid NSAIDs and angiotensin-converting enzyme inhibitors.

Table 5. Indications for Dialysis in Acute Renal Failure

Oliguria or anuria

Creatinine increases >0.5 mg/dL daily for 2 consecutive days

BUN >100

Pulmonary edema unresponsive to diuretics—*urgent dialysis*

Hyperkalemia (potassium >6.5), unresponsive to medical therapy—*urgent dialysis*

Symptomatic uremia such as pericarditis, bleeding, encephalopathy—*urgent dialysis*

Severe metabolic acidosis unresponsive to medical therapy—*urgent dialysis*

Prevention of Contrast-Induced Nephropathy
- Prehydrate patient with IV fluids at 1-1.5 mg/kg per hour for 8-12 hours before radiocontrast study.
- Consider two doses of acetylcysteine 600 mg PO the day before and the day of the radiocontrast study along with the IV fluids.
- Ultrafiltration before and after contrast exposure

ASTHMA

Augustine S. Lee, M.D.
Jason Persoff, M.D.
Stephen F. Grinton, M.D.

DEFINITION

- A chronic inflammatory disorder of the airways characterized clinically by the following:
  - ▲ Intermittent, frequently entirely reversible, obstruction of the airways
  - ▲ Generalized airway hyperreactivity
  - ▲ Absence of other diagnoses to account for these findings
- Classification
  - ▲ Asthma is subdivided into several classes, or steps, based on the following:
    - • Subjective severity of patient's symptoms
    - • Objective measurements of lung function
  - ▲ A classification of asthma severity is given in Table 1.

ETIOLOGY

- The epidemiologic features of asthma are listed in Table 2.

Risk Factors

- Several different associations place persons at risk for the development of asthma.
- Known risk factors
  - ▲ Bronchial hyperresponsiveness
  - ▲ Atopy
  - ▲ Rhinitis with or without postnasal drip
  - ▲ Exposure to indoor allergens (particularly dust mites, animal dander, mice, cockroaches, and fungi)
  - ▲ Exposure to outdoor allergens (particularly particulate pollution)

Special abbreviation used in this chapter: PEF, peak expiratory flow.

Table 1. Classification of Asthma Severity*†

	Symptoms‡	Nocturnal symptoms	Lung function
Step 4: severe persistent	Continuous symptoms Limited physical activity Frequent exacerbations	Frequent	FEV_1 or PEF ≤60% predicted PEF variability >30%
Step 3: moderate persistent	Daily symptoms Daily use of inhaled short-acting β_2-agonist Exacerbations affect activity Exacerbations ≥2 times a week, may last days	>1 time per week	FEV_1 or PEF >60% to <80% predicted PEF variability >30%
Step 2: mild persistent	Symptoms >2 times a week but <1 time a day	>2 times per month	FEV_1 or PEF ≥80% predicted PEF variability 20%–30%
Step 1: mild intermittent	Symptoms ≤2 times a week Asymptomatic & normal PEF between exacerbations Exacerbations brief (from few hours to few days), intensity may vary	≤2 times per month	FEV_1 or PEF ≥80% predicted PEF variability <20%

FEV_1, forced expiratory volume in 1 second; PEF, peak expiratory flow.

* A person should be assigned to the most severe grade in which any feature occurs.

† A person's classification may change over time.

‡ Patients at any level of severity can have mild, moderate, or severe exacerbations.

From the National Asthma Education and Prevention Program Expert Panel report 2: guidelines for the diagnosis and management of asthma. National Heart, Lung, and Blood Institute [cited 2005 Aug 4]. Available from http://www.nhlbi.nih.gov/guidelines/asthma/asthgdln.htm.

Table 2. Epidemiology of Asthma

Prevalence
>   Age-adjusted rate between ages 5 and 32 years—49.4 per 1,000
>   persons in the general U.S. population

Incidence
>   Bimodal distribution
>>   First peak between 4 & 10 years old
>>   Second peak after 40 years old

Demographics
>   Sex
>>   Age <20 (particularly during puberty), male predominance
>>   Age 20-40, male ≈ female
>>   Age >40, female predominance
>   Race
>>   Blacks & Hispanics (especially in inner cities of U.S.) have
>>   a greater prevalence of asthma than other ethnic groups

Geography
>   Countries with better housing construction have higher rates of
>   asthma
>>   Link between asthma & airtight housing seen in industri-
>>   alized areas
>>   Higher rates in the U.S., U.K., New Zealand, & Australia
>>   Lower rates in eastern and southern Europe, China
>   Atopy
>>   Presence of IgE to specific allergens

Associated diseases
>   Rhinitis
>>   Found in 80%-90% of patients with asthma regardless of
>>   atopy status
>>   Allergic rhinitis frequently precedes diagnosis of asthma
>   Aspirin sensitivity
>   Nasal polyps
>   Churg-Strauss syndrome
>>   Patients have pulmonary infiltrates, peripheral eosino-
>>   philia, & asthma
>   Gastroesophageal reflux disease

Genetics
>   Parental atopy & bronchial hyperresponsiveness
>>   Increased risk of asthma in offspring of parents with atopy
>>   (who do not have asthma)
>>   If 1 parent has atopy and the other bronchial hyperrespon-
>>   siveness, the risk of asthma increases substantially

Table 2 (continued)

Genes
> Chromosome 5—serum IgE level, eosinophil activation & survival, bronchial hyperresponsiveness, & steroid responsiveness
>
> Chromosome 11—β-chain high-affinity IgE receptor

Mortality
> Death rates
>> 18.8 per 1 million people in general U.S. population
>>
>> Higher rates & increasing rates in blacks

- ▲ Respiratory syncytial virus
- ▲ Maternal smoking during the in utero and childhood periods

Acute Asthma Exacerbations
- ■ Causes
  - ▲ Exposure to sensitizers at home or work
  - ▲ Respiratory infections
  - ▲ Cigarette smoke
  - ▲ Other environmental factors (e.g., cold or humidity)
  - ▲ Strong emotions
  - ▲ Menses
  - ▲ Inadequate asthma treatment
  - ▲ Ineffective asthma medication
  - ▲ Precipitating medications (e.g., aspirin or β-blockers)

CLINICAL PRESENTATION
- ■ The classic triad of wheezing, cough, and dyspnea or worsening exercise tolerance lack sensitivity and specificity for the diagnosis of asthma.
- ■ Objective testing is essential to confirm the diagnosis.
- ■ Increased risk for severe exacerbations
  - ▲ Known diagnosis of asthma
  - ▲ History of multiple asthma hospitalizations (particularly ICU admissions)
  - ▲ History of refractory or steroid-dependent asthma
  - ▲ History of intubation and mechanical ventilation from a previous asthma attack is the most powerful predictor of the future severity of an asthma exacerbation.

- All that wheezes is not asthma; look for other life-threatening causes (Tables 3-5)

COMPLICATIONS
Acute Complications
Status Asthmaticus
- Definition—severe asthma attack, poorly responsive to aggressive bronchodilator therapy, with a high probability of progressing to respiratory failure

Table 3. Differential Diagnosis of Wheezing*

Upper airway obstruction		Local airway obstruction
Extrathoracic causes	**Intrathoracic causes**	**Local airway obstruction**
Postnasal drip	**Foreign body**	**Asthma**
Gastroesophageal	**aspiration**	**COPD**
reflux	Tracheal stenosis	**Pulmonary edema**
Epiglottitis	**or tracheo-**	**Pulmonary embo-**
Obesity	**malacia**	**lism**
Vocal cord dysfunc-	**Endobronchial**	**Pneumonia**
tion or paralysis	**lesion**	**Bronchiectasis**
Retropharyngeal	**Intrathoracic goiter**	**Cystic fibrosis**
edema, abscess, or	Herpetic tracheo-	Adult respiratory
hemorrhage	bronchitis	distress syndrome
Irritant inhalants	Mediastinal tumor	Bronchiolitis oblit-
Anaphylaxis	or hemorrhage	erans
Factitious	Postpneumonec-	Bronchiolitis oblit-
Amyloidosis	tomy syndrome	erans organizing
Relapsing poly-	*Vascular compres-*	pneumonia
chondritis	*sion from a right-*	Eosinophilic infil-
Cricoarytenoid	*sided aortic arch*	tratration[†]
arthritis	*or from a thoracic*	*Angioedema*
Wegener granulo-	*aortic aneurysm*	*Carcinoid syndrome*
matosis		

*Boldface, common conditions; italics, rare conditions and should be considered only after a standardized work-up fails to disclose an obvious cause.
[†]Loeffler syndrome, eosinophilic pneumonia, polyarteritis nodosa, Churg-Strauss syndrome, helminth infection, allergic bronchopulmonary aspergillosis.

- Work-up—a clinical diagnosis (see above)
- Treatment—is unchanged from that outlined below except that most patients with status asthmaticus require endotracheal intubation

Pneumothorax
- Definition—a collection of gas within the pleural space with or without shifting of the mediastinum (tension pneumothorax)
- Work-up

Table 4. Some Historical Clues to the Cause of Wheezing

Historical clue	Possible cause
Scratchy throat, constant throat clearing	Postnasal drip
Recent intubation	Tracheal stenosis
Wheezing during or immediately after a meal	Aspiration, foreign body, gastroesophageal reflux, anaphylaxis
Sore throat out of proportion to exam findings	Epiglottitis; retropharyngeal edema, abscess, or hemorrhage
Paroxysmal nocturnal dyspnea, orthopnea, acute weight gain	Congestive heart failure, cor pulmonale from COPD
Connective tissue disease	Bronchiolitis obliterans, bronchiolitis obliterans organizing pneumonia, pulmonary fibrosis
Acute dyspnea (vs. insidious onset)	Pulmonary embolism, aspiration, foreign body, pneumothorax, gastroesophageal reflux
Urticaria, hypotension, abdominal pain	Anaphylaxis or angioedema
Flushing with diarrhea	Carcinoid syndrome
Recurrent infections of upper respiratory tract	Wegener granulomatosis, cystic fibrosis, bronchiectasis
Fevers	Pneumonia, bronchitis, malignancy, eosinophilic infiltration
Immunocompromised host	Herpetic tracheobronchitis
Young female with psychiatric history with normal PFTs & radiographic findings	Paroxysmal vocal cord motion (also called "Munchausen stridor")
Wheezing during exercise	Vocal cord dysfunction
Wheezing immediately after exercise	Exercise-induced bronchospasm

PFT, pulmonary function test.

Table 5. Physical Exam Pearls and Pitfalls Regarding Wheezing Patients

Pearls	Pitfalls
"Unilateral wheezing is pathologic and requires further investigation to exclude mechanical obstruction (such as endobronchial lesions)" (True)	"Wheezing during expiration is characteristic of asthma whereas wheezing during inspiration is not" (False)
"The use of accessory muscles (scalenes, sternocleiodomastoids, etc.); the presence of suprasternal or intercostal retractions; the presence of paradoxical movement of the thorax and abdomen (one rises while the other falls); or the inability to lie flat is suggestive of severe airway obstruction" (True)	"The degree of wheezing correlates with the degree of airway obstruction" (False)
	"A patient who is not wheezing does not have asthma" (False)
	"The absence of pulsus paradoxus excludes the possibility of severe airway obstruction" (False)
"The presence of digital clubbing is not typical of asthma—even severe asthma—and mandates a work-up for other diseases such as interstitial lung disease, COPD, hypertrophic osteopathy, etc." (True)	"The presence of hypoxia in a person with asthma suggests that asthma is the primary cause." (False—hypoxia in particularly young asthma patients is a very late finding; rarely in seniors or those with considerable comorbidities will asthma prove to be the primary cause of hypoxia)
"The presence of a pulsus paradoxus of >10 mm Hg during inspiration is seen in patients with severe airway obstruction" (True)	

- ▲ An upright inspiratory posteroanterior chest X-ray can detect a pneumothorax as small as 50 mL.
- ▲ Supine chest X-rays require as much as 500 mL of air to detect a pneumothorax.
- ■ Treatment—a thoracostomy tube is required for the following:
  - ▲ Tension pneumothorax

- ▲ Pneumothorax >3 cm from the lateral wall to the edge of the visceral pleura *or*
- ▲ Pneumothorax >4 cm from the apex to the visceral pleura
- ▲ A smaller pneumothorax in a nonventilated patient may be treated with oxygen, thoracentesis, or observation.

Metabolic Complications
- ■ Monitor potassium (hyperkalemia from β-agonist inhalers) and glucose (hyperglycemia from corticosteroids).
- ■ Osteoporosis occurs with long courses of systemic (not inhaled) corticosteroid therapy.

Chronic Complications
- ■ Progression to *irreversible* airway obstruction (COPD)
- ■ Decreased quality of life
- ■ Complications from long-term treatment with oral corticosteroids in patients with refractory asthma

DIAGNOSTIC STRATEGIES
- ■ When approaching a patient with suspected asthma always
  - ▲ Assess the severity of the patient's respiratory status
  - ▲ Exclude alternative diagnoses
  - ▲ Confirm airway obstruction

Assessing Respiratory Status
- ■ The following signs suggest potential impending respiratory failure and should prompt intensive monitoring and consideration of mechanical ventilation:
  - ▲ Obtundation
  - ▲ Suprasternal or intercostal retractions
  - ▲ Weak respiratory effort
  - ▲ Paradoxical respiratory pattern (chest rises while abdomen falls; chest falls while abdomen rises)
  - ▲ Respiratory rate >28 breaths/minute
  - ▲ Heart rate >130 beats/minute
  - ▲ Inability to lie flat
  - ▲ Arterial blood gases showing PaO_2 ≤60 mm Hg or $PaCO_2$ ≥40 mm Hg
- ■ Early in an asthma attack, tachypnea results in respiratory alkalosis. The development of a *normal* $PaCO_2$ suggests impending respiratory failure.

- Pulsus paradoxus (Table 6)
  - ▲ Abnormal when >10 mm Hg
  - ▲ Associated with severe asthma

Excluding Alternative Diagnoses
- Chest X-ray—may show hyperinflation but is most helpful to exclude other diseases
- Bronchoscopy—suspected foreign body aspiration, endobronchial lesions
- Ventilation-perfusion scanning—pulmonary embolism

Table 6. How To Manually Calculate Pulsus Paradoxus (PP)

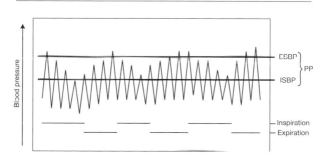

The patient must be in sinus rhythm

Have the patient breathe normally throughout the procedure

Inflate a sphygmomanometer 30 mm Hg above the systolic blood pressure

Slowly deflate the cuff until first Korotkoff sound is heard, then stop deflating the cuff

Gently increase cuff pressure until the first Korotkoff sound is heard intermittently. The pressure is the "expiratory systolic blood pressure" (ESBP)

Now slowly deflate the cuff until the first Korotkoff sound is heard regularly, then stop deflating the cuff. This pressure is the "inspiratory systolic blood pressure" (ISBP)

The pulsus is the difference between ISBP and ESBP

- Computed tomography of the chest—pulmonary embolism, interstitial lung disease, mediastinal tumors
- Serologic, sputum, or urine studies—eosinophilic infiltration, Wegener granulomatosis, carcinoid syndrome, Churg-Strauss syndrome, eosinophilic bronchitis
- Pulmonary function tests—not usually recommended in acute exacerbations of asthma but full pulmonary function tests are helpful in showing the following:
  - Flow loops suggestive of intrathoracic, extrathoracic, or fixed airway obstruction
  - Impaired diffusion capacity of carbon monoxide suggesting interstitial lung disease
  - Presence of a restrictive process
- Methacholine challenge—contraindicated as a diagnostic test during an exacerbation. It is helpful in outpatient work-up when the diagnosis of asthma is questionable.
- Consider occupational asthma.
- Consider reactive airway dysfunction syndrome with history of acute inhalation injury.

Confirming Airway Obstruction
Peak Expiratory Flow (PEF)
- PEF testing
  - Have the patient exhale as hard and fast as possible into the peak flow meter. The final measurement is the average of the best three readings. Compare this with the patient's known baseline.
  - Generally, patients having a severe exacerbation of asthma
    - Have a PEF <120 L/minute *or*
    - Have a PEF <50% of known personal best PEF or of standardized PEF *or*
    - Are too dyspneic to perform PEF assessments
- Limitations of PEF testing
  - Correlation between PEF and FEV_1 has had limited validation.
  - PEFs are better for excluding airway obstruction than for confirming it.
  - A low PEF has a positive predictive value for a low FEV_1 of 46.5% but a negative predictive value for a low FEV_1 of 95%.

▲ PEF does not distinguish among causes of airway obstruction, neuromuscular weakness, poor patient effort, and asthma.

MANAGEMENT
Goals
- Relieve bronchospasm
- Maintain oxygenation and ventilation
- Suppress airway inflammation
- Prevent subsequent exacerbations

Acute Management (Accepted Therapy)
Oxygen
- Give oxygen nasally or by mask to maintain oxygen saturation >92%.
- Objective measurement of ventilation (with arterial blood gases) is critical to prevent delayed intubation of patients at risk for respiratory failure (see above).

Albuterol
- Metered dose inhaler, 4-6 puffs every 20 minutes, or nebulizers, 2.5-5.0 mg every 20 minutes, until relief or onset of side effects (tachyarrhythmias or severe tremors)
- No difference in clinical response between nebulizers and metered dose inhalers with spacers in acute exacerbations of asthma, but nebulizers are associated with a high frequency of tachyarrhythmias.
- Continuous albuterol administration via a nebulizer (10 mg/hour) has been advocated in severe cases.

Corticosteroids
- Methylprednisolone, 125 mg IV, followed by 40-60 mg every 6 hours for 24-48 hours, then switch to prednisone, 60 mg PO
- Corticosteroid tapers are not necessary if corticosteroids are used for <10 days.
- Corticosteroid use reduces relapses after hospitalization or emergency department presentation, rapidly improves airway obstruction (by FEV_1), and possibly reduces the likelihood of death from asthma.

ATRIAL FIBRILLATION

Garvan C. Kane, M.D.
Arshad Jahangir, M.D.

DEFINITION

- Atrial fibrillation (AF)
  - ▲ Irregular, disorganized electrical activity of the atria with an irregular ventricular response
  - ▲ On ECG, P waves are absent and irregular waveforms continuously change in shape, duration, amplitude, and direction.

CLASSIFICATION

- Paroxysmal—Episodes terminate spontaneously, recur, and last <48 hours.
- Persistent—Continuous AF that can be converted to sinus rhythm
- Permanent—Ongoing AF refractory to reversion or allowed to continue

ETIOLOGY

- Common—ischemic heart disease, dilated cardiomyopathy, familial, chronic hypertension, valvular disease (particularly rheumatic mitral stenosis), advanced age, postcardiac surgery
- Other cardiac predictors—presence of left atrial enlargement, left ventricular hypertrophy, ventricular dysfunction, acute myocardial infarction (10% of persons with acute myocardial infarction have an associated episode of AF and up to 20% if they develop congestive heart failure), sinus node dysfunction, hypertrophic cardiomyopathy, Wolff-Parkinson-White syndrome
- Noncardiac precipitators—hyperthyroidism, alcohol (holiday heart syndrome), severe infection, pulmonary embolism

Special abbreviation used in this chapter: AF, atrial fibrillation.

- Lone AF—AF in the absence of recognizable heart disease or precipitating illnesses
- Note: Every patient who presents only with acute onset of AF does not need to be "ruled out for a myocardial infarction or screened for an occult pulmonary embolus." Although AF may be associated with these conditions, it is quite uncommon in the absence of other clinical clues (symptoms, ECG changes, hypoxia)

EPIDEMIOLOGY
- AF affects 2.3 million Americans and results in 75,000 strokes annually.
- The incidence of AF is estimated at 0.4% of the general population and increases with age: 2%-5% at age 65 and 9% by age 80.
- Prevalence of paroxysmal AF is 22%-65%, about one-fourth of cases will progress to persistent form.
- Presence of valvular heart disease, left atrial or left ventricular enlargement, left ventricular hypertrophy, or ventricular systolic dysfunction increases the risk of progression to permanent AF.

CLINICAL PRESENTATION
- Many patients may be asymptomatic or complain of malaise or palpitations.
- The elderly or those with compromised coronary or cerebral circulation may present with dizziness or angina.
- Heart failure may occur because of rapid rates or loss of atrial contribution to ventricular filling.
- Thromboembolic stroke often can be the first presentation of AF (1 of every 6 strokes occurs in patients with AF).
- Some patients complain of episodic polyuria, probably secondary to increased production of atrial natriuretic peptide.

DIAGNOSTIC STRATEGIES
Clinical Signs of AF
- Irregularly irregular rhythm with variable intensity of the first heart sound
- No "a" wave in the jugular venous pressure and no fourth heart sound

- Absent presystolic accentuation of mitral stenosis murmur
- Pulse varies in amplitude because of differing diastolic filling times.
- The apical rate exceeds the radial rate (pulse deficit).

Signs of Complications
- What is the degree of patient distress?
- Presence or absence of chest pain or altered level of consciousness?
- Check blood pressure yourself.
- Signs of congestive heart failure (increased jugular venous pressure, third heart sound, pulmonary crackles)

ECG Clues
- Absent P waves, fibrillatory waves may be seen (especially in V_1, V_2).
- Irregularly irregular, normal-looking QRS complexes; aberrant ventricular conduction (wide QRS) of atrial impulses may be present, usually with long-short cycle (Ashman phenomenon) or with very rapid rates.
- Watch for presence of delta waves on ECG (if irregular wide QRS complexes with varying duration).

Investigations
- CBC, electrolytes, magnesium, sTSH, chest X-ray
- CK-MB, troponin T (depending on history)

PATIENT WITH UNSTABLE AF
- Signs and plan of action are indicated in Figure 1.

FIVE-STEP MANAGEMENT OF PATIENTS WITH AF
Step 1—Treat Underlying Cause
- Rule out ischemia, hypoxia (pulmonary embolism), congestive heart failure, or other primary conditions such as hyperthyroidism, myocarditis, acute pulmonary decompensation.
- AF reverts spontaneously to normal sinus rhythm in 68% of patients within 72 hours.

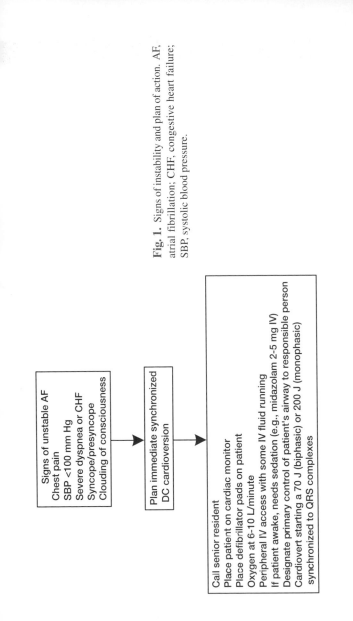

Signs of unstable AF
Chest pain
SBP <100 mm Hg
Severe dyspnea or CHF
Syncope/presyncope
Clouding of consciousness

Plan immediate synchronized
DC cardioversion

Call senior resident
Place patient on cardiac monitor
Place defibrillator pads on patient
Oxygen at 6-10 L/minute
Peripheral IV access with some IV fluid running
If patient awake, needs sedation (e.g., midazolam 2-5 mg IV)
Designate primary control of patient's airway to responsible person
Cardiovert starting a 70 J (biphasic) or 200 J (monophasic)
synchronized to QRS complexes

Fig. 1. Signs of instability and plan of action. AF, atrial fibrillation; CHF, congestive heart failure; SBP, systolic blood pressure.

Step 2—Control Ventricular Rate

- The fast ventricular response rate is the cause of predominant symptoms in patients with AF and even within a few weeks can result in a tachycardia-induced cardiomyopathy.
- If the patient is stable but the heart rate is >150 beats/minute, use IV medications for rate control in a monitored setting (Table 1).
- Aim for a ventricular rate <80 beats/minute at rest and <120 beats/minute with activity.

Calcium Channel Blockers

- Caveats
    - ▲ Avoid in severe left ventricular dysfunction or Wolff-Parkinson-White syndrome.

Table 1. Drugs for Controlling Ventricular Rate

Drug	Loading dose	Maintenance dose
Metoprolol	5 mg IV push every 5 minutes ×3	5-10 mg IV every 6 hours or 25-100 mg PO every 12 hours
Propranolol	0.5-1 mg IV push every 5 minutes to maximum of 6 mg (0.1 mg/kg)	Propranolol LA 60-320 mg PO daily
Esmolol	500 µg/kg (over 1 minute)	50-300 µg/kg per minute IV
Diltiazem	0.25 mg/kg over 2 minutes (10-20 mg) followed by 0.35 mg/kg over 5 minutes if needed	IV 5-15 mg/hour 90-240 mg/day PO
Verapamil	5-10 mg IV over 2 minutes, repeat in 10 minutes, then 0.005 mg/kg per minute for 30-60 minutes	120-360 mg daily
Digoxin	1 mg over 24 hours in 3-4 divided doses	0.125-0.5 mg IV or PO daily

LA, long acting.

- ▲ Diltiazem usually is well tolerated and can be administered in an infusion that is easily titrated to effect. It has replaced digoxin as a first-line agent for patients with a normal ejection fraction.
- ▲ Diltiazem PO is a good alternative to IV, with an onset of action at 30 minutes.

β-Blockers
- Best choice in high catecholamine states (ischemia, postoperatively)
- Caveats
  - ▲ Avoid in severe left ventricular dysfunction, moderate to severe asthma, or Wolff-Parkinson-White syndrome.
  - ▲ Use cautiously in patients with COPD.
  - ▲ β-Blockers are safe for diabetic patients except for a small number who are insulin-dependent and have poor hypoglycemic awareness.
  - ▲ There is no evidence for avoiding β-blockers in patients with peripheral vascular disease.
  - ▲ Esmolol is safer than other β-blockers because of a shorter half-life (10 minutes); it is ineffective without a bolus and is expensive.

Digoxin
- This traditionally has been the first-line agent.
- Caveats
  - ▲ Avoid in Wolff-Parkinson-White syndrome.
  - ▲ First choice for severe left ventricular dysfunction or aortic stenosis
  - ▲ Compared with drugs mentioned above, digoxin has less efficacy, slower onset of action, and more side effects (heart block, ventricular dysrhythmias, nausea and vomiting, yellow-green visual hallucinations).
  - ▲ It is ineffective at slowing heart rate in the setting of increased sympathetic tone (e.g., hyperthyroidism, fever, hypoxia, hypovolemia, exercise, or other form of stress).
  - ▲ Often good as an adjunct to β-blockers or calcium channel blockers
  - ▲ Reduce dose in the elderly and those with renal impairment.
  - ▲ Ideally, the dose should be withheld before cardioversion.

▲ Dose needs to be reduced by half if propafenone, amiodarone, or quinidine is added for rhythm control.

Clonidine

- Decreases sympathetic tone
- Not widely used
- Give 0.075 mg PO and repeat in 2 hours if no important effect

Step 3—Convert to Normal Sinus Rhythm

- An attempt to restore sinus rhythm should be considered for all patients with AF.
- Longer duration of AF (particularly >3 years) and certain causes, such as those associated with a dilated left atrium (>60 mm), make successful cardioversion or maintenance of sinus rhythm unlikely.
- Calcium channel blockers, digoxin, and β-blockers usually do not cause reversion to normal sinus rhythm.
- Electrical cardioversion is effective 80% (monophasic) and up to 95% (biphasic) of the time and pharmacologic cardioversion, 40%-80%.

Elective Electrical Cardioversion

- Patient should be fasting for 6 hours.
- Withhold preceding digoxin dose, and make sure potassium and magnesium levels are normal.
- Monophasic defibrillator—start at 200 J, 300 J, 360 J
- Biphasic defibrillator—70 J, 120 J, 150 J
- If unsuccessful, infuse ibutilide and then cardioversion

Pharmacologic Cardioversion

- Include IV procainamide or ibutilide (avoid ibutilide in patients with severe systolic dysfunction or prolonged QT intervals; 3% develop torsades de pointes after receiving ibutilide).
- Oral options include sotalol (only proven effective in AF after open-heart surgery), flecainide, propafenone, quinidine, dofetilide (characteristics similar to IV ibutilide).
- In patients with tachycardia-bradycardia syndrome, long

pauses could be observed after cardioversion before resumption of normal sinus rhythm.

Step 4—Maintain Sinus Rhythm
- Recurrence 50%-75% of the time
- Antiarrhythmic agents maintain sinus rhythm in up to 50%-65% of patients at 1 year.
  - However, these agents could cause life-threatening ventricular tachycardia or fibrillation in 2%-3.5% of patients with normal hearts and up to 15% of those with a history of ventricular dysfunction or arrhythmias.
- All patients with structurally abnormal hearts are monitored in hospital until they have had 5 doses of the drug (5 half-lives). For amiodarone, the loading dose is generally 5-6 g (600 mg twice daily).
- With the use of class III (sotalol, dofetilide, ibutilide) or class IA (quinidine, procainamide, disopyramide) antiarrhythmics, QTc duration needs to be monitored, as does the QRS duration with class IC antiarrhythmics.
- Sotalol and amiodarone because of the additional antiadrenergic effect have the added advantage of slowing the ventricular response when AF occurs.
- Maintaining sinus rhythm in high-risk patients with AF with the use of antiarrhythmic agents does not improve survival compared with those treated for rate control alone. The rate control approach resulted in fewer complications (AFFIRM trial) in high-risk AF patients.
- Maze procedure
  - Surgical technique resulting in up to 90% success of maintaining normal sinus rhythm
  - However, up to 2% of patients need pacemakers.
  - A variety of percutaneous catheter-based procedures are available, including ablation for pulmonary vein isolation or atrioventricular node (with pacemaker insertion for rate control)

Step 5—Prevent Embolic Complications
Anticoagulation for Chronic AF
- AF causes 14% of all strokes in patients older than 60 years.
- The risk of stroke for patients with AF is highest during the first few months after onset of the arrhythmia.

- Risk factors for thromboembolic events in AF
  - ▲ Risk factors are listed in Table 2.
  - ▲ Risk of embolization per year is given in Table 3.
- Recommendations for anticoagulation are outlined in Table 4.

Anticoagulation for Acute AF

- If patient has been in AF for ≥48 hours, the risk of pericardioversion embolization is 5.5%.
- This is reduced to 1% if the patient is anticoagulated, with therapeutic INR (2-3) for at least 3 weeks before and 4 weeks after cardioversion.

Table 2. Risk Factors for Thromboembolic Events in Atrial Fibrillation

History of previous emboli
Hypertension
History of congestive heart failure
Age >75 years
Diabetes mellitus
Left ventricular ejection fraction <0.40
Left atrial size >2.5 cm/m^2

Table 3. Risk of Embolization Per Year

No. of risk factors	Risk, %
0	1
1 or 2	5-6
3 or more	8-19

Table 4. Recommendations for Anticoagulation*

Age, years	No risk factors	>1 risk factor
<65	Aspirin 325 mg daily/no therapy	
65-75	Aspirin/warfarin	Warfarin
>75	Warfarin	

*Note: Warfarin to goal INR 2-3 (INR <1.8 offers no protection).

- Alternatively, transesophageal echocardiography stratifies patients with AF according to embolization risk.
  - No evidence of atrial thrombus or spontaneous echogenic "smoke"—Cardiovert with IV heparin and warfarin for 4 weeks, with therapeutic INR (2-3).
  - Atrial stunning—Delayed onset of effective atrial contractions after normal electrical activity has been reestablished may increase thrombogenic potential. Thus, 4 weeks of anticoagulation after cardioversion is indicated. Stunning occurs with both electrical and pharmacologic cardioversion.

CHRONIC OBSTRUCTIVE PULMONARY DISEASE

Rendell W. Ashton, M.D.
Paul D. Scanlon, M.D.

DEFINITIONS

- American Thoracic Society's official statement on COPD:
  - ▲ COPD—a disease state characterized by airflow obstruction due to chronic bronchitis or emphysema, which is generally progressive, may be accompanied by airway hyperreactivity, and may be partially reversible
  - ▲ Chronic bronchitis—the presence of chronic productive cough for 3 months in each of two successive years in a patient in whom other causes of chronic cough have been excluded. Definition is clinical.
  - ▲ Emphysema—abnormal permanent enlargement of the airspaces distal to the terminal bronchioles, accompanied by destruction of their walls and without obvious fibrosis. "Destruction" is defined as lack of uniformity in the pattern of respiratory airspace enlargement; the orderly appearance of this acinus and its components is disturbed and may be lost. Definition is pathologic.
  - ▲ COPD exacerbation—acute flare or worsening of chronic COPD symptoms; not attributable to other confounding conditions (pneumonia, congestive heart failure) with demonstrable decline in pulmonary function. Triggered by various stimuli, including infections and environmental exposures. More frequent in patients with comorbid conditions.
    - Cardinal features
      - Worsening dyspnea
      - Increased sputum purulence
      - Increased sputum volume

Classification

- The classification of COPD is given in Table 1.

Table 1. Classification of COPD

Classification*	Diagnosis is based on	
Emphysema	Pathologic demonstration of destruction of alveolar architecture	Overlap is common; often best to designate as "predominantly" emphysema or bronchitis
Chronic bronchitis	Clinical features, including productive cough	

*The distinction between emphysema and chronic bronchitis is somewhat arbitrary and has little clinical value.

ETIOLOGY

- Smoking tobacco in at least 85%-90% of patients
- Others: α_1-antitrypsin deficiency, environmental (second-hand) tobacco smoke, occupational and environmental exposures
- Airway hyperresponsiveness may be a predisposing factor.
- Infections are the most common identifiable cause of acute exacerbations.
  - ▲ The most common organisms implicated are *Haemophilus influenzae*, *Streptococcus pneumoniae*, *Moraxella catarrhalis*, *Mycoplasma pneumoniae*, influenza virus, and adenovirus (Table 2).

EPIDEMIOLOGY

- In the U.S., 16 million people have COPD.
- COPD is the fourth leading cause of death, after heart disease, cancer, and stroke.
- Prevalence and mortality of COPD are increasing, especially among women.
- The majority of patients with COPD are long-time smokers.
- Symptoms usually appear in the fifth or sixth decade.

CLINICAL PRESENTATION

- Patients with an acute exacerbation present with (usually) the following:
  - ▲ Known underlying COPD
  - ▲ One or more of three cardinal characteristics:
    - • Worsening dyspnea

- • Increased sputum purulence
- • Increased sputum volume
- ▲ Often one or more identifiable trigger(s)
- ■ Complications
  - ▲ The most common causes of death of persons with COPD are cardiovascular disease and lung cancer.
  - ▲ The major complication of a COPD exacerbation is respiratory failure.

Table 2. Triggers for COPD Exacerbation

Bacterial respiratory tract infection or colonization
    Haemophilus influenzae
    Pseudomonas aeruginosa
    Streptococcus pneumoniae
    Moraxella catarrhalis
    Mycoplasma pneumoniae
    Chlamydia pneumoniae
Viral respiratory tract infection
    Rhinovirus
    Adenovirus
    Influenza virus
    Other viruses
Environmental exposures
    Particulate pollutants (<10 μm, especially <2 μm)
    Ozone
    Nitrogen dioxide
    Sulfur dioxide
Exacerbations of comorbid conditions
    Heart failure
    Nonpulmonary infections
    Pulmonary thromboembolism
    Bronchospasm
    Pneumothorax (often secondary to underlying COPD)
Iatrogenic
    Excessive sedation from medication
    Anesthesia, especially with prolonged surgery of thorax or
      upper abdomen
    Electrolyte disturbances causing decreased ventilatory drive
Unexplained (a large proportion of cases)

▲ Clinical measures to follow include respiratory rate, use of accessory muscles, evidence of respiratory distress, paradoxical breathing, oxygen saturation determined with pulse oximetry, and evidence of hypoxia or hypercapnia as determined with arterial blood gases.

EVALUATION
- The initial evaluation is outlined in Table 3.
- Relevant lab and imaging tests are listed in Table 4.

DIAGNOSTIC STRATEGIES
- Chronic COPD
  - ▲ The diagnosis of advanced COPD suspected clinically, based on historical and physical findings at the time of evaluation.
  - ▲ The likelihood of advanced COPD in a patient who is or has been a smoker and who has consistent symptoms and signs is extremely high.
  - ▲ Assessment of severity—Spirometry is mandatory for staging severity (Table 5)

MANAGEMENT OF ACUTE EXACERBATIONS
General Measures
- See Table 3
- Decide whether the patient's condition warrants hospital stay (Table 6) or admission to the ICU (Table 7).
- The goals of treatment for COPD exacerbation are
  - ▲ To remove any ongoing triggers
  - ▲ To restore the patient's baseline work of breathing through aggressive supportive measures
- Many therapies are empiric. Of these, many have data to support their use (Table 8).
- Consult a pulmonary specialist when COPD exacerbation is complicated with any of the following:
  - ▲ Hemoptysis
  - ▲ Pneumothorax
  - ▲ Severe pneumonia
  - ▲ Respiratory failure requiring mechanical ventilation
  - ▲ Anatomic airway obstruction
  - ▲ Undefined lung disease
  - ▲ Large or recurrent pleural effusion

PROPHYLAXIS

- Therapeutic considerations for the time of hospital discharge, including guidelines for home oxygen therapy, are outlined in Tables 8 and 9.

Table 3. Initial Evaluation of Patients With Suspected COPD Exacerbation

History
    Smoking history (past & current, amount)
    Environmental & occupational exposures
        Residence in or travel to heavily polluted areas
        Exposure to environmental (second-hand) tobacco smoke
    Acute & chronic pulmonary illnesses
    Cough
        Daily cough & sputum production 3 months out of each of 2 successive years defines chronic bronchitis
    Wheezing
    Dyspnea (note severity & any change from baseline)
Physical exam
    Signs of hyperinflation (severe emphysema)
        Increased anteroposterior diameter
        Low diaphragmatic position
        Faint breath & heart sounds
        Inspiratory retraction of lower ribs from flattened diaphragm (Hoover sign)
    Signs of obstruction
        Prolonged expiratory phase of respiration
        Wheezing
        Pursed-lip breathing
        Hypertrophy of scalene muscles
    Signs of cor pulmonale (pulmonary hypertension in setting of lung disease)
        Increased jugular venous pressure
        Right ventricular heave
        Third/fourth heart sound or prominent pulmonic second sound, tricuspid regurgitation murmur (sign of advanced disease)
        Edema, hepatomegaly
    Plethora or cyanosis (clubbing not associated with COPD—think of cystic fibrosis, lung cancer, interstitial pulmonary fibrosis, asbestosis)

Table 4. Lab and Imaging Tests

Blood & sputum cultures, Gram stain (include *Legionella* and atypical organisms)

CBC & electrolytes

Chest X-ray—may show hyperinflation, oligemia, & bullae; helps rule out other lung disease

Peak flow measurements—help to quantify bronchospasm & follow condition objectively

Arterial blood gases—important in severe exacerbations to identify hypoxic (PaO_2 <60 mm Hg) or hypercapnic (>50 mm Hg, with pH <7.35) respiratory failure

Table 5. Staging of COPD*

Stage	Features
Mild (at risk)	FEV_1/FVC >0.7, FEV_1 ≥80% predicted
	Minimal symptoms with normal or near-normal exam
Moderate	FEV_1 50%-80% predicted
	Cough with or without sputum
	Dyspnea on exertion
	May have wheezing
Severe	FEV_1 30%-50% predicted
	Prominent cough
	Dyspnea on exertion or at rest, hyperinflation, wheezing, cyanosis, edema
Very severe	FEV_1 <30% predicted

FEV_1, forced expiratory volume in 1 second; FVC, forced vital capacity.
*Not at time of acute exacerbation.

Table 6.   Criteria for Hospital Admission for COPD Exacerbation

Progressive symptoms leading to concern of impending respiratory failure

Failure of outpatient management, with worsening symptoms and/or respiratory lab values

Difficulty with activities of daily life, eating, or sleeping because of dyspnea

Coexisting pulmonary or respiratory muscle disease with limited respiratory reserve

Worsening hypoxia or acute respiratory acidosis

Cor pulmonale with evidence of worsening right-heart failure

Coexisting respiratory depression

    Intoxication

    Excess sedation from analgesics or other psychotropic medications

    Need for procedure requiring anesthesia

Patient support not available for required home care

Table 7.   Criteria for ICU Admission for COPD Exacerbation

Need for intubation or noninvasive positive pressure ventilation

    Respiratory muscle fatigue or respiratory failure

    Hypoxia

    Uncompensated respiratory acidosis

    Inability to protect & maintain airway integrity

Poor response to initial therapies

    Persistent, severe dyspnea

    Worsening respiratory lab values despite treatment

    Persistent mental status changes due to respiratory failure

Table 8. Therapies for COPD Exacerbation, With Strength of Supporting Evidence

Therapy	Result and dose
Supported by randomized, controlled clinical trials	
Oral corticosteroids	Outcomes—shorter length of hospital stay, lower rates of treatment failure & repeat hospitalization
	Usual dose: prednisolone 25-125 mg IV/PO 2-4 times daily initially, then tapered over 14 days (longer taper not beneficial)
Inhaled anticholinergic drugs	Ipratropium showed significant FEV_1 improvement vs. placebo (effect size not calculable)
	Tiotropium 18 µg daily (long-acting anticholinergic) improved FEV_1 significantly better than placebo, slightly better than ipratropium
Inhaled β_2-agonist drugs	More variable response than with anticholinergics; may depend on degree of airway hyperresponsiveness
	Significant improvement in FEV_1 and/or symptoms in up to 50% of patients vs. placebo
	No difference in outcome between nebulized & metered dose inhaler preparations; correct inhaler technique critical
Combination of anticholinergic & β_2-agonist drugs	Significant improvement in FEV_1 in most patients, compared with either drug alone
Supported by some evidence from poor studies; not proven; benefits probably outweigh risks	
Antibiotics	Accelerated improvement in FEV_1 & lower relapse rates
	Positive Gram stain & culture results not necessary—start empiric therapy with trimethoprim-sulfamethoxazole, doxycycline, or a quinolone with strep coverage (levofloxacin, gatifloxacin, etc.) for 10 days
Supported by some evidence; usefulness limited because of adverse effects	
Theophylline	Variable improvement in FEV_1 from 0%-20%
	Narrow therapeutic range; common adverse effects even in therapeutic range: nausea, diarrhea, headache, seizures, arrhythmia

Table 8 (continued)

Therapy	Result and dose
	No evidence of benefit
Inhaled cortico-steroids	No benefit in acute exacerbation
Mucolytics (*N*-acetylcysteine, iodides)	Little evidence of benefit May worsen bronchospasm
Chest physiotherapy	Extrapolated from evidence in cystic fibrosis literature Little benefit in COPD exacerbation May worsen bronchospasm
	Experimental therapies
Cilomilast (non-theophylline phosphodiesterase-4 antagonist)	Currently in phase III trials; improved FEV_1 & fewer exacerbations in some trials
Zanamivir	Faster resolution of influenza symptoms & fewer complications in some trials No effect on pulmonary function Rare case reports of causing exacerbations of asthma & COPD
Anabolic steroids (androgens)	Speculative, no published studies Prohibitive adverse effects in women

FEV_1, forced expiratory volume in 1 second.

Table 9. Strategies for COPD Maintenance After Stabilization of Acute Exacerbation

Therapy	Comment
Accepted as standard of care; some evidence to support recommendation	
Establish diagnosis & stage (severity) of disease	Wait until acute episode resolves to assess baseline lung function & assign to a stage
Encourage lifestyle changes	Critical to slow progression of disease & reduce exacerbations
Reduce adverse exposures, including	
Smoking cessation	Help patient move through stages of cessation: precontemplation, contemplation, preparation, action, maintenance. Use encouragement, continued social support systems, nicotine replacement, bupropion, etc.
Immunizations	Pneumococcal and influenza vaccines
Exercise	Improves quality of life; fewer hospitalizations; no effect on FEV_1
Inhaled anticholinergic/β_2-agonist combination	Better than either drug alone; bronchodilation and symptomatic improvement; does not improve survival
Home oxygen therapy if indicated (Table 10)	Improves survival of patients with hypoxemia
Lung volume reduction surgery	Offered at certain centers as result of the National Emphysema Treatment Trial; beneficial only for some patients
Evidence equivocal; recommendations debated	
Inhaled corticosteroids	Some studies suggest fewer exacerbations & readmissions; improvement in lung function is small, early, and noncumulative; systemic adverse effects occur
Theophylline	Trade-off between benefit and harm; small improvement in lung function, but frequent adverse effects
Mucolytic agents	Showed decreased number of exacerbations & modest improvement in lung function
No evidence to support recommendation	
Antibiotics	No well-designed studies; no clear indication for long-term use
Oral corticosteroids	Only 20%-30% of patients have short-term response; no evidence of slowed progression of disease, multiple adverse effects

Table 10. Oxygen Therapy After Hospital Discharge of Patients With COPD Exacerbation

PaO_2	SaO_2 or SpO_2	O_2 indicated
<55 mm Hg	<88%	Yes
55-59 mm Hg	≥88%	If cor pulmonale, erythrocytosis, or congestive heart failure
≥60 mm Hg	≥88%	If documented nocturnal hypoxia despite CPAP or coexisting severe lung disease

CPAP, continuous positive airway pressure; SaO_2, arterial oxygen saturation; SpO_2, oxygen saturation determined by pulse oximetry.

CONGESTIVE HEART FAILURE

Guilherme H. M. Oliveira, M.D.
Joseph G. Murphy, M.D.

DEFINITIONS

- Congestive heart failure is a clinical syndrome characterized by
  - ▲ Impairment of cardiac contraction or relaxation or both
  - ▲ Increased left ventricular end-diastolic pressure (frequently measured by its surrogate, pulmonary capillary wedge pressure) >18 mm Hg
  - ▲ Neurohormonal activation, fluid retention, pulmonary congestion, decreased exercise tolerance, and reduced survival
- Systolic dysfunction
  - ▲ Decreased left ventricular ejection fraction
  - ▲ Asymptomatic or detected incidentally
  - ▲ Classic signs and symptoms of heart failure
- Diastolic dysfunction (stiff ventricle)
  - ▲ Increased resistance to ventricular filling resulting in increased left ventricular filling pressures
  - ▲ May result in congestive symptoms in the absence of systolic dysfunction

DIAGNOSIS AND TYPES

- The criteria for diagnosing congestive heart failure are listed in Table 1.
- The types of congestive heart failure are compared in Table 2.
- Acute and chronic congestive heart failure are compared in Table 3.

Special abbreviations used in this chapter: ACE, angiotensin-converting enzyme; ARB, angiotensin II receptor blocker; S_3, third heart sound; S_4, fourth heart sound.

Table 1. Framingham Criteria for Diagnosis of Congestive Heart Failure*

Major criteria
Paroxysmal nocturnal dyspnea or orthopnea
Neck vein distension
Rales
Cardiomegaly
Acute pulmonary edema
S_3 gallop
Increased venous pressure >16 cm H_2O
Circulation time >25 seconds
Hepatojugular reflux
Minor criteria
Ankle edema
Night cough
Dyspnea on exertion
Hepatomegaly
Pleural effusion
Vital capacity decrease 1/3 from maximum
Tachycardia (rate >120 beats/minute)
Major or minor criterion
Weight loss >4.5 kg in 5 days in response to treatment

S_3, third heart sound.
*Diagnosis requires 2 major or 1 major and 2 minor criteria.

ETIOLOGY

Systolic Dysfunction

- Ischemic cardiomyopathy (60% of patients)—myocardial infarction, unstable angina, left ventricular aneurysm, hibernating myocardium, myocardial stunning
- Dilated cardiomyopathies (18% of patients)—alcohol-induced, viral, idiopathic, peripartum, tachycardia-induced, drugs (Table 4)
- Advanced valvular heart disease (12%)—mitral regurgitation, aortic regurgitation, aortic stenosis
- Congenital—atrial septal defect, ventricular septal defect
- Hypertensive heart disease (<10% of patients)
- Sepsis and systemic inflammatory response syndrome
- Inflammatory diseases—systemic lupus erythematosus, Wegener granulomatosis
- Endocrine disorders—hyperthyroidism, hypothyroidism, acromegaly
- Genetic disease—Duchenne and other muscular dystrophies

Table 2. Comparison of Types of Congestive Heart Failure

Type	Symptoms	Signs	Ejection fraction	Causes
Left-sided	DOE, PND, OR	S_3, HJR, rales	↓	CAD, myocarditis, HTN, valve disease, congenital
Right-sided	± DOE, ↑ weight	Right ventricular lift, ↑ liver enzymes, edema	↔ ↓	MS, left ventricular failure, PHTN
Low output	DOE, ↑ weight	Congestive signs	↓	CAD, valvular, myocarditis
High output	DOE	S_3, ↑ pulse pressure	↗	↑ T_4, AR, beriberi, Paget disease
Systolic	DOE, PND, OR	Congestive signs	↑	CAD, myocarditis, valvular
Diastolic	DOE, FND	S_4, sustained PMI	↑ ↔	Acute myocardial infarction, HTN crisis, amyloidosis, hemochromatosis

AR, aortic regurgitation; CAD, coronary artery disease; DOE, dyspnea on exertion; HJR, hepatojugular reflux; HTN, hypertension; MS, mitral stenosis; OR, orthopnea; PHTN, portal hypertension; PMI, point of maximum impulse (apex); PND, paroxysmal nocturnal dyspnea; S_3, third heart sound; S_4, fourth heart sound; T_4, thyroxine.

Table 3. Comparison of Acute and Chronic Congestive Heart Failure

Feature	Acute	Decompensated chronic	Compensated chronic
Symptom severity	++++	++++	++/+++
Pulmonary edema	++++	++++	+
Peripheral edema	±	++++	+++
Weight gain	+	++++	+++
Whole-body fluid load	±	++++	++++
Cardiomegaly	±	++++	++++

Table 4. Drugs Associated With Cardiomyopathy

Antibiotics—AZT (zidovudine), chloroquine, ddI (didanosine)
Antipsychotics—lithium, phenothiazines
Antineoplastics—bleomycin, busulfan, cisplatin, doxorubicin, methotrexate, vincristine
Others—alcohol, cocaine

Diastolic Dysfunction

- Myocardial ischemia—occurs earlier than systolic dysfunction
- Hypertension
- Valvular diseases—aortic stenosis
- Primary restrictive cardiomyopathies—idiopathic, endomyocardial fibrosis, eosinophilic (Löffler endocarditis)
- Secondary restrictive cardiomyopathies—amyloidosis, hemochromatosis, Gaucher disease, Hurler syndrome, sarcoidosis
- Hypertrophic obstructive cardiomyopathy

High-Output Failure

- Anemia
- Hyperthyroidism
- Thiamine deficiency (beriberi)
- Arteriovenous fistulas
- Paget disease
- Multiple myeloma
- Pregnancy

Isolated Right-Heart Failure

- Congenital—isolated secundum atrial septal defect, sinus venosus atrial septal defect, pulmonary stenosis, Ebstein anomaly
- Right ventricular infarction—associated with 1/3 of inferior myocardial infarctions
- Cor pulmonale
- Pulmonary hypertension—primary, chronic thromboembolic disease, mitral regurgitation
- Arrhythmogenic right ventricular dysplasia
- Uhl anomaly

EPIDEMIOLOGY

- Framingham Heart Study estimates of prevalence of heart failure:
  - ▲ Age 50-59—8/1,000 men, 8/1,000 women
  - ▲ Age 80-89—66/1,000 men, 79/1,000 women
  - ▲ Higher prevalence for African Americans
- These values likely represent underestimates because Framingham Heart Study included only symptomatic cases of systolic or diastolic dysfunction based on exam, chest X-rays, ECGs.

CLINICAL PRESENTATION

- After establishing the clinical diagnosis of congestive heart failure, always look for a treatable cause (Table 5).

History

- Dyspnea on exertion is earliest and most constant symptom in all forms of heart failure.
- Orthopnea and paroxysmal nocturnal dyspnea occur later and tend to disappear after the right ventricle fails.
- Weakness, fatigue, edema, and weight gain (most often in legs and abdomen)
- Look for precipitating factors
  - ▲ Dietary salt load—most common factor but is diagnosis of exclusion
  - ▲ Medication noncompliance—second most common factor

Table 5. Treatable Causes of Congestive Heart Failure

Surgical treatment
    Coronary artery disease—better myocardial perfusion may
    occasionally improve congestive heart failure
    Valvular disease—mitral regurgitation, aortic regurgitation,
    mitral stenosis, aortic stenosis
    Atrial septal defect
    Left atrial myxoma
    Arteriovenous fistulas
    Constrictive pericarditis
Medical cure
    Thyrotoxicosis
    Acromegaly
    Beriberi

(lack of diuretics or excess digitalis; use of other drugs, e.g., NSAIDs; negative inotropics; alcohol)

- ▲ Infection—viral, pneumonia, urinary tract, skin, sinus
- ▲ Ischemia—always needs to be ruled out
- ▲ Arrhythmia—Anything other than sinus rhythm may decompensate congestive heart failure (15%-20% of patients with congestive heart failure have atrial fibrillation).
- ▲ Other organ dysfunction—renal insufficiency, hypothyroidism, hyperthyroidism, anemia, COPD
- ▲ Pericardial disease
- ▲ Hypertension

Physical Exam
- ■ Classic signs of systolic heart failure—bilateral basal lung rales (crackles), third heart sound (S_3), lower extremity or sacral edema, elevated jugular venous pressure
- ■ A right-sided S_3 increases with respiration.
- ■ A loud fourth heart sound (S_4) may indicate a diastolic cause.
- ■ A prominent v wave is found in tricuspid regurgitation.
- ■ Hepatojugular reflux in the absence of other signs of congestive heart failure may be an early sign of a fixed stroke volume and asymptomatic left ventricular dysfunction (more commonly, occurs in association with florid congestive heart failure when pulmonary wedge pressure is >18 mm H_2O).

- A sustained left ventricular impulse suggests left ventricular hypertrophy and a diastolic cause.
- Bounding carotid pulses suggest aortic regurgitation, thyrotoxicosis, arteriovenous fistula, or beriberi as cause of failure.
- A prominent right ventricular lift suggests cor pulmonale, pulmonary hypertension, thromboembolic disease, or mitral regurgitation as cause of failure.
- A systolic murmur that increases with the Valsalva maneuver suggests hypertrophic obstructive cardiomyopathy.
- Although rare, ascites can present without pronounced peripheral edema.

DIAGNOSTIC STRATEGY

ECG
- Rate
  - ▲ In florid congestive heart failure, usually tachycardia, more worrisome if bradycardia
- Rhythm
  - ▲ Look for rhythms that need to be cardioverted or paced.
- Ischemia
  - ▲ Inverted T wave
  - ▲ ST-segment abnormalities
  - ▲ New Q waves
  - ▲ New bundle branch block
- Microvoltage (<5 mm in frontal leads and <10 mm in precordial leads)
  - ▲ Suggests large pericardial effusion
  - ▲ Low voltage and a pseudoinfarction pattern in anterior leads suggest cardiac amyloidosis.
- Look for signs of electrolyte disorders and digitalis toxicity.

Chest X-ray
- Dilatation of upper lobe pulmonary vessels
- Kerley B lines (the only other differential diagnosis is lymphangitic carcinomatosis)
- Butterfly alveolar infiltrate (may be unilateral) with prominent hila
- Pleural effusions (initially on the right, then bilateral)

- Cardiomegaly (not on an anteroposterior view!)
  - ▲ Suggests biventricular or left ventricular failure
- Pulmonary infiltrates
  - ▲ Pneumonia
- Normal-size cardiac silhouette does not rule out systolic or diastolic heart failure!

Echocardiogram
- Left ventricular ejection fraction and size
  - ▲ Normal ejection fraction is about 0.55.
- Four-chamber enlargement suggests dilated cardiomyopathy.
- Regional wall motion abnormalities suggest ischemia.
- Diastolic dysfunction is suggested by enlarged atria and left ventricular hypertrophy with a long deceleration time and abnormal E/A ratio.
- Valvular lesions and intracardiac structures
- Pericardial diseases
  - ▲ Fluid
  - ▲ Thickening
  - ▲ Calcification

Blood Tests
- CBC and differential—infection, anemia
- Electrolytes—sodium, potassium, magnesium, calcium, phosphorous (hypophosphatemia can cause congestive heart failure)
- Serial troponins and CK-MB (every 6 hours × 4)
- BUN, creatinine, glucose

Always Consider the Following:
- Amyloidosis (cardiac amyloidosis can occur without systemic amyloidosis)
- Hemochromatosis
- HIV
- Myocarditis
- Postpartum cardiomyopathy
- Tachycardia-induced congestive heart failure

CONDITIONS THAT MIMIC CONGESTIVE HEART FAILURE
Mimic Congestive Heart Failure Clinically
- COPD

- Acute respiratory distress syndrome
- Pneumonia
- Lung cancer
- Portal hypertension
- Nephrotic syndrome
- Hypothyroidism

Mimic Congestive Heart Failure Radiographically

- Pneumonia
- Acute respiratory distress syndrome
- Lymphangitic carcinomatosis
- Noncardiac pulmonary edema—allergic, high altitude, high intracranial pressure
- Alveolar proteinosis

MANAGEMENT

Emergency Management of Heart Failure

- Always consider
  - Does the patient need to go to the catheter lab emergently?
  - Does the patient need emergency echocardiography?
  - Does the patient need emergency cardiac surgery?

What To Do

- Sit the patient upright
- Administer
  - Oxygen
  - Morphine
  - Furosemide
  - Nitrates
  - Intra-aortic balloon pump

All Patients With Chronic Congestive Heart Failure

- Sodium restriction— <5 g of NaCl or 2 g of sodium daily
- Physical activity based on individual exercise capacity
- Daily weight assessment
- Stop alcohol consumption
- Angiotensin-converting enzyme (ACE) inhibitors or angiotensin II receptor blockers (ARBs)—increased survival

- β-Blockers—increased survival
- Digoxin—no increased survival but symptomatic improvement
- Diuretics—for symptomatic relief

Hospitalized Patients Not In Cardiogenic Shock
- Bed rest if in New York Heart Association functional class IV
- Oxygen 2 L nasally
- Heparin—5,000 U SQ (or low-molecular-weight heparin) twice daily for deep venous thrombosis prophylaxis
- Intravenous diuretics—every 4-6 hours (target is weight reduction of 0.5-1.0 kg/day)
- ACE inhibitors or ARBs
- Spironolactone if ejection fraction is <0.35 or patient in New York Heart Association functional class IV
- Nitrates if ischemic origin
- Aspirin if ischemic
- Digoxin—drug of choice for patients with atrial fibrillation
- Consider hemodynamically tailored therapy for refractory or difficult-to-manage cases (see below).

Hospitalized Patients With Cardiogenic Shock or Refractory Congestive Heart Failure
- Send to catheter lab
- Intensive care setting
- Invasive hemodynamic monitoring—targets are the following:
  - Adequate right atrial pressure, >5 mm Hg
  - Adequate pulmonary capillary wedge pressure, >15 mm Hg (measure of preload and filling pressures)
  - Systemic vascular resistance 1,000-1,200 dynes/second per cm^2 (measure of afterload)
  - Cardiac index >2.5 L/min per m^2
  - Optimum mean arterial pressure (defined as minimally acceptable blood pressure to support renal and central nervous system function and not cause orthostatism)
- Nitroprusside
  - For combined preload and afterload reduction desired (high systemic vascular resistance, high pulmonary capillary wedge pressure, low cardiac index)
  - Use only if mean arterial pressure is ≥65 mm Hg, then start at 0.1-0.2 μg/kg per minute
- Nitroglycerin

- ▲ For primary reduction of preload (high pulmonary capillary wedge pressure), e.g., acute pulmonary edema
  - ▲ Start at 0.2-0.3 µg/kg per minute.
- ■ Dobutamine
  - ▲ For both inotropic effects and afterload reduction (high systemic vascular resistance, low cardiac index, normal pulmonary capillary wedge pressure)
  - ▲ Start at 2.5 µg/kg per minute, maximal dose <20 µg/kg per minute
- ■ Dopamine
  - ▲ When mean arterial pressure is inadequate or as coadjuvant with dobutamine
  - ▲ Start at 5 µg/kg per minute.
- ■ Milrinone
  - ▲ For combined preload and afterload reduction (high SVR, low cardiac index, high pulmonary capillary wedge pressure)
  - ▲ Start at 0.5 µg/kg per minute.
- ■ Intra-aortic balloon counterpulsation
  - ▲ If medical therapy is not sufficient
  - ▲ Increases mean arterial pressure, cardiac index, coronary perfusion, and reduces afterload.
  - ▲ Absolute contraindications
    - • Severe aortic insufficiency
    - • Aortic dissection
  - ▲ Valuable bridge to definitive therapy but not an answer in itself
- ■ Ventricular assist devices
  - ▲ May be short- or long-term bridge to cardiac transplant
- ■ Diuretics
  - ▲ Not usually indicated for cardiogenic shock, except in association with acute pulmonary edema
  - ▲ They decrease organ perfusion and lower mean arterial pressure.
- ■ ACE inhibitors
  - ▲ Not during acute shock
  - ▲ May be started if patient becomes stable on intra-aortic balloon pump
- ■ Heart transplant

CONNECTIVE TISSUE DISEASES

Kenneth J. Warrington, M.D.
Steven R. Ytterberg, M.D.

SYSTEMIC LUPUS ERYTHEMATOSUS (SLE)

Definition

- A chronic, immune-mediated multisystem disease
- The American College of Rheumatology revised classification criteria for SLE, developed primarily for research purposes, require that 4 of 11 criteria be met (Table 1).

Etiology

- An unknown trigger in a genetically predisposed host results in a sustained and injurious autoimmune response.

Epidemiology

- Strong female predominance
  - ▲ Female:male ratio is 9:1.
  - ▲ Peak age at onset is 20s-30s.
- Incidence rates in U.S. vary from 2.0 to 7.6/100,000 cases per year.
- Potential triggers—UV light, estrogen therapy, smoking, viral infections, drugs, environmental toxins

Clinical Presentation

- General
  - ▲ Fever, lymphadenopathy, Raynaud phenomenon
- Skin
  - ▲ Facial erythema is more common than classic "butterfly" rash.
  - ▲ Malar rash, discoid lupus, photosensitivity, aphthous ulceration

Special abbreviations used in this chapter: ANA, antinuclear antibody; BOOP, bronchiolitis obliterans with organizing pneumonia; ENA, extractable nuclear antigen; SLE, systemic lupus erythematosus; TNF, tumor necrosis factor.

Table 1. Criteria for Diagnosis of Systemic Lupus Erythematosus

Criterion	Definition
Malar rash	Fixed malar erythema, flat or raised
Discoid rash	Erythematous raised patches with keratotic scaling & follicular plugging
Photosensitivity	Skin rash as an unusual reaction to sunlight
Oral ulcers	Oral or nasopharyngeal ulcers, usually painless
Arthritis	Nonerosive arthritis involving 2 or more peripheral joints
Serositis	Pleuritis *or* pericarditis
Renal disorder	Persistent proteinuria (>0.5 g/day) *or* Cellular casts of any type
Neurologic disorder	Seizures (in absence of other causes) *or* Psychosis (in absence of other causes)
Hematologic disorder	Hemolytic anemia *or* Leukopenia (<4 × 10^9/L on 2 or more occasions) *or* Lymphopenia (<1.5 × 10^9/L on 2 or more occasions) *or* Thrombocytopenia (<100 × 10^9/L in absence of offending drugs)
Immunologic disorder	Anti–double-stranded DNA (dsDNA) *or* Anti-Smith (Sm) *or* Antiphospholipid antibodies
Antinuclear antibody (ANA)	Positive ANA in absence of drugs known to be associated with "drug-induced lupus syndrome"

- ▲ Also assess for alopecia and cutaneous vasculitis.
- ■ Musculoskeletal
  - ▲ Arthritis—symmetric, small and large joint, nonerosive arthritis that can lead to deformity (Jaccoud arthropathy)
  - ▲ Myositis—uncommon
- ■ Renal (glomerulonephritis)
  - ▲ Presents as proteinuria and/or cellular casts: red cell, hemoglobin, granular, tubular
  - ▲ Renal biopsy is basis for diagnosis and classification (Table 2).
- ■ Pulmonary
  - ▲ Pleurisy and pleural effusion (exudate) are common (50%-70% of cases).

Table 2. Classification of Systemic Lupus Erythematosus According to Biopsy Findings

WHO class	Biopsy findings	Prognosis
I	Normal	Excellent
II	Mesangial GN	Good
III	Focal proliferative GN	Moderate
IV	Diffuse proliferative GN	Poor, may respond to immunosuppression
V	Membranous GN	Nephrotic-range proteinuria, often with normal creatinine
VI	Chronic sclerosing changes	Irreversible, likely progression to renal failure

GN, glomerulonephritis; WHO, World Health Organization.

- ▲ Lupus pneumonitis is rare; rule out infection first.
- ▲ Other—pulmonary hemorrhage, bronchiolitis obliterans with organizing pneumonia (BOOP), shrinking lungs syndrome
- ■ Cardiovascular
  - ▲ Pericarditis and pericardial effusion (exudate) are common; tamponade is rare.
  - ▲ Myocardial disease—Premature atherosclerosis is a common cause of coronary artery disease, *especially in young females*; coronary arteritis and myocarditis are rare.
  - ▲ Libman-Sacks endocarditis can cause embolic events.
  - ▲ Other—pulmonary hypertension, systemic hypertension
- ■ Neurologic
  - ▲ First, rule out infection, drug reaction, metabolic causes, malignancy.
  - ▲ Headache—lupus meningitis, dural sinus thrombosis, stroke
  - ▲ Stroke
    - Infarct or hemorrhage from small-vessel vasculopathy
    - Embolic (Libman-Sacks endocarditis)
    - Antiphospholipid antibody–mediated
    - Other causes—hypertension, atherosclerosis

- • Rare—vasculitis
- ▲ Seizures, psychosis, cognitive function deficits
- ▲ Other—transverse myelitis, optic neuritis, peripheral neuropathy
- ■ Gastrointestinal
  - ▲ Abdominal pain
    - • Secondary to medications (e.g., NSAIDs, azathioprine)
    - • Secondary to lupus—serositis (lupus peritonitis), intestinal vasculitis, pancreatitis, infarcts (liver, spleen, bowel)
  - ▲ Other—protein-losing enteropathy
- ■ Hematologic
  - ▲ Anemia—of chronic disease (common), autoimmune hemolytic anemia
  - ▲ Leukopenia, lymphopenia
  - ▲ Thrombocytopenia—idiopathic thrombocytopenic purpura, antiphospholipid antibody–associated, thrombotic thrombocytopenic purpura, drugs

Complications
- ■ Infections
  - ▲ Major cause of morbidity and mortality
  - ▲ Disease activity can be difficult to distinguish from infection.
  - ▲ Always exclude infection before making diagnosis of "lupus flare."
- ■ Accelerated atherosclerosis
- ■ Secondary antiphospholipid antibody syndrome

Diagnostic Strategies
- ■ For initial SLE diagnosis
  - ▲ CBC, ESR, antinuclear antibody (ANA) (>99% positive, low specificity)
  - ▲ dsDNA antibodies—60%-80% positive, high specificity; associated with lupus nephritis, active disease
  - ▲ Extractable nuclear antigens (ENAs)
    - • Anti-Sm—specific but only 7%-30% of SLE patients are positive; associated with membranous glomerulonephritis
    - • Anti-U_1RNP—low specificity
    - • Anti-Ro/SSA—10%-50% positive, low specificity
    - • Anti-La/SSB—10%-20% positive, low specificity

- Anti–Scl-70—uncommon, may indicate scleroderma overlap
- ▲ Complement (total, C3, C4)—depressed with active disease
- ▲ Urinalysis, creatinine
- ▲ aPTT, antiphospholipid antibodies, lupus anticoagulant
- ▲ Assess organ involvement, depending on clinical presentation (e.g., echocardiography, MRI of head)
- ■ To assess disease activity in patient with known SLE
  - ▲ CBC—Look for decrease in hemoglobin, WBCs, or platelets.
  - ▲ ESR, dsDNA, urinalysis, creatinine, complement (total, C3, C4)
  - ▲ Assess organ involvement, depending on clinical presentation.
  - ▲ Note: Low complement and high dsDNA *may* predict disease flare.
    - Decrease in dsDNA can occur with active disease because of tissue deposition.
    - ANA value *does not* vary with disease activity and does not need to be repeated after SLE diagnosis is established.

Management

Principles of Therapy

- ■ Treatment depends on the pattern and severity of organ involvement.
- ■ Drug therapy according to disease manifestations is listed in Table 3.

Major Drug Complications

- ■ Hydroxychloroquine—retinal toxicity
- ■ Methotrexate—hepatotoxicity, cytopenias, pneumonitis
- ■ Corticosteroids—exogenous Cushing syndrome, hypertension, diabetes mellitus, osteoporosis, cataracts, avascular necrosis of bone, adrenal suppression (give steroid prep for major illness or surgery)
- ■ Cyclophosphamide—hemorrhagic cystitis, bladder cancer, infertility, bone marrow suppression
- ■ Mycophenolate mofetil—cytopenias

Table 3. Drug Therapy for SLE According to Disease Manifestations

Disease manifestation	Drug	Typical dose
Arthritis	NSAIDs	
	Hydroxychloroquine	200 mg twice daily
	Methotrexate	7.5-20 mg/week
	Prednisone	5-15 mg daily
Serositis	Prednisone	20-40 mg daily
	NSAIDs	
Neurologic	Prednisone	60 mg daily
	Pulse cyclophospha-mide IV	0.5-1.0 g/m^2 monthly
Hematologic		
Hemolytic anemia	Prednisone	60 mg daily
Thrombocytopenia	Prednisone	60-100 mg daily
	IV immunoglobulin	0.4 g/kg daily × 5 days
	Consider danazol, cytotoxics	
Lupus nephritis		
WHO class III-IV or mixed V/III-IV	Pulse methylpred-nisolone IV	1 g/day × 3 days, then
	Prednisone	1 mg/kg daily
	Pulse cyclophospha-mide IV	0.5-1.0 g/m^2 monthly
	Consider mycophe-nolate mofetil as alternative	1 g twice daily

SLE, systemic lupus erythematosus; WHO, World Health Organization.

- Azathioprine—cytopenia, pancreatitis, hepatotoxicity, neoplasia
- Note: Stopping hydroxychloroquine can result in minor and even major disease flares.

SJÖGREN SYNDROME
Definition
- A chronic inflammatory, autoimmune disease characterized by progressive inflammatory infiltration of exocrine glands, particularly lacrimal and salivary glands
- Primary Sjögren syndrome occurs alone.
- Secondary Sjögren syndrome occurs in association with

other connective tissue diseases (rheumatoid arthritis, SLE, or scleroderma).

Etiology
- Unknown, but genetic factors contribute and viral infection may be involved

Epidemiology
- Strong female predominance
  - Female:male ratio is 9:1.
  - Age at onset is usually >40 years.

Clinical Presentation
- Musculoskeletal—arthralgia, myalgia, myositis
- Sicca manifestations
  - Enlargement of parotid and/or submandibular glands
  - Dry eyes (xerophthalmia), corneal ulceration
  - Dry mouth (xerostomia), difficulty chewing, dysphagia, dental caries
- Pulmonary
  - Cough, tracheobronchitis sicca due to dry secretions
  - Bronchitis, bronchiolitis
  - Interstitial pulmonary fibrosis
- Hepatic—primary biliary cirrhosis, cryptogenic cirrhosis
- Renal—renal tubular acidosis type I (due to tubulointerstitial nephritis), glomerulonephritis (uncommon)
- Gastrointestinal
  - Dyspepsia, dysphagia
  - Chronic atrophic gastritis
  - Pancreatitis
- Neurologic
  - Peripheral neuropathy, mononeuritis multiplex
  - Central nervous system (rare)—focal motor deficits, seizures, movement disorders, encephalopathy
- Cutaneous vasculitis

Complications
- Non-Hodgkin lymphoma

- ▲ Relative risk in Sjögren syndrome is 44 times expected incidence.
- ▲ Patients with enlarged salivary glands and lymphadenopathy are at greatest risk.

Diagnostic Strategies
- ■ Lab abnormalities
  - ▲ Anemia, leukopenia, high ESR, high C-reactive protein
  - ▲ Positive ANA (50%), rheumatoid factor (44%), ENA (anti-Ro/SSA [70%], anti-La/SSB [50%-70%])
- ■ Ocular signs
  - ▲ Positive Schirmer test, rose bengal staining
- ■ Lip salivary gland biopsy—if positive, specificity 86.2%, sensitivity 82.4%

Management
- ■ Symptomatic (this often is all that is necessary)
  - ▲ Artificial tears, lacrimal duct occlusion, artificial saliva, pilocarpine, cevimeline
- ■ Immunomodulators
  - ▲ Hydroxychloroquine
  - ▲ Corticosteroids and cytotoxics are reserved for severe extraglandular disease.

ANTIPHOSPHOLIPID ANTIBODY SYNDROME
Definition
- ■ This syndrome is defined as the association of the following:
  - ▲ Autoantibodies directed against one or more phospholipid-binding plasma proteins and/or complexes of these proteins with phospholipids *and*
  - ▲ Venous or arterial thrombosis, recurrent fetal loss, or thrombocytopenia
- ■ Primary antiphospholipid antibody syndrome occurs in isolation.
- ■ Secondary antiphospholipid antibody syndrome occurs in patients with SLE or other connective tissue disease.

Epidemiology
- ■ The prevalence of primary antiphospholipid antibody syndrome is not known.
- ■ Clinically significant antiphospholipid antibody syndrome occurs in 10% to 15% of patients with SLE.

Clinical Presentation
- Thrombosis
  - ▲ Any part of the vascular tree can be affected
  - ▲ Common sites
    - • Arterial—stroke, myocardial infarction, extremity gangrene
    - • Venous—lower limb (often with pulmonary embolus), hepatic (Budd Chiari syndrome), portal vein
- Recurrent fetal loss—usually from the late first trimester onward
- Thrombocytopenia—usually moderate (platelets $\geq 50 \times 10^9$/L)
- Cardiac
  - ▲ Noninfective verrucous vegetations (Libman-Sacks endocarditis)
  - ▲ Myocardial infarction
- Skin
  - ▲ Cutaneous ulcers
  - ▲ Livedo reticularis
- Neurologic
  - ▲ Migraine
  - ▲ Stroke
  - ▲ Transient ischemic attack
  - ▲ Transverse myelitis
- Catastrophic antiphospholipid antibody syndrome
  - ▲ Multisystem vascular occlusion with poor prognosis (rare)
  - ▲ Can be precipitated by surgery, infection, stopping anti-coagulation

Diagnostic Strategies
- False-positive VDRL (not done at Mayo, syphilis serology is not helpful)
- Lupus anticoagulant—antibodies in patient's serum that prolong certain phospholipid-dependent coagulation reactions (e.g., aPTT and dilute Russel viper venom time are prolonged and do not correct after equal mix with normal plasma)
- Anticardiolipin antibodies—detected with ELISA
- Both lupus anticoagulant and anticardiolipin antibodies should be checked if antiphospholipid antibody syndrome is suspected.

- The strongest clinical associations have been seen with IgG anticardiolipin antibodies; however, IgM or IgA antibodies may be associated with the syndrome.
- A positive test for antiphospholipid antibody syndrome should be confirmed by repeating in 6-8 weeks.
- Diagnosis requires one of the clinical criteria (vascular thrombosis or pregnancy morbidity) and one of the lab criteria (lupus anticoagulant or anticardiolipin antibodies).

Management
- Therapy for various clinical scenarios of antiphospholipid antibody syndrome is listed in Table 4.

DIFFUSE SCLERODERMA (SYSTEMIC SCLEROSIS)
Definition
- Chronic systemic disorder characterized by microvascular injury, inflammation, and fibrosis

Etiology
- Unknown
- Environmental exposures in a genetically susceptible host may contribute.

Epidemiology
- Incidence—10-20 cases per million per year
- Female:male ratio is 3:1.
- Peak age at onset is 30-50 years.

Clinical Presentation
- Raynaud phenomenon (>95% of patients)
  - ▲ Usually severe
  - ▲ Assess for fingertip ischemia, necrosis, ulceration, pitted scars.
  - ▲ Nail fold capillaroscopy is typically abnormal.
- Skin
  - ▲ Tight, shiny, thickened skin is the hallmark feature (extending proximally above knees and elbows).
  - ▲ Also, telangiectasia, pigment changes, calcinosis
- Pulmonary
  - ▲ Interstitial lung disease—dyspnea, cough, "Velcro" crackles

Table 4. Therapy for Various Clinical Scenarios of Antiphospholipid Antibody Syndrome

Clinical scenario	Therapy
Thrombosis (arterial or venous)	Anticoagulation with warfarin Keep INR ≥3.0 (may require life-long therapy)
Fetal loss	5,000 U unfractionated heparin SQ twice daily & low-dose (81 mg) aspirin during pregnancy
Prophylaxis (no event with positive serologic test)	Consider low-dose aspirin (81 mg daily)
Catastrophic antiphospho-lipid antibody syndrome	IV heparin, high-dose corticosteroids, cyclophosphamide, plasmapheresis (>50% mortality)

- ▲ Pulmonary hypertension, usually secondary to interstitial lung disease
- ■ Renal
  - ▲ Hypertension
  - ▲ Hypertensive renal crisis occurs in 20% of patients.
    - • Manifests as accelerated hypertension and rapidly progressive renal failure, possibly with microangiopathic hemolysis.
    - • Can be precipitated by moderate to high doses of corticosteroids
- ■ Gastrointestinal
  - ▲ Upper tract—esophageal dysmotility, gastroesophageal reflux, erosive esophagitis, esophageal strictures, gastroparesis
  - ▲ Small bowel—intestinal hypomotility, pseudo-obstruction, bacterial overgrowth, malabsorption
  - ▲ Colon—wide-mouthed diverticula
- ■ Cardiac
  - ▲ Arrhythmias, myocardial fibrosis
  - ▲ Pericarditis (uncommon)
- ■ Musculoskeletal

▲ Tendon friction rubs are typical.
▲ Symmetric polyarthralgia, joint stiffness, finger swelling (early)
▲ Joint contractures (late)
▲ Myopathy

Diagnostic Strategies
- Scleroderma is a clinical diagnosis based on typical findings.
- Nonspecific findings—hypergammaglobulinemia, positive ANA (>90%), positive rheumatoid factor
- Helpful serology—anti–Scl-70 (specific but only present in 30%)
- Assess for organ involvement according to presentation, e.g., pulmonary function tests, high-resolution chest CT, echocardiography, gastrointestinal motility studies, renal function variables.

Management
- No known disease-modifying agent for scleroderma
  ▲ Each disease manifestation requires specific management.
- General
  ▲ Avoid smoking.
  ▲ Avoid cold exposure.
- Raynaud phenomenon—calcium channel blockers (nifedipine and amlodipine work best), angiotensin-converting enzyme inhibitors, α-blockers
- Gastrointestinal—proton pump inhibitor, prokinetic agents (e.g., metoclopramide)
- Musculoskeletal—low-dose corticosteroids, NSAIDs, methotrexate for synovitis
- Renal
  ▲ Patients with rapidly progressive skin thickening are at greatest risk for renal crisis.
  ▲ Close monitoring of blood pressure and urinalysis
  ▲ Aggressive use of angiotensin-converting enzyme inhibitors
  ▲ May need dialysis
- Pulmonary disease—cyclophosphamide for alveolitis documented by bronchoalveolar lavage and/or high-resolution chest CT
- Pulmonary hypertension—calcium channel blockers, bosetan prostacyclin analogues (e.g., epoprostenol), anticoagulation

LIMITED SCLERODERMA (CREST SYNDROME)

Definition

- A variant of scleroderma
- However, skin involvement *does not* extend proximally above knees and elbows (although face and neck can be involved).

Clinical Presentation

- C, calcinosis
- R, Raynaud phenomenon
- E, esophageal dysmotility
- S, sclerodactyly
- T, telangiectasia
- Not all five features need to be present for diagnosis of limited scleroderma.

Complications

- Pulmonary hypertension (usually in the absence of pulmonary parenchymal disease)
- Renal disease is rare in this subset of patients.

Diagnostic Strategies

- Limited scleroderma is a clinical diagnosis based on typical findings.
- Helpful serologic test is anti-centromere antibody (specific, present in 50%).
- Assess for organ involvement according to presentation, e.g., pulmonary function tests, echocardiography for pulmonary artery pressure, and gastrointestinal evaluation.

Management

- Disease manifestations are treated individually (see DIFFUSE SCLERODERMA, Management).

RHEUMATOID ARTHRITIS

Definition

- Chronic, autoimmune, inflammatory disorder characterized by erosive, symmetric arthritis with a variable degree of extra-articular involvement

- Presence of four of the seven following criteria have 90% sensitivity and specificity:
  - Morning stiffness >1 hour × 6 weeks
  - Arthritis >3 joints simultaneously × 6 weeks
  - Hand joint arthritis × 6 weeks
  - Symmetric joint involvement × 6 weeks
  - Rheumatoid nodules
  - Positive rheumatoid factor
  - Radiologic findings

Etiology
- Unknown
- Genetic factors (HLA genes in particular) are important.

Epidemiology
- Prevalence rate is about 1%.
- Female:male ratio is 2-3:1.
- Age at onset is 40-60 years.

Clinical Presentation
- Systemic—fatigue, myalgias
- Musculoskeletal
  - Symmetric, erosive, small and large joint polyarthritis, which is often progressively deforming
  - Assess for ulnar deviation, swan neck, boutonnière deformity.
  - Tenosynovitis, bursitis
- Extra-articular disease
  - Skin
    - Subcutaneous nodules (20%-30% of rheumatoid factor–positive patients)
    - Nail-fold infarcts
  - Eyes—secondary Sjögren syndrome, scleritis, scleromalacia
  - Pulmonary—pleurisy, pleural effusion, rheumatoid lung nodules, BOOP, fibrosis
  - Cardiac—pericarditis, myocarditis, rheumatoid nodules (valve, myocardium)
  - Felty syndrome—splenomegaly, large granular lymphocytosis, neutropenia
  - Neurologic—entrapment neuropathy (e.g., carpal tunnel), mononeuritis multiplex

Complications

- Infection—Rheumatoid arthritis and its treatment predispose to infection.
  - ▲ If infection is suspected or documented, consider withholding immunosuppressive agents.
  - ▲ Always rule out septic arthritis if one joint is inflamed out of proportion to other joints.
  - ▲ Carefully assess any prosthetic joints if infection is suspected.
  - ▲ Tumor necrosis factor (TNF) blockade can predispose to TB reactivation, opportunistic lung infection.
- Atlantoaxial subluxation
  - ▲ Spinal cord compromise
  - ▲ Obtain lateral flexion and extension cervical spinal films.
  - ▲ Careful neurologic assessment for evidence of radiculopathy or myelopathy
- Vasculitis
  - ▲ Polyarteritis nodosa-like illness, usually in patients with chronic, severe, deforming, nodular rheumatoid arthritis
  - ▲ Can present as mononeuritis multiplex, leg ulcers, mesenteric ischemia
  - ▲ Treat with high-dose corticosteroids and cytotoxic agents.
- Premature mortality—mainly cardiovascular and infectious causes
- Amyloidosis
  - ▲ Rheumatoid arthritis is a major cause of secondary amyloidosis.
- Adrenal suppression
  - ▲ If patient is receiving long-term corticosteroid therapy, steroid prep may be needed during major illness/surgery (50-100 mg hydrocortisone every 8 hours for 1-2 days or until stable, then resume usual dose).
- Osteoporosis

Diagnostic Strategies

- Rheumatoid arthritis is a clinical diagnosis, based on history and physical exam.
- Nonspecific lab abnormalities—anemia, high ESR, high C-reactive protein, thrombocytosis

- Positive rheumatoid factor—75%-80% of patients with rheumatoid arthritis are positive, but test is not specific
- Radiology—hand and foot X-rays to look for erosive changes

Management
- Needs to be individualized depending on patient characteristics, disease course, drug tolerability, drug toxicity, concurrent illness
- Disease-modifying antirheumatic drugs commonly used to treat rheumatoid arthritis and their major toxic effects are listed in Table 5.

SERONEGATIVE SPONDYLOARTHROPATHIES

Definition
- Group of disorders that includes the following:
  - Ankylosing spondylitis
  - Enteropathic arthritis (inflammatory bowel disease–associated arthropathy)
  - Reiter syndrome (reactive arthritis)
  - Psoriatic arthritis
- Common features of seronegative spondyloarthropathies
  - Absence of rheumatoid factor
  - Association with HLA-B27
  - Axial skeletal involvement with sacroiliitis and spondylitis
  - Asymmetric oligoarthritis of large weight-bearing joints
  - Dactylitis (inflammation of a digit)
  - Enthesitis (inflammation of bony insertions for tendons and ligaments)

Specific Disease Features
Ankylosing Spondylitis
- Needs to include the skeletal manifestations and radiographic findings
- Cause not known (exclude other causes of spondyloarthropathy listed above)
- Male:female ratio is 3:1; age at onset is adolescence to 35 years.
- Extraskeletal manifestations
  - Aortic valve regurgitation (~5% of patients), complete heart block
  - Apical lung fibrosis (1% of patients)

Table 5. Disease-Modifying Antirheumatic Drugs (DMARDs) Used to Treat Rheumatoid Arthritis

DMARD	Typical dose	Toxic effect
Hydroxychloro-quine	400 mg/day	Retinal damage
Methotrexate	7.5-25 mg weekly	Hepatotoxicity, acute interstitial pneumonia, cytopenias
Sulfasalazine	500-2,000 mg/day	Leukopenia
Azathioprine	2-2.5 mg/kg daily	Leukopenia, hepatotoxicity, lymphoma
Gold (injectable)	25-50 mg/week IM	Leukopenia, thrombocytopenia, pneumonitis, glomerulonephritis
Cyclosporine	3-4 mg/kg daily	Renal dysfunction, hypertension
Leflunomide	100 mg/day × 3 days, 20 mg/day	Hepatotoxicity
Infliximab	3 mg/kg at 0, 2, 6 weeks, then IV infusion every 8 weeks	Infusion reactions, TB reactivation, opportunistic lung infections
Etanercept	25 mg SQ twice weekly	Injection site reactions, infection, demyelinating disease
Adalimumab	40 mg SQ every other week	Injection site reactions, infection, demyelinating disease
Anakinra	100 mg/day SQ	Injection site reactions, neutropenia

- ▲ Thoracic cage restriction from costovertebral fusion
- ▲ Uveitis (25% of patients)
- ▲ Renal amyloidosis
- ■ Complications
  - ▲ Vertebral fractures—even after minimal trauma (because of spine rigidity and osteopenia)
  - ▲ Cauda equina syndrome—presents as sensory loss in lum-

bar and sacral dermatomes, lower limb weakness and pain, and loss of urinary and rectal sphincter tone
- Management
  - ▲ Physical therapy
  - ▲ NSAIDs
  - ▲ Sulfasalazine
  - ▲ TNF blockade

Enteropathic Arthritis
- Associated with inflammatory bowel disease (Crohn disease and ulcerative colitis)
- Sex ratio is equal; age at onset is 25-44 years.
- Arthritis occurs in 2%-20% of patients with inflammatory bowel disease.
- Peripheral arthritis often correlates with activity of gut inflammation; axial disease does not.
- Axial disease is clinically and radiographically identical to idiopathic ankylosing spondylitis.
- Management
  - ▲ Treat gastrointestinal disease.
  - ▲ Consider sulfasalazine, methotrexate, TNF blockade.

Reiter Syndrome (Reactive Arthritis)
- Acute inflammatory arthropathy arising after an infectious process, but at a site remote from the primary infection
- Common pathogens associated with the syndrome include *Shigella*, *Salmonella*, *Yersinia*, *Campylobacter* (enteric infections), *Chlamydia*, *Ureaplasma*, and HIV (genitourinary infection).
- Classic triad of urethritis, conjunctivitis, and arthritis occurs in 33% of patients.
- Other extraskeletal manifestations include circinate balanitis, keratoderma blennorrhagicum, and mucosal ulcers.
- Management
  - ▲ Physical therapy
  - ▲ NSAIDs
  - ▲ Immunosuppression for chronic disease
- Majority of patients have self-limiting disease.

Psoriatic Arthritis
- Occurs in 5%-7% of patients with psoriasis; sex ratio is equal.

- May manifest as
  - Spondyloarthropathy
  - Symmetric polyarthritis resembling rheumatoid arthritis
  - Distal interphalangeal joint arthritis
  - Arthritis mutilans (associated with osteolysis of affected joints)
  - Oligoarticular arthritis
- Assess for characteristic nail changes, including pitting, onycholysis, and subungual hyperkeratosis.
- Management
  - NSAIDs
  - Methotrexate
  - TNF blockade
  - Other agents used for rheumatoid arthritis

DIABETES MELLITUS

Gunjan Y. Gandhi, M.D.
Pierre Theuma, M.D.
Victor M. Montori, M.D.

DEFINITION

- Fasting plasma glucose— >126 mg/dL (7 mmol/L) and confirmed at least once on repeat measurement (normal if <100 mg/dL)
- Random glucose— >200 mg/dL plus symptoms of diabetes mellitus

CLASSIFICATION

- Type 1
- Type 2
- Secondary diabetes—drugs, endocrinopathies, exocrine pancreatic disease, infections, genetic syndromes
- Gestational diabetes

ETIOLOGY

- Type 1—results from immune-mediated destruction of insulin-producing β-cells of endocrine pancreas, could be idiopathic
- Type 2—results from insulin resistance and some degree of defective insulin production related to visceral obesity and sedentary lifestyle

EPIDEMIOLOGY

- Diabetes affects 6% of U.S. population, and 18% of population older than 60
  - Diabetes is more common among American Indians, Alaska Natives, and African Americans; prevalence is similar for Hispanics and non-Hispanic whites
- No difference between sexes

CLINICAL PRESENTATION

- Common clinical presentations of type 1 and type 2 diabetes are compared in Table 1.

MANAGEMENT

Routine Management of Diabetic Patients on Hospital Service

- In acutely ill patients or during immediate perioperative period, normoglycemia is the currently recommended ideal.

Perioperative

- Goals of hospital care
  - ▲ Maintain normoglycemia
  - ▲ Prevent hypoglycemic episodes and ketoacidosis.
  - ▲ Patients on oral agents or diet control may need insulin therapy during the acute stress of major surgery and critical illness.
  - ▲ IV insulin infusions are preferred to SQ route during the immediate postoperative period (e.g., after cardiac and vascular surgery). This ensures adequate insulin delivery in case of peripheral shutdown in the perioperative period and also makes it possible to carefully titrate insulin to frequently measured blood glucose levels.
  - ▲ Tight glycemic control with insulin improves outcomes of patients in ICU.
  - ▲ Currently, there is no consensus on intraoperative management of hyperglycemia.
  - ▲ Note: Measure glucose every half hour during the operation and in postanesthesia recovery room. An insulin infusion may be used intraoperatively. Goal has not been established.

Table 1. Comparison of Common Clinical Presentations of Type 1 and Type 2 Diabetes

Type 1	Type 2
Fatigue	Asymptomatic or incidental finding
Weight loss	End-organ damage
Polyuria	Recurrent infections
Polyphagia	Visual blurring
Polydipsia	
Severe dehydration	
Diabetic ketoacidosis	

- ▲ Measure immediate postoperative glucose level.
  - • If >80 mg/dL, see Table 2 for insulin infusion algorithm (your hospital may have implemented a different algorithm), especially in cardiac surgery patients.
- ▲ On day of surgery, omit sulfonylurea
- ▲ Stop metformin before any contrast study
- ▲ Current guidelines recommend that patients not restart metformin any sooner than 48 hours after contrast study or surgery and only if renal function is stable and normal, i.e., creatinine <1.5 mg/dL in men, <1.4 mg/dL in women (potential risk of lactic acidosis)
- ■ The common practice of sliding scale administration of regular insulin doses every 6 hours based on reflectance meter glucose results does not provide proper control.
  - ▲ Insulin-treated patients could receive the usual insulin dose on the day before the operation.
  - ▲ On the day of the operation, give half the usual morning dose of NPH or Lente insulin SQ.
  - ▲ If the patient is on Ultra-Lente insulin, the entire dose may be given the evening before the operation.
- ■ The algorithm in Table 2 *should not* be used for patients with diabetic ketoacidosis or hyperosmolar states.
  - ▲ A typical insulin infusion is 250 U Human Regular insulin in 250 mL of 0.45% sodium chloride.

DIABETIC EMERGENCIES

- ■ Check blood glucose levels in patients with glycosuria, in any ill diabetic patient, and in any patient with a clinical state in which derangement of blood glucose must be excluded (Table 3).

Hypoglycemia
Diagnosis

- ■ Whipple triad
  - ▲ Suggestive symptoms
  - ▲ Low plasma glucose level (<50 mg/dL in men, <40 mg/dL in women)
  - ▲ Prompt symptomatic relief with glucose administration

Table 2. Insulin Infusion Protocol

Column 1		Column 2		Column 3	
Start in this column		Patient has not reached glucose range of 80-100 mg/dL within 2 hours using column 1 and glucose has decreased by <50 mg/dL over preceding 1 hour		Patient has not reached glucose range of 80-100 mg/dL within 2 hours using column 2 and glucose has decreased by <50 mg/dL over preceding 1hour	
Restart in this column when insulin infusion had to be discontinued for glucose <80 mg/dL					
Serum glucose, mg/dL	**Insulin infusion rate, units/hour**	**Serum glucose mg/dL**	**Insulin infusion rate, units/hour**	**Serum glucose, mg/dL**	**Insulin infusion rate, units/hour**
>400	18	>400	25	>400	30
351-400	16	351-400	22	351-400	27
301-350	14	301-350	20	301-350	24
251-300	12	251-300	18	251-300	21
201-250	10	201-250	15	201-250	18
176-200	8	176-200	12	176-200	15
151-175	6	151-175	9	151-175	12
121-150	4	121-150	7	121-150	9
101-120	2	101-120	4	101-120	6
80-100	1	80-100	2	80-100	3
<80	Off	<80	Off	<80	Off

- When glucose is <60 mg/dL, stop insulin infusion and initiate 50 mL/h of 10% dextrose in water.
- Check glucose every 30 minutes until glucose is ≥80 mg/dL. Discontinue D10W. Resume insulin infusion, always in column 1.
- If glucose is <60 mg/dL, initiate Treatment of Hypoglycemia Protocol (MC1156-30).
- Restart insulin infusion in column 1 when glucose ≥80 mg/dL.
- Check arterial blood glucose every 1 hour in the ICU once insulin infusion has been started.

Etiology
- Causes of hypoglycemia are listed in Table 4.

Management
- If the patient is not able to take oral feeding safely, then NPO
  - ▲ Administer 25 mL of 50% dextrose in water IV over 3-5 minutes in a large vein immediately and repeat every 15-20 minutes if needed.
  - ▲ If this is not feasible, give glucagon 1 mg SQ (preferred) or IM.

Table 3. Clinical States in Which Glucose Derangements Should Be Excluded

Acute confusion
Seizures
Suspected stroke
Decreased level of consciousness
Sepsis
Hypothermia
Liver failure
Metabolic acidosis
Salicylate poisoning
Severe hyponatremia
High-dose corticosteroid use

Table 4. Causes of Hypoglycemia

Common mismatch between hypoglycemic agent and caloric intake
    Insulin excess (decreased renal function, erratic absorption)
    Oral hypoglycemic agent excess
    Severe liver disease
    Severe sepsis
    Alcohol excess, especially after a binge
Less common causes
    Adrenal failure
    Salicylate poisoning
    Insulinoma
    Hypopituitarism

- ▲ Recheck blood glucose level by capillary stick test after 15 minutes of initial treatment.
- ▲ Repeat treatment if blood glucose is <80 mg/dL and monitor. Repeat until blood glucose is >80 mg/dL.
- ■ If patient is alert and can swallow, give 15 g of carbohydrates:
  - ▲ Half cup of fruit juice, 2 packets of sugar dissolved in half cup of water, or glucose oral gel 15 g PO
  - ▲ Then provide a snack to prevent recurrence
- ■ Consider and treat the underlying cause (Table 4).
- ■ Exclude artifactual hypoglycemia or possibility of lab error. *Do not rely only on blood glucose measurements by glucose-monitoring devices.*
- ■ If hypoglycemia recurs or is likely to recur (sepsis, excessive sulfonylurea therapy, or long-acting insulin)
  - ▲ Start 5% or 10% dextrose infusion at 75 mL/hour in a large peripheral or central vein.
  - ▲ Check the reflectance meter glucose regularly, and adjust the infusion rate to keep the blood glucose level in normal range.
  - ▲ In sulfonylurea excess (especially long-acting preparations such as glyburide or chlorpropamide), maintain glucose infusion for 24 hours, then taper off over the next 2-3 days.
  - ▲ If alcohol excess is suspected, add thiamine IV to the infusion to prevent Wernicke encephalopathy.
  - ▲ If the response to 10% glucose is not sufficient, give more 50% dextrose, preferably in a central vein.

Diabetic Ketoacidosis
- ■ Consider the diagnosis in any ill patient who has diabetes.
- ■ Exclude this diagnosis for patients with confusion, coma, or metabolic acidosis who have increased anion gap.

Pathophysiology
- ■ Severe insulin deficiency with or without excess counter-regulatory hormones (glucagon, epinephrine)

Diagnosis
- ■ Hyperglycemia >250 mg/dL (13.9 mmol/L)
- ■ Ketonemia/ketonuria (check β-hydroxybutyrate if available)
- ■ Metabolic acidosis with increased anion gap

Etiology
- In diabetic patients
  - ▲ Insulin deficiency (missed doses, failure to increase dose with illness)
  - ▲ Infection
  - ▲ Inflammation
  - ▲ Myocardial ischemia, infarction
  - ▲ Glucocorticoid administration
- Presenting feature in patients with previously undiagnosed type 1 diabetes

Clinical Presentation
- Often characterized by a gradual deterioration, sometimes over days
- Anorexia, nausea, vomiting, polyuria, and subsequent dehydration
- Abdominal pain may be present.
- Kussmaul respiration (deep and rapid), acetone breath
- If untreated, altered consciousness or frank coma

Diagnostic Strategies
- Order priority
  - ▲ Blood glucose level (reflectance meter glucose and lab)
  - ▲ Ketones (plasma and urine)
  - ▲ Electrolyte panel
  - ▲ Arterial blood gases
  - ▲ Blood cultures
  - ▲ ECG
  - ▲ Chest X-ray
  - ▲ Urinalysis and Gram stain
  - ▲ Evaluate anion gap (sodium, chloride, bicarbonate)

Management
- Consider transfer to medical ICU.
- Fluids
  - ▲ Deficit is usually 5-8 L, and both free water and salt are required.
  - ▲ Aggressive hydration needs to be initiated (may require

boluses, depending on clinical assessment of hydration state)
- Rate initially, 10-14 mL/kg per hour of 0.9 normal saline
- May need to titrate based on cardiovascular status
- Insulin
  - Immediately give 10-20 U (0.15 U/kg body weight) regular insulin as IV bolus.
  - Start insulin infusion at 0.1 U/kg body weight per hour, and titrate to blood glucose level of 200-250 mg/dL.
  - Adjust infusion rate to decrease glucose by 50 mg/dL per hour.
  - Aim to reverse ketosis in the first 24 hours, avoid hypoglycemia, and avoid cerebral edema from too rapid a decrease in osmolality.
  - Stop insulin infusion when the anion gap has resolved. Overlap the infusion with SQ insulin by 2-3 hours. Monitor reflectance meter glucose every 4 hours.
  - When glucose is ≤250 mg/dL, change to 5% dextrose plus 0.45 NaCl with insulin coverage (e.g., 200 mL/hour infusion with 0.05 U/kg per hour IV or 5-10 U SQ every 2 hours). Goal is 150-200 mg/dL glucose until metabolic control is achieved.
- Monitor electrolytes.
  - Potassium deficit is about 300-500 mEq independently of serum potassium; the total body stores are low and will decrease further with therapy. If renal perfusion and urinary flow are adequate, add 40 mEq of potassium to each liter of IV fluid.
  - Replace phosphate if <1 mg/dL. Give 20-30 mEq/L of potassium phosphate IV over 6 hours.
  - Bicarbonate may be given if pH is <7.1 and systolic blood pressure is <90 mm Hg despite fluid replacement. Avoid excess bicarbonate because it will exacerbate hypokalemia and lead to paradoxical CSF acidosis.
  - Hyponatremia may be present because of osmotic water shifts or as pseudohyponatremia due to hyperglycemia (for every increase in glucose of 100 mg/dL over 100 mg/dL, sodium decreases by 1.6 mmol).
- Treat underlying cause
  - Check for a focus of infection, including the feet and perineum.

- ▲ Fever may be absent despite infections.
- ▲ Consider empiric antibiotic therapy, including anaerobic cover.
- ▲ Leukocytosis does not necessarily imply infection but may be due to diabetic ketoacidosis itself.
- ■ Monitor pH, bicarbonate, anion gap, ketones (including β-hydroxybutyrate), glucose, potassium, and urine output every 1-2 hours, keeping track of vital signs, IV fluid rate and composition, and insulin infusion.

HYPEROSMOLAR NONKETOTIC HYPERGLYCEMIC COMA

- ■ Consider the diagnosis for any patient with hyperglycemia, hyperosmolality, change in mental status, and no ketoacidosis.

Etiology

- ■ Same as for diabetic ketoacidosis; in addition, dehydration and renal failure

Clinical Presentation

- ■ Mostly affects elderly patients who have type 2 diabetes. Circulating insulin prevents ketogenesis.
- ■ Features
  - ▲ Mental obtundation, polyuria, nausea, vomiting
  - ▲ Extreme dehydration, orthostatic hypotension, tachycardia
  - ▲ Reversible hemiplegia, focal seizures

Diagnosis

- ■ Order priority—serum osmolality, blood cultures, LDH, CBC, electrolyte panel (including magnesium), phosphate, urine culture and stain, urinalysis, arterial blood gases, ECG, chest X ray
- ■ Often, the blood glucose level is >600 mg/dL (>33.3 mmol/L), serum osmolality >340 mOsm/L, BUN 60-90 mg/dL. Lactic acidosis may be present.
- ■ Sodium is decreased (normal or increased, if severe dehydration) —correct by 2.4 mEq/L per 100 mg/dL glucose over 100 mg/dL.

- Bicarbonate is usually >12 mEq/L (average, 17), pH >7.2 (average, 7.26).
- Decreased calcium, magnesium, potassium, and inorganic phosphorus

Management
- Consider transfer to medical critical care unit.
- Coma rarely occurs unless the calculated effective osmolality is >320 mOsm/L
- Serum osmolality = 2 (sodium + potassium) + (plasma glucose/18) + (BUN/2.8)

Fluids
- Mean fluid loss is ≈ 9L, thus, aggressive hydration (1 L normal saline per hour)
  - ▲ Start normal saline infusion if hypotensive
  - ▲ Change to 5% dextrose plus 0.45 normal saline after blood glucose level reaches 300 mg/dL
  - ▲ Maintain blood glucose at 250-300 mg/dL until osmolality is ≤315 mOsm/kg and patient is alert.

Insulin
- Use same insulin algorithm for diabetic ketoacidosis.

Potassium
- Correct hypokalemia (serum potassium level <3.3 mEq/L)
  - ▲ Withhold insulin.
  - ▲ Administer 40 mEq potassium (2/3 potassium chloride, 1/3 potassium phosphate)
- If potassium level is
  - ▲ 3.3-5.5 mEq/L, give 20 mEq/L potassium IV
  - ▲ >5.5 mEq/L, recheck every 2 hours.

EPILEPTIC SEIZURES

Yoon-Hee K. Cha
Gregory A. Worrell, M.D.
Gregory D. Cascino, M.D.

DEFINITIONS

- Seizure—transient episode of disturbed cerebral function caused by abnormal excessive synchronous electrical discharge of cortical neurons
- Provoked seizures—a symptomatic seizure caused by a precipitating factor (e.g., fever, drugs, ethanol withdrawl, electrolyte abnormalities)
- Epilepsy—chronic medical condition characterized by recurrent unprovoked seizures
- Status epilepticus—life-threatening condition defined by continuous seizures for ≥5 minutes or ≥2 seizures with incomplete recovery of consciousness between seizures (older definition of status epilepticus: seizures lasting >30 minutes)

CLASSIFICATION OF EPILEPSY

The International Classification of Epileptic Seizures is given in Table 1, and the features distinguishing secondarily generalized from primarily generalized seizures are listed in Table 2.

EPIDEMIOLOGY OF SEIZURES, EPILEPSY, AND STATUS EPILEPTICUS

- Seizures
  - 10% lifetime risk
  - Account for 1% of emergency department visits
- Epilepsy
  - 3%-4% lifetime risk, with 0.5%-1% prevalence
- Status epilepticus

Special abbreviations used in this chapter: AED, antiepileptic drug; CNS, central nervous system.

Table 1. International Classification of Epileptic Seizures

Partial seizures (focal onset)
    Simple partial seizures (normal consciousness)
        Motor signs
        Somatosensory or special-sensory symptoms (olfactory,
          visual, taste)
        Autonomic symptoms or signs (e.g., epigastric rising
          sensation)
        Psychic symptoms (e.g., déjà vu, jamais vu, fear)
    Complex partial seizures (impaired consciousness)
        No impairment of consciousness at onset
            Without automatisms
            With automatisms (picking at clothes, lip smacking,
              complex motor behaviors)
        With impairment of consciousness at onset
            Without automatisms
            With automatisms
    Partial seizures secondarily generalized (see Table 2)
Generalized seizures (bihemispheric at onset)
    Absence or atypical absence seizures (may have mild clonic,
      atonic, tonic, or autonomic activity or automatic behavior)
    Myoclonic seizures
    Clonic seizures
    Tonic seizures
    Tonic-clonic seizures
    Atonic seizures
Unclassified epileptic seizures

Modified from Mosewich RK, So EL. A clinical approach to the classification of seizures and epileptic syndromes. Mayo Clin Proc. 1996;71:405-14. By permission of Mayo Foundation for Medical Education and Research.

- ▲ 50/100,000 persons, with 22% mortality
- ▲ Incidence is highest for patients <1 year old, patients >60 years make up largest group.
- ■ Mortality from status epilepticus
  - ▲ Pediatric, 2.5%
  - ▲ Adults, 14%
  - ▲ Adults >60 years, 38%

CAUSE OF SEIZURES

- ■ Vascular—subarachnoid hemorrhage, venous sinus thrombosis, ischemic stroke, intracranial hemorrhage, hypertensive encephalopathy, arteriovenous malformation

Table 2. Evidence for Secondarily Generalized Versus Primarily Generalized Seizure

Preceeding aura (e.g., epigastric rising sensation, tastes, smells, psychic)

Preceeding motionless period with unresponsiveness and staring

Preceeding automatisms (e.g., lip smacking, chewing, picking, complex patterned movements)

Preceeding focal or asymmetric motor phenomena (e.g., tonic or dystonic posturing, clonic jerking, head or eye deviation)

Any of the above occurring occasionally in isolation without generalization or loss of consciousness

Focal abnormalities on neurologic exam

Focal epileptiform activity on EEG

Focal abnormality on MRI (e.g., hippocampal atrophy, tumor, infarct, vascular malformation, hamartoma, cortical dysplasia, encephalomalacia)

Modified from Mosewich RK, So EL. A clinical approach to the classification of seizures and epileptic syndromes. Mayo Clin Proc. 1996;71:405-14. By permission of Mayo Foundation for Medical Education and Research.

- Infection—meningitis, encephalitis (e.g., California virus, herpes simplex), abscess
- Toxic—drugs/drug withdrawal, ethanol, carbon monoxide, lead, strychnine, mercury (review patient's medicines for ability to provoke seizures)
- Autoimmune/inflammatory—thrombotic thrombocytopenic purpura, central nervous system (CNS) vasculitis, multiple sclerosis
- Metabolic—hypoglycemia, nonketotic hyperglycemia, hyponatremia, hypocalcemia, hypomagnesemia, hypoxia, pyridoxine deficiency
- Trauma—penetrating head trauma, subdural or epidural hematoma
- Neoplasm—primary CNS tumor (e.g., astrocytoma, meningioma, oligodendroglioma, lymphoma), metastatic lesion (e.g., lung, breast, melanoma, lymphoma)
- Genetic and congenital—primary idiopathic epilepsy, tuberous sclerosis, Sturge-Weber syndrome, neurofibromatosis, perinatal injury (infection, hypoxia, birth trauma)

- Epilepsy—patient with known epilepsy and a subtherapeutic antiepileptic drug level, infection, or other underlying medical condition
- Common causes of symptomatic seizures by age are listed in Table 3.

CLINICAL PRESENTATION
- Clinical presentation—can range from obvious (e.g., generalized tonic-clonic seizure) to subtle changes in awareness, behavioral, emotional, or psychic symptoms
- Alteration of consciousness—associated with both generalized seizures (e.g., absence and tonic-clonic) and complex partial seizures
- Nonconvulsive status epilepticus—varied presentations ranging from alterations of consciousness to coma

DIAGNOSTIC STRATEGY
- Simultaneous EEG and clinical observation of the seizure provide the definitive diagnosis of seizure type. The most common situation is a patient who has had a seizure without a physician observing the clinical event. For this reason, the most important diagnostic tool is the history.
- The history should be taken from an eyewitness observer if possible. When necessary, telephone persons who have witnessed the patient's clinical events.

Table 3. Common Causes of Symptomatic Seizures by Age

Age, years	Cause
5-15	CNS infection
	Head trauma
15-35	Ethanol withdrawal
	Head trauma
	Eclampsia
35-64	Ethanol withdrawal
	CNS tumor
	Trauma
	Stroke
≥65	Stroke
	Metabolic

CNS, central nervous system.

History

- Ask about the common risk factors for epilepsy, including:
  - Family history (genetic predisposition to seizure disorder)
  - Birth history and complications, cognitive and motor development
  - Infant or childhood seizures (e.g., febrile seizures are associated with temporal lobe epilepsy)
  - Past history of CNS infections, stroke, head trauma, cancer (see causes listed above)
- Detailed description of the event— Seizures are generally brief and have stereotyped patterns.
  - What was patient doing at time of the event, e.g., did the seizure occur during sleep?
  - Were there any warning symptoms/aura and were they focal (Table 2)?
  - Did the patient lose consciousness?
  - What other symptoms were present (e.g., shortness of breath or chest pain may suggest a different diagnosis)?
  - How long did the event last (most seizures last <3 minutes)?
  - Description of the movements—Did patient fall to the ground?
  - Did patient lose bowel/bladder control or bite the tongue?
  - Was there postictal confusion?
- The history can suggest other possible diagnoses for transient neurologic symptoms and loss of consciousness, including:
  - Syncope (presyncopal symptoms, precipitating maneuvers, orthostatic blood pressure, abnormal ECG)
  - Sleep disorders such as narcolepsy
  - Stroke (posterior circulation)
  - Migraine
  - Paroxysmal vertigo
  - Transient global amnesia
  - Ethanol/drug-related "blackouts"
  - Movement disorder (myoclonus, dyskinesias)
  - Psychiatric (nonepileptic seizures, panic attacks, hyperventilation)

Physical Exam

- Vital signs, including oxygenation status
- Detailed exam with attention to the following:
  - ▲ Level of consciousness—In unresponsive patients, subtle rhythmic movements of limbs or eyes may indicate ongoing seizure activity.
  - ▲ Head—signs of trauma
  - ▲ Cranial bruits—vascular malformation
  - ▲ Cervical bruit—carotid stenosis
  - ▲ Focal neurologic deficits may indicate a structural lesion—hemiparesis, asymmetric reflexes, sensory deficit, visual field defect, memory deficit
  - ▲ Cardiac arrhythmia and/or murmurs
  - ▲ Skin—stigmata of neurocutaneous syndromes

Lab Testing

- Baseline CBC, sodium, potassium, calcium, magnesium, BUN, creatinine, glucose, liver function tests, PT, PTT, arterial blood gases, VDRL, toxin screen, antiepileptic drug (AED) levels, chest X-ray, and ECG
- Same night
  - ▲ Head CT (without contrast)—to rule out structural lesions, head trauma, or bleeding
  - ▲ Lumbar puncture if infection is suspected (perform CT first if neurologic exam is abnormal, patient is >60 years old or is immunocompromised)
  - ▲ EEG if ongoing subclinical seizure activity is suspected (consider nonconvulsive status epilepticus for patients with persistent mental status alterations)
- Outpatient evaluation
  - ▲ MRI—the imaging modality of choice for evaluation of seizure disorders
  - ▲ EEG—sleep and awake EEG (diagnostic yield is increased with sleep deprived recording)

COMPLICATIONS

- The most common complication associated with seizures is physical trauma suffered during the event (e.g., falling, automobile accident, drowning).
- Hypoxia, hyperthermia, hypotension, and hypoglycemia can complicate prolonged seizures and status epilepticus.

- Generally, the longer that status epilepticus continues, the more difficult it is to control.

MANAGEMENT (ADULTS)
- General indications for AEDs are listed in Table 4.

Acute Management
- Seizures are usually self-limited (<3 minutes) and rarely require emergency intervention.
- Overly aggressive therapy with benzodiazepines and other AEDs can have dangerous consequences (e.g., hypotension, respiratory depression, cardiac arrhythmia).

Table 4. General Indications for Antiepileptic Drugs (AEDs)

Seizure type	AED		
	First line	Second line	Third line
Partial—simple, complex, with/ without secondary generalization	Carbamazepine Phenytoin	Lamotrigine Levetiracetam Topiramate Gabapentin	Felbamate Phenobarbital
Generalized			
Classic absence	Ethosuximide	Valproic acid Lamotrigine	Felbamate
Atypical absence	Valproic acid Lamotrigine	Topiramate	Felbamate
Tonic-clonic	Valproic acid	Carbamazepine Phenytoin Lamotrigine Topiramate	Felbamate Clonazepam
Myoclonic	Valproic acid Lamotrigine		Felbamate Clonazepam Phenobarbital
Tonic, atonic, akinetic, clonic, or mixed	Valproic acid	Lamotrigine	Phenytoin Felbamate Clonazepam
Infantile spasms	ACTH	Prednisone	Clonazepam

ACTH, adrenocorticotropic hormone.

- Procedure
  - Position patient on his/her side and in location where no harm is likely during a convulsion (e.g., falling out of bed, injury from sharp furniture).
  - Maintain an airway and ensure adequate oxygenation (face mask oxygen if needed).
  - Monitor vital signs (oxygen saturation, blood pressure, pulse, respiratory rate, temperature).
  - Check finger stick glucose.
  - Draw blood sample for routine lab tests and AED levels; establish IV line if needed.
  - Record accurate time of duration of seizure.
    - If a generalized tonic-clonic or tonic seizure lasts >3 minutes, begin treatment with IV lorazepam (2 mg initial dose) and consider loading with fosphenytoin (20 mg/kg) (Fig. 1).
    - If the seizure continues, follow algorithm in Figure 2.
  - Seizure precautions should be implemented, including padding the bed rails; restraints should not be used.

Long-Term Management
- General guidelines for starting long-term AED therapy are given in Table 5.
- Not all patients require an AED after a seizure.
- If the evaluation is normal and no risk factors are identified, the risk of a second seizure is approximately 25%.
- The risk of recurrence after a second seizure is 65%-80%.
- Discuss the following with all patients:
  - Risk of injury if they have a seizure while driving, operating dangerous equipment, or swimming; driving laws vary by state (see Epilepsy Foundation Web site http://efa.org)
  - Women with epilepsy
    - AED therapy is associated with teratogenesis.
    - All women require folic acid supplementation of ≥0.4 mg/day.
    - Attempt to plan pregnancy with help of physicians (neurologist and obstetrician)
    - Some AEDs decrease the effectiveness of oral contraceptives.

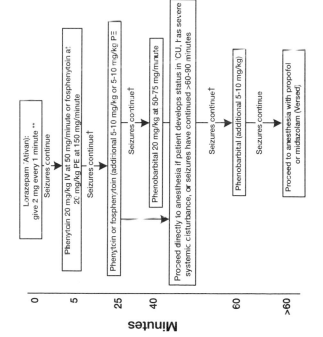

Fig. 1. Acute management for seizures lasting more than 3 minutes. PE, phenytoin equivalents. *More lorazepam can be given. **If emergent IV access cannot be obtained, use rectal diazepam 0.5 mg/kg. (Modified from Lowerstein DH, Alldredge BK. Current concepts. Status epilepticus. N Engl J Med. 1998;338:970-6. Used with permission.)

Lorazepam (Ativan); give 2 mg every 1 minute **
Seizures continue

Phenytoin 20 mg/kg IV at 50 mg/minute or fosphenytoin at: 20 mg/kg PE at 150 mg/minute
Seizures continue†

Phenytoin or fosphenytoin (additional 5-10 mg/kg or 5-10 mg/kg PE
Seizures continue†

Phenobarbital 20 mg/kg at 50-75 mg/minute

Proceed directly to anesthesia if patient develops status in ICU, has severe systemic disturbance, or seizures have continued >60-90 minutes
Seizures continue†

Phenobarbital (additional 5-10 mg/kg)
Seizures continue

Proceed to anesthesia with propofol or midazolam (Versed)

Minutes

0
5
25
40
60
>60

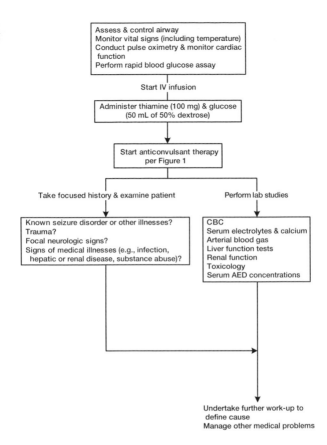

Fig. 2. Emergency management of status epilepticus. AED, antiepileptic drug. (From Lowenstein DH, Alldredge BK. Current concepts. Status epilepticus. N Engl J Med. 1998;338:970-6. Used with permission.)

Table 5. Guidelines for Starting Long-term Therapy With Antiepileptic Drugs

Treat	Maybe treat	Do not treat
Status epilepticus as a first seizure	Uncomplicated single seizure if history suggests that one occurred earlier	Ethanol withdrawal or other provoked seizure
MRI/CT lesion		Substance abuse (if due to barbiturate abuse, should replace the drug & taper slowly)
Clear-cut epileptic focus on EEG	Single seizure in someone at risk if seizure recurs (drivers, home alone, etc.)	
Active or previous CNS infection		
Abnormal neurologic exam findings		Sleep deprivation
Head injury with loss of consciousness		Febrile seizures
History of epilepsy in siblings/parents		Seizures due to acute illness that is resolving
		Nonepileptic spells
		Epilepsy with centrotemporal spikes

CNS, central nervous system.

FULMINANT HEPATIC FAILURE

Thomas C. Sodeman, M.D.
J. Eilene Hay, M.B., Ch.B.

DEFINITION
- Hepatic dysfunction—jaundice, increased PT, low albumin
- Encephalopathy
- No previous history of liver disease

CLASSIFICATION
- Hyperacute—within 1 week after development of jaundice
- Acute—within 1-4 weeks after development of jaundice
- Subacute—within 5-12 weeks after development of jaundice

ETIOLOGY
Common Causes
- Drugs—acetaminophen most common (up to 40% of cases)
- Viral—hepatitis B > hepatitis A
  - ▲ Consider hepatitis E with appropriate travel history.

Uncommon Causes
- Wilson disease—Kayser-Fleischer rings (uncommon); ALT < AST; serum uric acid and phosphate low; serum, hepatic, and urine copper high; ceruloplasmin low (5% normal)
- Vascular problems—Budd-Chiari syndrome (rapid onset ascites and/or jaundice, preexisting hypercoagulable state, post–bone marrow transplant)
- Fatty liver of pregnancy—second half of pregnancy, increased PT, mildly increased ALT and AST
- Ischemia—prolonged code, severe hemorrhage
- Reye syndrome
- Toxins—*Amanita phalloides* (recent camping trip)
- Malignant infiltration
- Autoimmune hepatitis—positive for antinuclear antibodies, increased gamma globulins

Unknown

- Cause is undetermined in up to 40% of cases (i.e., viral markers negative, drug levels undetectable, no other history).

EPIDEMIOLOGY

- Associated with underlying conditions

CLINICAL PRESENTATION

Classic Presentation

- Encephalopathy, jaundice, synthetic defects (flapping, yellow, and bleeding)

Common Presentation

- Early
  - ▲ Subtle mental changes (stage 1 encephalopathy)
  - ▲ Mildly increased ALT and AST levels
  - ▲ History of drug intake is often unclear (i.e., patient does not volunteer information without being asked).
  - ▲ Synthetic function may be intact or only slightly abnormal.
- Late
  - ▲ Can include multiorgan dysfunction

COMPLICATIONS

- Encephalopathy (coma), coagulopathy (bleeding), hypoalbuminemia (edema), ascites, jaundice, renal failure, increased intracranial pressure, infection (bacterial, viral, and fungal), hypotension, hypoglycemia
- Predictors of poor outcome—age >40, cause not acetaminophen or hepatitis A or B, encephalopathy stage 3 or 4, PT >50 seconds, bilirubin >17.5 mg/dL

DIAGNOSTIC STRATEGIES

- Rule out treatable causes.
  - ▲ Hepatitis A virus IgG, IgM (HBsAg), anti-HBsAg, hepatitis B virus DNA, hepatitis C virus RNA, hepatitis E virus, cytomegalovirus, Epstein-Barr virus, ceruloplasmin, urine and serum copper levels, drug screen, antinuclear antibodies, and gamma globulins.
- Establish baselines.
  - ▲ CBC, electrolytes, creatinine, BUN, uric acid, calcium, phosphorus, AST, ALT, bilirubin, alkaline phosphatase,

PT, PTT, fibrinogen, factor V level (indicator of short-term synthetic function), albumin, arterial blood gases
- ▲ Iron studies can be misleading.
- ▲ Increased liver enzymes with no encephalopathy or synthetic defect is not fulminant liver failure.

MANAGEMENT

- ■ Transplant candidate vs. nontransplant candidate
  - ▲ Transplant candidacy—age <65, no malignancy, no sepsis, no HIV, no active cardiac disease, good family and social support
    - • Spontaneous bacterial peritonitis not a contraindication.
- ■ Contact a transplant center *early* with questions; the center will request age, sex, blood type, diagnosis (if known), comorbidities, current medications, past surgical history, social history, alcohol and drug history, current treatment.
- ■ Management either while awaiting transplant or transport or if transplant is not an option
  - ▲ Supportive care—blood products, intubation, maintenance of low intracranial pressure (intracranial pressure monitor, mannitol, hyperventilation, elevation of head), prophylactic antimicrobials (amphotericin 10 mg IV and valganciclovir 900 mg IV twice daily [high mortality from fungal and cytomegalovirus infections]), nutrition, bowel decontamination (neomycin), IV glucose, *N*-acetylcysteine (consider use in all cases of fulminant hepatic failure)
  - ▲ Experimental—bioartificial perfusion devices, charcoal hemoperfusion, xenoperfusion

HIV DISEASE COMPLICATIONS

Kiran M. Bambha, M.D.
Stacey A. R. Vlahakis, M.D.

DEFINITION

- Immunodeficiency—the hallmark of HIV
- In 1993, the Centers for Disease Control and Prevention described clinical AIDS that results from infection with 23 opportunistic infections (e.g., *Pneumocystis carinii* pneumonia) and neoplasms (e.g., Kaposi sarcoma).
  - ▲ Also included in this definition
    - HIV seropositive patients with weight loss, diarrhea, or dementia
    - HIV seropositive patients who ever had a CD4 count <200 cells/µg or a CD4 percentage <14%

ETIOLOGY

- AIDS is caused by the human retroviruses HIV-1 and HIV-2 (HIV-1 is the more common virus in the U.S.)
- The virus can infect all cells expressing the CD4 and chemokine coreceptors, which act as entry receptors for HIV.
- The CD4 helper T cell is the primary cell affected, but other cells that may be involved include B lymphocytes, macrophages, and glial cells.
- HIV induces both qualitative and quantitative changes in CD4 cells.
- Most of the disorders caused by the virus can be explained by one of the following three mechanisms:
  - ▲ Immunodeficiency as a direct result of the effect of the virus on immune cells
  - ▲ Autoimmune phenomena secondary to disordered cellular or B-lymphocyte function
  - ▲ Neurologic impairment caused by direct effects of the virus or, more commonly, release of cytokines and neurotoxins by infected macrophages capable of disseminating HIV to multiple organ systems.

FEATURES

- HIV is transmitted by
  - ▲ Sexual contact with an infected person
  - ▲ Parenteral exposure to infected blood or blood products by needle sharing or transfusion
  - ▲ Occupational exposure in health care workers
  - ▲ Perinatal exposure
- The illness induced by the infection may be characterized by
  - ▲ Constitutional complaints including weight loss, sweats, wasting
  - ▲ Opportunistic infections
  - ▲ Aggressive cancers such as Kaposi sarcoma and extra-nodal lymphoma
  - ▲ Neurologic disorders

DIAGNOSIS AND EVALUATION

- Complications related to HIV may affect almost any organ system. A useful approach is to evaluate the organ system(s) involved.
- Important measure—the patient's CD4 lymphocyte count
  - ▲ The relation between the CD4 count and development of certain complications and opportunistic infections is outlined in Table 1.
  - ▲ The major diagnoses to be considered for an HIV patient according to organ system involved and presenting symptoms are listed in Table 2.
  - ▲ The diagnosis and treatment of specific disease entities are provided in Table 3.
  - ▲ Prophylactic regimens for opportunistic infections in AIDS patients are summarized in Table 4.
  - ▲ Current treatment of HIV infection is not discussed. For the most current information on HIV/AIDS, the reader should refer to the most recent literature on the subject.

Table 1. Relation of CD4 Cell Count to Opportunistic Infections and Other Complications

CD4 cell count	Infections	Noninfectious complications
>500 cells/mm^3	Acute retroviral syndrome, *Candida* vaginitis	Persistent generalized lymphadenopathy, myopathy, aseptic meningitis, Guillain-Barré syndrome
200-500 cells/mm^3	Pneumococcal & other bacterial pneumonias, pulmonary TB, Kaposi sarcoma, herpes zoster, thrush, cryptosporidia (self-limited), oral hairy leukoplakia	Cervical intraepithelial neoplasia, cervical cancer, B-cell lymphoma, Hodgkin lymphoma, lymphocytic interstitial pneumonitis, mononeuropathy multiplex, anemia, idiopathic thrombocytopenic purpura
<200 cells/mm^3	*Pneumocystis carinii* pneumonia, toxoplasmosis, disseminated histoplasmosis, disseminated coccidioidomycosis, progressive multifocal leukoencephalopathy, miliary/extrapulmonary TB	Wasting, cardiomyopathy, peripheral neuropathy, HIV-associated dementia, vacuolar myelopathy, progressive polyradiculopathy, non-Hodgkin lymphoma
<100 cells/mm^3	Disseminated herpes simplex, toxoplasmosis, cryptococcosis, cryptosporidiosis, microsporidiosis, *Candida* esophagitis	
<50 cells/mm^3	Disseminated CMV, disseminated *Mycobacterium avium* complex	Central nervous system lymphoma

CMV, cytomegalovirus.
From Bartlett JG. The Johns Hopkins Hospital 2000-2001 guide to medical care of patients with HIV infection. 9th ed. Philadelphia: Lippincott Williams & Wilkins; 2000. p. 51-4. Used with permission.

Table 2. Diagnostic Considerations for Complications in HIV According to Involved Organ System

Organ system	Complications, findings	Potential causes
Sinopulmonary	Sinusitis	*Streptococcus pneumoniae, Haemophilus influenzae, Pseudomonas aeruginosa, Staphylococcus aureus, Legionella pneumophilia, Klebsiella pneumoniae, Cryptococcus, other fungi, Alternaria, CMV*
	Pneumonia	Consider both infectious and noninfectious causes: PCP, TB, *S. pneumoniae, H. influenzae*, gram-negative rods, *Staph. aureus, Nocardia, P. aeruginosa, Legionella* (uncommon), MAC, *Cryptococcus*, histoplasmosis, *Candida, Aspergillus* (uncommon), *Coccidioides immitis, Rhodococcus*, CMV, influenza, HSV, VZV, Kaposi sarcoma, lymphoma, lymphocytic interstitial pneumonia, aspiration, nonspecific interstitial pneumonitis
	Radiologic abnormalities (nodules, cavitary lesions)	TB, *Cryptococcus, Nocardia*, MAC, histoplasmosis, PCP, *Rhodococcus, Aspergillus*, Kaposi sarcoma, lymphoma, *Staph. aureus* (especially IV drug abusers)
	Pneumothorax	PCP, aerosolized pentamidine

Table 2 (continued)

Organ system	Complications, findings	Potential causes
Oral cavity	Visible oral lesions that may or may not be symptomatic, plaques, erythema, dysphagia, odynophagia, bleeding gums, unpleasant taste, dry mouth, salivary gland enlargement (usually benign cystic enlargement)	Thrush, oral hairy leukoplakia, aphthous ulcers, CMV, HSV, Kaposi sarcoma, gingivitis/periodontitis
Esophagus	Esophagitis, dysphagia, odynophagia, ulcers, chest pain	*Candida*, CMV, HSV, aphthous ulcers, Kaposi sarcoma
Liver	Hepatitis, right upper quadrant pain, nausea, vomiting, elevated liver enzymes with/without symptoms, hepatomegaly, hepatic steatosis & development of lactic acidosis may complicate treatment with NRTIs due to mitochondrial toxicity induced by these medications	Medications (all antiretrovirals, sulfonamides, imidazoles, antituberculous medications, pentamidine, clarithromycin, ddI), mycobacterial infections, CMV, hepatitis B or C virus, lymphoma, disseminated bacterial & fungal infections, fatty liver due to malnutrition, ETOH
Biliary tree	Cholecystitis	More likely to be acalculous than in non-HIV patients
	AIDS, cholangiopathy & papillary stenosis	CMV, *Cryptosporidium* & Microsporidia have been implicated, papillitis, isolated bile duct stricture

Table 2 (continued)

Organ system	Complications, findings	Potential causes
Pancreas	Pancreatitis, pancreatic insufficiency, nausea, vomiting, abdominal pain	Medications (ddI, ddC, sulfonamides, corticosteroids, pentamidine, INH, 3TC, rifampin, erythromycin, paromomycin), HIV, CMV, mycobacteria, toxoplasmosis, Candida, Cryptosporidium, Cryptococcus, ETOH, hypertriglyceridemia, cholelithiasis, lymphoma, Kaposi sarcoma
		Treatment should focus on the most likely cause; may institute pancreatic supplements as needed
Spleen	Splenomegaly	Lymphoma, MAC, HIV, cirrhosis, fungal infections (histoplasmosis), PCP
Bowel	Enterocolitis, diarrhea (acute or chronic), abdominal pain, anal dysplasia/squamous cell carcinoma	Medication effect (including protease inhibitors), Campylobacter jejuni, Clostridium difficile, Salmonella, Shigella, CMV, adenovirus, calicivirus, astrovirus, Giardia, Entamoeba histolytica, Cryptosporidium, Isospora, Microsporidia, HIV, small-bowel overgrowth, MAC, Cyclospora cayetanensis, idiopathic diarrhea (diagnosis of exclusion); HPV is associated with anal squamous neoplasia; Kaposi sarcoma or lymphoma may involve bowel

Table 2 (continued)

Organ system	Complications, findings	Potential causes
Skin	Papules, pustules, pruritus, nodules, ulcerative lesions, vesicles, plaques, macules, petechiae, purpura	Drug reaction (TMP-SMX, dapsone, nevirapine, delavirdine, efavirenz), abacavir has been associated with severe hypersensitivity reaction (fever, rash [maculopapular or urticarial], GI symptoms, dyspnea, arthralgias) in 2%-3% of patients, HSV, herpes zoster, Kaposi sarcoma, bacillary angiomatosis, nodular prurigo, cryptococcosis, *Staphylococcus aureus*, eosinophilic folliculitis, molluscum contagiosum, seborrhea (*Malassezia furfur*), psoriasis, ITP, TTP, eczema
Central nervous system	Meningitis, encephalitis, dementia, focal neurologic deficits, altered mental status, paraparesis, retinitis, visual changes, headache, myelopathy, mononeuropathy multiplex, seizures	Toxoplasmosis, *Cryptococcus*, lymphoma, TB, bacterial infection/abscess, *Nocardia*, CMV, neurosyphilis, HSV, VZV, PML due to JC virus, AIDS dementia complex; other causes of mental status changes (hypoglycemia, hyponatremia, medications, hypoxemia, other metabolic abnormalities/nutritional deficiencies), depression

Table 2 (continued)

Organ system	Complications, findings	Potential causes
Central nervous system (continued)	Brain imaging abnormalities (solitary vs. multiple lesions, punctate lesions, enhancing vs. nonenhancing lesions)	(See Table 3, Central Nervous System)
Peripheral nervous system	Inflammatory demyelinating polyneuropathy, progressive polyradiculopathy, sensory neuropathy, myopathy, mononeuropathy multiplex	CMV, HIV, drug-induced (zidovudine, ddI, ddC, d4T), ETOH, vitamin B_{12} deficiency, thyroid disorders, syphilis, diabetes, acute & chronic inflammatory demyelinating polyradiculoneuropathies & may be seen in early HIV presumed due to immune dysregulation; distal symmetric polyneuropathy may be seen in advanced HIV (cause is uncertain); also case reports of peripheral neuropathy presumed due to lactic acidosis induced by NRTIs
Cardiac	Dilated cardiomyopathy, pericardial effusion, pericarditis, tamponade, endocarditis, drug-related toxicity, pulmonary hypertension, cardiac neoplasms (including Kaposi sarcoma & lymphoma), echocardiography may show dilated cardiomyopathy in up to 8% of HIV patients, may require myocardial biopsy for diagnosis, cardiomyopathy may be treated	Drug toxicity (zidovudine, NRTIs, doxorubicin, interferon, amphotericin B, TMP-SMX, pentamidine), HIV, other viral & fungal infections (myocarditis), other immunologically mediated effects; causes of pericardial effusions include *Staph. aureus*, TB, myocardial infarction, endocarditis, lymphoma, *Cryptococcus, Nocardia*, MAC, toxoplasmosis, & others

Table 2 (continued)

Organ system	Complications, findings	Potential causes
Cardiac (continued)	with standard heart failure regimens if indicated, some patients with dilated cardiomyopathy respond to HAART	
Renal	HIV- or heroin-associated nephropathy; acute tubular necrosis; rising creatinine & BUN, electrolyte abnormalities; decreased urine output; check urinalysis & Gram stain; check urine electrolytes if low urine output; urine eosinophils; renal ultrasound; correct any reversible factors for possible prerenal, intrinsic, postrenal causes; HIV nephropathy may respond to HAART & prednisone taper	Most common renal lesion in HIV is collapsing focal glomerulosclerosis (may progress rapidly to end-stage renal disease) Renal failure in AIDS is usually multifactorial & addressed similarly to patients without HIV: **prerenal** (hypovolemia, hypotension, reduced circulating arterial blood volume), **intrinsic** (acute tubular necrosis, rhabdomyolysis, acute interstitial nephritis, hemolytic uremic syndrome, TTP, postinfectious glomerulonephritis), **postrenal** (crystalluria—due to acyclovir, indinavir, saquinavir, ritonavir, sulfadiazine; extrinsic or intrinsic obstruction in urinary tract) Medications may contribute to renal failure (pertamidine, foscarnet, cidofovir, aminoglycosides, indinavir, contrast)

Table 2 (continued)

Organ system	Complications, findings	Potential causes
Hematopoietic	Anemia	Bleeding, hemolysis, iron deficiency, renal insufficiency, infection (MAC); if none of these is causative, may consider a trial of erythropoietin
	Neutropenia	Medications (zidovudine, ganciclovir, 3TC, ddI, d4T, foscarnet, ribavirin, flucytosine, amphotericin, sulfonamide, pyrimethamine, interferon); may treat with filgrastim (granulocyte colony-stimulating factor) (controversial)
	Thrombocytopenia	ITP, TTP, medication-induced thrombocytopenia
	Pancytopenia	Medication effect, infiltrative process involving bone marrow (infection, neoplasm)
Lymphatic	Lymphoma (non-Hodgkin, Hodgkin)	
	Adenopathy	Lymphoma, TB, MAC, Kaposi sarcoma, syphilis, HIV, toxoplasmosis, histoplasmosis, pneumocytosis, acute retroviral syndrome, isolated infection with *Bartonella henselae* may cause local adenopathy
Gynecologic	Vaginitis	*Candida*, bacterial vaginosis
	Pelvic inflammatory disease	*Neisseria gonorrhoeae*, *Chlamydia trachomatis*, anaerobes, *H. influenzae*, enteric gram-negative rods, streptococci
	Cervical dysplasia/cancer	HPV

CMV, cytomegalovirus; ddC, zalcitabine; ddI, didanosine; d4T, stavudine; ETOH, ethanol; HAART, highly active antiretroviral therapy; HPV, human papillomavirus; HSV, herpes simplex virus; ITP, idiopathic thrombocytopenic purpura; MAC, *Mycobacterium avium* complex; NRTI, nucleoside reverse transcriptase inhibitor; PCP, *Pneumocystis carinii* pneumonia; PML, progressive multifocal leukoencephalopathy; 3TC, lamivudine; TMP-SMX, trimethoprim-sulfamethoxazole; TTP, thrombotic thrombocytopenic purpura; VZV, varicella-zoster virus.

Table 3. Diagnosis and Treatment of Specific Diseases

Condition	Findings, associations*	Diagnosis	Treatment
Sinopulmonary disease Sinusitis	Frontal headache, fever, sinus congestion & pain, purulent nasal discharge postnasal drip; some patients may be only mildly symptomatic; chronic sinusitis is especially common with CD4 <200	Sinus X-rays (air-fluid levels, opacification of sinuses) or sinus CT/MRI scans (sinus mucosal thickening)	Appropriate antimicrobial coverage If nonsmoker, amoxicillin 500 mg tid If smoker, cover for *Haemophilus influenzae* with amoxicillin-clavulanate 500 tid or ciprofloxacin 500 bid Recommended treatment duration 10-14 days Refer refractory cases to ear, nose, & throat
Pneumonia *Streptococcus pneumoniae*	Common cause of pneumonia, acute onset, seen in all stages of HIV, may be associated with bacteremia	Chest imaging shows lobar or bronchopneumonia with/without pleural effusions, blood cultures, sputum Gram stain & culture, quellung-lung reaction	Azithromycin 500 mg PO × 1 dose, then 250 mg qd to complete a total of 5 days *or* Clarithromycin 500 mg PO bid *or* Levofloxacin 500 mg PO qd *or* Amoxicillin-clavulanate 875 mg PO bid *or* 2nd-Generation cephalosporin Except where noted, recommended treatment duration is 10-14 days;

Table 3 (continued)

Condition	Findings, associations*	Diagnosis	Treatment
Streptococcus pneumoniae (continued)			note that antimicrobial resistance is ever increasing, resistant strains should be treated with newer quinolones or vancomycin
Haemophilus influenzae	Common, acute onset, seen in all stages of HIV	Chest imaging shows bronchopneumonia, sputum Gram stain & culture	2nd-Generation cephalosporin *or* fluoroquinolone *or* macrolide (not erythromycin) *or* TMP-SMX DS 1 PO bid (note increasing incidence of resistance to TMP-SMX) Recommended treatment duration 10–14 days
Gram-negative rods	Acute onset, usually a nosocomial infection or with neutropenia, prolonged antimicrobial use or late-stage HIV (especially *Pseudomonas aeruginosa*)	Chest imaging shows lobar or bronchopneumonia; cavitary lesions; sputum Gram stain & culture	Appropriate antimicrobial coverage for specific organisms; adjust according to sensitivities; 3rd-generation cephalosporin with antipseudomonal coverage or 4th-generation cephalosporin or extended spectrum 4th-generation penicillin with antipseudomonal coverage
Staphylococcus aureus	Acute onset, uncommon cause, may be a superinfection in setting of influenza, may be seen in IV drug abusers (with septic emboli from endocarditis)	Chest imaging shows bronchopneumonia, multiple nodules, or cavitary lesions; blood cultures, sputum Gram stain & culture	Adjust coverage according to sensitivities, β-lactam antimicrobials for MSSA (nafcillin or 1st-generation cephalosporin), vancomycin for MRSA, recommended treatment duration 10–14 days

Table 3 (continued)

Condition	Findings, associations[=]	Diagnosis	Treatment
Nocardia	May be chronic or asymptomatic, uncommon infection, seen in late-stage HIV	Chest imaging may show nodules or cavitary lesions; sputum or bronchoscopy, Gram stain, modified AFB stain & culture	Sulfisoxazole 2 g PO q 6 hours *or* TMP-SMX 1 PO bid *or* Minocycline 200 mg PO bid Recommend treatment duration 6 months If patient has AIDS, lifelong treatment recommended
Legionella	Acute onset, consider diagnosis in patient in endemic region or in setting of epidemic (may be seen with exposure to contaminated environmental water sources)	Chest imaging shows bronchopneumonia in multiple, noncontiguous segments; culture on selective media; urinary *Legionella* antigen	Azithromycin 500 mg PO × 1 dose then 250 mg qd *or* Clarithromycin 500 mg PO bid *or* Levofloxacin 500 mg PO qd Recommended treatment duration 10-14 days based on clinical improvement
Aspiration	Subacute onset, suspect it in patients with depressed mental status, neurologic disorders, or poor oral control	Chest imaging shows patchy infiltrates without consolidation, usually involves dependent segments of lung (posterior segments of	β-Lactam or quinolone, include anaerobic coverage (clindamycin or metronidazole) if necessary; recommended treatment duration of 2-3 weeks depending on patient's condition & degree of aspiration

Table 3 (continued)

Condition	Findings, associations*	Diagnosis	Treatment
Aspiration (continued)		upper lobes, superior segments of lower lobes), may see necrosis & cavitation if infection is advanced	
Mycobacterium tuberculosis	May be chronic, subacute, or asymptomatic; marked increased risk in all stages of HIV; mean CD4 count 200–300; usually represents reactivation of prior infection rather than new exposure; extrapulmonary manifestations may be present	Chest imaging may show focal infiltrates, cavitary lesions, hilar adenopathy, reticular infiltrates, pleural effusions; the lower & middle lobes may be more commonly involved; perform multiple induced sputums and/or bronchoscopy; sputum AFB stain & culture, if sputum show AFB, must distinguish TB	Multidrug-resistant TB is a problem; perform sensitivities on all cultures; multiple regimens available—tailor according to patient's needs; patients from areas with multidrug-resistant TB need 4-drug regimen; isoniazid, rifampin, pyrazinamide, ethambutol are available drug options; rifabutin is alternative to rifampin; streptomycin-based therapy is available; check CDC Web site for detailed recommendations on treatment of TB in HIV (*http://www.cdc.gov/mmwr/PDF/rr/rr4720.pdf*); patients receiving HAART may need adjustment of dosing of rifampin & other TB medications or adjustment of dosing of HAART because of altered drug

Table 3 (continued)

Condition	Findings, associations*	Diagnosis	Treatment
Mycobacterium tuberculosis (continued)		from other mycobacteria; cultures provide definitive identification, but a more rapid identification may be obtained with DNA probes; if TB is suspected, treat accordingly until organism is identified	metabolism; for patients with drug-resistant strains of TB, consult an infectious diseases specialist
Mycobacterium avium complex	Chronic, uncommon cause, usually seen when CD4 count <50, important to note that MAC may be present as a colonizer only	Chest imaging findings may vary, sputum, bronchoscopy; AFB stain & culture	Clarithromycin 500 mg PO bid or Azithromycin 600 mg PO qd + ethambutol 15-25 mg/kg qd = rifabutin 300 mg PO qd. Treat indefinitely unless immune reconstitution occurs
Mycobacterium kansasii	Chronic or asymptomatic infection, uncommon, seen in late-stage HIV with CD4 counts <50	Chest imaging may show infiltrates, nodules, cysts, cavitary lesions; perform sputum analysis with AFB stain & culture	Isoniazid 300 mg PO qd + rifampin 600 mg PO qd + ethambutol 25 mg/kg qd × 2 months, then 15 mg/kg qd; treat for 15 months. All strains are resistant to pyrazinamide, recommend substituting rifabutin for rifampin if patient is on HAART

Table 3 (continued)

Condition	Findings, associations*	Diagnosis	Treatment
Pneumocystis carinii	Subacute or chronic, most common pulmonary infection in HIV, CD4 count <200, median CD4 counts with (without) prophylaxis are 30 (130), commonly seen in late-stage HIV	Chest imaging findings may vary: diffuse or perihilar infiltrates in 66%, atypical infiltrates in 30%, but chest X-ray is negative in 5%–10% of cases; apical infiltrates may be present in patients receiving aerosolized pentamidine Pneumothorax may occur; pleural effusions are uncommon; LDH elevated in 95% of cases but has a low specificity; low Po_2, low Sao_2, low diffusing capacity; perform induced sputum with Wright-Giemsa	Multiple alternative regimens available: 1. TMP-SMX DS 1 PO bid × 21 days; adverse reactions are common (rash, fever) 2. Clindamycin 300-450 mg q 6 hours + primaquine 15-30 mg base PO qd × 21 days 3. Atovaquone 750 mg PO bid with food × 21 days 4. Pentamidine 4 mg/kg qd IV × 21 days (usually reserved for severe cases of PCP) Patients with moderately severe to severe disease (i.e., Po_2 <70 mm Hg or A–a gradient >35 mm Hg) should be given course of steroids (prednisone 40 mg PO bid × 5 days, then 40 mg PO qd × 5 days, then 20 mg PO qd until treatment completed)

Table 3 (continued)

Condition	Findings, associations*	Diagnosis	Treatment
Pneumocystis carinii (continued)		stain or Calcoflour White; if negative for PCP & suspicion is still high, perform bronchoscopy (sensitivity ~95%)	
Cryptococcus	Chronic, subacute, or asymptomatic; fairly common; seen in late-stage HIV; CD4 <50; up to 80% of patients with cryptococcal pneumonia also have cryptococcal meningitis	Chest imaging shows nocules, cavitary lesions, or diffuse infiltrates; sputum or bronchoscopy; stain & culture; cryptococcal antigen titers in serum; cryptococcal antigen titers in bronchoalveolar lavage fluid with titer ≥1:8 indicating infection; LP should be performed to evaluate for coexisting meningitis	Treat disseminated cryptococcosis with meningeal involvement with amphotericin B 0.7–1.0 mg/kg qd IV + flucytosine 100 mg/kg qd × 14 days PO, then fluconazole 400–800 mg qd × 10 weeks, then maintenance therapy with fluconazole 200 mg PO qd indefinitely Treat disseminated cryptococcosis without meningeal involvement with fluconazole 200–400 mg PO qd indefinitely See IDSA Web site (*http://www.journals.uchicago.edu/IDSA/guidelines/*) for treating cryptococcosis in HIV

Table 3 (continued)

Condition	Findings, associations*	Diagnosis	Treatment
Histoplasma capsulatum	Subacute or chronic, consider in patients living in an endemic area (Mississippi and Ohio river valleys), advanced HIV, CD4 <50, disease may be disseminated at diagnosis	Chest imaging shows various lesions (diffuse or nodular infiltrates, nodules, focal infiltrates, cavities, hilar adenopathy), perform sputum analysis or bronchoscopy, stains & cultures, stains & cultures of bone marrow if suspicion warrants, serum or urine antigen may be positive in 80%-90% of patients	Treat disseminated histoplasmosis with amphotericin B 0.7-1.0 mg/kg qd IV × 14 days, followed by maintenance therapy & lifelong suppression with itraconazole See IDSA Web site (*http://www.journals.uchicago.edu/IDSA/guidelines/*) for treating histoplasmosis in HIV
Coccidioides immitis	Subacute or chronic, consider in patients living in endemic region (Southwestern U.S.), CD4 count <50	Chest imaging shows various lesions (diffuse or nodular infiltrates, nodules, focal infiltrates, cavities, hilar adenopathy), perform	Treat diffuse pneumonia with amphotericin B until clear clinical improvement, then treat with fluconazole indefinitely Treat disseminated extrapulmonary coccidioidomycosis with/without meningitis with fluconazole 400 mg qd

Table 3 (continued)

Condition	Findings, associations*	Diagnosis	Treatment
Coccidioides immitis (continued)		sputum analysis or bronchoscopy, stains & cultures, *Coccidioides* serology	See the IDSA Web site (*http://www.journals.uchicago.edu/IDSA/guidelines/*) for treating coccidioidomycosis in HIV
Candida	Chronic or subacute, may cause bronchitis, *Candida* is frequently isolated from respiratory secretions but rarely causes the illness, CD4 <50	Chest imaging rarely shows infiltrate, diagnosis requires demonstrating the organisms in biopsy specimen, sputum analysis is not useful in diagnosis	Fluconazole, amphotericin B See the IDSA Web site (*http://www.journals.uchicago.edu/IDSA/guidelines/*) for treating candidiasis in HIV
Aspergillus	Acute or subacute illness, predisposing factors include neutropenia with absolute neutrophil count <500 & corticosteroids, may be seen in advanced HIV	Chest imaging may show focal infiltrates, cavitary lesions; lesions seen on chest X-ray or CT can be highly suggestive of diagnosis; sputum stains & cultures may be associated with high rate of	Amphotericin B, itraconazole, caspofungin may be used in refractory cases See the IDSA Web site (*http://www.journals.uchicago.edu/IDSA/guidelines/*) for treating aspergillosis in HIV

Table 3 (continued)

Condition	Findings, associations*	Diagnosis	Treatment
Aspergillus (continued)		false-negatives and false-positives; most reliable diagnosis is with biopsy showing invasion	
CMV	Subacute or chronic, CMV is frequently isolated from respiratory secretions but is uncommon cause of pulmonary disease, CMV pneumonia may occur in advanced HIV, CD4 <20	Chest imaging may show interstitial infiltrates, most reliable diagnosis is biopsy showing CMV inclusions	Ganciclovir or oral valganciclovir
Influenza	Acute illness; common cause of respiratory infection (upper respiratory tract infection, pharyngitis, bronchitis) but pneumonia is not common unless due to bacterial super-infection, may occur with any stage of HIV	Influenza culture or rapid stain of respiratory secretions	Within first 48 hours of illness, consider zanamivir (ramantadine or amantadine if influenza A only); treat any superinfection according to cause

Table 3 (continued)

Condition	Findings, associations*	Diagnosis	Treatment
Varicella	Acute, varicella pneumonia usually follows cutaneous exanthem within 1-7 days	Chest imaging may show interstitial infiltrates with peribronchiolar distribution; cytology, biopsy, or culture of respiratory secretions/tissue may show VZV as intranuclear inclusions & multinucleated giant cells	Acyclovir
Kaposi sarcoma	Chronic or asymptomatic	Chest imaging may show interstitial, alveolar, or nodular infiltrates, hilar adenopathy, pleural effusions; bronchoscopy may yield endobronchial lesion, but yields of parenchymal lesions may be as low as 10%-30%	Chemotherapy for systemic disease, radiotherapy

Table 3 (continued)

Condition	Findings, associations*	Diagnosis	Treatment
Lymphoma	Chronic or asymptomatic, un-common cause of pneumonia	Chest imaging may show various lesions (interstitial, alveolar, nodular infiltrates, cavitary lesions, pleural effusions, hilar adenopathy); perform bronchoscopy with transbronchial biopsy; VATS or open lung biopsy if needed; biopsy of extrapulmonary sites	Chemotherapy
Lymphocytic interstitial pneumonia	Subacute or chronic, CD4 <200 commonly	Chest imaging shows diffuse reticular or focal infiltrates; bronchoscopy with biopsy may give diagnosis 30%–50% of time, but may need to perform VATS or open lung biopsy	HAART, prednisone

Table 3 (continued)

Condition	Findings, associations*	Diagnosis	Treatment
Nonspecific interstitial pneumonia	Subacute or chronic	No specific radiologic findings. biopsy shows diffuse alveolar damage with interstitial inflammatory infiltrate consisting of macrophages & lymphocytes	HAART, prednisone
GI disorders Diarrhea			
Salmonella	Gastroenteritis or enteric fever	Blood & stool cultures, may have fecal WBCs	Ciprofloxacin 500-750 mg PO bid × 14 days *or* TMP-SMX DS 1-2 PO bid × 14 days
Shigella	Dysentery, fever. colitis	Stool cultures, fecal WBCs	Ciprofloxacin 500 mg PO bid × 3 days *or* TMP-SMX DS 1 PO bid × 3 days
Campylobacter jejuni	Watery stools or dysentery, may be associated with fever. colitis	Blood & stool cultures, may have fecal WBCs	Ciprofloxacin 500 mg PO bid × 3-5 days *or* Azithromycin 500 mg PO qd × 3-5 days

Table 3 (continued)

Condition	Findings, associations*	Diagnosis	Treatment
Clostridium difficile	Watery stools, fever, leukocytosis, colitis, almost always associated with antimicrobial use (cephalosporins, clindamycin, ampicillin)	*C. difficile* toxin assay, may have fecal WBCs	Metronidazole 500 mg PO tid × 10-14 days *or* Vancomycin 125 mg PO qid × 10-14 days
Small-bowel overgrowth	Watery stools, malabsorption, afebrile	Small-bowel aspirate for quantitative culture, hydrogen breath test, no fecal WBCs	Doxycycline *or* metronidazole *or* amoxicillin-clavulanate
MAC	Watery stools; enteritis; commonly associated with MAC bacteremia & fever, abdominal pain; CD4 <50	Small-bowel biopsy with AFB stain/culture	Clarithromycin 500 mg PO bid + ethambutol 15 mg/kg qd ± rifabutin 300 mg/day
Cryptosporidia	Enteritis, profuse watery stools, commonly afebrile, CD4 <200	Stool-modified AFB stain shows oocytes, no fecal WBCs	No treatment is consistently effective, paromomycin may be helpful, treat symptomatically, octreotide may be useful
Isospora	Watery stools, enteritis, usually afebrile, CD4 <100	Stool AFB, no fecal WBCs	TMP-SMX DS 1 PO qid × 10 days, then bid × 3 weeks *or* Pyrimethamine 50-75 mg PO qd + folinic acid 10 mg qd × 14 days

Table 3 (continued)

Condition	Findings, associations*	Diagnosis	Treatment
Microsporidia	Watery stools, enteritis, usually afebrile, CD4 <50	Stool trichrome stain, electron microscopy or Giemsa stain of small-bowel biopsy	Albedazole 400–800 mg PO bid for at least 3 weeks, best results if combined with HAART
Giardia	Watery diarrhea, may be associated with malabsorption, afebrile, enteritis, bloating, flatulence, especially seen in travelers & homosexual men	Stool ova & parasite studies, Giardia antigen assay	Metronidazole 250 mg PO tid × 5 days *or* Albendazole 400 mg PO qd × 5 days
Entamoeba histolytica	If symptomatic, may have bloody diarrhea, fever, & colitis; asymptomatic carriage common, particularly in homosexual men; may be more frequent in travelers & homosexual men	Stool ova & parasite studies, yield of studies may vary with technical expertise; fecal RBCs; endoscopy with biopsy; elevated IFA titer	Metronidazole 750 mg PO tid × 10 days, followed by paromomycin 500 mg PO tid × 7 days *or* Iodoquinol 650 mg PO tid × 20 days
Cyclospora cayetanensis	Watery diarrhea	Circular organisms seen on AFB staining	TMP-SMX DS 1 PO qid × 10 days, then 1 PO 3×/week

Table 3 (continued)

Condition	Findings, associations*	Diagnosis	Treatment
CMV	Seen in disseminated CMV, fever, abdominal pain, colitis, enteritis, may be complicated by colonic perforation or GI bleed, CD4 <50	Flexible sigmoidoscopy or colonoscopy with intestinal biopsy showing CMV inclusions	Ganciclovir
Enteric viruses	Watery stools, enteritis	Most common causes are adenovirus, calciviruses, picorna-virus, astrovirus	Symptomatic
Idiopathic	Watery stools, wasting, protein-losing enteropathy	No pathogens identi-fied, small-bowel biopsy may show villous atrophy	Symptomatic, TPN if needed
Liver disease	May present with nausea, vomiting, RUQ pain, elevated aminotransferases & alkaline phosphatase	Ultrasound, CT, liver biopsy if needed	Tailor treatment to cause of disorder

Table 3 (continued)

Condition	Findings, associations*	Diagnosis	Treatment
Biliary disease			
Cholangiopathy	May present with nausea vomiting, RUQ pain, markedly elevated alkaline phosphatase compared to aminotransferases	Ultrasound shows dilated ducts, ERCP shows "pruning" of terminal ducts & irregularities of proximal intrahepatic ducts, stenosis of distal common bile duct	Sphincterotomy may help, but symptoms frequently recur; endoscopic stenting
Oral disease			
Thrush (*Candida*)	White plaques that are easily scraped off; may present as erythematous, friable lesion; dry mouth, bad taste in mouth	Usually clinical diagnosis; KOH shows yeast & pseudohyphae	Clotrimazole PO troches *or* nystatin *or* fluconazole PO until lesions resolve
			Thrush frequently relapses in absence of immune reconstitution, but concern about maintenance therapy is development of azole-resistant strains of *Candida*
Oral hairy leukoplakia	Usually asymptomatic; well-demarcated verrucous plaque	Usually clinical diagnosis, does not rub off,	Acyclovir, frequently recurs if not on maintenance therapy with

Table 3 (continued)

Condition	Findings, associations*	Diagnosis	Treatment
Oral hairy leukoplakia (continued)	with white hair-like projections on lateral or inferior aspect of tongue; associated with Epstein-Barr virus	does not respond to anticandidal therapy	high-dose acyclovir Topical podophyllin 25%
Aphthous ulcers	Painful ulcerations on mucosa	Exclusion of HSV, CMV, VZV as cause	Mile's solution (hydrocortisone, nystatin, tetracycline, viscous lidocaine mixture), dexamethasone solution, topical fluocinonide with orabase, thalidomide is experimental, prednisone may be used for severe cases
HSV	Small, painful vesicles on erythematous base	May be clinical diagnosis in patients with history of similar lesions, Tzanck smear shows multinucleate giant cells & intranuclear inclusions	Acyclovir or famciclovir or valacyclovir
Kaposi sarcoma	Purple, red, black, or brown firm nodules, especially on hard palate	Biopsy may be needed	Local therapy (laser, chemotherapy, radiotherapy), systemic chemotherapy for extensive disease

Table 3 (continued)

Condition	Findings, associations*	Diagnosis	Treatment
Gingivitis/ periodontitis	Painful bleeding gums, cratered ulcers, red marginal gum line, necrosis of interdental papillae, due to bacterial overgrowth		May require professional cleaning & debridement; topical antiseptic mouth rinses; severe cases may require antimicrobials (metronidazole or clindamycin) to cover anaerobes
Esophageal disease	Usually presents as dysphagia, odynophagia, chest pain		
Candida	Usually (not invariably) associated with thrush; afebrile, CD4 <100, white plaques	Usually clinical diagnosis; endoscopy shows typical white plaques, with microscopic exam showing yeast. In patient with esophageal pain, it is reasonable to treat empirically for Candida and evaluate further if no improvement	Fluconazole

Table 3 (continued)

Condition	Findings, associations*	Diagnosis	Treatment
CMV	Often febrile; localized, severe pain; CD4 <100; ulcerative lesions	Endoscopy shows ulcerations, biopsy shows CMV inclusions	Ganciclovir
HSV	Afebrile, focal pain, vesicles on erythematous base, patients often have coexisting vesicles in the oral cavity, CD4 <100	Endoscopy shows small, confluent ulcerations; biopsy shows HSV inclusions	Acyclovir *or* valacyclovir *or* famciclovir
Aphthous ulcers	Afebrile, localized pain	Endoscopy, no evidence of other pathogens	Prednisone taper, thalidomide (experimental)
CNS disorders			
Toxoplasmosis	Headache, focal neurologic signs, fever, lethargy, seizures, mental status changes, CD4 usually <200	Characteristic contrast-enhancing lesions on CT, with nodular or ring-enhancing structure with mass effect; usually multiple lesions; MRI may be more sensitive than CT for detecting toxoplasmosis; a positive serum toxoplasmosis titer may	Pyrimethamine, folate, & sulfadiazine; should see response within 1 week (clinically) & 2 weeks (radiographically); if not, consider other diagnoses Patients require life-long suppressive therapy with pyrimethamine, folate, & sulfadiazine Control cerebral edema with dexamethasone

Table 3 (continued)

Condition	Findings, associations*	Diagnosis	Treatment
Toxoplasmosis (continued)		be found in absence of disease, thus cannot be used in diagnosis; toxoplasmosis serology may be negative in up to 15% of patients with disease	
Primary CNS lymphoma	Headache, focal neurologic deficits, seizures, mental status changes usually occurs with CD4 <100	CT or MRI shows single or multiple contrast-enhancing lesions; may be difficult to distinguish from toxoplasmosis based on imaging & symptoms alone; definitive diagnosis for focal brain lesions may need stereotactic biopsy; PCR for Epstein-Barr virus in CSF may help make diagnosis	Radiotherapy may improve neurologic outcome, quality of life, & survival

Table 3 (continued)

Condition	Findings, associations*	Diagnosis	Treatment
Non-Hodgkin lymphoma	Metastatic lymphoma to brain; may present with mental status changes, cranial neuropathies, spinal root lesions; more than 70% of cases in HIV patients tend to be extranodal & fairly aggressive tumors	Repeated LP for CSF analysis, including cytology; bone marrow biopsy; CT of chest, abdomen, pelvis, head	Systemic chemotherapy (CHOP or MBACOD) For CNS involvement, therapy may include cranial irradiation or intrathecal chemotherapy
Progressive multifocal leukoencephalopathy	Due to the JC virus; infection of white matter; may present as altered mental status, speech, visual & gait disturbances, hemiparesis, cortical blindness, incoordination; aphasia; usually in advanced HIV; CD4 <200	CT may show single or multiple confluent, hypodense, nonenhancing lesions, primarily in parieto-occipital white matter without mass effect MRI may be superior to CT Definitive diagnosis requires biopsy PCR for JC virus may have false-negative rate of up to 40%-50%	HAART, cidofovir (currently experimental)

Table 3 (continued)

Condition	Findings, associations*	Diagnosis	Treatment
Cryptococcal meningitis	Due to *Cryptococcus neoformans*; CD4 usually <100; classic signs of meningitis (photophobia & neck stiffness) are often absent; presentation may include malaise, fever, nausea, vomiting, headache; less commonly patient may have cranial nerve palsies, psychiatric disorder, speech abnormalities, & seizures	CSF India ink stain; CSF cryptococcal antigen titer >1:8; CSF culture positive for *Cryptococcus*; opening pressure should be recorded when performing LP; usually no focal lesions on CT; positive cryptococcal antigen titer may be noted in blood in >90% of cases	Treat disseminated cryptococcosis with meningeal involvement with amphotericin B 0.7-1.0 mg/kg IV qd + flucytosine 100 mg/kg qd × 14 days PO, then fluconazole 400-800 mg qd × 10 weeks, then maintenance therapy with fluconazole 200 mg PO qd indefinitely CSF, not serum, cryptococcal antigen titers may be useful for monitoring response to treatment; unfavorable prognostic factors include elevated opening pressure, altered mental status, elevated CSF cryptococcal antigen titer, low CSF WBC count See the IDSA Web site (*http://www.journals.uchicago.edu/IDSA/guidelines*) for treating cryptococcosis in HIV

Table 3 (continued)

Condition	Findings, associations*	Diagnosis	Treatment
CMV encephalitis	Usually seen with CD4 <50; often associated with CMV involvement of other organ systems, including adrenals (which may present as hyponatremia); presentation is characterized by fairly abrupt onset of mental status changes, patient may be afebrile	CT shows hydrocephalus & periventricular or meningeal enhancement, perform ophthalmoscopy to evaluate for retinitis, CMV PCR of CSF	Ganciclovir Prognosis of CMV encephalitis is poor, therapy not shown to improve survival
HSV encephalitis	HSV frequently affects temporal lobe orbitofrontal cortex & limbic structures; may present with fever, focal neurologic symptoms (especially referable to temporal lobe), focal seizures (especially of temporal lobe), depressed consciousness, personality changes, altered mental status	Most sensitive test is detection of HSV DNA in CSF by PCR (may be negative during first 24-48 hours after infection); MRI of head (T_2-weighted) may show high-intensity signal lesions in temporal lobe CSF with high opening pressure & mild-to-moderate	Acyclovir or foscarnet or valacyclovir

Table 3 (continued)

Condition	Findings, associations*	Diagnosis	Treatment
HSV encephalitis (continued)		increase in protein & lymphocyte predominance & normal or mildly decreased glucose; CSF viral cultures nearly always negative Diagnosis may also be based on detection of HSV antigen, HSV DNA, or HSV replication in brain biopsy tissue (brain biopsy usually not needed for diagnosis)	
VZV encephalitis	May occur with/without recent history of characteristic vesicular rash; depressed consciousness, headache, vomiting, altered mental status, fever, seizures	Lymphocyte predominance in CSF; VZV antibody detected by indirect immunofluorescence in CSF in titer of 1:2; detection of VZV DNA in CSF	Acyclovir or foscarnet (preferred treatment for acyclovir-resistant VZV) or cidofovir

Table 3 (continued)

Condition	Findings, associations*	Diagnosis	Treatment
VZV encephalitis (continued)		by PCR; radiologic evidence of multifocal ischemic & hemorrhagic infarctions of white matter > gray matter, often at the gray-white matter junction	
Neurosyphilis	Due to *Treponema pallidum*; presentation may vary, including asymptomatic infection, meningitis, tabes dorsalis, general paresis, meningovascular disease, ocular disease	Positive CSF VDRL is diagnostic (but sensitivity of 30%–70%), CSF may show increased protein & pleocytosis	If patient with positive serum VDRL, symptoms consistent with neurosyphilis, & CSF profile compatible with *Treponema* infection, treat presumptively for neurosyphilis even if CSF VDRL is negative
Treatment is aqueous penicillin G 12-24 million units qd × 10 days; serum & CSF VDRL levels & CSF fluid analysis should be followed serially 1-2 years
AIDS dementia complex	May occur with CD4 <100; patient is generally alert & afebrile; symptoms/signs may include forgetfulness, difficulty concentrating,	Neuropsychiatric testing may show cognitive dysfunction; no imaging studies are specific for AIDS dementia (may show	High-dose zidovudine is effective; calcium channel blockers are being investigated

Table 3 (continued)

Condition	Findings, associations*	Diagnosis	Treatment
AIDS dementia complex (continued)	loss of balance, leg weakness, slowed mentation, social withdrawal; seizures, incontinence, tremor, & paraparesis may occur with advanced dementia	cerebral atrophy, ventricular enlargement, white matter changes); it is diagnosis of exclusion; perform imaging & LP to evaluate other causes of neurologic change; presence of β_2-microglobulin, neopterin, & quinolinate in CSF may correlate with presence of AIDS dementia complex.	
TB	May present as altered mental status, fever, cranial nerve palsies (TB has predilection for skull base)	CT may show intracerebral enhancing lesions (tuberculoma; abscess, tuberculomas in 50%-70% of cases, brain biopsy may be needed	See the CDC Web site (*http://www.cdc.gov/mmwr/PDF/rr/rr4720.pdf*) for treating TB in HIV

Table 3 (continued)

Condition	Findings, associations*	Diagnosis	Treatment
TB (continued)		to idenfity the mass; obtain chest X-ray, positive TB culture from any site suggests the diagnosis, CSF culture may be positive in 20% of cases	
HIV meningitis	Common in early HIV infection, may present with fever & headache	No focal abnormalities on CT, CSF has a mild mononuclear pleocytosis (<200 cells/mm³) & elevated protein; all cultures are negative for other pathogens Note: HIV is associated with mild mononuclear pleocytosis (<100 cells/mm³) with/without elevated protein even in absence of neurologic symptoms; this may confound interpretation of CSF results in HIV patients	HAART

Table 3 (continued)

Condition	Findings, associations*	Diagnosis	Treatment
HIV myelopathy	Slowly progressive gait disturbance, sensory changes in lower extremities, sphincter dysfunction, hyperreflexia, spastic paraparesis Causes of myelopathy may include vacuolar myelopathy (most common cause in AIDS patients), toxoplasmosis, lymphoma, VZV, HSV, CMV, vitamin B$_{12}$ deficiency	MRI or CT of spinal cord & LP to evaluate for potentially treatable causes of myelopathy	No effective treatment for AIDS-associated vacuolar myelopathy; symptomatic relief may be achieved with antispasticity agents & physical therapy
Retinitis	May be due to CMV or HIV (less commonly, HSV, syphilis, fungal infections, herpes zoster, toxoplasmosis); with CMV retinitis, patients usually asymptomatic until lesions involve fovea, optic nerve, or cause retinal detachment; patients may complain	Ophthalmoscopy may show cotton-wool spots without associated hemorrhage or exudate in HIV retinitis (lesions may remit spontaneously & are benign); may show perivascular hemorrhage & fluffy	IV foscarnet or IV ganciclovir or IV cidofovir; life-long maintenance therapy with foscarnet, ganciclovir, or cidofovir is recommended for patients without immune reconstitution; ganciclovir implants are an option but provide no protection against systemic CMV & no protection for uninvolved eye

Table 3 (continued)

Condition	Findings, associations*	Diagnosis	Treatment
Retinitis (continued)	of floaters, blurry vision, visual field deficits; CMV retinitis not generally associated with pain or light sensitivity	exudates, opaque retinal lesions	
PNS disorders			
Inflammatory demyelinating polyneuropathies	May be acute or chronic; tend to occur early in HIV; acute illness resembles Guillain-Barré syndrome; patients may present with progressive weakness, areflexia, sensory signs; thought to be autoimmune-related process	Mild mononuclear pleo-cytosis & elevated protein in CSF (nonspecific finding in HIV), EMG may show demyelination & axon loss	Variable clinical course, but most patients improve; may respond to corticosteroids, plasmapheresis, IV immunoglobulin
Distal symmetric polyneuropathy	Most common polyneuropathy in HIV, incidence increases with advanced HIV; cause not known; may present with symmetric paresthesias, pain, numbness, dysesthesia of	Must rule out other causes of distal symmetric poly-neuropathy, including vitamin B_6 & B_{12} deficiencies, diabetes, alcoholism, medications	Treatment is symptomatic relief with tricyclic antidepressants, anticonvulsants, analgesics, or topical capsaicin; antiretro-viral therapy has no efficacy If medication is suspected cause, a drug holiday may benefit

Table 3 (continued)

Condition	Findings, associations*	Diagnosis	Treatment
Distal symmetric polyneuropathy (continued)	feet; decreased or absent ankle reflexes; decreased sensation to pain & vibration in lower limbs; upper limb involvement less common & may occur later in disease	(vincristine, ddI, ddC, d4T); EMG may show predominant axonal loss with demyelination	
Progressive polyradiculopathy	Likely due to CMV infection of nerve roots; findings include lower limb & sacral paresthesias or pain, rapidly progressive flaccid paralysis, areflexia, sphincter disturbances, urinary retention, sensory loss; less common causes are neurosyphilis, leptomeningeal lymphoma, TB	CSF shows marked pleocytosis with predominance of PMNs; CMV identified in culture in ~50% of cases	Ganciclovir or foscarnet; it is important to treat early in disease course to prevent irreversible nerve root damage
Mononeuropathy multiplex	Sensory & motor deficits in distribution of multiple spinal, peripheral, cranial nerves (may include facial or	Nonspecific CSF findings (pleocytosis, elevated protein); EMG may show axonal	

595

Table 3 (continued)

Condition	Findings, associations*	Diagnosis	Treatment
Mononeuropathy multiplex (continued)	laryngeal palsy, wrist or foot drop); symptoms may resolve spontaneously in early HIV but progress rapidly to quadraparesis in late HIV, especially if CD4 <50	neuropathy; sometimes nerve biopsy shows necrosis	
Myopathy	Most common causes are presumed direct HIV-virally-induced myopathy (may occur at all stages of disease) & zidovudine-associated myopathy; may present with proximal muscle weakness (especially thighs), myalgia, weight loss	HIV-associated myopathy: mild to moderate CK elevation, myopathic EMG abnormalities, up to 50% may have nerve conduction abnormalities Zidovudine-associated myopathy: muscle tenderness & weakness may be preceded by increased CK; muscle biopsy may show ragged-red fibers (mitochondrial dysfunction)	HIV-associated myopathy may respond to corticosteroids Zidovudine-associated myopathy may, but not always, respond to drug withdrawal

Table 3 (continued)

Condition	Findings, associations*	Diagnosis	Treatment
Dermatologic disorders			
Eosinophilic folliculitis	Idiopathic, pruritic, edematous follicular papules & pustules usually on trunk or face; seen in advanced HIV; CD4 <100–200	Biopsy shows perifollicular & perivascular infiltrates with eosinophils no evidence of other pathogenic organisms, may be associated with peripheral eosinophilia	Antihistamines, topical corticosteroids, or permethrin cream; prednisone may resolve folliculitis but recurrence is common after treatment cessation; isotretinoin
Kaposi sarcoma	Multisystem vascular neoplasia; human herpesvirus 8 is implicated; may present as violaceous, red, pink, brown, or black macules, papules, plaques, or nodules; lesions may have greenish hemosiderin halo; Kaposi sarcoma may cause bulky lymphedema; distribution is widespread, including oral lesions, common on hard palate	Skin biopsy needed for diagnosis; may be confused with bacillary angiomatosis; approximately 40% of patients with dermatologic Kaposi sarcoma develop visceral disease (GI, pulmonary)	May respond to local therapy (radiotherapy, cryosurgery, laser surgery); intralesional chemotherapy with vincristine and/or bleomycin; systemic chemotherapy for extensive mucocutaneous disease with visceral involvement

Table 3 (continued)

Condition	Findings, associations*	Diagnosis	Treatment
Bacillary angiomatosis	Due to *Bartonella henselae* or *B. quintana*; usually seen in more advanced HIV, CD4 <200; red or violaceous, firm papules or nodules; may resemble Kaposi sarcoma; infection may spread hematologically & involve liver (peliosis hepatis) or spleen (parenchymal bacillary peliosis)	Biopsy showing *Bartonella* on silver stain	Avoid contact with cats; treat with erythromycin *or* doxycycline *or* ciprofloxacin *or* azithromycin; may benefit from maintenance therapy if relapse occurs
Herpes simplex virus	Grouped vesicles or erosions on erythematous base; painful; may be oral, genital, perirectal or generalized disease; with increasing immunocompromise, lesions may be more severe with marked ulceration & erosions	Diagnosis based on clinical appearance & possible history of recurring lesions; Tzanck smear, cultures, antigen detection, or PCR shows HSV	Acyclovir; if no response, may require higher doses of acyclovir or foscarnet (if acyclovir-resistant strain suspected)

Table 3 (continued)

Condition	Findings, associations*	Diagnosis	Treatment
Herpes zoster	Vesicles on erythematous base may progress to crusting lesions; usually has dermatomal distribution; painful; disseminated disease in some patients	Usually based on clinical findings; Tzanck smear shows giant & multinucleated cells (as in HSV); antigen detection; VZV serology shows rising titers; viral culture (difficult)	Acyclovir PO or IV depending on disease severity
Molluscum contagiosum	Viral infection; pearly white or skin-colored, round or oval umbilicated papules or nodules; hundreds of lesions usually asymptomatic; may occur in HIV patients; may be on face, neck, trunk, or anogenital regions; severity may increase with increasing immunodeficiency	Usually clinical diagnosis; may require biopsy to distinguish from other nodular lesions	Curettage, cryosurgery, electrodessication, or laser ablation

Table 3 (continued)

Condition	Findings, associations*	Diagnosis	Treatment
Staphylococcus aureus	Most common cutaneous bacterial infection in HIV; may present as folliculitis, furuncles, carbuncles; lesions may be pruritic; localized infection may progress to bacteremia or disseminated infection	Gram-positive cocci on microscopy; culture positive for *S. aureus*	Dicloxacillin *or* cephalexin *or* other penicillinase-resistant antistaphylococcal agents
Human papillomavirus	Warts may range from papules to cauliflower-like masses on anogenital or oral mucosa or skin; lesions may be extensive, difficult to treat in advanced HIV; associated with squamous cell carcinoma of cervix, penis, vulva, perineum, anus	Usually clinical diagnosis, biopsy if necessary	Cryosurgery, podofilox, podophyllin, trichloroacetic acid, electrodessication
Dermatophytosis	Causes include *Trichophyton, Microsporum, Epidermophyton;* infection may be extensive,	Microscopy, KOH preparation, Wood lamp, fungal cultures	Topical or systemic antifungal agents

Table 3 (continued)

Condition	Findings, associations*	Diagnosis	Treatment
Dermatophytosis (continued)	difficult to treat in HIV; proximal white subungual onychomycosis is common presentation of *T. rubrum* tinea unguium in HIV		
Drug reactions	Rashes may be erythematous, papular, or pruritic; less common are urticaria, erythema multiforme, photosensitivity; common offending drugs are TMP-SMX, dapsone, nevirapine, delaviridine, efavirenz	Diagnosis confirmed by resolution of rash after offending drug discontinued	Discontinue offending drug
Syphilis	Primary: painless chancre usually in genital region Secondary: pink macules or pink or brown-red papules; condyloma lata in moist body regions; may have papulo-squamous lesions	Dark field exam, direct fluorescent antibody test, serologic testing for VDRL, rapid plasma reagin, FTA-ABS	Penicillin

Table 3 (continued)

Condition	Findings, associations*	Diagnosis	Treatment
Syphilis (continued)	Tertiary: brown, firm plaques & nodules with/without scales or ulceration; gumma—rubbery lump that may ulcerate		
Histoplasmosis	Erythematous, necrotic or hyperkeratotic papules or nodules; macules; folliculitis; pustules; ulcers; lesions may be widely distributed; mucous membranes are commonly involved; disseminated disease may be associated with lymphadenopathy & hepatosplenomegaly	Biopsy shows *Histoplasma capsulatum*; culture	Treat disseminated disease with amphotericin B 0.7-1.0 mg/kg IV qd × 14 days, followed by maintenance therapy & life-long suppression with itraconazole See the IDSA Web site (*http://www.journals.uchicago.edu/IDSA/guidelines/*) for treating histoplasmosis in HIV
Cryptococcosis	Papules or nodules; may resemble molluscum contagiosum; may also present as vesicles, pustules, cellulites, ulcers; lesions usually on face & scalp in HIV	Skin biopsy, cultures	Treat disseminated disease *with* meningeal involvement with amphotericin B 0.7-1.0 mg/kg IV qd + flucytosine 100 mg/kg PO qd × 14 days, then fluconazole 400-800 mg qd × 10 weeks, then maintenance therapy with fluconazole 200 mg PO qd indefinitely

Table 3 (continued)

Condition	Findings, associations*	Diagnosis	Treatment
Cryptococcosis (continued)			Treat disseminated disease *without* meningeal involvement with fluconazole 200–400 mg PO qd indefinitely
Coccidioidomycosis	May initially present as papule with evolution to pustules, plaques, nodules, ulcers, abscesses; usually involves central face (especially nasolabial folds)	Detection of *Coccidioides immitis* in skin biopsy	Treat disseminated extrapulmonary coccidioidomycosis with/without meningitis with fluconazole 400 mg qd See the IDSA Web site (*http://www.journals.uchicago.edu/IDSA/guidelines/*) for treating coccidioidomycosis in HIV
Blastomycosis	Initial lesion may be inflammatory nodule that grows & ulcerates; SQ nodule; pustules; verrucous, crusted plaques with well-demarcated borders	Microscopy; detection of *Blastomyces* antigen or antibody; culture	Treat with amphotericin B 0.7–1.0 mg/kg IV qd for total dose of 1.5–2.5 g, continue suppressive therapy with itraconazole 200–400 mg qd, consider fluconazole 800 mg/day for suppression if CNS disease present

Table 3 (continued)

Condition	Findings, associations*	Diagnosis	Treatment
Blastomycosis (continued)			See the IDSA Web site (*http://www.journals. uchicago.edu/IDSA/guidelines/*) for treating blastomycosis in HIV
Psoriasis	Well-demarcated plaques with silvery scale, propensity for extensor surfaces, may be associated with nail pitting or arthritis	Usually clinical diagnosis	Topical corticosteroids; phototherapy (may be poorly tolerated due to photosensitivity of some HIV patients); retinoids; tar preparations
Seborrheic dermatitis	May vary from fine white scales without erythema to plaques & patches of erythema with yellow, greasy scale; may be found on scalp, face, chest, upper back; pruritis	Usually clinical diagnosis	Topical corticosteroids; UV radiation; ketoconazole cream or shampoo

AFB, acid-fast bacillus; bid, twice daily; CNS, central nervous system; CMV, cytomegalovirus; ddC, zalcitabine; ddI, didanosine; d4T, stavudine; ERCP, endoscopic retrograde cholangiopancreatography; GI, gastrointestinal; HAART, highly active antiretroviral therapy; HSV, herpes simplex virus; IDSA, Infectious Diseases Society of America; IFA, immunofluorescent antibody; LP, lumbar puncture; MAC, *Mycobacterium avium* complex; MRSA, methicillin-resistant *Staphylococcus aureus*; MSSA, methicillin-sensitive *Staphylococcus aureus*; PCP, *Pneumocystis carinii* pneumonia; PCR, polymerase chain reaction; PNS, peripheral nervous system; q, every; qd, daily; qid, four times daily; RUQ, right upper quadrant; tid, three times daily; TMP-SMX, trimethoprim-sulfamethoxazole; TPN, total parenteral nutrition; VATS, video-assisted thoracic surgery; VZV, varicella-zoster virus.

*CD4 counts are cells/mm^3.

Table 4. Prophylaxis for Opportunistic Infections

Disease	Indications	Regimen	Comments
TB	Positive PPD (≥5 mm induration), history of prior positive PPD without INH prophylaxis, high-risk exposure	INH 300 mg qd with pyridoxine 50 mg qd for 9 months	
Pneumocystis carinii pneumonia	Prior bout; CD4 <200 cells/mm³; thrush; FUO	TMP-SMX 1 DS qd or 1 DS 3×/week or one SS qd *or* Dapsone 200 mg PO qd *or* Aerosolized pentamidine 300 mg q 3 weeks	May be discontinued if immunologic reconstitution is achieved, with CD4 >200 cells/mm³ for 3-6 months
Toxoplasmosis	CD4 <100 cells/mm³ with presence of IgG	TMP-SMX 1 DS qd	May be discontinued if immunologic reconstitution is achieved, with CD4 >100 cells/mm³ for 3-6 months
Mycobacterium avium complex	CD4 <50 cells/mm³	Azithromycin 1,200 mg weekly or clarithromycin 500 mg bid	May be discontinued if immunologic reconstitution is achieved, with a CD4 >100 cells/mm³ for 3-6 months

Table 4 (continued)

Disease	Indications	Regimen	Comments
Varicella	Exposure to chickenpox or zoster in person with no history of either or negative VZV antibody	Varicella-zoster immuno-globulin 625 units IM given within 96 hours of exposure	
Streptococcus pneumoniae	All patients	Pneumococcal vaccine	May have a suboptimal response in patients with CD4 <200 cells/mm³
Influenza	All patients	Influenza vaccine	No definitive evidence supporting its utility; has been associated with a transient elevation in HIV viral load in patients with CD4 <200 cells/mm³
Hepatitis A	For patients with antibody to HCV, test for HAV; if anti-HAV negative, administer HAV vaccine	HAV vaccine × 2 doses	
Hepatitis B	All negative anti-HBs & anti-HBc patients	HBV vaccine × 3 doses	May require booster dose if no response to initial 3 doses
CMV			Prophylaxis not generally recommended; no clear guidelines or proven efficacy; concern over promotion of drug-resistant strains

Table 4 (continued)

Disease	Indications	Regimen	Comments
Candida			Prophylaxis not generally recommended
Cryptococcosis			No evidence of survival benefit with prophylaxis
Histoplasmosis	CD4 <100 cells/mm³ in patient living in endemic area & at high risk for exposure to histoplasmosis	Itraconazole 200 mg qd	Effective (not much supporting data)
Coccidioidomycosis			Prophylaxis—efficacy unknown & not routinely recommended
Neutropenia	Absolute neutrophil count <500 cells/mL		Prophylaxis with filgastrim (granulocyte colony-stimulating factor) not routinely recommended

bid, twice daily; CMV, cytomegalovirus; FUO, fever of unknown origin; HAV, hepatitis A virus; HBc, hepatitis B core; HBs, hepatitis B surface; HCV, hepatitis C virus; PPD, purified protein derivative (tuberculin); q, every; qd, daily.
Data from the Practice Guidelines from the Infectious Diseases Society of America. [cited 2005 Oct 7]. Available from: http://www.journals.uchicago.edu/IDSA/guidelines and modified from Bartlett JG. The Johns Hopkins Hospital 2000-2001 guide to medical care of patients with HIV infection. 9th ed. Philadelphia: Lippincott Williams & Wilkins; 2000. p. 51-4. Used with permission

HYPERTENSIVE CRISIS

Guilherme H. M. Oliveira, M.D.
Alexander Schirger, M.D.

DEFINITION

- Hypertensive crisis—acute, severe increase in blood pressure, with or without end-organ damage, that occurs in a setting in which rapid control is necessary: coronary artery disease, aortic dissection, bleeding intracranial aneurysm, postoperative state, or heart failure

CLASSIFICATION

Hypertensive Emergency

- Increased blood pressure to systolic pressure >210 mm Hg and/or diastolic pressure >130 mm Hg causing symptoms of severe target-organ impairment: headache, papilledema and blurred vision, acute renal failure, acute coronary syndromes, pulmonary edema, encephalopathy, aortic dissection

Hypertensive Urgency

- Sudden increase in blood pressure, with systolic pressure >180 mm Hg and/or diastolic pressure ≥130 mm Hg, without overt evidence of end-organ damage but in a clinical setting in which it is urgent to prevent progression to hypertensive emergency

Malignant Hypertension

- Hypertensive urgency characterized by rapidly progressive vasospastic disorder with increased peripheral resistance; cerebral vessel dilatation; high plasma levels of renin, angiotensin, and aldosterone; generalized arteriolar fibrinoid necrosis; and target-organ damage

Special abbreviation used in this chapter: ACE, angiotensin-converting enzyme.

ETIOLOGY

The causes of hypertensive crisis are listed in Table 1.

EPIDEMIOLOGY

- Of all patients with hypertension, <1% develop malignant hypertension during the illness, whereas 2%-7% develop accelerated hypertension.
- Blacks are more susceptible than whites and males more than females.
- Increased risk is between ages 40 and 60.

CLINICAL PRESENTATION

- Central nervous system—headache, confusion, convulsions, stupor, coma; generally referred to as "hypertensive encephalopathy"
- Cardiovascular—acute coronary syndromes, aortic dissection, flash pulmonary edema
- Renal—oliguria, microscopic hematuria, acute renal failure
- Visual—papilledema, transient blindness (reversible with adequate decrease in blood pressure), retinal hemorrhages and exudates

DIAGNOSTIC STRATEGIES

- Acute evaluation should include a focused physical exam to look for the following:

Table 1. Causes of Hypertensive Crisis

Neglected or inappropriately treated essential hypertension
Abrupt discontinuation of antihypertensive medications (usually β-blockers & clonidine) leading to rebound hypertension
Renal artery stenosis
Coarctation of the aorta
Use of MAO inhibitors & subsequent ingestion of tyramine-containing foods or Chianti wine
Intracerebral or subarachnoid hemorrhage
Pheochromocytoma crisis
Collagen vascular diseases, especially systemic sclerosis
Glomerulopathies
Acute head injury or stroke
Eclampsia

MAO, monoamine oxidase.

- ▲ New third heart sound (acute or worsened congestive heart failure)
- ▲ New aortic regurgitation murmur (aortic dissection)
- ▲ Wet rales and orthopnea (flash pulmonary edema)
- ▲ Focal neurologic signs (hemorrhagic stroke, encephalopathy)
- ▲ Papilledema (defines malignant hypertension)
- ▪ Additional tests should include
  - ▲ ECG—ischemic changes and left ventricular hypertrophy (poor prognostic sign)
  - ▲ Chest X-ray—heart size, aortic dilatation, pulmonary venous hypertension
  - ▲ Urinalysis—microhematuria, RBC casts, proteinuria
  - ▲ Creatinine, BUN, glucose, potassium, and sodium
- ▪ The above tests are diagnostic for end-organ damage. Evaluation of the cause should be deferred until after blood pressure is stable.
- ▪ Further testing should include
  - ▲ Renal artery ultrasound—abnormal Doppler flow patterns to suggest renal artery stenosis
    - • If equivocal, consider magnetic resonance angiography or angiography.
  - ▲ Urinary metanephrines—screening for increased catecholamine production in pheochromocytoma
    - • If abnormal, confirm with 24-hour urinary catecholamines.
  - ▲ Aldosterone-to-renin ratio
    - • A ratio >20 should alert to hyperaldosteronism (patients may have normal serum potassium levels while receiving treatment with angiotensin-converting enzyme [ACE] inhibitors).

MANAGEMENT

Hypertensive Emergencies

- ▪ Decrease in mean arterial pressure by 25% within 2 hours, and then over 6 hours further decrease to systolic pressure ≤160 mm Hg and diastolic pressure <100 mm Hg. The major goal is to halt progressive organ damage.
- ▪ In acute aortic dissection, the goal is to decrease systolic

pressure to 120 mm Hg within 20 minutes; nitroprusside and labetolol should be used (see below).

- Drug of choice is sodium nitroprusside given in ICU with blood pressure monitoring through an arterial catheter.
  - ▲ Initial dose is 0.5-10.0 µg/kg per minute, titrated to a maximal dose of 500 µg/kg per hour.
  - ▲ Monitor thiocyanate levels every 48 hours, discontinue if blood level is >12 mg/dL
  - ▲ If toxicity develops, give sodium nitrate or hydroxocobalamin.
- Labetalol (especially in postoperative hypertension and pregnancy)—IV miniboluses of 20-80 mg every 5-10 minutes or at an infusion of 0.5-2 mg/minute
- Nitroglycerin (especially in acute congestive heart failure and coronary syndromes)—infused IV at 5-100 µg/kg per minute.
- Esmolol (useful in setting of tachyarrhythmias, migraine, acute coronary syndromes) 500 µg/kg IV bolus, then 25-100 µg/kg per minute
- Nicardipine (calcium channel blocker, useful in COPD patients) 5-15 mg/h IV infusion
- Fenoldopam (dopamine D_1 and α_2-agonist) 0.25-1.6 µg/kg per minute

Hypertensive Urgencies
- Without evidence of end-organ damage, immediate control of blood pressure is seldom needed, but control should be obtained within 12-24 hours with blood pressure <160/100 mm Hg.
- Sublingual nifedipine is detrimental. *Do not use*!
- Addition of furosemide should be tried if patient has difficult-to-control hypertension.
- ACE inhibitors can be given safely to patients with chronic renal insufficiency and creatinine level as high as 3 mg/dL who do not have bilateral renal artery stenosis. Follow creatinine and potassium levels. Discontinue ACE inhibitors if creatinine increases more than 1.0 mg/dL.
- Amlodipine, α-blockers, and reserpine are safe and useful drugs.
- Clonidine or labetalol PO can be used for a more gradual decrease to a target diastolic pressure of 95 mm Hg.

- α-Methyldopa and hydralazine are the drugs of choice for hypertensive crisis of pregnancy.
- If fluid overload state exists, loop diuretics should be considered for cautious use. Monitor both by chemical and hemodynamic parameters.

INFECTIVE ENDOCARDITIS

Axel Pflueger, M.D.
Walter R. Wilson, M.D.

DEFINITION
- Infective endocarditis—results from infection primarily of valvular endocardium and occasionally mural endocardium

CLASSIFICATION AND ETIOLOGY
- Endocarditis can be classified according to
  ▲ Microorganisms involved (Table 1)
  ▲ Type of valve affected (native vs. prosthetic)
  ▲ Clinical course (acute vs. subacute)

EPIDEMIOLOGY
- Incidence/prevalence in U.S.—1.7-4.2/100,000 population; 0.32-1.3/1,000 hospital admissions
- Predominant age—all ages, increased incidence among elderly patients (>70 years)
- Predominant sex
  ▲ Male—aortic valve
  ▲ Female—mitral valve

CLINICAL PRESENTATION
Signs and Symptoms
- Generally due to cytokine release, microemboli, congestive heart failure, and other organ involvement
- Look for
  ▲ Fever
    • May be high, low, or absent
    • May be only symptom in prosthetic valve endocarditis
  ▲ Heart murmur

Special abbreviations used in this chapter: TEE, transesophageal echocardiography; TTE, transthoracic echocardiography.

Table 1. Classification of Infective Endocarditis

Class	Course/comments	Underlying cardiac disease	Organism
Acute	Aggressive	May or may not have preexisting valve disease	*Staphylococcus aureus*, group B streptococci, *Streptococcus pneumoniae*, *Neisseria gonorrhoeae*
Subacute	Indolent	Structural valve disease	Viridans streptococci, enterococci, *Streptococcus bovis*, HACEK group
Intravenous drug abusers	Aggressive	Tricuspid valve (most common), may involve left-sided valves	*Staphylococcus aureus*, *Pseudomonas aeruginosa* or other gram-negative bacilli, *Candida* species
Early prosthetic valve	≤60 days after valve implant	Prosthesis	*Staphylococcus epidermidis*, *Staphylococcus aureus*, gram-negative bacilli, *Candida*, *Aspergillus* species
Late prosthetic valve	>60 days after valve implant	Prosthesis	Viridans streptococci, *Staphylococcus epidermidis*, enterococci
Culture-negative	5%–10% patients on antibiotics		*Bartonella quintana* (homeless people), *Brucella*, fungi, *Coxiella burnetii* (Q fever), *Chlamydia trachomatis*, *Chlamydia psittaci*, *Tropheryma whippelii*

HACEK, *Haemophilus parainfluenzae*, *H. aphrophilus*, *Actinobacillus actinomycetemcomitans*, *Cardiobacterium hominis*, *Eikenella corrodens*, and *Kingella kingae*.

▲ Roth spots—lymphocytes surrounded by edema and hemorrhage in nerve fiber layer of retina

▲ Osler nodes—small, tender, purplish erythematous skin lesions from infected microemboli or hypersensitivity reaction in pads of fingers or toes, in palms of hands or soles of feet

▲ Janeway lesions—macular raised, nontender hemorrhagic lesions in palms of hands and soles of feet

▲ Splenomegaly

▲ Signs of congestive heart failure—chest pain, shortness of breath, neck vein distension, gallops, rales, cardiac arrhythmia

▲ Symptoms related to embolization—stroke, splenic pain, coronary artery embolism

▲ Symptoms of intracranial mycotic aneurysm

▲ Other features are listed in Table 2.

Complications

■ Congestive heart failure and neurologic embolic events have the greatest influence on prognosis.

■ The complications are listed in Table 3.

DIAGNOSTIC STRATEGIES
Lab Findings

■ Positive blood cultures

Table 2. Additional Signs and Symptoms of Infective Endocarditis

Pallor	Cough
Pleural friction rub (from pulmonary emboli)	Paralysis, hemiparesis, aphasia
	Numbness, muscle weakness
Night sweats, chilly sensation	Cold extremity with pain (embolism)
Malaise, myalgia, joint pain	
Back pain (may be severe)	Bloody urine (may be gross or microscopic)
Anorexia, weight loss	
Stiff neck	Bloody sputum (from septic pulmonary emboli)
Delirium, headache	

Table 3. Complications of Infective Endocarditis

Congestive heart failure	Brain abscess
Ruptured valve	Ruptured mycotic aneurysm
Sinus of Valsalva aneurysm	(intracranial hemorrhage)
Aortic root abscess	Septic pulmonary infarcts
Myocardial abscess	Splenic infarcts
Myocardial infarction	Arterial emboli and infarcts
Pericarditis	Arthritis
Cardiac arrhythmia	Myositis
(conduction defects)	Glomerulonephritis
Meningitis	Acute renal failure
Cerebral emboli	Mesenteric infarct

- Leukocytosis in acute endocarditis
- Anemia in subacute endocarditis
- Increase in ESR and C-reactive protein
- Presence of valvular vegetations on echocardiography
- Decreased C3, C4, CH50 in subacute endocarditis
- Hematuria (microscopic or macroscopic)
- Rheumatoid factor in subacute endocarditis
- Serologic tests (IgG, IgA) for *Chlamydia*, Q fever (*Coxiella*), *Brucella*, and *Bartonella* may be useful in "culture-negative" endocarditis.

Lab Result Variations
- Antibiotics may make blood cultures falsely negative.
- Endocarditis caused by *Aspergillus*, *Chlamydia trachomatis*, *C. psittaci*, *Coxiella burnetii*, *Tropheryma whippelii*, *Bartonella* species may be associated with negative blood cultures.
- Prolonged incubation of blood cultures is needed in endocarditis caused by fastidious organisms, e.g., HACEK group (*Haemophilus*, *Actinobacillus*, *Cardiobacterium*, *Eikenella*, *Kingella*), *Abiotrophia* species, nutritionally variant *Streptococcus viridans*, *Brucella* species.

Pathology Findings
- Vegetations consist of platelets, fibrin, and colonies of microorganisms.
- Destruction of valve endocardium, perforation of valve leaflets, rupture of chordae tendineae, myocardial abscesses, rupture of sinus of Valsalva

- Pericarditis may occur.
- Emboli and/or infarction may be found in various body organs, as may abscesses and microabscesses.
- Kidneys may show embolic and/or immune-complex glomerulonephritis.

DIAGNOSTIC PROCEDURES
Echocardiography
- For vegetations, abscess, new prosthetic valve dehiscence, new regurgitation
  - ▲ Transthoracic echocardiography (TTE)
    - • 98% specificity, <60% sensitivity
    - • Inadequate 20% of time if obesity, prosthetic valves, COPD, chest wall deformity
  - ▲ Transesophageal echocardiography (TEE)
    - • 94% specificity, 70%-100% sensitivity
    - • Does not require antibiotic prophylaxis
  - ▲ TEE is preferred with prosthetic valve endocarditis or *Staphylococcus aureus* infection
  - ▲ When TTE and TEE are negative, negative predictive value is 95%.

Very Rarely Indicated
- Cardiac catheterization may be indicated to ascertain degree of valvular damage.
- Aortic root injection may be useful when aortic root abscess or rupture of sinus of Valsalva is suspected.

Pulmonary Ventilation Perfusion Scan
- May be useful in right-sided endocarditis

Axial CT
- May be useful in locating metastatic abscesses

Duke Criteria for Diagnosis
- The criteria are listed in Table 4.
- Diagnosis requires two major criteria, or one major and three minor criteria, or five minor criteria.

Table 4. Duke Criteria for Diagnosis of Infective Endocarditis

Major criteria

1. Positive blood culture

   Typical microorganism for infective endocarditis from 2 separate blood cultures—viridans streptococci, *Streptococcus bovis*, HACEK group, or community-acquired *Staphylococcus aureus* or enterococci, in the absence of a primary focus *or*

   Persistently positive blood culture—defined as recovery of a microorganism consistent with infective endocarditis from a) blood cultures drawn more than 12 hours apart or b) all of 3 or a majority of 4 or more separate blood cultures, with first and last drawn at least 1 hour apart

2. Evidence of endocardial involvement

   Positive echocardiogram

   Oscillating intracardiac mass on valve or supporting structures, in the path of regurgitant jets, or on implanted material and in the absence of an alternative anatomic explanation *or*

   Abscess *or*

   New partial dehiscence of prosthetic valve

   New valvular regurgitation (worsening or change in pre-existing murmur not sufficient)

3. Positive serologic tests for *Brucella*, *Bartonella*, or *Coxiella*

Minor criteria

1. Predisposition—predisposing heart condition or IV drug use
2. Fever 38.0°C (100.4°F)
3. Vascular phenomena—major arterial emboli, septic pulmonary infarcts, mycotic aneurysm, intracranial hemorrhage, conjunctival hemorrhage, Janeway lesions
4. Immunologic phenomena—glomerulonephritis, Osler nodes, Roth spots, rheumatoid factor
5. Microbiologic evidence—positive blood culture, but not meeting major criterion as noted above or serologic evidence of active infection with organism consistent with infective endocarditis
6. Echocardiogram—consistent with infective endocarditis but not meeting major criterion as noted above
7. C-reactive protein, ESR increased

HACEK (see Table 1).

MANAGEMENT

General Measures

- Initial hospitalized care
- Intensive care may be needed for critically ill patients.
- Outpatient home IV antibiotic therapy may be used for selected patients who are stable and reliable.
- Blood cultures—two sets at three different times (12 hours apart)
- CBC, serum creatinine, BUN, electrolytes, ESR, rheumatoid factor, urinalysis, C3, C4, CH50, ECG, chest X-ray
- Start antibiotics (see below)
- Consider indwelling central venous catheter line for IV antibiotics.
- Keep patient NPO for TEE
- Echocardiography—TTE and TEE
- Consult infectious diseases, cardiology, cardiac surgery, oral surgery if dentulous
- Treatment for congestive heart failure
- Oxygen treatment may be indicated.
- Hemodialysis may be used if renal failure develops.

Drug Therapy of Choice

- Therapy for endocarditis of various causes is outlined in Tables 5-10.

Precautions

- Patients with renal impairment—Dosage adjustment should be made for penicillin G, ampicillin, gentamicin, cefazolin, and vancomycin.
- Rapid infusion of vancomycin (<1 hour) may cause "red man syndrome," an intense redness or rash over upper half of the body.
  - ▲ This is due to histamine release and not an allergic reaction.
  - ▲ It disappears when the rate of infusion is decreased.
- The combination of vancomycin and gentamicin may cause increased incidence of renal toxicity.

Table 5. Therapy for Native Valve Endocarditis Caused by Highly Penicillin-Susceptible (MIC ≤0.12 μg/mL) Viridans Group Streptococci and *Streptococcus bovis*

Regimen	Dosage & route*	Duration, weeks	Strength of recommendation	Comments
Aqueous crystalline penicillin G sodium *or*	12-18 million U/24 hours IV continuously or in 6 equally divided doses	4	IA	Preferred for most patients >65 years or patients with impaired CN VIII or renal function
Ceftriaxone sodium	2 g/24 hours IV or IM in 1 dose Pediatric dose† Penicillin: 200,000 U/kg per 24 hours IV in 4-6 equally divided doses Ceftriaxone: 100 mg/kg per 24 hours IV or IM in 1 dose	4		

Table 5 (continued)

Regimen	Dosage & route*	Duration, weeks	Strength of recommendation	Comments
Aqueous crystalline penicillin G sodium *or* Ceftriaxone sodium *plus* Gentamicin sulfate‡	12-18 million U/24 hours IV continuously or in 6 equally divided doses 2 g/24 hours IV or IM in 1 dose 3 mg/kg per 24 hours IV or IM in 1 dose Pediatric dose† Penicillin: 200,000 U/kg per 24 hours IV in 4-6 equally divided doses Ceftriaxone: 100 mg/kg per 24 hours IV or IM in 1 dose Gentamicin: 3 mg/kg per 24 hours IV or IM in 1 dose or 3 equally divided doses§	2 2	IB	2-Week regimen is not intended for patients with known cardiac or extracardiac abscess or for those with creatinine clearance <20 mL/min, impaired CN VIII function, or *Abiotrophia*, *Granulicatella*, or *Gemella* species infection Gentamicin dosage should be adjusted to achieve a peak serum concentration of 3-4 µg/mL & trough serum concentration <1 µg/mL when 3 divided doses are used A nomogram is used for single daily dosing

623

Table 5 (continued)

Regimen	Dosage & route*	Duration, weeks	Strength of recommendation	Comments
Vancomycin hydrochloride‖	30 mg/kg per 24 hours IV in 2 equally divided doses, not to exceed 2 g/24 hours unless serum levels are inappropriately low Pediatric dose:† 40 mg/kg per 24 hours IV in 2-3 equally divided doses	4	IB	Vancomycin therapy is recommended only for patients unable to tolerate penicillin or ceftriaxone Vancomycin dosage should be adjusted to obtain peak (1 hour after completion of infusion) serum level of 30-45 µg/mL and trough level of 10-15 µg/mL

CN, cranial nerve; MIC, minimum inhibitory concentration.

*Dosages recommended are for patients with normal renal function.

†Note that pediatric dose *should not exceed that for a normal adult.*

‡Other potentially nephrotoxic drugs (e.g., NSAIDs) should be used with caution in patients receiving gentamicin therapy.

§Although data are available for once-daily dosing of aminoglycosides for children, none are available for treatment of infective endocarditis

‖Vancomycin dosages should be infused over at least 1 hour to reduce risk of histamine release red-man syndrome.

Table 6.   Therapy for Native Valve Endocarditis Caused by Strains of Viridans Group Streptococci and *Streptococcus bovis* **Relatively Resistant (MIC >0.12 µg/mL to ≤0.5 µg/mL) to Penicillin***

Regimen	Dosage & route	Duration, weeks	Strength of recommendation	Comments
Aqueous crystalline penicillin G sodium *or*	24 million U/24 hours IV continuously or in 4-6 equally divided doses	4		Patients with endocarditis caused by penicillin-resistant (MIC >0.5 µg/mL) strains should be treated with a regimen recommended for enterococcal endocarditis (Table 7)
Ceftriaxone sodium *plus*	2 g/24 hours IV or IM in 1 dose	4	IB	
Gentamicin sulfate†	3 mg/kg per 24 hours IV or IM in 1 dose	2		
	Pediatric dose‡			
	Penicillin: 300,000 U/24 hours IV in 4-6 equally divided doses			
	Ceftriaxone: 100 mg/kg per 24 hours IV or IM in 1 dose			
	Gentamicin: 3 mg/kg per 24 hours in 1 dose or 3 equally divided doses			

Table 6 (continued)

Regimen	Dosage & route*	Duration, weeks	Strength of recommendation	Comments
Vancomycin hydrochloride§	30 mg/kg per 24 hours IV in 2 equally divided doses, not to exceed 2 g/24 hours unless serum level is inappropriately low Pediatric dose:‡ 40 mg/kg per 24 hours in 2 or 3 equally divided doses	4	IB	Vancomycin therapy is recommended only for patients unable to tolerate penicillin or ceftriaxone

MIC, minimum inhibitory concentration.
*Dosages recommended are for patients with normal renal function.
†See Table 5 for appropriate dosage of gentamicin.
‡Note that pediatric dose *should not exceed that for a normal adult.*
§Vancomycin dosages should be infused over at least 1 hour to reduce risk of histamine release red-man syndrome.

Table 7. Therapy for Endocarditis Due to Enterococci

Regimen	Dosage & route	Duration, weeks	Comments
Aqueous crystalline penicillin G sodium	18–30 million U/24 hours IV continuously or in 6 equally divided doses		4 weeks for patients with symptoms <3 months
With gentamicin sulfate	1 mg/kg IM or IV every 8 hours	4–6	6 weeks for patients with symptoms >3 months
Ampicillin sodium	12 g/24 hours IV continuously or in 6 equally divided doses		
With gentamicin sulfate	1 mg/kg IM or IV every 8 hours		
Vancomycin hydrochloride	30 mg/kg per 24 hours IV in 2 equally divided doses, not to exceed 2 g/24 hours unless serum levels are monitored	4–6	Recommended for patients allergic to β-lactams
With gentamicin sulfate	1 mg/kg IM or IV every 8 hours	4–6	Cephalosporins not acceptable alternatives for patients allergic to penicillin

Table 8. Therapy for Endocarditis Caused by Staphylococci in Absence of Prosthetic Materials*

Regimen	Dosage & route*	Duration	Strength of recommendation	Comments
	Oxacillin-susceptible strains			
Nafcillin sodium *or* oxacillin†	12 g/24 hours IV in 4-6 equally divided doses	6 weeks	IA	For uncomplicated right-sided IE (i.e., 2 weeks)
With optional addition of gentamicin sulfate‡	3 mg/kg per 24 hours IV or IM in 2 or 3 equally divided doses	3-5 days	IB	For complicated right-sided IE and for left-sided IE Clinical benefit of aminoglycosides has not been established
	Pediatric dose§			
	Nafcillin or oxacillin: 200 mg/kg per 24 hours IV in 4-6 equally divided doses			
	Gentamicin: 3 mg/kg per 24 hours IV or IM in 3 equally divided doses			

Table 8 (continued)

Regimen	Dosage & route*	Duration	Strength of recommendation	Comments
For penicillin-allergic (non-anaphylactoid type) patients				Consider skin testing for oxacillin-susceptible staphylococci and questionable history of immediate-type hypersensitivity to penicillin
Cefazolin	6 g/24 hours IV in 3 equally divided doses	4-6 weeks	IB	Cephalosporins should be avoided in patients with anaphylactoid-type hypersensitivity to β-lactams; vancomycin should be used in these cases§
With optional addition of gentamicin sulfate‡	3 mg/kg per 24 hours IV or IM in 2 or 3 equally divided doses Pediatric dose:§ Cefazolin: 100 mg/kg per 24 hours IV in 3 equally divided doses Gentamicin: 3 mg/kg per 24 hours IV or IM in 3 equally divided doses	3-5 days		Clinical benefit of aminoglycosides has not been established

Table 8 (continued)

Regimen	Dosage & route*	Duration	Strength of recommendation	Comments
Oxacillin-resistant strains				
Vancomycin^//	30 mg/kg per 24 hours IV in 2 equally divided doses Pediatric dose: 40 mg/kg per 24 hours IV in 2 or 3 equally divided doses	6 weeks	IB	Adjust vancomycin dosage to achieve 1-hour serum level of 30-45 µg/mL and trough level of 10-15 µg/mL

IE, infective endocarditis.

*Dosages recommended are for patients with normal renal function.

^†Penicillin G 24 million U/24 hours may be used in place of nafcillin or oxacillin if strain is penicillin-susceptible (minimum inhibitory concentration ≤0.1 µg/mL).

^‡Gentamicin should be administered in close temporal proximity to vancomycin, nafcillin, or oxacillin dosing.

^§Note that pediatric dose *should not exceed that for a normal adult.*

^//Vancomycin dosages should be infused over at least 1 hour to reduce risk of histamine release red-man syndrome.

Table 9.   Therapy for Prosthetic Valve Endocarditis Caused by Staphylococci (Oxacillin-Susceptible Strains)*

Regimen	Dosage & route	Duration, weeks	Strength of recommendation	Comments
Nafcillin or oxacillin *plus*	12 g/24 hours IV in 6 equally divided doses	≥6	IB	Cefazolin may be substituted for nafcillin or oxacillin
Rifampin *plus*	900 mg IV or PO in 3 equally divided doses	≥6		Penicillin G 24 million U/24 hours may be used in place of nafcillin or oxacillin if strain is penicillin-susceptible (MIC ≤0.1 µg/mL) and does not produce β-lactamase
Gentamicin†	3 mg/kg per 24 hours IV or IM in 2 or 3 equally divided doses	2		Vancomycin should be used in patients with immediate-type hypersensitivity reactions to β-lactam antibiotics (see Table 5 for dosing guidelines)
	Pediatric dose‡ Nafcillir or oxacillin 200 mg/kg per 24 hours IV in 4-6 equally divided doses Rifampin: 20 mg/kg per 24 hours PO or IV in 3 equally divided doses Gentamicin: 3 mg/kg per 24 hours IV or IM in 3 equally divided doses			

Table 9 (continued)

Regimen	Dosage & route*	Duration, weeks	Strength of recommendation	Comments
Vancomycin *plus*	30 mg/kg per 24 hours in 2 equally divided doses	≥6	IB	Adjust vancomycin to achieve 1-hour serum level of 30-45 μg/mL and trough level of 10-15 μg/mL
Rifampin *plus*	900 mg/24 hours IV or PO in 3 equally divided doses	≥6		
Gentamicin†	3 mg/kg per 24 hours IV or IM in 2 or 3 equally divided doses	2		
	Pediatric dose:‡			
	Vancomycin: 40 mg/kg per 24 hours IV in 2 or 3 equally divided doses			
	Rifampin: 20 mg/kg per 24 hours IV or PO in 3 equally divided doses (up to the adult dose)			
	Gentamicin: 3 mg/kg per 24 hours IV or IM in 3 equally divided doses			

MIC, minimum inhibitory concentration.

*Dosages recommended are for patients with normal renal function.

†Gentamicin should be administered in close proximity to vancomycin, nafcillin, or oxacillin dosing.

‡Note that pediatric dose *should not exceed that for a normal adult.*

Table 10. Therapy for Both Native Valve and Prosthetic Valve Endocarditis Caused by HACEK Microorganisms

Regimen	Dosage & route	Duration, weeks	Strength of recommendation	Comments
Ceftriaxone sodium *or*	2 g/24 hours IV or IM in 1 dose*	4	IB	Cefotaxime or another 3rd- or 4th-generation cephalosporin may be substituted
Ampicillin-sulbactam† *or*	12 g/24 hours IV in 4 equally divided doses	4	IIaB	
Ciprofloxacin‡‡	1,500 mg/24 hours PO or 800 mg/24 hours IV in 2 equally divided doses Pediatric dose§ Ceftriaxone: 100 mg/kg per 24 hours IV or IM once daily	4	IIbC	Fluoroquinolone therapy is recommended only for patients unable to tolerate cephalosporin & ampicillin Levofloxacin, gatifloxacin, or moxifloxacin may be substituted Fluoroquinolones are generally not recommended for patients <18 years

Table 10 (continued)

Regimen	Dosage & route*	Duration, weeks	Strength of recommendation	Comments
	Ampicillin-sulbactam: 300 mg/kg per 24 hours IV in 4 or 6 equally divided doses			Prosthetic valve: Patients with endocarditis involving a prosthetic cardiac valve or other prosthetic cardiac material should be treated for 6 weeks
	Ciprofloxacin: 20-30 mg/kg per 24 hours IV or PO in 2 equally divided doses			

HACEK (see Table 1).

*Patients should be informed that IM injection of ceftriaxone is painful.

†Dosage recommended for patients with normal renal function.

‡Fluoroquinolones are highly active in vitro against HACEK microorganisms. Published data on use of fluoroquinolone therapy for endocarditis caused by HACEK are minimal.

§Note that the pediatric dose *should not exceed that for a normal adult.*

- Rifampin may increase the requirement for warfarin oral anticoagulant and oral hypoglycemic agents.
- Gentamicin blood levels should be determined if treatment is >5 days and for patients with renal dysfunction.
  - ▲ Peak gentamicin level should be about 3 µg/mL and trough <1 µg/mL.
- Vancomycin blood levels should be determined in patients with renal dysfunction.
  - ▲ Desired peak level is 30-45 µg/mL and trough <10 µg/mL.
- BUN and serum creatinine should be measured twice weekly while patient is receiving gentamicin.
- Consider audiometry baseline and follow-up during long-term aminoglycoside therapy.
- Gentamicin should be used with caution or avoided if possible in pregnant women.

Alternative Drugs for Patients Allergic to Penicillin
- Endocarditis due to penicillin susceptible viridans streptococci and *Streptococcus bovis*
  - ▲ Ceftriaxone 2 g IM or IV every 24 hours (*not* for patients with immediate-type hypersensitivity to penicillin) *or*
  - ▲ Vancomycin 15 mg/kg (usual dose, 1 g) IV infused over 1 hour every 12 hours for 4 weeks (6 weeks for prosthetic valve endocarditis)
- Endocarditis due to enterococci
  - ▲ Desensitization to penicillin should be considered.
  - ▲ Vancomycin 15 mg/kg (usual dose, 1 g) IV infused over 1 hour every 12 hours plus gentamicin (3 mg/kg/day in divided doses q 8-12 hours, depending on renal function and results of peak and trough measures) for 4-6 weeks (6 weeks for prosthetic valve endocarditis)

Surgical Measures
- Cardiac surgery to replace infected valve may be performed before the course of antibiotic treatment is completed when one of the following occurs:
  - ▲ Evidence of congestive heart failure due to valve incompetence

- ▲ Multiple major systemic emboli
- ▲ Infection caused by resistant organisms, e.g., *Aspergillus*, *Candida*, other fungi, *Pseudomonas aeruginosa*
- ▲ Dehiscence of infected prosthetic valve
- ▲ Relapse of prosthetic valve endocarditis
- ▲ Persistent bacteremia despite antibiotic treatment

RISK FACTORS

- ■ High-risk category—antimicrobial prophylaxis recommended for invasive procedures (dental work, genitourinary tract, some endoscopic procedures)
  - ▲ Prosthetic cardiac valves, including bioprosthetic and homograft valves
  - ▲ Previous bacterial endocarditis, even in the absence of heart disease
  - ▲ Complex cyanotic congenital heart disease (e.g., single-ventricle states, transposition of great arteries, tetralogy of Fallot)
  - ▲ Surgically constructed systemic pulmonary shunts or conduits
- ■ Moderate-risk category—prophylaxis recommended
  - ▲ Most other congenital cardiac malformations (other than those listed above and below)
  - ▲ Acquired valvular dysfunction (e.g., rheumatic heart disease)
  - ▲ Hypertrophic cardiomyopathy
  - ▲ Mitral valve prolapse with valvular regurgitation and/or thickened leaflets
- ■ Negligible-risk category (not greater than that of the general population)—prophylaxis not recommended
  - ▲ Isolated secundum atrial septal defect
  - ▲ Surgical repair of atrial septal defect, ventricular septal defect, or patent ductus arteriosus (without residual beyond 6 months)
  - ▲ Previous coronary artery bypass graft surgery
  - ▲ Mitral valve prolapse without valvular regurgitation
  - ▲ Physiologic, functional, or innocent heart murmurs
  - ▲ Previous Kawasaki disease without valvular dysfunction
  - ▲ Previous rheumatic fever without valvular dysfunction
  - ▲ Cardiac pacemakers (intravascular and epicardial) and implanted defibrillators

PREVENTION AND PROPHYLAXIS

- Who should receive antibiotic prophylaxis?
  - *All* patients with high- and moderate-risk factors undergoing
    - Dental extractions
    - Periodontal procedures, including surgery, scaling and root planing, probing, and recall maintenance
    - Dental implant placement and reimplantation of avulsed teeth
    - Endodontic (root canal) instrumentation or surgery only beyond the apex
    - Subgingival placement of antibiotic fibers or strips
    - Initial placement of orthodontic bands but not brackets
    - Intraligamentary local anesthetic injections
    - Prophylactic cleaning of teeth or implants when bleeding is anticipated
    - Respiratory tract procedures
      - Tonsillectomy and/or adenoidectomy
      - Surgical operations involving respiratory mucosa
      - Bronchoscopy with rigid bronchoscope
    - Genitourinary tract procedures
      - Prostatic surgery
      - Cystoscopy
      - Urethral dilation
  - *All* patients with high-risk factors (optional for those with moderate-risk factors) undergoing gastrointestinal tract procedures
    - Sclerotherapy for esophageal varices
    - Esophageal stricture dilation
    - Endoscopic retrograde cholangiography for biliary obstruction
    - Biliary tract surgery
    - Surgical operations involving intestinal mucosa
- Endocarditis prophylaxis is not recommended for
  - Patients with negligible risks
  - The following dental procedures:
    - Restorative dentistry (operative and prosthodontic) with or without retraction cord
    - Local anesthetic injections (nonintraligamentary)

- Intracanal endodontic treatment; postplacement and build-up
- Placement of rubber dams
- Postoperative suture removal
- Placement of removable prosthodontic or orthodontic appliances
- Taking of oral impressions
- Fluoride treatments
- Taking of oral X-rays
- Orthodontic appliance adjustment
- Shedding of primary teeth
▲ The following respiratory tract procedures:
- Endotracheal intubation
- Bronchoscopy with flexible bronchoscope, with or without biopsy
- Myringotomy tube insertion
▲ The following gastrointestinal tract procedures:
- TEE
- Endoscopy with or without gastrointestinal biopsy
▲ The following genitourinary tract procedures:
- Vaginal hysterectomy
- Vaginal delivery
- Cesarean section
- In uninfected tissue
  - Urethral catheterization
  - Uterine dilatation and curettage
  - Therapeutic abortion
  - Sterilization procedures
  - Insertion or removal of intrauterine devices
▲ The following other procedures:
- Cardiac catheterization, including balloon angioplasty
- Implanted cardiac pacemakers, implanted defibrillators, and coronary stents
- Incision or biopsy of surgically scrubbed skin
- Circumcision
■ Antibiotic prophylaxis
▲ Antibiotics administered more than 4 hours after the procedure probably have no prophylactic effect.
▲ Generally, prophylaxis should be administered PO 1 hour and IM/IV within 0.5 hour before the procedure in adults and children (Tables 11 and 12)

▲ Prophylaxis should not be extended more than 24 hours postoperatively.

COURSE AND PROGNOSIS

■ In staphylococcal endocarditis, fever may persist up to 5 days and positive blood cultures may persist up to 5 days after appropriate treatment is started

■ In streptococcal endocarditis, clinical response should occur within 48 hours after starting antibiotic treatment and blood cultures should be negative soon after antibiotic treatment is started.

■ Prognosis depends largely on the possible complications.

▲ Prognosis is worse for elderly persons.

Table 11. Prophylactic Regimens for Dental, Oral, Respiratory Tract, or Esophageal Procedures

Situation	Agent	Regimen
Standard	Amoxicillin	A: 2.0 g PO
		C: 50 mg/kg PO
Unable to take PO	Ampicillin	A: 2.0 g IM/IV
		C: 50 mg IM/IV
Allergic to penicillin	Clindamycin *or*	A: 600 mg PO
		C: 20 mg/kg PO
	Cephalexin *or*	A: 2.0 g PO
	Cefadroxil *or*	C: 50 mg/kg PO
	Azithromycin *or*	A: 500 mg PO
	Clarithromycin	C: 15 mg/kg PO
Allergic to penicillin & unable to take PO	Clindamycin *or*	A: 600 mg IV
		C: 20 mg/kg IV
	Cefazolin	A: 1.0 g IM/IV
		C: 25 mg/kg IM/IV

A, adult; C, child.

Table 12. Prophylactic Regimens for Genitourinary or Gastrointestinal Procedures

Situation	Agent	Regimen
High-risk patients	Ampicillin plus gentamicin	Ampicillin Adults: 2 g Children: 50 mg/kg Gentamicin—adults & children: 1.5 mg/kg 30 Minutes before procedure & ampicillin 1 g 6 hours later
High-risk patients allergic to ampicillin	Vancomycin plus gentamicin	Vancomycin Adults: 1 g Children: 20 mg/kg Gentamicin—for adults & children: 1.5 mg/kg Complete infusion 30 minutes before proce- dure
Moderate-risk patients	Same regimens as in Table 11	

INFLAMMATORY BOWEL DISEASE

Conor G. Loftus, M.D.
Edward V. Loftus, Jr., M.D.

DEFINITION

- Inflammatory bowel disease (IBD) encompasses at least two forms of idiopathic intestinal inflammation (ulcerative colitis and Crohn disease).
- Absence of a specific underlying etiologic agent sets IBD apart as a cause of intestinal inflammation.

CLASSIFICATION

- Classification is based on typical clinical, pathologic, endoscopic, radiologic, and lab features.
- The broad classification of IBD
  - ▲ Ulcerative colitis—confined to colon
  - ▲ Crohn disease (regional enteritis, regional ileitis, Crohn ileitis, and granulomatous colitis)—may involve any portion of the gastrointestinal tract
  - ▲ Indeterminate colitis—cases in which it is impossible to distinguish with confidence between ulcerative colitis and Crohn disease affecting the colon by using any conventional diagnostic criteria

ETIOLOGY

- Exact cause of ulcerative colitis and Crohn disease is unknown.
- They may result from interaction between genetically determined host susceptibility and acquired environmental influences

Genetic Factors

- Frequency of disease in first-degree relatives of patients with IBD is 5%-10%.

Special abbreviation used in this chapter: IBD, inflammatory bowel disease.

- High concordance of disease in monozygotic twin pairs (Crohn disease > ulcerative colitis)
- Identical twin of a patient does not uniformly develop IBD, so nongenetic factors are also involved.

Infection
- Atypical mycobacteria, cell-wall deficient bacteria, and previous exposure to measles (rubeola) are implicated as potential causes, but this is controversial.
- Bacterial or viral gastroenteritis may serve as an "environmental trigger" for IBD.

Smoking
- Ulcerative colitis
  - More common in nonsmokers
  - Risk is particularly high for ex-smokers, especially within first 2 years after cessation.
- Crohn disease
  - Smoking increases the risk.

Psychosocial Factors
- Environmental stress may have a role in IBD "flares."

Medications
- Ulcerative colitis and Crohn disease are frequently exacerbated by NSAIDs.
- Role of oral contraceptive pills in exacerbations of IBD is not clear.

EPIDEMIOLOGY
- Epidemiologic features of IBD are listed in Table 1.

CLINICAL PRESENTATION
Ulcerative Colitis
- Symptoms
  - Classic—bloody diarrhea
  - Common—fatigue, fever, abdominal pain, rectal pain, tenesmus, rectal urgency
- Signs
  - Mild disease—mild abdominal tenderness
  - Severe disease—hypotensive, tachycardic, febrile, dry

Table 1. Epidemiologic Features of Inflammatory Bowel Disease

Incidence/100,000	CD 1-10
	UC 2-18
Prevalence/100,000	CD 20-150
	UC 40-250
Race	White>black>Hispanic>Asian
Sex	UC M>F
Age at onset, years	CD peak 15-30
	UC peak 20-40
Ethnic	Jewish>non-Jewish
Smoking	Predisposes CD
	Protective UC
Relapse association	NSAIDs

CD, Crohn disease; UC, ulcerative colitis.

mucosae, pallor, marked abdominal tenderness (often rebound), guarding, hypertympanism (consider toxic megacolon), decreased bowel sounds

Crohn Disease
- Symptoms
  - Classic—diarrhea, abdominal pain, weight loss
  - Common—fatigue, weight loss, diarrhea, steatorrhea, cramping right lower abdominal pain, bloating, nausea, vomiting, epigastric pain
- Signs
  - Pale, ill-appearing, cachectic, muscle-wasting, clubbing, abdominal distension, right lower quadrant tenderness or mass, perianal fistulous opening or abscess
  - Compared with ulcerative colitis, Crohn disease has a more varied presentation because of the
    - Diversity of anatomic involvement
    - Transmural nature of the inflammatory process

Differential Diagnosis for Fulminant Colitis and Toxic Megacolon
- The differential diagnosis is listed in Table 2.

Table 2. Differential Diagnosis for Fulminant Colitis and Toxic Megacolon

Ulcerative colitis
Crohn colitis
Infectious colitis
    Shigella
    Salmonella
    Aeromonas hydrophila
    Campylobacter
    E. coli O157:H7
    Clostridium difficile
    Amoeba
    Cytomegalovirus (immunosuppressed)
Medication-related
    Gold
    Methotrexate
    NSAIDs
    Estrogen
Ischemic colitis
Kaposi sarcoma
Neutropenic colitis

Complications

- Emergent complications in IBD are classified as shown in Figure 1.

Intestinal Complications

- The incidence of fulminant colitis is approximately 5%-10%; incidence of toxic dilatation in ulcerative colitis in the modern era is lower.
- Perforation occurs in up to one-third of patients with toxic megacolon.
  - ▲ Perforation may also occur in fulminant colitis without colonic dilatation.
  - ▲ Free perforation with generalized peritonitis is rare in Crohn disease; microperforation with localized peritonitis is more common, especially right lower quadrant.
- Bloody diarrhea occurs in 95% of patients with ulcerative colitis.
- Intra-abdominal abscesses complicate Crohn disease in 12%-25% of patients and are more common in ileocolitis than in isolated ileitis or colitis.

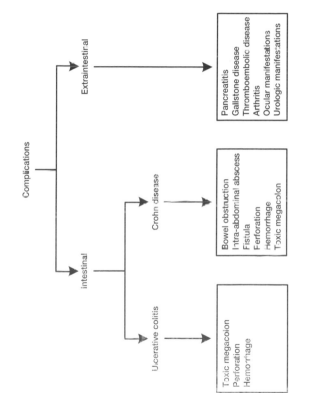

Fig. 1. Emergent complications of inflammatory bowel disease.

Extraintestinal Complications
- Pancreatitis
  - Duodenal Crohn disease may obstruct the pancreatic duct or render the sphincter of Oddi incompetent.
  - In IBD, bile is lithogenic, predisposing to biliary sludge or stones and secondary pancreatitis.
  - IBD medications—azathioprine, 6-mercaptopurine, sulfasalazine, mesalamine, olsalazine, and metronidazole—have been implicated in development of pancreatitis.
- Gallstone disease
  - Extensive ileal disease or resection decreases bile acid pool, rendering bile lithogenic.
- Thromboembolic disease
  - Hypercoagulable state in IBD is caused by increased factors V and VIII, thrombocytosis, abnormal platelet activity, and decreased antithrombin III.
  - Patients may present acutely with deep venous thrombosis or pulmonary embolism.
  - Dilemma—when patients have active colitis with pronounced bleeding. In this setting, anticoagulation with heparin is well tolerated, but colectomy may be required for bleeding or recurrent thromboembolism.
  - Patients with IBD rarely present with cerebrovascular accidents due to arterial thrombosis.
- Seronegative arthritis
  - IBD may be associated with both peripheral and axial arthritis.
  - Patient may present with acute arthritis; aspirate synovial fluid to rule out septic arthritis.
  - Treatment is directed at the intestinal disease; use NSAIDs with caution because they may exacerbate IBD.
  - Axial arthropathy (sacroiliitis and spondylitis) is independent of intestinal activity.
  - Peripheral arthritis follows activity of intestinal disease, axial arthropathy does not.
- Dermatologic disease
  - Erythema nodosum
  - Pyoderma gangrenosum
  - Aphthous ulcers
- Ocular manifestations

- ▲ Ocular emergencies include episcleritis and anterior uveitis.
- ▲ Episcleritis parallels intestinal disease activity; anterior uveitis does not.
- ▲ Consult ophthalmology.
- ■ Urologic manifestations
  - ▲ Urolithiasis
    - Uric acid stones are common because of chronic dehydration, the metabolic acidosis induced by diarrhea, and hypercatabolic state associated with IBD.
    - Crohn patients with extensive disease or resection who have malabsorption develop calcium oxalate stones.
  - ▲ Urosepsis
    - This may result from chronic enterovesical fistula, and patient may complain of pneumaturia or fecaluria.
    - Pyelonephritis can occur from obstructive uropathy.
    - Crohn disease can fistulize posteriorly, encasing the ureter and causing obstruction. This is more likely to occur on the right side, with consequent hydroureter, hydronephrosis, and complicating urosepsis.

DIAGNOSTIC STRATEGIES
- ■ Diagnosis of IBD relies on
  - ▲ Clinical and lab data
  - ▲ Imaging (barium studies or CT)
  - ▲ Endoscopy (esophagogastroduodenoscopy, colonoscopy, flexible sigmoidoscopy, capsule endoscopy)
  - ▲ Pathology
- ■ Stepwise approach for diagnosing ulcerative colitis and Crohn disease is provided in Table 3.

Physical Exam
- ■ Ill-appearing, febrile, orthostatic, tachycardic, abdominal guarding, absent bowel sounds, tympanic percussion note

Investigations
- ■ Stool samples for ova, parasites, bacterial culture, and *Clostridium difficile* toxin

Table 3. Stepwise Approach to Diagnosis of Ulcerative Colitis and Crohn Disease According to Type of Investigation

Investigation	Ulcerative colitis	Crohn disease
Clinical	Bloody diarrhea	Diarrhea
		Weight loss
		Abdominal pain
		Right lower quadrant mass
		Perianal disease
Lab		
CBC	Anemia (iron, TIBC), leukocytosis, thrombocytosis	Anemia (iron, TIBC, vitamin B_{12}, folate), leukocytosis, thrombocytosis
Electrolytes	Hypokalemia	Hypokalemia
Inflammatory markers	ESR, CRP	ESR, CRP
Albumin	Low in severe disease	Low in severe disease
Other	Elevated p-ANCA	Elevated ASCA
Radiologic		
Distribution	Continuous, symmetric	Discontinuous, asymmetric
Ulceration	Fine, superficial	Deep, submucosal extension
Fissures	Never	Often
Strictures or fistulas	Rare	Common
Ileal involvement	Dilated, backwash iliitis (uncommon)	Narrowed, nodular, erosions, ulcers (common)
Endoscopic		
Friability	Characteristic	Occasional
Aphthous & linear ulcers	Rare	Common
Cobblestone appearance	Never	Common
Pseudopolyps	Common	Occasional
Rectal involvement	95%	50% of cases
Distribution	Continuous, distal	Discontinuous, skip lesions

Table 3 (continued

Investigation	Ulcerative colitis	Crohn disease
Pathologic		
Focal granulo-mas	Never	Common
Transmural inflammation	Rare	Common
Deep fissures, fistulas	Never	Common
Macroscopic thickening	Rare	Common
Narrowing of bowel lumen	Rare	Common

ASCA, anti-*Saccharomyces cerevisiae* antibody; CRP, C-reactive protein; p-ANCA, perinuclear antineutrophil cytoplasmic antibody; TIBC, total iron-binding capacity.

- Abdominal supine and upright X-rays—loss of colonic haustra, "thumbprinting" indicating bowel-wall edema, colonic dilatation (especially transverse colon)

Severity
- Criteria for assessing severity of ulcerative colitis are listed in Table 4.

MANAGEMENT
General
- NPO
- Fluid and electrolyte replacement, transfusion of blood products as required
- Nasogastric tube if toxic megacolon
- Corticosteroids— methylprednisolone, 20-40 mg IV every 12 hours
- Antibiotics—cefotaxime, 1 g IV every 8 hours + metronidazole, 500 mg IV every 8 hours if patient is toxic, febrile, has leukocytosis, etc.
- Serial abdominal X-rays, especially if toxic megacolon

Table 4. Criteria for Assessing Severity of Ulcerative Colitis

Variable	Mild	Moderate	Severe
Bowel movements	<4/day	4-6/day	>6/day
	Minimal blood	Bloody	Bloody
Fever	None	±	>99.5°F
Pulse, beats/minute	<90	90-100	>100
Hemoglobin, g/L	>12	9-12	<9
ESR, mm/1 hour	<10	10-30	>30
Albumin, g/dL	>3.5	3-3.5	<3

Data from Truelove SC, Witts LJ. Cortisone in ulcerative colitis: final report on a therapeutic trial. Br Med J. 1955;2:1041-8.

- Surgical consultation
- Colectomy if unresolving with medical therapy or clinical deterioration

Medical Management if IBD
5-Aminosalicylates
- Oral
  - ▲ Sulfasalazine (Azulfidine)—4-6 g daily in 4 divided doses
  - ▲ Sulfa-free agents
    - • Mesalamine (Asacol, Pentasa)—2-4 g daily in divided doses
    - • Balsalazide (Colazal)—6.75 g daily in divided doses
    - • Olsalazine (Dipentum)—1.5-3 g daily in divided doses
- Rectal
  - ▲ Mesalamine suppository (Canasa)—500 mg twice daily (proctitis)
  - ▲ Mesalamine enema (Rowasa)—4 g daily (for distal colitis)
- 5-Aminosalicylates for mild or moderate disease and maintenance therapy
- Sulfa-free agents
  - ▲ Efficacy in ulcerative colitis comparable with sulfasalazine
  - ▲ Fewer undesirable effects

Corticosteroids
- Classic
  - ▲ Prednisone—40-60 mg PO daily, taper by 5 mg/week over 2-3 months

- ▲ Methylprednisolone (Solu-Medrol)—IV 40-60 mg daily (for severe IBD flares)
- ▲ Hydrocortisone enema (Cortenema)—100 mg twice daily (for acute management of distal colitis)
- ■ Novel
  - ▲ Budesonide (Entocort EC)
    - • 6-9 mg PO daily (controlled ileal release formulation)
    - • High potency and low bioavailability for minimizing adverse systemic effects

Immunomodulators

- ■ Azathioprine/6-mercaptopurine
  - ▲ For patients resistant to or dependent on corticosteroids
  - ▲ Azathioprine—a prodrug yielding 6-mercaptopurine
  - ▲ Azathioprine, 2.0-2.5 mg/kg body weight, and 6-mercaptopurine, 1-5 mg/kg body weight
  - ▲ Monitor for myelosuppression, especially leukopenia.
- ■ Methotrexate
  - ▲ IM or SQ for Crohn disease, not for ulcerative colitis
  - ▲ Induction dose—25 mg/week
  - ▲ Maintenance dose—15 mg/week
  - ▲ Time to onset of response may be more rapid than for azathioprine/6-mercaptopurine.
- ■ Cyclosporine
  - ▲ May be used for IBD flares refractory to other treatments
  - ▲ Administered as a continuous infusion—2-4 mg/kg daily
  - ▲ Mean response time of 7 days
  - ▲ Monitor for hypertension, renal insufficiency

Antibiotics

- ■ Metronidazole (Flagyl)
  - ▲ Beneficial for
    - • Mild to moderate Crohn disease
    - • Perianal and fistulous Crohn disease
    - • Postoperative prophylaxis
    - • "Pouchitis" following ileoanal pouch surgery
- ■ Ciprofloxacin (Cipro)
  - ▲ In Crohn disease, it has been used as a single agent or in

combination with metronidazole for active disease and fistulas.

Biologic Response Modifiers
- Infliximab (Remicade)
  - ▲ Chimeric monoclonal antibody to tumor necrosis factor α
  - ▲ Approved for treating refractory or fistulizing Crohn disease
  - ▲ For moderate to severe Crohn disease, 5 mg/kg IV infusion on weeks 0, 2, and 6, followed by every 8 weeks
  - ▲ For fistulizing Crohn disease, 5 mg/kg on weeks 0, 2, and 6, followed by every 8 weeks
  - ▲ Acute infusion reactions are rare.
  - ▲ Delayed hypersensitivity reactions after 3-10 days because human antichimeric antibodies develop
  - ▲ Perform PPD (tuberculin test) and chest X-ray before initiating therapy (reactivation of latent TB can occur).

CANCER SURVEILLANCE
- After 10 years of extensive ulcerative colitis, cancer risk is about 0.5%-1%/year.
- Patients with left-sided colitis reach similar levels of cumulative risk after 3-4 decades.
- After 8-10 years of colitis, surveillance colonoscopy with multiple biopsies should be performed every 1 to 2 years.
- Definite dysplasia of any grade, confirmed by expert pathologist, is indication for colectomy.

MYASTHENIA GRAVIS AND DISORDERS OF THE NEUROMUSCULAR JUNCTION

Guilherme H. M. Oliveira, M.D.
Kathleen M. McEvoy, M.D.

DEFINITION

- Myasthenia gravis is an acquired autoimmune disorder in which pathogenic autoantibodies destroy acetylcholine receptors (AChRs) at the neuromuscular junction.
- It is a pure motor syndrome characterized by weakness and fatigue of extraocular, pharyngeal, facial, cervical, proximal limb, and respiratory musculature.
- Onset may be sudden and severe, but more typically is mild and intermittent over many years.

CLASSIFICATION

- Clinical classification is based on distribution and severity of symptoms, as follows:
    - Type 1 (20% of cases)—confined to extraocular muscles
    - Type 2A (30%)—mild generalized weakness (cranial, trunk, limb)
    - Type 2B (20%)—moderately severe generalized weakness
    - Type 3 (11%)—acute fulminating (early respiratory involvement)
    - Type 4 (9%)—late severe

ETIOLOGY

- Humoral and cellular immune mediated destruction of postsynaptic AChRs at neuromuscular junction
- Weakness results from decreased number of functional AChRs at neuromuscular junction secondary to destruction by pathogenic autoantibodies.
    - Thymic abnormality is believed to be involved in the

Special abbreviation used in this chapter: AChR, acetylcholine receptor.

pathogenesis of autoimmune myasthenia gravis, perhaps by triggering recognition of self AChR as nonself.
- Neonatal myasthenia gravis—10%-15% of infants born to myasthenic mothers develop neonatal myasthenia gravis from transplacental transfer of AChR antibodies.
  - ▲ It typically presents as feeble cry, feeding and respiratory difficulty, general or facial weakness, and ptosis, which may resolve completely in several weeks.

EPIDEMIOLOGY
- Myasthenia gravis—the most common disorder of the neuromuscular junction
- Prevalence, 3/100,000 (13-64 per million)
- Incidence, 2-5/million people annually
- Female:male ratio, 3:2
- May present at any age
  - ▲ Incidence in women peaks in third decade.
  - ▲ Incidence in men peaks in fifth to seventh decades.
- Familial predisposition (5% of cases) with an increased frequency of HLA-B8 and DR3
  - ▲ HLA studies show increased association with other autoimmune disorders (Hashimoto thyroiditis, rheumatoid arthritis, and pernicious anemia).
    - • Thymoma—in 10%-15% of patients, especially if older than 40
    - • Thymic hyperplasia—in 85% of patients younger than 40

CLINICAL PRESENTATION
Classic Presentation
- Clinical hallmark is fluctuating muscle weakness of ocular, cranial, and bulbar muscles producing diplopia, ptosis, and dysphagia.

Common Presentation
- May include generalized weakness, fatigue with chewing, dysarthria, dysphonia, neck weakness, proximal limb weakness, and respiratory weakness

Exacerbating Factors
- May include emotional stress, exercise and heat, illness and infection, fever, hormonal imbalance, drug-induced

(corticosteroids, aminoglycosides, tetracyclines, quinidine, procainamide, β-blockers, lidocaine, narcotics, and psychotropics)

Complications
Crisis (Myasthenic vs. Cholinergic)

- In myasthenia gravis, severe muscle weakness and respiratory failure can result from not enough functional acetylcholine receptors (myasthenic crisis) or too much acetylcholine (cholinergic crisis).
  - ▲ Cholinergic crisis
    - Typically caused by overdose of anticholinergic medications
    - Suspect cholinergic crisis when other signs of cholinergic overactivity (excessive secretions, diarrhea, bradycardia) are present.
    - Treat with atropine, 0.4 mg IV.
  - ▲ Myasthenic crisis
    - Most likely cause is infection with undertreatment of myasthenia gravis.
    - A potential respiratory emergency!
  - ▲ Myasthenic vs. cholinergic
    - Distinguish the two types of crisis by a test dose of edrophonium (Tensilon)—2 mg IV of edrophonium usually increases muscle weakness if the patient is on the verge of a cholinergic crisis. If no change in muscle activity occurs after the initial dose, an additional 8 mg of edrophonium, for a total of 10 mg, may be administered.
    - Patients experiencing a myasthenic crisis typically improve with edrophonium.

Corticosteroids

- Acute complications—Administration of corticosteroids can cause a transient exacerbation of weakness within the first 5-7 days after administration (lasting 1-20 days).
- Chronic complications—Long-term corticosteroid use can cause a myriad of adverse effects.

DIAGNOSTIC STRATEGIES

- Diagnosis is based on history, physical exam, anti-cholinesterase testing, and lab studies.

Physical Exam

- Examine using provocative maneuvers to induce weakness by asking the patient to do the following:
  - ▲ Look up without closing the eyes for 1 minute
  - ▲ Count loudly from 1 to 100
  - ▲ Hold the arms elevated for 3 minutes
  - ▲ Perform repeated deep knee bends (normal, 10-20)

Anticholinesterase Tests

- Edrophonium (Tensilon) test—initial dose is 2 mg IV. If no response or side effects, give 8 mg IV. A positive test shows improvement of strength within 30 seconds after administration. (Use atropine 0.4 mg IV as antidote for severe bradycardia.)
- Atropine-neostigmine test—0.5 g atropine IM (control), then 1.5-2.0 mg neostigmine IM. A positive test shows improvement within 10 minutes after administration.

Lab Studies

Electrophysiology Testing

- Repetitive motor stimulation at 2-3 Hz—A decrease >15% in amplitude of the compound muscle action potential is highly suggestive of myasthenia gravis.
- Single fiber EMG—This assesses the temporal variability between two muscle fibers within the same motor unit (jitter) commonly seen in myasthenia gravis. It is highly sensitive but less specific than repetitive stimulation and technically difficult to perform.

Anti-AChR Antibodies

- Diagnostic test of choice
- Detection of anti-AChR antibodies is positive in
  - ▲ Nearly 100% of patients with moderately severe disease
  - ▲ 80% with mild generalized disease
  - ▲ 50% with ocular myasthenia gravis
  - ▲ Only 25% of those in remission
- Highly sensitive and specific assay

Other Studies

- MRI, CT of mediastinum to detect thymoma

MANAGEMENT OF ACUTE AND CHRONIC CONDITION

Acute Crisis

- Weakness sufficient to cause respiratory failure

General Measures

- Temporarily stop anticholinesterase drugs to rule out cholinergic crisis.
- Most common cause of myasthenic crisis is infection: look for it!
- Myasthenic patient with fever and infection should be treated the same way as any immunocompromised patient.
- Manage respiratory assistance in ICU.

Supportive Management

- May include intubation, tracheostomy, artificial ventilation, respiratory therapy, antibiotics, and nasogastric tube and/or gastrostomy.

Medical Therapy

- Pyridostigmine bromide (Mestinon)—first-line treatment
  - ▲ For daytime use, 60-mg tablets and for nighttime use, 180-mg sustained release tablets. Elixir is available.
  - ▲ Titrate dosage to symptoms (average dose, 600 mg/day).
  - ▲ Initial dose, 60 mg every 3-4 hours
  - ▲ Effects are apparent within 15-30 minutes and peak 1-2 hours after administration.
  - ▲ Increase dose 30 mg every several days as tolerated.
  - ▲ Watch for muscarinic side effects (diarrhea, abdominal cramps, salivation, nausea).
- Neostigmine methylsulfate (Prostigmin)
  - ▲ Concentrations of 0.25, 0.5, and 1 mg/mL
  - ▲ Titrate dosage to clinical need (starting dosages, 0.5 mg SQ or IM every 3 hours or continuous IV infusion at 1/45 of the total daily dose of pyridostigmine over 24 hours if unable to take oral medications).

- Plasmapheresis
  - ▲ Indication—severe generalized or fulminating myasthenia gravis refractory to other forms of treatment
  - ▲ Three to four daily exchanges of 2 L of plasma result in objective improvement and decreased AChR antibody titer.
- Prednisone
  - ▲ Initial dose, 60-80 mg daily

Long-Term Therapy
General Management
- Encourage patients to listen to their bodies!
- Advise them to avoid intense exercise and sick contacts.
- Update immunizations with Pneumovax and influenza vaccines.

Medical Therapy
Prednisone
- Alternate-day prednisone treatment induces remission or markedly improves the disease in >50% of patients (average time, 5 months).
- After improvement reaches a plateau, gradually lower the dose over several months to establish minimal maintenance dose (typically 35 mg every other day).

Azathioprine
- 150-200 mg daily (2-3 mg/kg daily) induces remissions in >50% of patients in 3-12 months.
- Survey for side effects (pancytopenia, leukopenia, serious infection, and hepatocellular injury).
- Azathioprine as adjunct to alternate-day prednisone reduces maintenance dose of prednisone required, lessening side effects.

Mycophenolate Mofetil
- 1,000 mg twice daily may control symptoms more quickly than azathioprine.
- Requires similar monitoring for side effects as azathioprine

Cyclophosphamide
- 150-200 mg daily

Immune Globulin

- IV immunoglobulin at 400 mg/kg for 5 consecutive days may improve severe disease within 2-3 weeks.

Cyclosporine

- Is equally effective as azathioprine, with more rapid onset of benefit
- Usual dose, 4-5 mg/kg daily, given in two divided doses
- Relatively high risk of renal dysfunction and hypertension

Thymectomy

- Increases remission rate and improves clinical course of disease
- Although controlled clinical studies of thymectomy according to age, sex, severity, and duration of disease have never been performed, there is general agreement that the best response occurs in young women with hyperplastic thymus glands and high antibody titer.
- Generally recommended routinely to patients with myasthenia who are younger than 40 years; rarely recommended if older than 60 years

NEUTROPENIA

Tait D. Shanafelt, M.D.
Rafael Fonseca, M.D.

IS THE PATIENT'S LIFE AT RISK?

- Common infections can be life threatening *in hours* in neutropenic patients.
- Neutropenia may be the first manifestation of acute leukemia that requires prompt evaluation and chemotherapeutic treatment.

ADDRESSING THE RISK

- It is critical to instruct patients who are or may become neutropenic (i.e., after chemotherapy) to *call immediately* when fever or symptoms of infection develop.
  - ▲ Instruct them *not* to take antipyretics and "wait until morning."
  - ▲ Neutropenic fever should always be treated as an emergency.
- Fever (>38.0°C) or symptoms of infection (cough, sore throat, rash, diarrhea) require immediate evaluation in neutropenic patients.

DIFFERENTIAL DIAGNOSIS

- Neutropenia is defined by an absolute neutrophil count <1.5 × 10^9/L.
  - ▲ Absolute neutrophil count = total WBCs × % neutrophils
- Severity of the neutropenia is clinically important, with risk of infection increasing substantially with neutrophil counts <0.5 × 10^9/L.
- Most patients with neutropenia have a known malignancy and experience neutropenia because of myelosuppressive effects of chemotherapy.

Special abbreviations used in this chapter: HSV, herpes simplex virus; MRSA, methicillin-resistant *Staphylococcus aureus*.

- A short differential of the causes of neutropenia is listed in Table 1.

DIFFERENTIATING THE DIFFERENTIAL

- Patients with de novo neutropenia (i.e., no recent chemotherapy)
  - ▲ Evaluate blood smear for blasts.
  - ▲ Stop offending medications (see list in Table 1).
  - ▲ Check vitamin B_{12}, folate, HIV, antinuclear antibody.
  - ▲ Consider bone marrow biopsy.
  - ▲ Perform peripheral blood T-cell gene rearrangement study, and consider flow cytometry to identify a large granular lymphocyte disorder.
  - ▲ Consult hematology.
- Differentiating the causes of neutropenic fever
  - ▲ General principle—Neutropenic patients have limited ability to mount an inflammatory response. Typical signs and symptoms of infection are often absent.
  - ▲ History
    - • Date of last chemotherapy? (Review expected timing and duration of neutropenia for a given chemotherapeutic protocol, often 7-14 days after treatment.)
    - • Does patient have indwelling catheter? (Raises question of line infection)
    - • Does patient have symptoms of cough, sore throat, rash, diarrhea, cold sores, abdominal pain?
    - • Does patient have history of cold sores? (Raises question of herpes simplex virus [HSV] infection)

Table 1. Causes of Neutropenia

Chemotherapy

Hematologic disorders—acute leukemia, lymphoma, myelodysplastic syndrome, aplastic anemia, myelofibrosis, congenital disorders

Infectious—Epstein-Barr virus, HIV, cytomegalovirus, TB, malaria

Medication—ticlopidine, propylthiouracil, olanzapine, clozapine, gold, penicillin, sulfa, ganciclovir, NSAIDs, carbamazepine, phenytoin, valproic acid, furosemide, thiazides, tricyclic antidepressants

Nutritional—vitamin B_{12} deficiency, folate

Other—systemic lupus erythematosus, Felty syndrome, myelophthisis, cyclic neutropenia

▲ Physical exam
  - Examine oropharynx, lungs, abdomen, skin (search for source of infection).
  - Inspect site of indwelling catheters for erythema or drainage (search for evidence of line infection).
  - Evaluate dentition (search for oral abscess and likelihood of anaerobic infection).
  - Inspect perineal region for abscess, and palpate perianal area. Standard practice is to avoid the rectal exam, but evidence supporting this practice is lacking.

TEST ORDERING

- CBC with differential and absolute neutrophil count
- Pan culture (blood, urine, sputum). Draw blood specimens from each lumen of indwelling lines for culture studies. Include fungal cultures of blood.
- Urinalysis (patients with neutropenia often do not have pyuria even if they have urinary tract infection)
- Liver function tests
- BUN, creatinine
- Chest X-ray (may fail to show consolidation when absolute neutrophil count is low)
- Directed imaging by symptoms (sinus CT if sinus pain or drainage; abdominal CT if abdominal pain, evaluate for typhlitis)
- If new murmur and bacteremic, consider echocardiography (possible secondary seeding of heart valves).

MANAGEMENT OF NEUTROPENIC FEVER

- Admit patient.
- Empiric treatment with broad-spectrum antibiotics for *all* patients
  - ▲ Imipenem-cilastatin, cefepime, ceftazidime, ticarcillin are all acceptable (select on basis of the formulary and local sensitivities).
- Add vancomycin empirically if evidence of line infection on physical exam or if preliminary culture grows gram-positive cocci.

- ▲ Many centers add vancomycin empirically for all neutropenic bone marrow transplant patients at onset of fever.
- ▲ Vancomycin should also be added empirically for nosocomial neutropenic fever if incidence of methicillin-resistant *Staphylococcus aureus* (MRSA) is high (>5%) in your facility.
- ■ Add acyclovir if cold sores or HSV-appearing lesions are present.
- ■ Add anaerobic coverage (metronidazole, clindamycin, imipenem-cilastatin) if abdominal pain is consistent with typhlitis (right lower or right upper quadrant tenderness on palpation).
- ■ Add oral fluconazole if patient has oral thrush.
- ■ Admit patient to monitored bed if systolic blood pressure is <100 mm Hg.
  - ▲ Neutropenic patients *do not* manifest typical signs of sepsis and require close monitoring.
- ■ Tunnel infections at site of indwelling catheter require removal of the line.
  - ▲ Some line infections can be treated through the line without removal (*Staphylococcus epidermidis*).
  - ▲ Consult hematology or infectious disease for assistance if line culture is positive.
- ■ If patient remains febrile without a source, consider what infections the antibiotics are not covering—possible abscess, viral infection (HSV, varicella-zoster virus), MRSA, *Clostridium difficile*, atypical bacteria, anaerobes, *Pneumocystis carinii* pneumonia, fungal infections.
- ■ If patient remains febrile without source on hospital day 4-5, add empiric antifungal coverage to cover *Candida* and *Aspergillus* (amphotericin, 1 mg/kg)
- ■ Fulminant sepsis >3-6 hours despite appropriate antibiotics should raise suspicion of *Clostridium septicum*.
  - ▲ Start anaerobic antibiotic coverage (metronidazole, clindamycin, imipenem-cilastatin) and perform physical exam to identify possible site of necrotizing fasciitis requiring surgical debridement.
- ■ If possible source of infection is identified, add specific antibiotic coverage for that infection but *do not* narrow broad-spectrum coverage.
- ■ Continue to reculture at least once every 24 hours if patient remains febrile.

Use of Growth Factors in Neutropenic Fever

- The value of routine use of growth factors (i.e., G-CSF, GM-CSF) is debatable and they cannot be recommended at this time.
  - ▲ Primary effect—to shorten the duration of neutropenia or hospitalization by approximately 24 hours without affecting mortality
  - ▲ Consult a hematologist before initiating growth factor therapy.

PANCREATITIS

Marina G. Silveira, M.D.
Suresh T. Chari, M.D.

DEFINITION AND PATHOGENESIS

- Acute or chronic inflammatory process of the pancreas, with variable involvement of other regional tissues or remote organ systems
- Pathogenetic mechanisms are not fully understood.
- Acute and chronic pancreatitis appear to involve different pathophysiologic processes (Table 1).
  - ▲ In most cases, acute pancreatitis probably does not lead to chronic pancreatitis.
  - ▲ Currently, the acute and chronic forms are differentiated on the basis of radiographic and histologic features.
  - ▲ Acute and chronic pancreatitis are compared in Table 2.

ACUTE PANCREATITIS

Etiology

- The etiology of acute pancreatitis is outlined in Table 3.

EPIDEMIOLOGY

- Incidence—4.8-24.2/100,000
- Incidence increases with age (peak age, 50-60 years).
- Gallstone disease—more common in women
- Alcoholic disease—more common in men
- Threefold more common in black men than white men

CLINICAL PRESENTATION

- The signs, symptoms, and severity of acute pancreatitis are listed in Tables 4, 5, and 6, respectively.

Special abbreviations used in this chapter: APACHE, acute physiologic assessment and chronic health evaluation; ERCP, endoscopic retrograde cholangiopancreatography.

Table 1. Pathophysiology of Acute and Chronic Pancreatitis

	Acute pancreatitis	Chronic pancreatitis
Presumed initiating event	Inappropriate intra-pancreatic activation of zymogens	Incompletely understood Hypotheses include: Duct obstruction due to protein plugs Toxic effects of chronic alcohol use Repeated episodes of pancreatitis lead to chronic scarring (necrosis-fibrosis sequence)
Aggravating events	Ischemia (transformation from mild edematous pancreatitis to severe necrotizing form)	Ischemia, free radicals, immune-mediated insult
Pancreatic morphology	Normal before attack Unless parenchyma is lost from necrosis, structure returns to normal after pancreatitis resolves	Usually associated with permanent, often progressive, alteration in pancreatic structure Changes include varying degrees of edema, acute inflammation, & necrosis superimposed on chronic changes, e.g., fibrosis, inflammation, loss of exocrine tissue

Complications
- Acute complications are listed in Table 7.

DIAGNOSTIC STRATEGIES
- Acute pancreatitis can be suspected clinically.
- Confirmation requires biochemical or radiologic evidence.
- All features must be considered together.
- Clinical
  - Acute upper abdominal pain

Table 2. Comparison of Features of Acute and Chronic Pancreatitis

	Acute	Chronic
Etiology (most common)	Alcohol, gallstones	Alcohol
Epidemiology	Men, women Age: 50-60s	Men Age: 35-45
Clinical presentation	Acute abdominal pain	Abdominal pain can be recurrent, continuous, or absent
Common diagnostic tests	Amylase/lipase, CT	Abdominal X-ray, CT, ERCP, pancreatic function tests
Management	Pain management Fluids Removal of precipitating factors (e.g., common bile duct stone)	Alcohol abstinence Pain management Treatment of pancreatic insufficiency (endocrine/exocrine) Treatment of complications
Common complications	Local—necrosis & infection Pancreatic fluid collections Systemic—organ failure	Pseudocysts Bile duct or duodenal obstruction
Prognosis	Excellent if mild disease High morbidity/mortality if necrotizing, especially if infected	Good long-term survival High morbidity due to complications Death often a complication of chronic alcohol & tobacco abuse

ERCP, endoscopic retrograde cholangiopancreatography.

Table 3. Etiology of Acute Pancreatitis*†

Obstruction	**Gallstones**, biliary sludge, microlithiasis Ampullary or pancreatic tumors (primary or metastatic) Less common—pancreas divisum with accessory-duct obstruction, choledochocele, periampullary duodenal diverticula, hypertensive sphincter of Oddi, worms or foreign bodies (occluded pancreatic duct stent) obstructing papilla
Toxins	**Ethanol**, methyl alcohol, scorpion venom, organophosphorus insecticides
Drugs	
Definite	**Didanosine**, pentamidine, metronidazole, stibogluconate, sulfonamides, tetracycline, furosemide, thiazides, sulfasalazine, 5-ASA, **azathioprine**, **6-mercaptopurine**, valproic acid, L-asparaginase, sulindac, salicylates, calcium, estrogen, tamoxifen
Probable	Nitrofurantoin, ethacrynic acid, diazoxide, warfarin, cimetidine, ranitidine, quinidine, acetaminophen, ACE inhibitors, methyldopa, clonidine
Metabolic abnormalities	**Hypertriglyceridemia** (hyperlipoproteinemia types I, II, VI or acquired causes, e.g., poorly controlled diabetes mellitus, obesity, drug-induced, nephrotic syndrome, hypothyroidism, pregnancy, glucocorticoid excess) **Hypercalcemia**
Infectious	
Parasitic	**Ascariasis**, clonorchiasis, toxoplasmosis, cryptosporidiosis
Viral	Mumps, rubella, hepatitis A & B, coxsackievirus, echovirus, adenovirus, CMV, HSV, varicella, EBV, HIV
Bacterial	*Mycoplasma, Campylobacter jejuni, Mycobacterium tuberculosis, M. avium* complex, *Legionella, Leptospira, Salmonella*
Fungal	*Aspergillus*
Inherited	Pancreas divisum, choledochocele type V, **hereditary gene mutations**
Vascular abnormalities	Ischemic pancreatitis (e.g., postoperative hypoperfusion) Atherosclerotic emboli Vasculitis (SLE, polyarteritis nodosa, malignant hypertension)

Table 3 (continued)

Trauma	
Accidental	Blunt or penetrating trauma to abdomen
Iatrogenic	**Post-ERCP** (especially after therapeutic intervention or manometry of sphincter of Oddi), postoperative
Miscellaneous	Penetrating peptic ulcer, Crohn disease, renal transplantation
Idiopathic	

ACE, angiotensin-converting enzyme; CMV, cytomegalovirus; EBV, Epstein-Barr virus; ERCP, endoscopic retrograde cholangiopancratography; HSV, herpes simplex virus.

*Gallstones and ethanol abuse account for 75% of cases.

†Items in bold are common causes for the category.

- Biochemical
  - Many tests are available but none has proved superior to amylase or lipase for diagnosis, although pancreatic isoamylase has the best sensitivity and specificity of all markers (Table 8).
  - For etiologic determination:
    - ALT— ≥3-fold increase from baseline specific for biliary pancreatitis
    - Serum triglycerides—usually >1,000 mg/dL to cause pancreatitis
    - Serum calcium—should be repeated after resolution of attack to avoid false-negative results
  - Biochemical tests available are listed in Table 9.
- For prognostic evaluation—CBC, fasting glucose, LDH, AST, BUN, serum calcium, arterial blood gases (see Ranson criteria below)
- Imaging—crucial for confirming diagnosis and determining cause
  - Plain films
    - Inexpensive and easy to obtain at bedside if necessary
    - Useful for ruling out life-threatening causes of abdominal pain, e.g., bowel obstruction or perforation

- Findings are nonspecific, and additional testing is usually needed.
- Abdominal X-ray—Findings are normal in mild disease; "sentinel" loop (small-bowel ileus) or colon "cut-off sign" (descending colon spasm due to severe inflammation) or diffuse ileus seen in severe disease.
- Chest X-ray—Findings are abnormal in about 1/3 of patients and include elevation of hemidiaphragm, pleural effusions, basal atelectasis, pulmonary infiltrates, and acute respiratory distress syndrome.

Table 4. Signs of Acute Pancreatitis

Systemic features	Fever, tachycardia; in severe cases, even shock and coma
	Jaundice (if obstruction present)
Abdominal exam	Mild—epigastric tenderness
	Severe—abdominal distension (especially epigastric), tenderness, guarding
Respiratory	Dyspnea, shallow breathing, pleural effusions
Hemorrhagic complications (uncommon)	Grey Turner sign (flank ecchymosis), Cullen sign (periumbilical ecchymosis)
Miscellaneous (rare)	Epigastric palpable mass (pseudocyst), SQ evidence of fat necrosis (panniculitis), thrombophlebitis of lower extremities, polyarthritis

Table 5. Symptoms of Acute Pancreatitis

Acute abdominal pain (90%-95% of patients)
Quality—steady
Location—midepigastrium, right upper quadrant, diffuse, left upper quadrant
Duration—up to days
Radiation—bandlike with radiation to back (50% of patients)
Provocative factors—postprandial (biliary), alcohol binge/cessation (alcoholic)
Relieving factors—bending forward and/or sitting upright
Nausea and vomiting (90% of patients)
Restlessness, agitation

Table 6. Severity of Acute Pancreatitis

Mild	Minimal or no organ dysfunction
	No local complications
	Uneventful recovery
Severe	Manifests as organ failure and/or local complications
	(e.g., necrosis, abscess, or pseudocyst)
	≥3 of Ranson's 11 criteria present
	APACHE-II score >8

APACHE, acute physiologic assessment and chronic health evaluation.

Table 7. Acute Complications of Pancreatitis

Local	Systemic	
Pancreatic necrosis— sterile or infected	Shock	SQ nodules
Pancreatic-fluid collections—pseudocysts or abscesses	Coagulopathy	Purtscher angiopathic retinopathy & acute blindness
Bowel necrosis & necrotizing obstruction or fistulization of colon	Respiratory failure & ARDS	
GI hemorrhage—ulceration, gastric varices, rupture of pseudoaneurysm	Acute renal failure	Pancreatic encephalopathy
Splenic vein thrombosis	Hyperglycemia	
Splenic rupture or hematoma	Hypocalcemia	
Hydronephrosis & hydroureter		

ARDS, acute respiratory distress syndrome; GI, gastrointestinal.

▲ Ultrasound
  • Not used routinely for diagnosis—Bowel gas obscures imaging of pancreas in 1/3 of patients, leading to incomplete examination.
  • Sensitive method for evaluating gallbladder, not as sensitive for common bile duct stones
  • Classic finding—diffusely enlarged, hypoechogenic pancreas.

Table 8. Current Diagnostic Approach

Test	Comments
Amylase	Increase ≥3 times upper limit of normal, cornerstone of diagnosis; returns to normal faster than lipase levels
	Many nonpancreatic diseases can also cause increased serum levels, especially <3 times elevated
	Combine with clinical and radiologic features for diagnosis
Lipase	Somewhat greater sensitivity & specificity than amylase
	Many nonpancreatic causes for elevation
	Useful for late presentation to physician
	Combination of amylase & lipase does not seem to improve diagnostic accuracy
	No prognostic role for serial measurement
	If amylase is increased without increase in lipase on repeated testing, consider macroamylasemia or nonpancreatic amylase increase
Pancreatic isoamylase	Not commonly ordered despite apparent superiority
	Useful when suspecting nonpancreatic amylase increase
Urinary amylase	Does not usually add important diagnostic information to serum enzyme levels except in macroamylasemia

▲ CT

- Most important test for diagnosis of acute pancreatitis and intra-abdominal complications and for assessment of severity of disease (see Balthazar-Ranson CT Severity Index below).
- In mild disease, CT may be normal.
- All patients whose condition is not improving or who have suspected complications should have CT.
- Contrast-enhanced CT—gold standard for noninvasive diagnosis of pancreatic necrosis (necrosis may not be apparent on CT in the first 24 to 48 hours after onset of pancreatitis)
- If infection is suspected, CT-guided aspiration can differentiate sterile pancreatic necrosis from infected necrosis.

Table 9. Biochemical Tests Available

Condition	Tests
Increased serum & urinary levels of pancreatic enzymes	Amylase, pancreatic isoamylase, lipase not clinically used
Increased serum levels of nonenzymatic pancreatic secretion	Pancreatitis-associated protein, trypsinogen activation peptide
Severity markers	Hematocrit, C-reactive protein

- Findings—edematous pancreas, areas of necrosis, peripancreatic inflammation, acute fluid collections, pseudocysts, abscess, hemorrhage into pancreas and surrounding areas
  ▲ MRI and magnetic resonance cholangiopancreatography
    - Increasing role in diagnosis and management of pancreatitis
    - Images are equal or superior to those of CT, without nephrotoxicity of contrast or invasive technique of endoscopic retrograde cholangiopancreatography (ERCP).
    - Limitations—higher cost and operator dependence
  ▲ ERCP
    - Diagnosis and treatment of common bile duct stones
    - Role when no definite cause of pancreatitis is found after initial investigation
    - Abnormalities shown—small pancreatic tumors, pancreatic ductal strictures, gallstones, pancreas divisum, choledochocele, hypertensive sphincter of Oddi.

MANAGEMENT
Mild Acute Pancreatitis
- ■ Supportive care
  - ▲ IV fluids
    - Generous fluid resuscitation because of third space loss, vomiting, diaphoresis
    - No "magic numbers," use clinical variables to guide amount of fluid.

- ▲ Pain control—parenteral narcotics usually required
  - • Fentanyl, morphine, meperidine, hydromorphone can be used (see Severe Acute Pancreatitis below)
- ▲ Oral intake is encouraged early and advanced from clear liquid diet to solid food as tolerated. Routine nasogastric tube is not necessary or beneficial (use only for gastric or intestinal ileus or intractable nausea and vomiting).
- ▲ Removal or management of factors that may have precipitated attack—cessation of alcohol use, cessation of drugs, insulin for poorly controlled diabetes with hypertriglyceridemia, reversal of hypercalcemia, early ERCP when indicated for gallstone disease (see Special Considerations—Gallstone Pancreatitis below)
- ▲ Not indicated—proton pump inhibitors or H_2-receptor blockers, prophylactic antibiotics

Severe Acute Pancreatitis
- ▪ ICU monitoring
- ▪ Fluid resuscitation
  - ▲ May need 5-10 L of fluid (normal saline or Ringer lactate) daily
  - ▲ Goal—keep hematocrit approximately 30%, may need packed RBCs if <30%
  - ▲ Unstable cardiovascular and pulmonary states may benefit from Swan-Ganz catheter placement to help guide fluid resuscitation.
- ▪ Pain control—IV narcotics, usually patient-controlled analgesia.
  - ▲ Fentanyl preferred
  - ▲ Hydromorphone for more severe pain
  - ▲ Morphine, despite theoretical increase in sphincter of Oddi pressure, no evidence of aggravating or causing pancreatitis or cholecystitis
  - ▲ Meperidine can be used but should be avoided because potentially toxic metabolites accumulate.
- ▪ Multiorgan support
  - ▲ Respiratory
    - • Oxygen for saturation <95% by nasal prongs or face mask
    - • Endotracheal intubation and assisted ventilation (in case of failure to correct hypoxemia or fatigue/respiratory insufficiency)

- Acute respiratory distress syndrome (serious complication)—endotracheal intubation with positive end-expiratory pressure ventilation and low tidal volume
- ▲ Cardiovascular
  - Complications such as congestive heart failure, acute myocardial infarction, arrhythmias, cardiogenic shock
  - Hypotension refractory to fluid resuscitation—dopamine drip
- ▲ Renal
  - Monitor urine output—adequate marker for tissue perfusion
  - Aggressive fluid resuscitation to prevent acute renal tubular necrosis
- ▲ Metabolic
  - Hyperglycemia—careful use of insulin (variable blood glucose with ongoing inflammation)
  - Hypocalcemia—only if decreased ionized calcium, supplementation with calcium gluconate/chloride
  - Hypomagnesemia—Supplementation may be enough to avoid symptomatic hypocalcemia.
- ■ Prevention of infection—IV prophylactic systemic antibiotics
  - ▲ Imipenem-cilastatin, quinolones, third-generation cephalosporins, piperacillin, mezlocillin, metronidazole
  - ▲ Prophylactic therapy for 5-10 days; after that, continue only if documented infection
  - ▲ Role for prophylactic antifungals is not clear, not routinely recommended.
- ■ Treatment of pancreatic necrosis
  - ▲ If sterile, no specific intervention is required
  - ▲ If infected, debridement (percutaneous, surgical, endoscopic) may be required.
  - ▲ Surgery consultation is recommended.
  - ▲ Usual approach is to initiate antibiotics once necrosis involving >30% pancreatic tissue is diagnosed by CT.
    - If no improvement after 1 week, perform CT-guided aspiration and necrosectomy or other debridement techniques if infection is present.

- If sterile, continue medical therapy for 4-6 weeks (patients usually do well medically).
- If suspicion for infection is high, consider repeating aspiration.
- Nutrition
  - Make every attempt to give enteral nutrition whenever possible to maintain intestinal barrier, to decrease bacterial translocation, and to avoid metabolic and catheter-related infectious complications associated with total parenteral nutrition.
  - Because of intolerance to oral intake, such patients usually require placement of jejunal feeding tube, either endoscopically or radiologically.
  - If goal rate is not achieved within 48-72 hours, provide supplemental parenteral nutrition.
  - Refeeding should be gradual once appetite returns and should not be dictated by lab studies such as CBC or amylase levels.
- Not proved to be beneficial—octreotide, somatostatin, calcitonin, gabexate mesilate, aprotinin, nasogastric decompression, H_2-receptor antagonists, anticholinergics, glucagon, fresh frozen plasma, peritoneal lavage

Special Considerations—Gallstone Pancreatitis
- Early ERCP and papillotomy for patients with severe acute biliary pancreatitis with obstructive jaundice (bilirubin >5 mg/dL) or cholangitis
- For patients without cholangitis or biliary obstruction, elective cholangiography (magnetic resonance cholangiopancreatography or intraoperative cholangiography) should be performed to exclude residual nonobstructing bile duct stones.
- Cholecystectomy—after recovery and preferably before hospital discharge for all patients with gallstone pancreatitis (delay of approximately 7 days for mild and at least 3 weeks for severe pancreatitis is reasonable)

COURSE AND PROGNOSIS
- Most attacks are mild; recovery is within 5-7 days. Death is unusual.
- Daily amylase or lipase tests to follow course of pancreatitis are not helpful. Patient's condition can worsen despite improving enzyme levels.

- Severe necrotizing pancreatitis—high rate of complications and marked mortality, especially when infection is present
- Risk of infection—increases with amount of necrosis and time from onset of acute pancreatitis (peaks at 3 weeks)
- Overall mortality in necrotizing pancreatitis, up to 30%.
  - ▲ Early deaths (<2 weeks) usually are due to severe systemic inflammatory response and multisystem failure.
  - ▲ Late deaths are due to local or systemic infections; 80% of these deaths are due to infected necrotizing pancreatitis.
- Mortality of infected necrotizing pancreatitis is approximately 30% compared with 10% for sterile necrotizing pancreatitis.
- Grading systems that combine clinical and lab data have been proposed to indicate the severity of pancreatitis and identify patients at risk for complications.
  - ▲ The most useful in practice are the Ranson criteria and acute physiologic assessment and chronic health evaluation (APACHE) II scores.
    - • Ranson criteria are based on 11 clinical signs with prognostic importance (Table 10).
    - • APACHE II is based on 12 physiologic variables, patient age, and any history of severe organ-system insufficiency or immunocompromised state.
    - • Advantages of APACHE II over Ranson criteria
      - – Can be used not only within first 48 hours after admission but throughout hospitalization
      - – May be the most accurate predictor of disease severity
- CT grading system—Balthazar-Ranson CT Severity Index (Table 11)
  - ▲ CT is probably the most helpful way to assess severity of acute pancreatitis, particularly when the results are combined with clinical scores.

CHRONIC PANCREATITIS
Classification

- Chronic calcifying pancreatitis—progressive disorder characterized by calcification and failure of pancreatic function, often despite removal of offending agent (e.g., abstinence in alcohol-induced pancreatitis)

Table 10. Ranson Criteria for Predicting Severity of Acute Pancreatitis*

Non-gallstone pancreatitis		Gallstone pancreatitis	
0 hour	**48 hours**	**0 hour**	**48 hours**
Age >55	Hematocrit ↓ by ≥10%	Age >70	Hematocrit ↓ by ≥10%
WBC >16 × 10^9/L	BUN ↑ ≥5 mg/dL despite fluids	WBC >18 × 10^9/L	BUN ↑ ≥2 mg/dL despite fluids
Blood glucose >200 mg/dL	Serum Ca <8 mg/dL	Blood glucose >220 mg/dL	Serum Ca <8 mg/dL
LDH >350 U/L	pO$_2$ <60 torr	LDH >400 U/L	
AST >250 U/L	Base deficit >4 mEq/L	AST >250 U/L	Base deficit >4 mEq/L
	Fluid deficit >6 L		Fluid deficit >4 L

*Presence of 1 or 2 criteria, mortality <1%; 3 or 4 criteria, 15%; 6 or 7 criteria, 100%.

- Chronic obstructive pancreatitis—result of pancreatic duct obstruction by any cause
  - ▲ Does not calcify
  - ▲ Cured by relief of obstruction

Etiology

- The causes of chronic pancreatitis are listed in Table 12.

Epidemiology

- True prevalence—not known
- Incidence—3-9/100,000
- Peak incidence—35-45 years
- Alcoholic disease—more common in men

Table 11. Balthazar-Ranson CT Severity Index (CTSI)*

Grade	Findings	Score
Grading based on findings on unenhanced CT		
A	Normal pancreas—normal size, sharply defined, smooth contour, homogeneous enhancement, retroperitoneal peripancreatic fat without enhancement	0
B	Focal or diffuse enlargement of pancreas, contour may show irregularity, enhancement may be inhomogeneous but there is no peripancreatic inflammation	1
C	Peripancreatic inflammation with intrinsic pancreatic abnormalities	2
D	Intrapancreatic or extrapancreatic fluid collections	3
E	Two or more large collections of gas in pancreas or retroperitoneum	4
Necrosis score based on contrast-enhanced CT		
Necrosis, %		
0		0
<33		2
33-50		4
>50		6

*CTSI = unenhanced CT score + necrosis score (maximum = 10). Severe disease ≥6.

Table 12. Causes of Chronic Pancreatitis

Chronic calcifying pancreatitis*
    Chronic alcohol use
    Hereditary pancreatitis
    Tropical pancreatitis
    Metabolic diseases (hyperlipidemia, primary hyperpara-
    thyroidism)
    Autoimmune (primary or associated with Sjögren syndrome,
    PSC, IBD)
    Idiopathic
Chronic obstructive pancreatitis
    Ductal obstruction (posttraumatic & postpancreatitis
    strictures, periampullary tumors, intraductal tumors)

IBD, inflammatory bowel disease; PSC, primary sclerosing cholangitis.
*Alcohol abuse accounts for 70%-90% of cases.

CLINICAL PRESENTATION

Signs and Symptoms

- Abdominal pain
  - ▲ Characteristics similar to those of acute pancreatitis
  - ▲ Early in disease course, may occur in discrete attacks but progressively tends to become more continuous
  - ▲ Absent in approximately 15% of cases
  - ▲ Findings may include epigastric or upper abdominal tenderness, fever, and epigastric mass (pseudocyst).
- Pancreatic insufficiency
  - ▲ Exocrine
    - Loss of >90% of pancreatic parenchyma leads to steatorrhea with malabsorption of fat, protein, and carbohydrates and malabsorption of vitamin B_{12} and fat-soluble vitamins.
    - Weight loss is usually prominent.
  - ▲ Endocrine
    - With >90% loss of tissue, glucose intolerance occurs.
    - Overt diabetes is rare, usually occurs in advanced disease.

Diagnosis

- Biochemical and imaging tests are listed in Tables 13 and 14, respectively.

Complications

- Complications of chronic pancreatitis are listed in Table 15.

Management

- General—abstinence from alcohol or other causative agents
- Pain management—guidelines recommend following step-wise approach:
  - ▲ Look for treatable causes of pain (e.g., pseudocyst) or pain unrelated to pancreatitis.
  - ▲ Abstinence from alcohol, nonnarcotics for pain
  - ▲ Eight-week trial of high-dose oral pancreatic enzymes with acid suppression (proton pump inhibitor or H_2-antagonists)
  - ▲ Consider celiac plexus block
  - ▲ Consider endoscopic treatment (preliminary evidence for endoscopic procedures, sphincterotomy, lithotripsy, pancreatic duct stenting)—At this point, consider narcotics and surgery.

Table 13. Biochemical Tests for Chronic Pancreatitis

Test	Comments
Amylase & lipase	Usually increased levels during acute flares but may be normal or only slightly elevated
Liver function tests	May be abnormal from alcoholic liver disease
	May be abnormal in 5%-10% of patients with intrapancreatic bile duct obstruction (edema/fibrosis)
72-Hour fecal fat	Increased if exocrine insufficiency present
Pancreatic function tests	Useful in cases of recurrent pain & negative imaging studies
	Negative results do not exclude chronic pancreatitis
	Usually done in combination with ERCP or endoscopic ultrasonography
	Most sensitive is secretin or CCK-stimulated pancreatic function test (requires approximately 60%-70% of tissue loss)

CCK, cholecystokinin; ERCP, endoscopic retrograde cholangiopancreatography.

Table 14. Imaging Tests for Chronic Pancreatitis

Test	Comments
Plain abdominal X-rays	Pancreatic calcifications (within ductal system, not in parenchyma) pathognomonic, present in up to 30% of cases
Transabdominal ultrasound	Pancreatic enlargement, ductal dilatation, pseudocyst
CT	Best noninvasive test
	May show calcifications & cysts not seen on plain X-rays
MRI/MRCP	Still under investigation
	Calcification often not seen
ERCP	Gold-standard for imaging diagnosis
	Not usually first test done
Endoscopic ultrasound	Operator dependent
	Picks up subtle changes in gland not seen on ERCP
	Role being evaluated

ERCP, endoscopic retrograde cholangiopancreatography; MRCP, magnetic resonance cholangiopancreatography.

- ▲ Usually short-term use of narcotics (preferably, long-acting fentanyl or morphine [MS Contin])
- ▲ Reserve surgical treatment for patients with severe pain not responsive to lesser tactics.
  - If duct dilatation is present (>6 mm)—surgical decompression and drainage (e.g., lateral pancreaticojejunostomy or Peustow procedure)
  - If absent—nerve ablation (unilateral or bilateral thoracoscopic splanchnic nerve resection or percutaneous celiac nerve block) or pancreatic resection (partial or complete, with or without pylorus and duodenum preservation)
- ■ Treatment of complications
  - ▲ PO pancreatic enzyme replacement for fat malabsorption
  - ▲ Resection, external drainage or internal drainage for pseudocysts that persist for >6 weeks, have signs of infection, or are rapidly enlarging or causing symptoms
  - ▲ ERCP with stenting of pancreatic duct leak for pancreatic ascites and pleural fistulas

Table 15. Complications of Chronic Pancreatitis

Pseudocysts	Splenic vein thrombosis	Endocrine insufficiency
Pancreatic ascites & pleural effusion	Bile duct or duodenal obstruction	Exocrine insufficiency
Hemosuccus pancreaticus	Pseudoaneurysm	Narcotic addiction
Pancreatic cancer		

▲ Relief of obstruction by pseudocyst decompression, endoscopic stenting, or surgical procedure for symptomatic bile duct or duodenal obstruction

Course and Prognosis
- Chronic pancreatitis leads to structural damage of pancreas and progressive loss of parenchymal tissue
  ▲ Chronic pain and exocrine and endocrine dysfunction may result.
- Association with pancreatic cancer—develops in about 4% of patients within 20 years, more frequent with tropical and hereditary pancreatitis
- Associated with various complications, of which pseudocyst and duodenal or bile duct obstruction are the most common
- Abstinence from alcohol may reduce frequency and severity of attacks.
  ▲ It also reduces risk of dying of alcohol-related nonpancreatic disease.
- Mortality
  ▲ Related mostly to lethal effects of alcohol and tobacco use
  ▲ About 15%-20% of patients die of complications of chronic pancreatitis.

PERICARDIAL DISEASES

Guilherme H. M. Oliveira, M.D.
James B. Seward, M.D.

DEFINITIONS

- Acute pericarditis—acute, painful inflammation of the pericardium that usually results in mild to moderate pericardial effusion
- Effusive-constrictive pericarditis—recurring bouts of acute pericarditis that eventually cause pericardial thickening and constrictive physiology
- Constrictive pericarditis—chronic pericarditis that causes global or localized thickening and loss of elasticity of the pericardium, with or without calcification, that leads to impaired ventricular filling and high intracavitary pressures, resulting in a syndrome of right-sided heart failure
- Pericardial effusion—abnormal amount of fluid in the pericardial space (>50 mL)
- Pericardial tamponade—acute hemodynamic compromise consisting of increased end-diastolic pressures, impediment to ventricular filling with low cardiac output, as a result of rapid and/or severe accumulation of pericardial effusion causing high intrapericardial pressures.

TYPES AND CAUSES OF PERICARDIAL DISEASE

- The types of pericardial diseases and their causes are listed in Table 1.

CLINICAL PRESENTATION

Acute Pericarditis

Clinical Setting

- Suspect acute pericarditis in patients who have
  - ▲ Low risk factor profile for coronary disease
  - ▲ Acute febrile illness

Table 1. Types and Causes of Pericardial Disease

Type	Cause	Acute symptoms	Effusion size	Constriction	Tamponade
Idiopathic	Up to 30% of cases	Very common	Small/moderate	Very rare	Almost never
Viral	Coxsackievirus, influenza, hepatitis A & B, HIV, enterovirus	Very common	Small/moderate	Very rare	Almost never
Bacterial	Staphylococci, streptococci, pneumococci, gram-negative bacteria	Infrequent	Variable	Common with staphylococci	Uncommon but possible
Mycobacterial	TB	Rare	Variable	Very common	Rare
Fungal	*Histoplasma*, coccidiodomycosis, *Candida*, *Aspergillus*	Variable	Variable	Uncommon	Uncommon
Metabolic/hemodynamic	Uremia, hypothyroidism, adrenal insufficiency, CHF, hypoalbuminemic states	Rare but common with uremia	Variable	Never	Possible with uremia
Rheumatologic	Rheumatoid arthritis, SLE, scleroderma, Wegener granulomatosis, sarcoidosis	Rare but common with SLE	Small but may be large with SLE	Rare	Rare but possible with SLE

Table 1 (continued)

Type	Cause	Acute symptoms	Effusion size	Constriction	Tamponade
Traumatic	Postcardiotomy syndrome, MI, radiation, blunt or perforating trauma, aortic dissection, esophageal fistula	Common postoperative cardiac and post MI	Variable	Uncommon, but common with radiation	Rare with Dressler syndrome & radiation, but common with dissection, myocardial rupture
Neoplastic	Primary tumors of pericardium (sarcoma, mesothelioma), metastatic tumors (renal cell, melanoma, lymphoma)	Uncommon	Large	Rare	Common
Drugs	Hydralazine, procainamide, amiodarone (drug-induced lupus)	Uncommon	Small to moderate	Rare	Rare

CHF, congestive heart failure; MI, myocardial infarction; SLE, systemic lupus erythematosus.

▲ Chest pain in the setting of another disease, e.g., upper respiratory tract illness, florid connective tissue disease, acute uremia

Symptoms
- Fevers
- Chest pain, pleuritic component—worsens in supine position and is relieved with leaning forward, may be indistinguishable from anginal pain

Signs
- Tachycardia
- 85% of patients have pericardial rubs.
- Atrial arrhythmias are not uncommon.
- Increase in jugular venous pressure depends on the physiologic significance of the effusion rather than on the size and should alert you to the possibility of tamponade.
- Distant heart sounds in very large effusions

Pericardial Tamponade
Clinical Setting
- Suspect tamponade in patients who
  - ▲ Acutely decompensate days after myocardial infarction (free wall rupture)
  - ▲ Have sudden onset of hypotension with high central venous pressure in the early post cardiac surgery period in the ICU
  - ▲ Have metastatic malignancy
  - ▲ Have had TB or systemic lupus erythematosus
  - ▲ Have aortic dissection or known thoracic aortic aneurysm
- Remember that the effusion does not need to be large for tamponade to occur: small effusions that develop in minutes to hours (e.g., myocardial puncture during right ventricular biopsy), very large effusions that develop over weeks to months (e.g., neoplastic effusions).

Symptoms
- Dyspnea is the main and most often the only complaint.
- Occasionally chest pressure or heaviness
- Light-headedness when progression is slow

Signs
- Tachycardia is universal.
- Most patients are hypotensive or relatively hypotensive compared with previous measurements of their blood pressure.
- Extremities are cold.
- Jugular venous pressure is invariably elevated.
- Tachypnea with borderline oxygen saturation
- Edema is present only if tamponade has been a very slow process.
- Fourth heart sound is usually present.
- Distant heart sounds are present only if progression is slow and effusion is very large.
- Pulsus paradoxus is the classic sign but is insensitive and a very late preterminal finding.

Constrictive Pericarditis
Clinical Setting
- Suspect constriction in patients who
  - Present with predominant right-sided heart failure
  - Had previous cardiac surgery
  - Present years after having radiotherapy to the chest
  - Have had several bouts of pericarditis in the past (effusive-constrictive)
  - Become rapidly prerenal when placed on diuretics without proportional fluid loss
  - Had TB

Symptoms
- Progressive dyspnea
- Increased abdominal girth
- Lower extremity swelling

Signs
- Increased central venous pressure
- Prominent x and y descent on jugular venous pulsations
- Kussmaul sign (increased jugular venous pressure with inspiration)
- Pericardial rub (15% of patients)

- Ascites
- Lower extremity edema
- Pericardial knock (protodiastolic dull sound, like a third heart sound but heard best in the left sternal border)

DIAGNOSTIC TESTS

Acute Pericarditis

Echocardiography
- Diagnostic gold standard in the right clinical setting
- Pericardial effusion
- "Sunburst" pattern of the pericardium (in pericarditis without effusion)

Lab Exam (Low Specificity, Low Sensitivity)
- Increased number of WBCs with lymphocytosis
- Increased ESR and C-reactive protein
- Mildly increased levels of cardiac enzymes
- Markers of other diseases—BUN, creatinine, antinuclear antibody, rheumatoid factor, antineutrophil cytoplasmic antibody, etc.

ECG (Low Sensitivity, Moderate Specificity)
- Sinus tachycardia or atrial arrhythmias (i.e., atrial fibrillation or flutter)
- Diffuse ST-segment elevation
  - In all walls
  - If in contiguous leads, suspect myocardial infarction or myocarditis.
- PR depression in inferolateral leads (II, III, aVF, V_5, V_6)
- Low voltage (in large effusion, insensitive)
- Electrical alternans (in very large effusions)
- Absence of Q waves, peaked T waves

Radiology
- Chest X-ray shows globular heart (low sensitivity, low specificity).
- CT of chest shows effusion (good sensitivity, useful to rule out other causes of chest pain, e.g., pneumonia, dissection, pulmonary embolism)

Cardiac Tamponade
Echocardiography
- The gold standard and only test necessary
- Pericardial effusion is usually circumferential but may be localized in patients after cardiac surgery.
- Right ventricular diastolic collapse (very specific, but may be insensitive in patients with very high right ventricular pressures, i.e., pulmonary hypertension)
- Atrial diastolic collapse (very sensitive but not very specific because it may occur in patients with normal hemodynamics)
- More than 25% respiratory variation of Doppler transmitral inflow velocities or >50% variation across the tricuspid valve (moderate sensitivity and good specificity)
- Hepatic vein and inferior vena cava dilatation with lack of inspiratory collapse (sensitive but not specific, has a high negative predictive value, i.e., if absent, makes tamponade unlikely even in the setting of a large effusion)

Lab Exam, ECG, Chest X-Ray
- No role in the diagnosis of tamponade—do not waste time!

Constrictive Pericarditis
Echocardiography
- The "gold standard"
- Respiratory septal displacement with ventricular interdependence (sensitive and good specificity)
- Thickened or calcified pericardium (insensitive)

Lab Exam and ECG
- Not helpful in the diagnosis

Radiology
- CT may show thickened pericardium (specificity increases with pericardial thickness and microcalcification).
- Chest X-ray, second-most helpful examination, may show pericardial calcification in 25% of cases.
- MRI shows thickened pericardium (will not show calcium).
- Constriction can occur with a normal pericardial thickness

Right and Left Heart Catheterization
- Only performed if necessary after echocardiography
- Ventricular interdependence (sensitive and specific)
- End-diastolic pressure equalization between the left and right ventricles (sensitive but not specific)
- Rapid descent, rapid increase, and plateauing of right ventricular diastolic pressure (square root sign)
- Prominent x and y descent on right atrial tracing
- The main difficulty in the diagnosis of constrictive pericarditis is differentiating it from restrictive cardiomyopathy.
  - ▲ It is usually necessary to use echocardiographic, hemodynamic, and radiologic data to establish either diagnosis.
  - ▲ At times, the diagnosis of constriction is so elusive that it can be confirmed only at surgery.

MANAGEMENT
Acute Pericarditis
- Idiopathic
- Viral—NSAIDs
- Bacterial—antibiotics with percutaneous or surgical drainage and pericardiectomy in some cases
  - ▲ Inadequate treatment may lead to constriction.
- Systemic lupus erythematosus, rheumatoid arthritis—corticosteroids
  - ▲ Effusions due to scleroderma do not respond to corticosteroids.
- Post-pericardiotomy syndrome—corticosteroids
- Dressler (late post-myocardial infarction) syndrome—corticosteroids or NSAIDs
- Early post-myocardial infarction revascularization
  - ▲ Avoid NSAIDs and corticosteroids for a week because they are associated with increased risk of myocardial rupture.
- Uremia—dialysis
- Hypothyroidism—thyroid hormone replacement

Tamponade
- Treatment is emergency echocardiography-guided pericardiocentesis for immediate pericardial decompression.
- Long-term strategy depends on the cause:
  - ▲ Malignant—prolonged drainage, window infrequently necessary

▲ Traumatic—surgical correction of trauma (i.e., dissection, rupture, perforation)
▲ Inflammatory—pericardiocentesis with pigtail catheter and treatment of underlying disease

Constrictive Pericarditis
■ Surgical pericardiectomy
  ▲ Surgical risk moderate
  ▲ Total pericardiectomy preferred
  ▲ Nerve injury complication (phrenic)

PNEUMONIA

David Allan Cook, M.D.
Randall S. Edson, M.D.

DEFINITION
- Pneumonia— cough, fever, and new infiltrate on chest X-ray (regardless of sputum production)
- Nosocomial pneumonia—new pulmonary infiltrate and fever developing after 48 hours of hospitalization

CLASSIFICATION AND ETIOLOGY
Community-Acquired Pneumonia
- "Typical" and "atypical" usually refer to organism causing disease; there is loose association with presentation (see below)

Typical
- *Streptococcus pneumoniae* most common (including AIDS)
- Other organisms—*Haemophilus influenzae*, *Moraxella catarrhalis*; occasionally *Klebsiella* sp or *Staphylococcus aureus*

Atypical
- *Mycoplasma pneumoniae* or *Chlamydia pneumoniae* (previously healthy, young)
- *Legionella* spp (elderly smoker)
- Viral (especially influenza depending on season)

Nosocomial Pneumonia
- Gram-negative rods (Enterobacteriaceae, *Pseudomonas aeruginosa*), *S. aureus*, *S. pneumoniae*, *Legionella*, anaerobes

Aspiration Pneumonia
- Often noninfectious chemical pneumonitis
  ▲ Develops within 2 hours after event

- ▲ Resolves in 4-5 days
- ■ True pneumonia is late development (>2 days after event), likely superinfection
    - ▲ Anaerobic bacteria are common—*Bacteroides*, *Peptostreptococcus*, *Fusobacterium*
    - ▲ Usual "bugs" (vary with clinical setting, i.e., community vs. nosocomial) are also still common (if infectious).

EPIDEMIOLOGY

Community-Acquired Pneumonia
- ■ 2,000,000 cases/year
- ■ 40,000-70,000 deaths/year
- ■ Major problem in geriatric population

Nosocomial Pneumonia
- ■ Most common hospital-acquired infection, complicating 0.3%-0.7% of hospitalizations
- ■ Risk factors
    - ▲ Intubation
    - ▲ Age >70 years
    - ▲ Chronic lung disease
    - ▲ Poor nutrition
    - ▲ Risk of aspiration (see below)
    - ▲ Thoracic or upper abdominal surgery
    - ▲ Immunosuppression

Aspiration Pneumonia
- ■ Risk factors
    - ▲ Altered consciousness—alcoholism, stroke, dementia, seizure, drug overdose, head trauma
    - ▲ Dysphagia—stroke, neuropathy, myopathy
    - ▲ Recent vomiting or gastroesophageal reflux disease
    - ▲ Nasogastric or endotracheal intubation

CLINICAL PRESENTATION
- ■ Classic presentation (often correlates with "typical" organisms) includes
    - ▲ Abrupt onset
    - ▲ High fever and chills
    - ▲ Cough productive of purulent sputum
    - ▲ Constitutional symptoms (malaise, fatigue), dyspnea

- Symptoms can be very nonspecific, especially among elderly or hospitalized patients
  - ▲ Nonspecific fever
  - ▲ Mental status change
  - ▲ Nonproductive cough
  - ▲ Pleuritic chest pain
- "Atypical" presentation—often, but not always, correlates with "atypical" organism
  - ▲ Often young, otherwise healthy (except for *Legionella* in elderly smoker)
  - ▲ Gradual onset and progression
  - ▲ Fever
  - ▲ Constitutional symptoms predominate
  - ▲ Nonproductive cough
  - ▲ "Chest X-ray worse than exam"
- Classic exam findings include
  - ▲ Fever
  - ▲ Abnormal vital signs—tachycardia, tachypnea, hypoxia
  - ▲ Abnormal lung exam—crackles, egophony, bronchial breath sounds

Complications
Respiratory
- No specific management
- Consider
  - ▲ Checking arterial blood gas values
  - ▲ Administering oxygen
  - ▲ Administering bronchodilators (albuterol, ipratropium) via metered dose inhaler or nebulizer
  - ▲ Invasive airway management

Empyema
- Purulent pleural effusion
- Often polymicrobial, multiple species of both aerobic and anaerobic bacteria (anaerobes found in up to 75% of cases)
- Diagnosis
  - ▲ Thoracentesis—cell count, LDH, culture, pH, glucose (in addition to whatever else you would order)

- ▲ Critical question—Does it need drainage? The answer is "yes" if
  - pH <7.1 (best single test)
  - LDH >1,000 U/L
  - Cell count >25,000/μL (>25 × 10⁹/L)
  - Glucose <40 mg/dL
- ■ Treatment
  - ▲ Drainage (chest tube)
  - ▲ IV antibiotics
    - Add clindamycin if not already in regimen (metronidazole is probably less effective).
    - Note that some antibiotics (aminoglycosides and some β-lactams) may be inactivated in presence of pus and low pH.

DIAGNOSTIC STRATEGIES

Community-Acquired Pneumonia

- ■ Outpatient
  - ▲ Chest X-ray (to make diagnosis)
  - ▲ CBC
  - ▲ Pulse oximetry
  - ▲ Decide whether to admit (see below)
- ■ Inpatient
  - ▲ Chest X-ray
  - ▲ Arterial blood gases
  - ▲ Lab—CBC, electrolytes, ALT, alkaline phosphatase, HIV if 15-54 years old and high prevalence in community
  - ▲ Blood cultures
  - ▲ Sputum—Gram stain is inexpensive and useful if positive.
    - Culture is less useful and in modern therapy has little effect on management.
  - ▲ Tap pleural effusion if present, send for cell count, pH, LDH, protein, glucose, Gram stain, and culture (acid-fast bacillus stain optional).
- ■ Determine severity of illness and triage according to the "Fine criteria" (Table 1).

Nosocomial Pneumonia

- ■ Evaluation
  - ▲ Blood culture for all patients
  - ▲ "Fine criteria" not validated on these patients—may not apply.

Table 1. "Fine Criteria" for Triage of Pneumonia

If all of the following are true:
    Age <50 years
    No history of CHF, cancer, stroke, renal disease, liver disease
    Vital signs: pulse <125, respirations <30, temperature <40°C
    & >35°C, SBP >90 mm Hg
    Mental status normal
Then triage to outpatient management ("Class 1")
Else, check BUN, sodium, glucose and use the following scoring
system:

	Score
Age	Age (years)
Female	−10
Nursing home resident	10
Active cancer	30
Liver disease	20
CHF, history of stroke, renal disease	10 each
Mental status change, respirations >30, or SBP <90 mm Hg	20 each
Temp >40°C or <35°C	15 each
Pulse >125	10
Presence of plural effusion	10
pH <7.35	30
BUN >30 mg/dL or sodium <130 mEq/L	20 each
Glucose >250 mg/dL, hematocrit <30%, pO_2 <60 mm Hg	10 each

CHF, congestive heart failure; SBP, systolic blood pressure.

▲ Consider obtaining sputum sample (deep suction, bronchoscopy, etc.).

Aspiration Pneumonia
- Evaluation—same as for community-acquired pneumonia
- Infiltrate is most common in superior segment (if patient was supine) or lower segments (if patient was erect) of right lower lobe.

MANAGEMENT
Community-Acquired Pneumonia
Outpatient
- Preferred

- ▲ Doxycycline is appropriate if patient is <50 years old and otherwise healthy.
- ▲ Erythromycin (most cost-effective), azithromycin, and clarithromycin are next choices.
- ▲ Levofloxacin, gatifloxacin, moxifloxacin (*not* ciprofloxacin) are extremely effective but expensive, and there is concern about encouraging resistance.
- ■ Alternative—amoxicillin-clavulanate (Augmentin), PO cephalosporin
- ■ Treat 7-10 days (afebrile at least 3 days), except azithromycin for 5 days total.

Inpatient
- ■ Standard—fluoroquinolone (levofloxacin, gatifloxacin)
  - ▲ First dose IV
  - ▲ Convert to PO dosing as soon as able.
- ■ Alternative—third-generation cephalosporin IV ± macrolide (if concern for "atypical")
- ■ Initiate antibiotics within 4 hours after admission
- ■ Treat 10-14 days (afebrile at least 3 days), except azithromycin for 5 days total.

Nosocomial Pneumonia
Nonneutropenic
- ■ Cefepime or ceftazidime or piperacillin-tazobactam (Zosyn)
- ■ If severely ill, add ciprofloxacin IV (or other antipseudomonal fluoroquinolone) or an aminoglycoside.
- ■ If question of aspiration, add clindamycin or metronidazole (not needed with piperacillin-tazobactam)

Neutropenic
- ■ Imipenem-cilastatin or as for nonneutropenic
- ■ Add vancomycin if line source is suspected.
- ■ If patient is still febrile on day 3, add amphotericin.

▶ Aspiration Pneumonia
- ■ Standard regimen (i.e., levofloxacin) + clindamycin or metronidazole
  - ▲ "Clindamycin above the diaphragm, metronidazole below the diaphragm" is quoted but is largely theoretical and based on scanty clinical evidence.

▲ Clindamycin is probably better in lung abscess.

■ Alternative—piperacillin-tazobactam or amoxicillin-clavulanate

General Measures for All Types of Pneumonia

Cough

■ Use combination expectorant (guaifenesin) or antihistamine (Phenergan) plus suppressant (codeine, dextromethorphan, benzonatate) –such as

▲ Robitussin AC 10 mL every 4 hours

▲ Robitussin DM 10 mL every 6 hours

▲ Phenergan with codeine 5 mL every 4 hours

▲ Tessalon Perles 3 times daily

Fever

■ Acetaminophen as needed

Hypoxia/Ventilation

■ Treat hypoxia! Oxygen as needed (saturation >89%)

■ Chest physiotherapy

■ Incentive spirometer

Dehydration or Inadequate Oral Intake

■ IV fluids as needed

Monitoring

■ Vital signs

▲ Rapid respirations and pulse can indicate decompensation.

▲ Fever should resolve in 48 hours with appropriate therapy.

■ Pulse oximetry (do not need to follow arterial blood gases for oxygenation)

■ Arterial blood gases if acidosis, hypercarbia

■ No need to monitor chest X-ray unless worsening of clinical status (takes weeks for infiltrate to resolve)

■ Initially, watch renal function, electrolytes, CBC daily and liver function tests if abnormal or every 3-4 days.

Pleural Effusion

■ Tap all effusions.

POISONINGS AND OVERDOSES

Geeta G. Gyamlani, M.D.
William F. Dunn, M.D.
Robert W. Hoel, Pharm. D.

DEFINITIONS
- Poisoning—harmful effects following exposure to chemicals
- Overdosage—exposure to excessive amounts of a substance normally intended for consumption

EPIDEMIOLOGY
- In the U.S., chemical exposures result in >5 million requests for medical advice or treatment annually.

DIAGNOSTIC APPROACH
History
- SATS (substance, amount ingested, time ingested, symptom)
- Obtain AMPLE (age and allergies, medications, past history of ingestions and past medical history, time of last meal because it may influence absorption, events leading to present condition) information
- Diagnosis of the exact substance involved in overdose or poisoning should never take precedence over stabilization of the patient.
- In case of self-ingestion, confirm the history by a second source whenever possible.
  - ▲ In suicide attempts, data provided by patient may be inaccurate or even contrived.

Physical Exam
- Vital signs should be recorded—heart rate, blood pressure, temperature, respiratory rate.
- Mental status should be categorized.
- Eyes—nystagmus, pupil size, pupil reactivity

Special abbreviations used in this chapter: CNS, central nervous system; D5W, 5% dextrose in water; GABA, γ-aminobutyric acid; NAC, N-acetylcysteine.

- Abdomen—bowel sounds, bladder size
- Skin—burns, bullae, color, warmth, puncture marks
- Breath—odor
- Physical exam findings may help characterize the poisoning as a classic "toxidrome," which can be extremely helpful, especially when the ingested agent is unknown (Table 1).

Lab Exam
- Will vary depending on individual scenario and clinical suspicions of an astute clinician
- The following studies may assist in the evaluation of selected patients:
  - Arterial blood gas—detects hypercarbia, hypoxemia, and important acid-base disorders
  - Anion gap—$Na^+ - (HCO_3^- + Cl^-)$ >12 mEq/L
  - Osmolar gap is the difference between measured and calculated osmolality.
    - $2 \times Na^+$ + glucose/18 + BUN/2.8
    - Osmolar gap >10 mOsm/L suggests presence of an osmotically active substance (ethanol, methyl alcohol, ethylene glycol, isopropyl alcohol, or acetone).
  - Drug screens for urine and plasma are necessary because many agents first detected in urine are then quantified in plasma.

Table 1. Classic Toxidromes

Poisoning	Symptoms
Cholinergic	SLUDGE—**s**alivation, **l**acrimation, **u**rination, **d**efecation, **g**astrointestinal upset, & **e**mesis
	Also bradycardia, confusion, miosis, & fasciculations
Anticholinergic	Dry skin, hyperthermia, mydriasis, tachycardia, delirium, thirst
Sympathomimetic	Hypertension, tachycardia, seizures, mydriasis, & CNS excitation
Narcotic	Miosis, respiratory depression, & depressed level of consciousness
Sedative, hypnotic	Depressed level of consciousness, respiratory depression, & hyporeflexia

CNS, central nervous system.

- ▲ Urine toxicology screens may detect agents not screened in plasma, including drugs of abuse.
- ▲ Plasma toxicology screens include drugs, many of which are tested quantitatively—acetaminophen, salicylates, carboxyhemoglobin, ethanol, methyl alcohol, ethylene glycol, theophylline, phenytoin, lithium, digoxin, barbiturates, and tricyclic antidepressants.
- ▲ Because of potential necessary alterations in drug extraction lab techniques (based on drug-specific dissociation constant [pKa, etc.]), the lab should be notified of the clinical suspicions about the type(s) of drug ingested.

MANAGEMENT (GENERAL)

- ■ Airway, breathing, and circulation
- ■ Patients with depressed level of consciousness should receive
  - ▲ 50% dextrose, 50 mL
  - ▲ Thiamine, 100 mg
  - ▲ Naloxone, 2-4 mg IV (especially with miosis and respiratory depression), repeated as necessary
  - ▲ Oxygen
- ■ Gastric lavage
- ■ Activated charcoal, 1 g/kg through orogastric or nasogastric tube
- ■ Enhanced elimination
  - ▲ Multiple doses of activated charcoal, 12.5 g/hour, for drugs with enterohepatic circulation (barbiturates, phenytoin, carbamazepine, tricyclic antidepressants, theophylline, digoxin).
  - ▲ Alkaline diuresis for barbiturate and salicylate toxicity
    - • 3 Ampules bicarbonate added to 1 L of 5% dextrose in water (D5W) IV starting at 2-3 mL/kg per hour adjusted to keep urine pH >7 and urine flow of 2-3 mL/kg per hour
  - ▲ Acidification of urine is controversial for ingestions involving amphetamines, quinine, and phencyclidine because risks outweigh benefits.
  - ▲ Hemodialysis
    - • Useful in elimination of water-soluble, low-molecular-

weight toxins (alcohols, amphetamines, phenobarbital, lithium, salicylates, theophylline, thiocyanate)
- Is most effective in removing drugs with low protein binding and low volume of distribution (VD)
  - VD = (amount drug ingested/plasma concentration) × 1/weight

SPECIFIC INTOXICATIONS

Acetaminophen
- Second leading cause of toxic prescription drug ingestion in the U.S.

Toxic Mechanism
- 95% of acetaminophen metabolism involves formation of sulfate and glucuronide conjugates that are then excreted by the kidney.
- 5% of the metabolism involves oxidation by cytochrome P450-dependent enzymes to *N*-acetyl-*p*-benzoquinoneimine (NAPQI), a toxic metabolite normally removed by conjugation with glutathione.
- Large doses of acetaminophen prompt increased use of the glutathione pathway, leading to depletion of glutathione and accumulation of the toxic metabolite.
- Predisposing conditions leading to toxicity are
  ▲ Depletion of glutathione (chronic alcohol ingestion, malnutrition, HIV infection)
  ▲ Drugs that enhance P450 microsomal enzymes (barbiturates, phenytoin, rifampin)

Clinical Features
- Nausea (first 24 hours)
- Evidence of liver toxicity—elevated aminotransferase levels, right upper quadrant tenderness (from 24 to 72 hours)
- Evidence of progressive hepatic injury and fulminant hepatic failure—encephalopathy, coagulopathy (after 72 hours)

Diagnosis
- The Rumack-Matthew nomogram is designed to determine potential acute hepatotoxicity and need for *N*-acetylcystein (NAC) treatment.
- A serum acetaminophen level above the lowest line on the

Rumack-Matthew nomogram between 4 and 24 hours after ingestion indicates possible hepatotoxicity and need for antidote therapy (Fig. 1).

- Ingestion of 150 mg/kg or more may be associated with acute hepatotoxicity; if 7.5 g or more is ingested, serum level should be measured.

Treatment

- Gastric lavage
- Activated charcoal
  - ▲ Interferes only slightly with NAC absorption
  - ▲ No dose adjustment needed for NAC
- NAC is a glutathione analogue that helps inactivate the toxic acetaminophen metabolite.

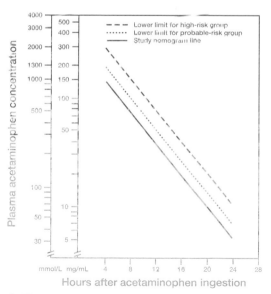

Fig. 1. Nomogram to define risk according to plasma concentration of acetaminophen. (Modified from Rumack BH, Matthew H. Acetaminophen poisoning and toxicity. Pediatrics. 1975;55:871-6. Used with permission.)

- Folic acid supplementation
- Lorazepam IV for seizures
- Lorazepam PO or IV for ethanol withdrawal syndrome

Ethylene Glycol
- Ethylene glycol is used as a solvent for plastics, paints, windshield cleaners, antifreeze, and deicer preparations.

Toxic Mechanism
- Ethylene glycol is oxidized by alcohol dehydrogenase to glycolic acid, glycoxylic acid, and oxalic acid, which cause CNS depression and interstitial and tubular damage to the kidney.

Clinical Features
- Nausea, vomiting, and abdominal pain
- Sweet aromatic odor to breath
- Slurred speech, ataxia, nystagmus, seizures, and coma
- Hypotension
- Pulmonary edema
- Oliguria, anuria, and acute renal failure

Diagnosis
- Serum ethylene glycol and glycolic acid levels
- Increased anion and osmolar gaps
- Oxalate crystals in urine
- Most commercial antifreeze preparations contain fluorescein, which causes urine to fluoresce under Wood lamp examination, thereby fostering a rapid presumptive diagnosis in the appropriate setting, pending confirmation by other studies.

Treatment
- Maintain a safe airway; intubate if necessary.
- Gastric lavage
- Activated charcoal if other substances are potentially ingested (does not absorb alcohols)
- 50% dextrose if indicated
- Thiamine, folic acid, and pyridoxine supplement
- Because alcohol dehydrogenase has a higher affinity for ethanol than for ethylene glycol or methanol, ethanol is administered orally or 5% or 10% ethanol in D5W IV to maintain ethanol blood level at 100-150 mg/dL.

- Fomepizole (methylpyrazole) inhibits the alcohol dehydrogenase enzyme, thereby slowing the metabolism of ethylene glycol or methanol.
- Hemodialysis for visual impairment (methyl alcohol), renal failure, pulmonary edema, significant or refractory acidosis, and ethylene glycol (or methyl alcohol) level >25 mg/dL

Methyl Alcohol
- Component of varnishes, paint removers, and windshield washer solutions and a denaturant that makes ethanol unfit for consumption

Toxic Mechanism
- Methyl alcohol is metabolized to formaldehyde and formic acid by alcohol dehydrogenase which injure the retina.

Clinical Features
- Nausea, vomiting, and abdominal pain
- Sweet aromatic odor to breath
- Slurred speech, ataxia, nystagmus, seizures, and coma
- Hypotension and bradycardia
- Ophthalmologic—clouding and diminished vision, flashing spots, dilated or fixed pupils, hyperemia of optic disc, retinal edema, and blindness

Diagnosis
- Serum levels of methyl alcohol
- Increased anion and osmolar gaps

Treatment
- Same as for ethylene glycol poisoning

Benzodiazepines
- Most commonly overdosed prescription drugs in the U.S.

Toxic Mechanism
- Potentiation of the inhibitory effects of γ-aminobutyric acid (GABA) on CNS by binding to the GABA receptors and

increasing frequency of opening of chloride channels in response to GABA stimulation

Clinical Features
- Dose-dependent depression in level of consciousness not usually accompanied by respiratory or cardiovascular depression
  - ▲ Airway protection, including intubation, may be necessary.

Diagnosis
- History
- Urine metabolites may be helpful, although a negative result does not exclude the diagnosis.

Treatment
- A benzodiazepine receptor antagonist (flumazenil) is available as a diagnostic and therapeutic tool.
- Flumazenil—0.2 mg over 15 seconds and 0.2 mg every minute up to a cumulative dose of 1 mg, titrated to effect
  - ▲ Doses from 3 to 10 mg have been necessary in some cases.
- Flumazenil reverses the sedative effects of benzodiazepines but is inconsistent in reversing the respiratory depression and should not be used as a substitute for intubation in patients with notable respiratory depression.
- Because of the risk of seizures, flumazenil is contraindicated for patients with mixed overdoses involving tricyclic antidepressants and patients physically dependent on benzodiazepines.
- Resedation is likely because of the short half-life of flumazenil compared with that of benzodiazepines.

Digoxin
- Of patients receiving digoxin, 25% develop toxic reactions, but most are non–life-threatening.

Toxic Mechanism
- Cardiac glycosides act by inhibiting sodium-potassium ATPase, leading to increased intracellular levels of sodium and calcium and a corresponding efflux of potassium, resulting in decreased intracellular potassium levels.

Clinical Features

- Nausea, vomiting, abdominal pain, and diarrhea
- Confusion, delirium, and hallucinations
- Blurred vision, xanthopsia (yellow vision), photophobia, and scotomata
- Premature ventricular contractions (most common), sinus arrhythmia, sinus bradycardia, all degrees of atrioventricular block, bigeminy, ventricular tachycardia, and ventricular fibrillation
- Acute toxicity is often exhibited by hyperkalemia, and in chronic toxicity, hypokalemia can be a predisposing feature.
- The combination of supraventricular tachyarrhythmia and atrioventricular block is highly suggestive of digitalis toxicity.

Diagnosis

- Increased serum levels of digoxin (3-5 ng/mL in chronic toxicity; very high levels, 50-60 ng/mL, usually seen with acute overdose)

Treatment

- Repeated activated charcoal doses to enhance elimination
- Hemodialysis, hemoperfusion, and diuresis are ineffective.
  - ▲ Patients with normal renal function clear ~30% of the total body amount and anuric patients, ~14%.
- Correct potassium, magnesium, and calcium abnormalities.
- Treat ventricular tachyarrhythmias with magnesium sulfate, phenytoin, or lidocaine.
- Immunotherapy with digoxin-specific Fab-fragment antibodies used for patients with potentially life-threatening toxicity not responsive to the above measures
  - ▲ Dose of Fab-fragment antibodies is calculated by estimating total body content of digoxin.
  - ▲ Each 40 mg (1 vial) of Fab-fragment antibodies binds to 0.6 mg of digoxin.
  - ▲ Usually 1-2 vials are sufficient for chronic digoxin toxicity, but 15-20 vials may be required for acute overdose.
  - ▲ Although free digoxin levels decrease rapidly to zero after antibody administration, routine methods used to measure

digoxin levels do not distinguish between bound and unbound drug; hence, drug levels do not correlate with toxicity after antibody therapy.
- ▲ May cause sensitization (to future doses) after administration
- ▲ Expensive

Salicylates
- Found in many over-the-counter drugs such as aspirin, bismuth salicylate (Pepto-Bismol), and oil of wintergreen.

Toxic Effects
- Increases sensitivity of the respiratory center to changes in PaO_2 and PCO_2, with an increase in rate and depth of respiration causing respiratory alkalosis
- Later causes uncoupling of oxidative phosphorylation and metabolic acidosis

Clinical Features
- Tinnitus, vomiting, diaphoresis, and hyperventilation
- Respiratory depression, convulsions, and coma
- Hepatotoxicity with prolonged PT
- Noncardiogenic pulmonary edema
- Cardiovascular collapse

Diagnosis
- Positive ferric chloride test in urine
- Serum salicylate levels
  - ▲ Mild— <40 mg/dL
  - ▲ Moderate— 40-100 mg/dL
  - ▲ Severe— >100 mg/dL
- Anion gap metabolic acidosis
- Respiratory alkalosis

Treatment
- Gastric lavage
- Activated charcoal
- Alkalization of urine to enhance elimination of salicylate if salicylate level >35 mg/dL
- Hemodialysis is indicated for salicylate levels >100 mg/dL, refractory seizures, alteration in mental status, or refractory acidosis.

Tricyclic Antidepressants
- Leading cause of death from pharmaceutical drug overdose in the U.S.

Toxic Mechanism
- Toxicity results from
  ▲ Anticholinergic actions
  ▲ Block of the reuptake of neurotransmitters such as norepinephrine

Clinical Features
- Pupillary dilatation, delirium, seizures, and coma
- Tachycardia, hypertension, hypotension, prolonged QRS interval (>0.10 second), and arrhythmias (ectopic beats) and wide complex tachycardia

Diagnosis
- Serum levels confirm ingestion but do not correlate well with clinical toxicity.
- Prolongation of QRS interval can be a prognostic sign of progression to seizures (QRS >0.10 second) and serious arrhythmias (QRS >0.16 second)

Treatment
- Maintain a secure airway.
- Stabilize vital signs.
- ECG monitoring
- Gastric lavage
- Activated charcoal
- Magnesium sulfate for torsades de pointes
- Benzodiazepines for seizures
- Norepinephrine or phenylephrine for refractory hypotension
- Alkalization of blood with sodium bicarbonate to a pH of 7.45-7.55 for prolonged QRS or wide complex tachycardia
- Bicarbonate is also useful for refractory seizures and hypotension.

PULMONARY THROMBOEMBOLISM

Ives R. De Chazal, M.D.
William F. Dunn, M.D.

DEFINITION

- Embolization of a thrombus (usually formed in deep veins of lower extremities, pelvis, or upper extremities) to pulmonary vasculature

CLASSIFICATION

- The clinical presentation may be classified as symptomatic, asymptomatic, or massive.

ETIOLOGY

- Pulmonary embolism (PE) most commonly results from deep venous thrombosis (DVT) of proximal deep veins of the lower extremities, including the popliteal veins.
- Hypercoagulability leading to the development of thrombosis occurs in patients with risk factors (Table 1):
  - ▲ Venous stasis, as with immobilization
  - ▲ Endothelial injury, as in surgery
  - ▲ Coagulopathy
  - ▲ Other risk factors include oral contraceptives or postmenopausal estrogen, pregnancy, and inherited or acquired hypercoagulable disorders (e.g., factor V Leiden).

EPIDEMIOLOGY

- Annually in the U.S., 250,000-300,000 patients are hospitalized with diagnosis of PE.
- One year mortality of up to 25% can be decreased to 2%-8% with treatment.
- Incidence doubles with each decade of life.

Special abbreviations used in this chapter: ABG, arterial blood gas; DVT, deep venous thrombosis; PE, pulmonary embolism; VTE, venous thromboembolism.

Table 1. **Hypercoagulable States**

Inherited
    Factor V Leiden mutation
    Antithrombin III deficiency
    Protein C deficiency
    Protein S deficiency
    Hyperhomocysteinemia
    Prothrombin 20210A
    Dysfibrinogenemia
    Impaired clot lysis
Acquired
    Disseminated intravascular coagulopathy
    Lupus anticoagulant
    Antiphospholipid antibody syndrome
    Myeloproliferative disorders
    Heparin-induced thrombocytopenia
    Hyperviscosity syndromes (e.g., Waldenström macroglobuli-
      nemia)
    Thrombotic thrombocytopenic purpura
    Malignancy

Data from Mateo J, Oliver A, Borrell M, Sala N, Fontcuberta J. Laboratory evaluation and clinical characteristics of 2,132 consecutive unselected patients with venous thromboembolism: results of the Spanish Multicentric Study on Thrombophilia (EMET-Study). Thromb Haemost. 1997;77:444-51.

- Estimate: clinically unsuspected PE occurs in 30%-50% of patients with DVT.
- In postoperative patients, asymptomatic PE occurs 4 times as often as symptomatic PE, thus the paramount importance of venous thromboembolism (VTE) prophylaxis.
- In up to 70% of patients who die of PE, diagnosis is not suspected before death; thus, a high index of suspicion must be maintained.

CLINICAL PRESENTATION
- Signs and symptoms are common but typically nonspecific.
- Most common presentation in symptomatic patients is unexplained dyspnea with or without chest pain.
- Symptoms—dyspnea (73% of patients), pleuritic chest pain (66%), cough (37%), and hemoptysis (13%)
- Signs—tachypnea (70% of patients), rales (51%), and tachycardia (30%)

DIAGNOSTIC STRATEGY

- Clinical approach to diagnosis of acute PE varies depending on
  - ▲ Patient factors (e.g., underlying lung disease)
  - ▲ Local institution-specific diagnostic and therapeutic capabilities
  - ▲ Hemodynamic status
- First, establish the degree of clinical suspicion (low, intermediate, or high) based on the risk factors, history, and physical exam and by excluding other conditions.
- Initial evaluation includes chest X-ray, arterial blood gases (ABGs), and ECG.
- ABGs—Patients with PE commonly have hypoxemia, hypocapnia, and thus increased alveolar-arterial gradient.
  - ▲ Although ABG findings are helpful in the evaluation, PE cannot be diagnosed based on these findings only because many conditions that mimic PE manifest with hypoxemia.
  - ▲ In PIOPED study, 8% of patients with PE had normal alveolar-arterial gradients.
- ECG—important for ruling out acute coronary syndrome and pericarditis.
  - ▲ Most common ECG finding is sinus tachycardia.
  - ▲ Classic S wave in lead I and Q and T waves in lead III findings and other signs of acute cor pulmonale (new right bundle branch block, P pulmonale, and right axis deviation) occur in <30% of patients with PE.
- Chest X-ray—Normal findings in setting of severe dyspnea and hypoxemia of acute onset strongly suggest PE.
  - ▲ Abnormal findings are common but nonspecific.
  - ▲ Classic findings such as focal oligemia (Westermark sign) and peripheral wedge-shaped density (Hampton hump) are suggestive but infrequent.
- Ventilation/perfusion (V/Q) lung scan—most useful initial evaluation tool, particularly in patients without preexistent lung disease
  - ▲ V/Q scan results are traditionally reported as normal, low probability, intermediate probability, and high probability.
  - ▲ Normal perfusion study result practically excludes PE, but a high-probability result warrants therapy.

- ▲ Combining the data of the degree of clinical suspicion and the results of the V/Q scan add to the accuracy of the evaluation (Table 2).
- ■ Venous ultrasonography—highly accurate study in patients with suspected DVT
  - ▲ A negative study cannot rule out PE.
- ■ Approximately 30% of patients with PE by pulmonary angiography have normal lower extremity ultrasound findings.
- ■ Positive lower extremity ultrasound findings require therapy.
- ■ Pulmonary artery angiography—"gold standard" for diagnosis of PE
  - ▲ Useful when clinical suspicion is low and other tests indicate PE
  - ▲ Also helpful in cases of high clinical suspicion of PE and nondiagnostic V/Q scan (and/or a negative ultrasound study of the extremities)
  - ▲ Complication rates have declined—mortality, 0.5%; major complications, 1%; minor complications, 5%
- ■ Other important diagnostic studies
  - ▲ D-dimer
    - • A fibrin degradation product that indicates activation of the coagulation pathway
    - • High in PE and DVT but also trauma, metastatic cancer, postoperative state, sepsis, late pregnancy, and advanced age
    - • When increased, its specificity ranges from 30% to 70%.
    - • A negative ELISA study virtually rules out PE, with a negative predictive value of 99%.

Table 2. Likelihood of Pulmonary Embolism in Settings of Various "Index of Suspicion" and Ventilation-Perfusion (V/Q) Scan Results

V/Q scan results	Clinical index of suspicion		
	Low	Intermediate	High
Normal	<2%	6%	<2%
Probability			
Low	4%	16%	40%
Intermediate	16%	28%	66%
High	56%	88%	96%

- ELISA is preferable to latex method.
▲ Spiral CT
  - Best for identifying PE in proximal pulmonary vasculature, may not identify distal emboli
  - With 70% sensitivity and 91% specificity, a negative study does not conclusively rule out PE
  - Allows study of lung parenchyma, possibly clarifying an alternative diagnosis
  - Has obviated the need for pulmonary artery angiography in many cases
▲ MRI
  - Preliminary studies suggest sensitivity of 75%-100% and specificity of 95%-100%.
  - May have the advantage in diagnosing DVT and PE at the same time and avoiding nephrotoxic contrast agents
▲ Echocardiography
  - Role in diagnosis of PE is undefined
  - May yield important information (i.e., with regard to right-sided heart strain) when evaluating acute hemodynamic compromise in patient with suspected massive PE

MANAGEMENT

- Start heparin promptly if clinical suspicion is moderate to high, in the absence of contraindications (e.g., gastrointestinal tract bleed), until definitive evaluation is complete.
- Warfarin should always be instituted within the course of heparinization.

Unfractionated Heparin

- Bolus of 80 U/kg and continuous infusion of 18 U/kg per hour
- aPTT goal—1.5-2 times normal value
- Adjustments are made according to aPTT results 4-6 hours later (Table 3).
- Complications—major bleeding, 2%-3% of patients; heparin-induced thrombocytopenia, 2.7%, with subsequent risk of thrombosis and osteoporosis

Table 3. Weight-Based Nomogram for Heparin Dosing

Initial dose	80 U/kg bolus, then 18 U/kg per hour
aPTT <35 seconds (<1.2 × control)	80 U/kg bolus, then 4 U/kg per hour
aPTT, 35-45 seconds (1.2-1.5 × control)	40 U/kg bolus, then 2 U/kg per hour
aPTT, 46-70 seconds (1.5-2.3 × control)	No change
aPTT, 71-90 seconds (2.3-3 × control)	Decrease infusion rate by 2 U/kg per hour
aPTT >90 seconds (>3 × control)	Hold infusion 1 hour, then decrease infusion rate by 3 U/kg per hour

From Raschke RA, Reilly BM, Guidry JR, Fontana JR, Srinivas S. The weight-based heparin dosing nomogram compared with a "standard care" nomogram: a randomized controlled trial. Ann Intern Med. 1993;119:874-81. Used with permission.

Low-Molecular-Weight Heparin

- May be as effective as unfractionated heparin in treating VTE with comparable major bleeding profile
- Advantages—conventional dosing and administration, no need to follow aPTT, thus facilitating outpatient treatment and potential for cost savings
- Heparin-induced thrombocytopenia can occur
- Disadvantages—higher drug cost and incomplete reversal by protamine
- Contraindicated in renal failure with creatinine clearance <30 mL/hour
- Enoxaparin sodium dose is 1 mg/kg SQ every 12 hours or 1.5 mg/kg SQ daily (not to exceed 180 mg daily).

Warfarin

- Warfarin can reduce protein C levels faster than factors II, IX, and X, creating a relative and transient (4 days) hypercoagulable state; thus, heparin is always started first.
- Heparin and warfarin should overlap until INR is 2.5-3 for 2-3 days.
- Load with warfarin 5 mg unless the patient weighs >85 kg, then use 7.5 mg.

- Duration of therapy
  - ▲ First event with time-limited risk factors—3-6 months
  - ▲ Idiopathic VTE—6 months
  - ▲ May treat with subtherapeutic warfarin (INR 1.5-2) life-long after check.
  - ▲ History of cancer, anticardiolipin antibodies, antithrombin deficiency, recurrent PE or thrombophilia—12 months to life

Thrombolytic Therapy
- Indicated for patients with massive PE and hypotension
- May improve pulmonary artery perfusion in 2 hours and be lifesaving
- Central administration offers no outcome advantage.
- If thrombolysis is contraindicated, catheter and/or surgical embolectomy may be considered.
- Incidence of intracerebral hemorrhage is 2%.
- Contraindicated in active bleeding and cerebral metastasis

Inferior Vena Cava Filters
- The two best filters are the Greenfield and Birds Nest
- Indicated in VTE when anticoagulation is contraindicated, VTE is recurrent despite anticoagulation, and when underlying cardiopulmonary status is so severe that recurrent PE may be fatal
- Filters do not halt DVT, and the incidence of DVTs distal to the filter may increase.
- Filters and anticoagulation do not decrease 2-year mortality compared with anticoagulation alone.

DVT Prophylaxis
- Approximately 2/3 of patients do not receive prophylaxis despite clear indications (Table 4).
- Incidence of DVT and fatal PE in orthopedic surgery patients (without prophylaxis) is reportedly as high as 30% and 14%, respectively.
- PE is the most common and preventable cause of hospital death.

Table 4. Examples of Level of Deep Venous Thrombosis Risk

Level of risk	Successful prevention strategies
Low—minor surgery in patients <40 years with no additional risk factors	No specific measures Aggressive mobilization
Moderate—minor surgery in patients with additional risk factors, non-major surgery in patients 40-60 years with no additional risk factors, major surgery in patients <40 years with no additional risk	LDUH* every 12 hours, LMWH,† ES, or IPC
High—Nonmajor surgery in patients >60 years or with additional risk factors, major surgery in patients >40 years or with additional risk factors	LDUH every 8 hours, LMWH,† or IPC
Highest—major surgery in patients >40 years plus prior VTE, cancer, or molecular hypercoagulable state; hip or knee arthroplasty, hip fracture surgery; major trauma; spinal cord injury	LMWH,† oral anticoagulants, IPC/ES plus LDUH*/LMWH,† or ADH

ES, elastic stockings; IPC, intermittent pneumatic compression; LDUH, low-dose unfractionated heparin; LMWH, low-molecular-weight heparin; VTE, venous thromboembolism.

*5,000 U SQ.

†For example, enoxaparin 30 mg SQ twice daily (orthopedic surgery) or 40 mg SQ daily (general surgery); dalteparin 2,500-5,000 anti-Xa units SQ daily.

SEPSIS

Axel Pflueger, M.D.
Timothy R. Aksamit, M.D.

DEFINITIONS AND CLASSIFICATION

- Standardization of terminology according to the 1992 American College of Chest Physicians/Society of Critical Care Medicine Consensus
  - ▲ Infection—inflammatory response to microorganisms
  - ▲ Bacteremia—presence of viable bacteria in blood
  - ▲ Systemic inflammatory response syndrome (SIRS)—inflammatory response to various insults
    - Is defined by ≥2 of the following:
      - Temperature >38°C or <36°C
      - Heart rate >90 beats/min
      - Respiratory rate >20 beats/min or $PaCO_2$ <32 mm Hg
      - WBC >10,000/mm³ (>10 × 10⁹/L) or <4,000/mm³ (>4 × 10⁹/L), >10% immature band forms
  - ▲ Sepsis—infection plus SIRS
  - ▲ Multiorgan dysfunction syndrome—inflammatory-mediated injury involving several organ systems in an acutely ill patient such that homeostasis cannot be maintained without intervention
  - ▲ Severe sepsis—sepsis plus multiorgan system dysfunction
  - ▲ Septic shock—severe sepsis plus hypotension refractory to fluids (systolic blood pressure <90 mm Hg or a decrease of ≥40 mm Hg from baseline in absence of other causes of hypotension plus hypoperfusion abnormalities, e.g., oliguria, lactic acidosis, acute change in mental status)

EPIDEMIOLOGY

- Incidence/prevalence in U.S.—176/100,000 persons/year
  - ▲ In U.S., at least 750,000 cases/year, and 225,000 are fatal.

Special abbreviations used in this chapter: ARDS, adult respiratory distress syndrome; SIRS, systemic inflammatory response syndrome.

- Mortality—30%-50%
- Ages affected—all
- Sex ratio—male = female
- Annual incidence increased 9% between 1979 and 2000
- Increased incidence contributions from aging population, increase and prevalence of immunocompromised patients, and more invasive support of critically ill patients

ETIOLOGY
Microorganisms
- Positive blood cultures—only in 30% of cases
- The predominant pathogens are listed below:
  - ▲ Gram-positive organisms in 25% of cases (most common)
    - *Staphylococcus aureus* in 14% of cases, including methicillin-resistant and methicillin-sensitive *S. aureus*
    - *Staphylococcus* sp in 6%
    - *Streptococcus pneumoniae* in 11%
    - *Streptococcus* sp in 9%
    - *Enterococcus* sp in 7%, including vancomycin-resistant and vancomycin-sensitive *Enterococcus*
    - Others in 4%
  - ▲ Gram-negative organisms in 17% of cases
    - *E. coli* in 17%
    - *Klebsiella* sp in 7%
    - *Pseudomonas* sp in 6%
    - *Enterobacter* sp in 5%
    - *Haemophilus influenzae* in 4%
    - *Bacteroides* sp in 3%
    - Others in 10%
  - ▲ Mixed organisms in 15% of cases
  - ▲ Fungi in 10% of cases
    - *Candida albicans* in 2%
    - Other *Candida* sp in 5%
    - Yeast in 1%
    - Other fungi, including *Pneumocystis carinii* (*P. jiroveci*), in 1%
  - ▲ Anaerobes
  - ▲ Viral disease—influenza, dengue, other hemorrhagic viruses, coxsackievirus B
  - ▲ Rickettsial disease—Rocky Mountain spotted fever, endemic typhus

▲ Spirochetal disease—leptospirosis, relapsing fever (*Borrellia* sp), Jarisch-Herxheimer reaction in syphilis
▲ Protozoal disease—*Toxoplasma gondii*, *Trypanosoma cruzi*, *Plasmodium falciparum*

Common Sources of Sepsis
- Lungs in 40%-50% of cases
- Bloodstream infections in 10%-30%
- Urinary tract in 10%-20%
- Intra-abdominal focus (biliary tree, abscess, peritonitis) in 10%-20%
- Soft tissue (e.g., in skin, cellulitis, decubitus ulcer, gangrene) in 1%-5%
- Other sites in 1%-5%
- Unknown source in 14%-20%

Nosocomial Sepsis
- Organisms responsible for nosocomial sepsis and their source are listed in Table 1.
- Nosocomial infection and sepsis are especially common in the ICU.

Table 1. Organisms Causing Nosocomial Sepsis and the Corresponding Sources

Organism	Source
Gram-negative enteric pathogens	Pneumonia, urinary tract
Coagulase-negative staphylococci	Bloodstream infection
Staphylococcus aureus	Pneumonia, bloodstream infection
Enterococci	Urinary tract, bloodstream infection
Streptococci	Pneumonia
Anaerobic organisms	Pneumonia, intra-abdominal, head and neck infection
Candida sp	Urinary tract, bloodstream infection, intra-abdominal

- Pulmonary, bloodstream, and urinary tract are most common sites of ICU nosocomial infection.

CLINICAL PRESENTATION
- Signs and symptoms of sepsis are listed in Table 2.

DIAGNOSTIC STRATEGIES
Differential Diagnosis of SIRS
- The differential diagnosis for SIRS is listed in Table 3.

Lab Findings
- Positive blood cultures
- Positive Gram stain or cultures from other sites (sputum, urine, CSF, abscess, ascites, pleural fluid, synovial fluid, bronchoalveolar lavage)
- Previous or concurrent antibiotic use may decrease Gram stain and culture sensitivity.
- Blood work abnormalities (hematologic, metabolic, and organ-specific) are listed in Table 4.
- Previous antibiotic use

Pathophysiology
- Clinical course driven by host factors (e.g., genetics, comorbidities, and indwelling devices) as well as organism factors (e.g., virulence and size of inoculum)

Table 2. Signs and Symptoms of Sepsis

General—chills, rigors, diaphoresis, myalgias
Fever (>38°C) or hypothermia (<36°C)
Respiratory—tachypnea, cough, sputum production, dyspnea, chest pain, cyanosis
Cardiovascular—tachycardia, hypotension, rales, gallops, murmur
Renal—oliguria, anuria, dysuria, urgency, flank pain
Central nervous system—stiff neck, headache, photophobia, focal neurologic deficits, mental status changes (restlessness, agitation, confusion, delirium, lethargy, stupor, coma)
Gastrointestinal—nausea, vomiting, diarrhea, abdominal pain, jaundice
Skin lesions—erythema, petechiae, ecthyma gangrenosum, embolic lesions, purpura fulminans, livedo reticularis
Hematologic—bleeding, petechiae, ecchymosis

Table 3. Differential Diagnosis for Noninfectious Causes of Systemic Inflammatory Response Syndrome

Pancreatitis
Gastric aspiration
Trauma and tissue injury including burns
Blood product support, transfusions
Hemorrhagic shock
Collagen vascular diseases and associated organ injury
Intestinal endotoxin translocation
Drug therapy
Thrombotic thrombocytopenic purpura/hemolytic uremic syndrome
Endocrine— thyrotoxicosis, adrenal insufficiency
Cardiovascular—vasculitides, dissecting aortic aneurysm, myocardial infarction (rare)
Anaphylaxis (rare)

Table 4. Hematologic, Metabolic, and Organ-Specific Blood Abnormalities

Leukocytosis or leukopenia	Hyperglycemia or hypoglycemia
Lactic acidosis	Proteinuria
Thrombocytopenia	Hypoxemia
Prolonged PT/INR	Hyperbilirubinemia
Hypofibrinogenemia	Hypercalcemia
Increased soluble fibrin monomers	Hypoferremia

- Complex cascade of inflammatory and anti-inflammatory mediators (e.g., cytokines), homeostatic factors (e.g., tissue factor, protein C, protein S, and plasminogen activation), and other extracellular mediators (e.g., nitric oxide, platelet activating factor, complement)
- Systemic inflammatory, epithelial, and local tissue factors are all important and interdependent

Pathology Findings
- Inflammation at primary site of infection and organ dysfunction

- Disseminated intravascular coagulation
- Noncardiogenic pulmonary edema and diffuse alveolar damage

TEST ORDERING
- Blood cultures—positive in only 30% of patients
- Serum lactate
- Antigen detection systems—counterimmunoelectrophoresis and latex agglutination tests (pneumococcus, *H. influenzae* type B, group B streptococcus, meningococcus, legionella, histoplasmosis) for select specimens (e.g., urine, CSF)
- Polymerase chain reaction on select specimens for select organisms
- Gram stain of buffy coat smears is useful in a very limited number of cases.
- Radiographic studies (e.g., chest X-ray, kidney-ureters-bladder, chest CT, abdominal CT)
- Ultrasound, CT, or MRI may be useful in delineating sites of infection.
  - ▲ Intra-abdominal, pleural, bone, joint, endovascular, and paranasal sinus infections can easily be overlooked.
- Aspiration of potentially infected body fluids (pleural, peritoneal, CSF, synovial)
- Hematologic, metabolic, and organ-specific blood tests (Table 4)
- Assessment of oxygenation (e.g., oximetry, arterial blood gas analysis, and mixed venous oximetry or blood gas analysis)
- When appropriate, biopsy and/or drainage of potentially infected tissues for diagnosis and source control (e.g., abscess, biliary tree) may be neccessary.

MANAGEMENT
General Measures
- Early and appropriate
  - ▲ Resuscitation
  - ▲ Antibiotics
  - ▲ Source control
- Time is important
- Clinical approach should be proportionate in time (urgency) and intensity to severity of presenting illness.
- Hospitalization for severe sepsis

- ICU admission for patients with shock, respiratory failure, or progressive multiorgan system dysfunction
- Review, clarify, and articulate treatment goals and resuscitative status of patient if not already documented.

Organ Failure
- Average risk of death increases by 15%-20% with failure of each additional organ.
- Shock—occurs early and resolves rapidly or is fatal
- Oliguria—occurs early and is followed by variable course, with some patients recovering early and some requiring dialysis
- Central nervous system and liver dysfunction—occurs hours to days after onset of sepsis and persists for intermediate periods
- Acute respiratory distress—occurs early and may persist

Initial Resuscitation and Management (Urgent: First 6 Hours)
- Within first hour (0-1 hour)
  - Obtain cultures (e.g., blood, urine, sputum, other).
  - Begin appropriate antibiotics with one or more drugs against likely bacterial or fungal pathogens with tailoring to community and health care-associated sensitivity profiles.
  - IV access with consideration of placement of central venous access
  - Fluid resuscitation started with boluses of crystalloid (250-1,000 mL, or 20 mL/kg) every 15-30 minutes, with repeat boluses pending clinical assessment and response.
  - Crystalloid: 0.9 normal saline or lactated Ringer solution (albumin and colloid not shown to be of clear benefit)
- Within first 6 hours (0-6 hours)
  - Fluid resuscitation continued and guided to end point of
    - Central venous pressure of 8-12 mm Hg
    - Mean arterial blood pressure ≥65 mm Hg
    - Urine output ≥0.5 mL/kg per hour and/or mixed venous oxygen saturation of ≥70%

- ▲ Vasopressors started for mean arterial pressure <65 mm Hg or hypoperfusion (e.g., dopamine or norepinephrine, then with consideration of vasopressin, phenylephrine, or epinephrine)
- ▲ Renal dose of dopamine has not been shown to be of benefit and is not recommended.
- ▲ Transfusion of packed RBCs to be considered if:
  - Central venous pressure is ≥8 mm Hg
  - Mean arterial pressure is >65 mm Hg
  - Mixed venous oxygenation is <70%, and
  - Hematocrit is <30%
- ▲ Inotropic support (e.g., dobutamine) if :
  - Central venous pressure is >8 mm Hg
  - Mean arterial pressure is ≥65 mm Hg
  - Hematocrit is >30% and
  - Mixed venous oxygenation is still <70%
- ▲ Consider bedside transthoracic echocardiography if refractory shock or lack of response is noted.
- ▲ May need to consider placing pulmonary artery catheter in setting of persistent shock
- ▲ Source control with drainage and surgery consultation if necessary

Continuation Phase and Support (<24 Hours After Diagnosis of "Sepsis")
- ■ Within first 24 hours
  - ▲ If hemodynamically unstable (pressor dependent), cosyntropin stimulation test and start of stress dose of corticosteroids, e.g., glucocorticoid (hydrocortisone 50-100 mg every 6-8 hours) and mineralocorticoid (fludrocortisone, 50 μg every day), pending test results (for relative adrenal insufficiency)
  - ▲ Continue stress dose of corticosteroids for 7 days if increase in serum cortisol is <9 μg/dL after cosyntropin stimulation test.
  - ▲ Consider infusion of activated protein C for severe sepsis or septic shock with dysfunction of two or more organ systems and no contraindications (*refer to activated protein C order set*).
  - ▲ Begin ventilatory support for respiratory failure with endotracheal intubation and low tidal volume protective

strategy for those at risk for or in the presence of acute lung injury or adult respiratory distress syndrome (ARDS).

- ▲ A limited trial of noninvasive positive pressure ventilation may be appropriate if a short duration of ventilatory assistance is expected.
- ▲ Elevate head of bed >30° for patients requiring mechanical ventilation as tolerated.
- ▲ Tight glucose control with avoidance of hyperglycemia; goal blood sugar of 80-110 mg/dL with use of insulin infusion (*refer to ICU insulin infusion protocol*)
- ▲ Nothing PO
- ▲ Begin deep venous thrombosis stress prophylaxis with specific treatment proportional to risk of venothromboembolic disease, comorbid medical conditions, and relative contraindications (e.g., active bleeding).
- ▲ Tube feedings should be initiated within 5-7 days or sooner (if patient is without PO intake).
- ▲ Placement of a postpyloric feeding tube may decrease gastric residuals and improve tolerance of enteral nutrition and medications.
- ▲ Pain (analgesia) and sedation management to be addressed based on short- (<48 hours) or long- (>48 hours) term anticipated needs, includes a daily drug holiday (*refer to pain and sedation order sets*)
- ▲ Consult physical medicine and physical therapy for patient mobilization and decubitus ulcer prophylaxis as tolerated.

Pulmonary Dysfunction
- ■ Sepsis places extreme demands on the lungs, requiring a high minute ventilation when the compliance of the respiratory system is diminished and muscle efficiency is impaired.
- ■ Respiratory failure may progress rapidly.
- ■ A sustained respiratory rate >30 breaths/minute (tachypnea) or paradoxical breathing may be a sign of impending ventilatory collapse, even if P_{CO_2} is normal.
- ■ Volume- or pressure-controlled mechanical ventilation with an initial low tidal volume strategy (5-6 mL/kg based on

ideal body weight, *not actual*) should be started for those at risk for or with evidence of acute lung injury or ARDS.
- ▲ Limit volumes and airway pressures to decrease volume- and pressure-related overstretching of the alveoli.
- ▲ Limit plateau pressure to <30-35 cm H_2O pressure if possible
- Positive end-expiratory pressure generally to start at 10 cm H_2O pressure
- Use of corticosteroids is controversial and has not clearly been shown to alter outcome related to ARDS or acute lung injury.
- Nitrous oxide, alprostadil, epoprostenol, surfactant, acetyl-cysteine, or ketoconazole has not been shown to be of clear benefit.
- Consider *early* tracheostomy for patients anticipated to require prolonged ventilator support or have difficulty with extubation.

Cardiovascular Failure
- Shock is caused by inadequate supply or inappropriate use of metabolic substrate (especially oxygen) and results in ischemia, lactic acidosis, and tissue damage.
- Circulatory adequacy is best assessed by mentation, urinary output, skin perfusion, blood pressure, measurements of oxygen delivery, oxygen consumption, and serum lactic acid levels.
- Blood pressure monitoring alone is insufficient for shock assessment and management.
- Value of monitoring central circulation through a pulmonary artery catheter is unclear (use only in patients with refractory shock, undetermined intravascular volume/hemodynamic, or serious myocardial, pulmonary, or renal comorbid conditions).
- Renal function decreases with mean arterial pressure generally <60 mm Hg.
- Septic shock (distributive) on presentation is characterized by a low pulmonary capillary wedge pressure (<8 mm Hg), normal to high cardiac index, and low systemic vascular resistance before intravascular volume repletion.
- Septic shock following intravascular volume resuscitation is characterized by normal pulmonary capillary wedge pressure, high cardiac index, and low systemic vascular resistance.

- Late septic shock with severe sepsis-related left ventricular systolic dysfunction may demonstrate high pulmonary capillary wedge pressure, low cardiac index, and normal or high systemic vascular resistance.
- Crystalloid intravascular volume resuscitation (including repeat boluses) is guided by clinical and objective measures, as noted above.

Renal Dysfunction
- Transient oliguria is common, but anuria is rare.
  - ▲ Obstructive uropathy has to be excluded.
  - ▲ Volume repletion often restores urinary output.
- Acute renal failure requiring dialysis occurs in a small fraction of patients.
  - ▲ Transient hemofiltration often supports renal function when necessary.
  - ▲ In most cases of sepsis-induced renal failure, renal function recovers.
- The benefit of dopamine, diuretics, or fluid loading to *prevent* renal dysfunction in patients with volume repletion in addition to volume repletion in normal blood pressure has not been shown.
- Patients with renal dysfunction who are to receive iodine contrast (e.g., for CT, angiography) should be given acetylcysteine 600 mg PO or IV twice daily the day before the contrast is administered and on the day it is given, with consideration also given to a bicarbonate infusion on the day of administration or a single dose of theophylline.

Gastrointestinal Dysfunction
- The liver is a mechanical and immunologic filter for portal blood and may be a major source of cytokines that promote the inflammatory cascade leading to the phenotypic SIRS response.
  - ▲ For patients with normal liver function before sepsis, an increase in liver enzymes is common, including mild hyperbilirubinemia.
  - ▲ Frank hepatic failure is rare.

- Septic shock usually causes ileus, which persists for 1-2 days and resolves after hypoperfusion has been corrected.
- Delayed gastric emptying is common, especially early in the natural course of diseases with sepsis
- For stress ulcer prophylaxis, histamine antagonists, proton pump inhibitors, or sucralfate is indicated, especially for patients who require ventilatory support, have multiorgan system failure, and cannot be fed enterally.

Coagulopathy
- Subclinical coagulopathies, signified by mild increase in PT or aPTT, decrease in platelet count, or moderate decrease in plasma fibrinogen level, are common, but overt disseminated intravascular coagulopathy is less common.
- Coagulopathy is caused by deficiencies of coagulation proteins, including protein C, antithrombin III, tissue-factor pathway inhibitor, and the kinin system.
- Laboratory findings are often a result of both a prothrombotic and thrombolytic intrinsic response to the SIRS response.
- Recombinant human activated protein C (drotrecogin alfa) decreases mortality of patients who have sepsis.
  - Relative reduction of death, 19.4% (95% confidence interval, 6.6-30.5); absolute reduction of death, 6.1% (P=.005)
  - Risk of bleeding with protein C is only mildly increased (3.5% vs. 2.0%, P=.06).
  - Dosage of drotrecogin alfa, 24 µg/kg per hour for 96 hours IV
  - Contraindications
    - Increased risk of bleeding
    - Profound thrombocytopenia

Drug Therapy
- Initially, antibiotic coverage should accommodate the most likely pathogens and include two or more agents with likely activity based on community or health care-associated susceptibility profiles.
- Dose adjustments are often required in renal and hepatic insufficiency.
- Be mindful of important interactions.
  - Aminoglycosides

- Increased nephrotoxicity with enflurane, cisplatin, and possibly vancomycin
- Increased ototoxicity with loop diuretics
- Increased paralysis with neuromuscular blocking agent
- ▲ Ampicillin—increased frequency of rash with allopurinol
- ▲ Fluoroquinolones—prolonged QTc interval in the context of electrolyte abnormality or other cardioactive medications (e.g., selective antipsychotics or antiarrhythmics)
- ■ After culture results are available, treatment should be more organism-specific
- ■ If cultures remain negative and clinical presentation is consistent with a noninfectious cause, antibiotics should be discontinued within 48-72 hours.

URINARY TRACT INFECTIONS

Kirby D. Slifer, D.O.
William F. Marshall, M.D.

DEFINITIONS

- Lower urinary tract (cystitis)—urgency, frequency, dysuria, and occasional suprapubic tenderness
- Upper urinary tract (pyelonephritis)—flank pain, chills, fever, and, occasionally, urgency, frequency, dysuria, nausea, and vomiting
- Uncomplicated urinary tract infection (UTI)—infection in a host who has normal urinary tract anatomy and normal neurologic function
- Complicated UTI—infection in a patient with structural abnormalities of the urinary tract or abnormal neurologic function (e.g., pregnant women, patients with spinal cord injury, men with prostate obstruction, children)
- Lower urinary tract symptoms alone do not rule out involvement of the upper urinary tract.

Classification

- Upper and lower UTIs are compared in Table 1.
- In studying Table 1, remember 2 important points:
  - ▲ There can be "crossover" of signs and symptoms between lower and upper UTIs.
  - ▲ The listed signs and symptoms may occur in the absence of any infection (e.g., symptomatic nephrolithiasis, nonspecific inflammation).
- A detailed history and physical exam should direct clinical suspicion.
- It is useful to classify adults with UTI into the following five groups:

Special abbreviations used in this chapter: DS, double strength; UTI, urinary tract infection.

- ▲ Young women with acute uncomplicated cystitis
- ▲ Young women with recurrent cystitis
- ▲ Young women with acute uncomplicated pyelonephritis
- ▲ All adults with complicated UTI
- ▲ All adults with asymptomatic bacteriuria (this chapter does not consider "young women with recurrent cystitis")

ETIOLOGY
- ▪ Table 2 gives representative species and their approximate rates of identification in UTIs in different classes of patients.
- ▪ In as many as 10%-15% of symptomatic patients, bacteriuria cannot be detected with routine lab methods:
  - ▲ Look for *Neisseria gonorrhoeae* and *Chlamydia trachomatis* and herpes simplex infection.
  - ▲ Anaerobes are rare.
  - ▲ *Lactobacilli* spp, *Corynebacterium* spp, and streptococci are debatable.

EPIDEMIOLOGY
- ▪ Risk factors for the development of UTI include
  - ▲ Recent sexual activity
  - ▲ Spermicidal or diaphragm use
  - ▲ History of recurrent UTI
  - ▲ Failure to urinate after sexual intercourse
- ▪ Approximately 10%-20% of adult females will experience symptomatic bacteriuria some time in their lifetime.
- ▪ Frequency of UTI after a single catheterization is 1% for outpatients and 10% for hospitalized patients.
- ▪ Incidence of bacteriuria is equal among races.

Table 1. Comparison of Lower and Upper Urinary Tract Infections (UTIs)

Lower UTI	Upper UTI
Suprapubic pain	Flank pain/tenderness
Dysuria	Fever
Frequency	Bacteriuria
Urgency	Nausea/vomiting
Bacteriuria	Dysuria
Fever	Frequency
Hematuria	Urgency

Table 2. Cause of Urinary Tract Infections

Lower urinary tract, uncomplicated infection, outpatient		
E. coli, % of cases		70-95
Staphylococcus saprophyticus,* % of cases		5-15
Upper urinary tract, complicated infection, inpatient		
E. coli	Pseudomonas aeruginosa	Candida spp†
Proteus mirabilis	Enterobacter spp	Morganella
Klebsiella spp	Enterococci	morganii

*Associated with spermicidal agents.
†Especially with long-term catheterization

- Frequency of significant bacteriuria (defined as >105 CFU) for adults and the elderly is listed in Table 3.

CLINICAL PRESENTATION
- Presenting signs and symptoms are listed in Table 1.
- Elderly patients are mostly asymptomatic.
- Confusion may be presenting sign in the elderly with UTI.
- The elderly tend to have a higher incidence of bacteremia in association with pyelonephritis than younger patients.
- Bilateral papillary necrosis and progressive destruction of the kidney occur more often in the elderly and in persons with diabetes.
- Be aware that bacteremia may occur in the absence of urinary tract symptoms, especially in patients with an indwelling urinary catheter.

Complications
- Recurrent infection—Once a woman develops UTI, she is more likely to develop subsequent infections than a patient who has had no previous infection.
- Uncomplicated or recurrent UTIs in adults, in the absence of obstruction, rarely if ever cause renal failure.
- Perinephric abscess
  - ▲ Suspect this when fever does not resolve within 5 days after IV antibiotic therapy.

Table 3. Prevalence of Significant Bacteriuria by Age Group

Age group	Frequency, %
Adults	
Young, nonpregnant women	1-3
Pregnant women	4-7
Men	0.1
Elderly	
Women	20-30
Men	10

- ▲ Most often, it is a contiguous infection with gram-negative bacteria.
- ■ Intrarenal abscess
  - ▲ Most often blood-borne *Staphylococcus aureus*
  - ▲ Look for infections elsewhere (e.g., endocarditis, osteomyelitis).
- ■ Emphysematous pyelonephritis
  - ▲ More common in diabetic patients
  - ▲ Almost always requires nephrectomy
  - ▲ 70% mortality rate
- ■ Urosepsis—more common in the elderly

DIAGNOSTIC STRATEGIES

- ■ Microscopic exam of urine for WBCs
  - ▲ Upper limit of normal—5-10 WBCs per high-power field
- ■ Microscopic exam of urine for bacteria
  - ▲ One bacterium per oil-immersion field in midstream, clean-catch, Gram-stained, urine specimen correlates with $\geq 10^5$ bacteria per 1 mL of urine.
- ■ Dipstick WBC esterase
  - ▲ For >10 WBCs/mm^3 urine, sensitivity of 75%-96% and specificity of 94%-98%
- ■ Urinary dipstick for nitrates—sensitivity, 27%; specificity, 94%; negative predictive value, 87%

Diagnosis

- ■ For patients requiring hospitalization, always obtain cultures of blood and urine before starting antibiotic therapy.

- Symptomatic infection—usually have at least 10^5 bacteria/mL urine
- Asymptomatic bacteriuria—two specimens to confirm the diagnosis of infection
  - ▲ One clean-catch specimen with 10^5 bacteria/mL has 80% positive predictive value for true infection.
  - ▲ Two specimens with 10^5 bacteria/mL of same organism have a 95% positive predictive value.
- Screen only for asymptomatic bacteriuria in adults before urologic surgery and in pregnancy.
- "Urethral syndrome"
  - ▲ Up to one-half of women with symptoms of lower UTI have <10^5 bacteria/mL of urine.
  - ▲ This may represent an early phase in the infectious process; genital herpes infection; chemical, allergic, or psychologic factors; fungi; urinary dilution before collection; gram-positive organisms; or fastidious organisms.
- No lab test reliably differentiates lower UTI from upper UTI
- Indwelling urinary catheters— $\geq 10^2$ CFU/mL of urine is evidence of infection.
  - ▲ Virtually 100% of patients with an indwelling urinary catheter will have bacteriuria within 30 days after catheter insertion.
  - ▲ Treat only when there are symptoms of infection (fever, chills, etc.).
  - ▲ Treating asymptomatic infection in chronically catheterized patients invariably results in colonization or infection with progressively more antibiotic-resistant organisms.

TREATMENT

- Aggressive hydration is *not recommended*.
- Urinary analgesics or antiseptics have no role in routine management of symptomatic UTIs.
- Empiric treatment should always be guided by Gram stain.
  - ▲ Gram-negative UTIs should be treated with fluoroquinolones, trimethoprim-sulfamethoxazone, or cephalosporins.
  - ▲ Gram-positive UTIs should be given ampicillin (IV) or amoxicillin (PO).

Acute Cystitis
- Three days of treatment is more effective than single-dose therapy and no different from 7-day therapy.
  - ▲ Fluoroquinolones are first choice of therapy—norfloxacin 400 mg twice daily, ciprofloxacin 250 mg PO twice daily, levofloxacin 500 mg PO daily.
  - ▲ Trimethoprim-sulfamethoxazole—1 double strength (DS) tablet PO twice daily in areas where prevalence of resistance is <20%

Acute Pyelonephritis
- Mild to moderate, with normal or slightly elevated peripheral WBC count, without nausea or vomiting, may begin oral antibiotic therapy with a fluoroquinolone such as ciprofloxacin 500 mg PO twice daily or levofloxacin 500 mg PO once daily for 7 days
  - ▲ If the organism is known to be sensitive, trimethoprim-sulfamethoxazole, 1 DS tablet PO twice daily for 14 days
- If enterococci are suspected (elderly men with prostate hypertrophy or obstruction) or known to be responsible, treat with amoxicillin 500 mg PO 3 times daily for 14 days.
- Severe, with increased peripheral WBC count, dehydration, vomiting, fever, or evidence of sepsis, start IV antibiotic therapy including a fluoroquinolone, a third-generation cephalosporin, or piperacillin-tazobactam.
  - ▲ If a gram-positive organism is known to be responsible, ampicillin-sulbactam or piperacillin-tazobactam with or without an aminoglycoside is a reasonable empiric choice.
  - ▲ Adjust antibiotic choices based on results of cultures and susceptibilities when available.

Complicated UTI
- Remove indwelling urinary catheter.
- Start piperacillin-tazobactam, a third-generation cephalosporin, or fluoroquinolone.
- Attempt to address underlying abnormalities such as obstruction or prostatitis.
  - ▲ If anatomic, functional, or metabolic abnormality cannot be corrected, infection often recurs; thus, repeat culture in 1-2 weeks.

Asymptomatic Bacteriuria and Bacteriuria of Pregnancy

- Therapy is not indicated for asymptomatic bacteriuria in an adult except in cases of urinary tract obstruction and/or pregnancy.
- Remember, there is no urgency to begin treatment and two cultures should be obtained to confirm the presence of bacteriuria before instituting antibiotic therapy.
- Generally, 7 days of amoxicillin, amoxicillin-clavulanate, cephalexin, or a sulfonamide eradicates bacteriuria in 70%-80% of patients.
- Sulfonamides should be avoided in the first trimester and the last few weeks of pregnancy.
  - ▲ Avoid tetracyclines and quinolones throughout pregnancy.
- If the isolated organism is resistant to all "nontoxic" antibiotics, treatment should not be instituted in nonobstructed patients.

VASCULITIS

Peter D. Kent, M.D.
Thomas G. Mason, M.D.

DEFINITION

- A group of diseases caused by inflammation of blood vessel walls

CLASSIFICATION

- An arbitrary classification is by the size of the vessel or vessels involved (Table 1).
- The predominantly pediatric vasculitic syndromes of Kawasaki disease and Henoch-Schönlein purpura are not considered in this chapter.

ETIOLOGY

- The cause is often unknown.
  - ▲ It may be secondary to infection or malignancy.
- Immune complexes or antibodies, such as antineutrophil cytoplasmic antibodies (ANCAs) may be pathogenic.
- Interaction of endothelial cells with lymphocytes and cytokines is integral in the pathogenesis of many vasculitic syndromes.

CLINICAL PRESENTATION

- Presentation varies greatly depending on type of vasculitis.
- Systemic constitutional symptoms such as fever, weight loss, night sweats, myalgias, arthralgias, and malaise are common.
- Patients with large- and medium-artery vasculitis may have large-artery bruits.
- Hypertension may reflect renal involvement.

Special abbreviations used in this chapter: ANCA, antineutrophil cytoplasmic antibody (c, cytoplasmic; p, perinuclear); CRP, C-reactive protein; MRA, magnetic resonance angiography.

Table 1. Vasculitic Syndromes According to Blood Vessel Size

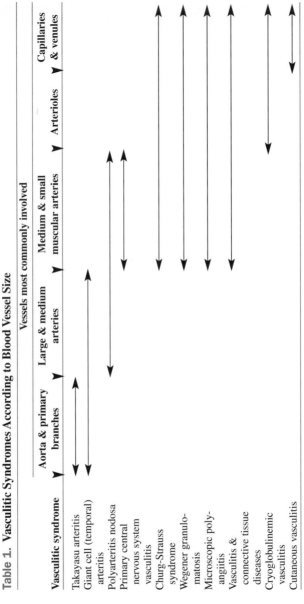

Vasculitic syndrome	Aorta & primary branches	Large & medium arteries	Medium & small muscular arteries	Arterioles	Capillaries & venules
			Vessels most commonly involved		
Takayasu arteritis	↕				
Giant cell (temporal) arteritis	↕	↑			
Polyarteritis nodosa		↕	↑		
Primary central nervous system vasculitis		↕	↕		
Churg-Strauss syndrome			↕		↑
Wegener granulomatosis			↕		↑
Microscopic polyangiitis			↕		↑
Vasculitis & connective tissue diseases			↕		↑
Cryoglobulinemic vasculitis				↕	↑
Cutaneous vasculitis					↕

Complications

- Vasculitis can cause many debilitating complications, including neuropathies, thromboses, tissue ischemia, hemorrhage, cognitive changes, and renal impairment.

DIAGNOSTIC STRATEGIES

- ESR and C-reactive protein (CRP) are increased in most vasculitic syndromes.
- Anemia of chronic disease, thrombocytosis, and low albumin are frequent.
- HIV testing and syphilis screening should be considered for patients with risk factors.
- Complement levels may be low in patients with immune complex–mediated vasculitis (cryoglobulinemia or vasculitis associated with connective tissue diseases).
- Complement levels are normal or high in giant cell arteritis, microscopic polyangiitis, and polyarteritis nodosa.
- Urinalysis may suggest renal involvement with microhematuria, proteinuria, or RBC casts.
- Chest X-ray may show pulmonary nodules with cavitation (often in Wegener granulomatosis), alveolar infiltrates of pulmonary hemorrhage, or chronic eosinophilic pneumonia in Churg-Strauss syndrome.
- EMG may be useful in the setting of mononeuritis multiplex or inflammatory myopathies.
- Many forms of large-vessel vasculitis can be diagnosed with arteriography.
  - ▲ Magnetic resonance angiography (MRA) may be a less invasive alternative.
- Biopsy is an excellent tool in the diagnosis of vasculitis.
  - ▲ The focal and segmental features of many types of vasculitis must be considered when evaluating biopsy specimens.
- Biopsy of symptomatically involved areas such as muscle, sural nerve, skin, or testis may be diagnostic.

MANAGEMENT

- Therapy depends on type and severity of vasculitis.
- Immunosuppressive medications are often used.

SPECIFIC DISEASE ENTITIES

Takayasu Arteritis

Definition
- Granulomatous arteritis of aorta and its major branches

Etiology
- Unknown

Epidemiology
- Young women <50 years, particularly of Asian or Eastern European background

Clinical Presentation
- Claudication in arms and legs and diminished or unequal peripheral pulses
- Bruits over large arteries
- Symptoms of central nervous system vascular insufficiency, including headaches, dizziness, amaurosis, transient ischemic attacks, and stroke
- Angina pectoris can occur if the ostia of the coronary arteries become narrowed.
- Mesenteric ischemia and hypertension can develop from narrowing of visceral and renal arteries.
- Complications
  - ▲ Ischemia of brain, viscera, and extremities
  - ▲ Aortic regurgitation or dissection

Diagnostic Strategies
- Assess acute phase reactants (ESR, CRP).
- Aortography shows long-segment smooth narrowings or complete occlusions.
- MRA detects increased arterial wall thickness.
- Histology shows focal panarteritis.

Management
- Corticosteroids and cytotoxic drugs (cyclophosphamide and methotrexate)
- Angioplasty, vascular bypass surgery, or aortic valve replacement may be necessary.

Giant Cell (Temporal) Arteritis

Definition
- Granulomatous arteritis of the aorta and its major branches, with predilection for extracranial branches of the carotid artery, particularly the temporal arteries

Etiology
- Unknown

Epidemiology
- Most patients are of Northern European descent.
- More common in women (2:1)
- Age at onset, ≥50 years (mean, 72 years)

Clinical Presentation
- Constitutional symptoms often with fever >39°C
- Polymyalgia rheumatica
  - ▲ Criteria for polymyalgia rheumatica
    - Age >50 years
    - ESR >40 mm/hour
    - Pain and morning stiffness for ≥30 minutes in at least 2 of the following: shoulder girdle, hip girdle, neck, or torso
    - Symptoms present for at least 1 month
- Headache, jaw claudication, scalp tenderness, visual symptoms, and cough or sore throat indicate cranial artery involvement by giant cell arteritis.
- Many patients have tender, nodular temporal arteries, sometimes without a pulse.
- Involvement of the aortic arch (aortic arch syndrome) and its primary branches may cause symptoms of arm claudication, diminished blood pressure, or cerebral ischemia.
- Complications
  - ▲ Visual loss, often permanent
  - ▲ Aortic arch syndrome, which involves smooth narrowing of the aorta or its primary branches
  - ▲ Acute aortic dissection or aortic aneurysms are uncommon and late complications.

Diagnostic Strategies
- ESR averages 80-100 mm/hour (Westergren)
- Diagnosis is confirmed with temporal artery biopsy specimen showing transmural inflammation with mononuclear cells, histiocytes, and multinucleated giant cells.
  - ▲ If the biopsy specimen from the first side is negative, a specimen should be obtained from the other side.

Management
- Giant cell arteritis generally is treated with oral prednisone, 40-60 mg/day in divided doses.
- Continue 40 mg/day for 2-4 weeks until the ESR is normal.
- Prednisone dose usually can be reduced by 5 mg every week until a 20-mg/day dose is reached, with careful monitoring of symptoms and ESR.
- If the dose is <20 mg/day, it is usually reduced by 2.5 mg per month as tolerated by symptoms and ESR.
- If the dose is <5 mg/day, it is reduced by 1 mg per month.

Polyarteritis Nodosa
Definition
- Necrotizing inflammation of medium-sized or small arteries without glomerulonephritis or vasculitis in arterioles, capillaries, or venules

Etiology
- May be a consequence of hepatitis B infection (7% of patients), HIV, cytomegalovirus, parvovirus B19, human T-lymphotropic virus 1, or hepatitis C infection

Epidemiology
- Occurs equally in men and women
- Age at onset, usually in 40s and 50s

Clinical Presentation
- Constitutional symptoms
- Neurologic—mononeuritis multiplex (70% of patients)
- Skin—livedo reticularis, skin ulcers, purpura
- Cardiac—congestive heart failure
- Gastrointestinal—abdominal pain, bleeding, perforation
- Renal—multiple infarcts

- Musculoskeletal—myalgias and arthralgias
- Orchitis is common.
- Pulmonary involvement is rare.
- Complications
  - ▲ Mononeuritis multiplex, intestinal ischemia, and renal infarcts, with the latter two being the leading causes of death
  - ▲ Aneurysms are at risk for rupture.
  - ▲ With treatment, 5-year survival is 60%-80%.

Diagnostic Strategies
- Hepatitis B surface antigen and antibody should be checked.
- ANCAs are rare.
- Mesenteric angiography often shows both microaneurysms and stenoses in medium-sized vessels.
- Biopsy specimens from skeletal muscle, sural nerve, kidney, testis, liver, or rectum show focal segmental necrotizing vasculitis.

Management
- Methylprednisolone, 30 mg/kg IV every 24 hours for 3 days, then prednisone at 1 mg/kg per day tapered over 9-12 months
- Pulse cyclophosphamide, 0.6 g/m^2, delivered monthly for 6-12 months and then every 2-3 months
  - ▲ Aggressive hydration and sodium 2-mercaptoethanesulfonate (mesna) are used during pulse therapy.
- Oral cyclophosphamide, 100-150 mg/day, may be used instead of pulse dosing for less severe cases, and it is steroid-sparing.
- In hepatitis B–related disease
  - ▲ Administer corticosteroids to stabilize life-threatening symptoms.
  - ▲ Administer antiviral therapy for hepatitis.

Primary Central Nervous System Vasculitis
Definition
- Necrotizing and/or granulomatous vasculitis affecting predominantly leptomeningeal and cortical vessels

Etiology
- Primary angiitis of the central nervous system has no known cause.
- Secondary angiitis of the central nervous system may result from another systemic vasculitic syndrome, an infection, a neoplasm, or a drug.

Epidemiology
- Age at onset, usually in the 20s or 30s

Clinical Presentation
- Headaches and focal and nonfocal neurologic deficits
- Decreased cognitive function or fluctuating level of consciousness
- Constitutional symptoms are uncommon.
- Complications
  - ▲ Strokes, seizures, cognitive decline

Diagnostic Strategies
- ESR is frequently normal.
- MRI may show multiple bilateral, supratentorial infarcts.
  - ▲ Leptomeninges may enhance with contrast.
- Angiography can show a beading pattern of alternating stenoses and dilatations.
- CSF may have increased opening pressure, mildly increased protein level, and pleocytosis.
- Pathology shows segmental necrotizing and frequently granulomatous vasculitis that affects predominantly leptomeningeal and cortical blood vessels.

Management
- PO or pulse cyclophosphamide in combination with corticosteroids

Churg-Strauss Syndrome
Definition
- Granulomatous arteritis of small- and medium-sized vessels associated with asthma, pulmonary infiltrates, and eosinophilia

Etiology
- Unknown

Epidemiology
- Mean age at onset, between 38 and 48 years.

Clinical Presentation
- Pulmonary—asthma (93% of patients) or allergic rhinitis, often present for years before onset of vasculitis
  - ▲ Infiltrates may be seen on chest X-ray.
- Neurologic—mononeuritis multiplex (53%-75% of patients)
- Skin—purpura and SQ nodules
- Cardiac—cardiomyopathy and pericarditis
- Gastrointestinal—diarrhea, bleeding, abdominal pain
- Renal—focal segmental glomerulonephritis with necrotizing features
- Musculoskeletal- -polyarthralgias and arthritis
- Complications
  - ▲ Neuropathy, cardiomyopathy, renal impairment
  - ▲ Five-year survival rate with treatment is about 82%.

Diagnostic Strategies
- Eosinophilia >10⁹/L on CBC
- Associated with ANCA (59% of patients), particularly antimyeloperoxidase positivity
- Eosinophils or extravascular eosinophilic granulomas in biopsy specimen

Management
- PO or pulse cyclophosphamide in combination with corticosteroids

Wegener Granulomatosis
Definition
- Granulomatous inflammation of upper and lower respiratory tract and necrotizing vasculitis of small- and medium-sized vessels, often causing glomerulonephritis

Etiology
- Unknown

Epidemiology

- Affects both sexes equally
- More common in whites
- Mean age at onset, 41 years; range, 9-78 years

Clinical Presentation

- Systemic constitutional symptoms
- Epistaxis, saddle nose deformity, nasal septal perforation or ulceration, pain over the sinuses
- Subglottic lesions and stenosis
- Hypertension or hematuria
- Pulmonary symptoms such as cough, dyspnea, hemoptysis, and chest pain (60%-80% of patients)
- Complications
  - ▲ Subglottic stenosis may require dilatation or tracheostomy
  - ▲ Renal failure
  - ▲ With treatment, 5-year survival rate is about 70%.

Diagnostic Strategies

- Assess acute phase reactants (ESR, CRP).
- Cytoplasmic ANCA (c-ANCA) and anti-proteinase 3 are both sensitive (80%) and specific (97%) for Wegener granulomatosis.
- The c-ANCA titer correlates with disease activity in about 2/3 of patients.
- Perinuclear ANCA (p-ANCA) is rarely associated with Wegener granulomatosis (1% of patients).
- Necrotizing granulomas are seen on biopsy specimens.

Management

- PO or pulse cyclophosphamide in combination with corticosteroids
- Trimethoprim-sulfamethoxazole, 160 mg/800 mg, twice daily decreases incidence of relapse.
- Methotrexate is another treatment option for selected patients.
  - ▲ It is used occasionally for cyclophosphamide sparing.

Microscopic Polyangiitis
Definition

- Necrotizing pauciimmune deposits (few or no immune

deposits) affecting small vessels, commonly causing glomerulonephritis

Etiology
- Unknown

Epidemiology
- Mean age at onset, about 50 years

Clinical Presentation
- Renal—Microscopic hematuria and proteinuria are nearly always present (>90% of patients).
- Unlike polyarteritis nodosa, pulmonary involvement may occur in microscopic polyangiitis.
  - ▲ Pulmonary hemorrhage and hemoptysis may occur (12%-29% of patients).
- Abdominal and musculoskeletal pain, gastrointestinal tract bleeding, or peripheral neuropathy may be present.
- Skin lesions (purpura, splinter hemorrhages) are found in 50% of patients.
- Complications
  - ▲ Pulmonary hemorrhage, renal failure
  - ▲ With treatment, 5-year survival is 65%
  - ▲ Relapse rate is 38%.

Diagnostic Strategies
- Eosinophilia in 14% of patients
- Normal whole complement and C3 and C4 levels
- Impaired renal function
- p-ANCA in 61% of patients and c-ANCA in 15%
- Most ANCAs are antimyeloperoxidase p-ANCA
- Positive predictive value of positive p-ANCA in these patients is only 12%.
- On arteriography, microaneurysms and/or stenoses are rare.
- Renal biopsy specimen may show segmental thrombosis and necrotizing crescenteric glomerulonephritis.
- Other possible biopsy sites include the skin and sural nerve.

- Small-vessel involvement is required and excludes the diagnosis of polyarteritis nodosa.

Management
- PO or pulse cyclophosphamide in combination with corticosteroids

Cryoglobulinemic Vasculitis
Definition
- Cryoglobulins are monoclonal or polyclonal immunoglobulins that precipitate at cold temperatures and may produce vasculitis.

Classification
- Cryoglobulin without underlying disease is "essential cryoglobulinemia."
- Type I—monoclonal cryoglobulin (IgM, IgG, etc.)
  - ▲ Usually associated with underlying lymphoproliferative or myeloproliferative disorder
  - ▲ Rarely causes vasculitis
- Type II—mixed cryoglobulins with a monoclonal (usually IgM) and polyclonal (usually IgG) component
  - ▲ Associated with lymphoproliferative diseases, autoimmune diseases, and infections
- Type III—mixed polyclonal cryoglobulins
  - ▲ Associated with lymphoproliferative diseases, autoimmune diseases, and bacterial infections

Etiology
- Cryoglobulins deposit in blood vessel walls and induce complement activation, causing tissue damage and recruitment of inflammatory cells.
- Hepatitis C infection, other infections, connective tissue diseases, and myeloproliferative and lymphoproliferative disorders can induce cryoglobulins.

Epidemiology
- Average age at onset, about 50 years
- Mixed cryoglobulins are present in >50% of patients with hepatitis C infection, but vasculitis occurs only in a small fraction of patients.

Clinical Presentation

- Purpura, cutaneous ulceration, and arthritis or arthralgia (>70% of patients)
- Peripheral neuropathy (40%-70%)
- Renal involvement (<40%)
  - ▲ Cryoglobulinemic glomerulonephritis occurs mainly with type II mixed cryoglobulinemia and causes chronic renal insufficiency in 50% of patients.
  - ▲ Renal vasculitis of small- and medium-sized renal arteries occurs in 33% of patients with cryoglobulinemic glomerulonephritis.
- Complications
  - ▲ Renal insufficiency
  - ▲ Prognosis is related to underlying disease.

Diagnostic Strategies

- Anti–hepatitis C antibodies (90% of patients), hepatitis C RNA (85%)
- Anti–hepatitis B antibodies (40%), hepatitis B surface antigen (4%)
- Aminotransferase levels are increased in 25%-40% of patients.
- Serum protein electrophoresis, immunofixation, and cryoglobulins
- Complement levels (hypocomplementemia in 90%)
- Rheumatoid factor in >70% of patients.
- Antinuclear antibody (20%), extractable nuclear antigen (8%), ANCA (<5%)
- With immunofluorescence, biopsy specimens show deposition of mixed cryoglobulins and complement in walls of small vessels.
- Bone marrow biopsy may be needed to rule out underlying myeloproliferative or lymphoproliferative disorder.

Management

- The underlying disease should be treated.
- If no underlying disease is found, treat with methotrexate, azathioprine, or interferon alfa.
- Acute exacerbations of hepatitis C–associated cryoglobu-

linemic vasculitis often require both corticosteroids and PO or pulse cyclophosphamide.

- ▲ Interferon alfa is not recommended for acute exacerbations.
- ▲ Interferon alfa should be used after remission has been achieved.
- ▲ Ribavirin may also be considered.
- Plasmapheresis may help in severe cases.

Cutaneous Vasculitis
Definition
- Vasculitis causing visible skin lesions

Classification and Etiology
- Leukocytoclastic vasculitis—necrotizing vasculitis with fibrinoid necrosis and leukocytolysis involving postcapillary venules
  - ▲ May be secondary to underlying systemic vasculitis, connective tissue disease, or malignancy
  - ▲ Hypersensitivity vasculitis
    - Usually secondary to drugs
    - Requires exclusion of other causes of leukocytoclastic vasculitis

Clinical Presentation
- Palpable purpura, often on lower extremities
- Urticaria, ulcerations, nodular lesions
- Complications
  - ▲ Related to underlying disease process

Diagnostic Strategies
- Skin biopsy can confirm leukocytoclastic vasculitis with involvement of dermal postcapillary venules.
- Immunofluorescence studies may show immunoglobulin and C3 deposition.
- Testing for systemic vasculitis, connective tissue disease, and malignancy should be done as clinically indicated.

Management
- Treat the underlying disease.
- With hypersensitivity vasculitis, discontinue the offending drug.
- Treat with prednisone or dapsone.

ANTIMICROBIAL AGENTS

John W. Wilson, M.D.
Lynn L. Estes, Pharm.D.

GENERAL PRINCIPLES

Factors to Consider Before Initiating Antimicrobial Therapy

- Define the "host"—many types of infection and rates of disease progression are influenced by host factors, including medical history, immunosuppression, patient age, absence of spleen, concurrent medications, recent or current hospitalization, contacts with infectious persons or animals and travel history.
- Define the infection "syndrome"—location of infection, rate of progression, severity of infection (i.e., localized vs. multiorgan involvement or hemodynamic instability)
- Define the "microbiology"—antimicrobial therapy (when possible) should be directed in a targeted fashion against identified or suspected organisms causing infection and should reach the site of infection.

Other Considerations

- Identify infections requiring emergent medical or surgical intervention: meningitis, septic shock, fasciitis, myonecrosis, others.
- Identify syndromes requiring prompt intervention: neutropenic gram-negative bacteremia, empyema, cholangitis biliary obstruction, complex vascular catheter infections
- Particular attention should be paid to the Gram stain, culture, and antimicrobial susceptibilities of fluid or tissue samples submitted to the microbiology laboratory to help direct antimicrobial therapy.

Special abbreviations used in this chapter: CMV, cytomegalovirus; CNS, central nervous system; GI, gastrointestinal; HHV, human herpesvirus; HSV, herpes simplex virus; VZV, varicella-zoster virus.

- Patient drug allergies and organ function are critical to identify and monitor for optimal selection and dosing of antimicrobial therapy.
- Infectious disease consultation should be obtained for all serious and complex infections.

ANTIBACTERIAL AGENTS
Penicillins (Table 1)
Prototypic Agents
- Natural penicillins—penicillin G
- Aminopenicillins—ampicillin, amoxicillin, ampicillin-sulbactam (Unasyn), amoxicillin-clavulanate (Augmentin)
- Penicillinase-resistant penicillins—nafcillin, oxacillin, dicloxacillin
- Carboxypenicillins/ureidopenicillins—ticarcillin, piperacillin, ticarcillin-clavulanate (Timentin), piperacillin-tazobactam (Zosyn)

Table 1. **Penicillins**

Drug	Usual adult dose with normal renal function	Elimination
Amoxicillin	250-500 mg tid, 875 mg bid	Renal*
Amoxicillin-clavulanate	250-500 mg tid, 875 mg bid	Renal*
Ampicillin IV	1-2 g q 4-6 hours	Renal*
Ampicllin-sulbactam	1.5-3 g q 6-8 hours	Renal*
Dicloxacillin	125-500 mg qid	Hepatic/biliary
Nafcillin	1-2 g q 4-6 hours	Hepatic/biliary
Oxacillin	1-2 g q 4-6 hours	Hepatic/biliary
Penicillin G IV	5-24 mU daily divided q 4 hours or continuous infusion	Renal*
Penicillin V PO	250-500 mg tid or qid	Renal*
Piperacillin	3-4 g q 4-6 hours	Renal*
Pipieracillin-tazobactam	3.375-4.5 g q 6 hours	Renal*
Ticarcillin-clavulanate	3.1 g q 4-6 hours	Renal*

bid, twice daily; q, every; qid, 4 times daily; tid, 3 times daily.
*Modify dose for renal dysfunction.

Spectrum of Activity

- Natural penicillins—most streptococci and enterococci; most *Neisseria gonorrhoeae*, susceptible anaerobes (*Clostridium* spp, most oral *Bacteroides*, *Fusobacterium*, *Peptostreptococcus*), *Listeria*, *Pasteurella*, *Treponema pallidum* (syphilis), *Borrelia burgdorferi* (the species for Lyme disease)
- Most staphylococci and gram-negative organisms produce β-lactamase that renders these agents inactive.
- Aminopenicillins—most streptococci, enterococci, many *Escherichia coli*, *Proteus mirabilis*, *Salmonella*, *Shigella*, β-lactamase–negative *Haemophilus influenzae*
  - ▲ Addition of a β-lactamase inhibitor (Augmentin, Unasyn) extends the spectra to include β-lactamase–producing but methicillin–sensitive staphylococci, *Bacteroides fragilis*, and β-lactamase–producing strains of *H. influenzae* and *Moraxella catarrhalis*.
- Penicillinase-resistant penicillins—narrow spectrum
  - ▲ Includes methicillin-susceptible staphylococcus and group A streptococci
  - ▲ Useful for serious staphylococcal infections and skin or soft tissue infections
  - ▲ No gram-negative, enterococcal, or anaerobic activity
- Carboxypenicillins/Ureidopenicillins
  - ▲ Many gram-negative bacteria, including most Enterobacteriaceae and most *Pseudomonas aeruginosa*
  - ▲ Compared with penicillin G, they are slightly less active against streptococci and enterococci.
  - ▲ Addition of a β-lactamase inhibitor (Zosyn and Timentin) extends the spectra to methicillin-sensitive staphylococci and *B. fragilis*; Timentin has activity against many *Stenotrophomonas*.
  - ▲ Used when broad-spectrum empiric therapy is needed and for gram-negative and mixed nosocomial infections

Toxicities

- Hypersensitivity reactions, gastrointestinal (GI) side effects (nausea, vomiting, diarrhea, and *Clostridium difficile*), phlebitis with IV therapy

- High-dose IV penicillin—can cause central nervous system (CNS) side effects, including seizures (especially without renal dose adjustment); hyperkalemia (potassium salt) or hypernatremia (sodium salt)
- Penicillinase-resistant penicillins—can cause interstitial nephritis, phlebitis, hepatitis, and neutropenia with prolonged use
- Ticarcillin and Timentin—can cause sodium overload, hypokalemia, platelet dysfunction

Cephalosporins (Table 2)
Prototypic Agents
- First generation: cefazolin, cephalexin
- Second generation: cefuroxime, cefoxitin, cefotetan, cefaclor, cefprozil, loracarbef

Table 2. Cephalosporins

Drug	Usual adult dose with normal renal function	Elimination
Cefaclor	250-500 mg tid	Renal*
Cefadroxil	500 mg-1 g bid	Renal*
Cefazolin	1-2 g q 8 hours	Renal*
Cefdinir	300 mg bid	Renal*
Cefepime	1-2 g q 8-12 hours	Renal*
Cefixime	400 mg daily	Renal*
Cefotaxime	1-2 g q 8 hours	Renal*
Cefotetan	1-2 g q 12 hours	Renal*
Cefoxitin	1-2 g q 6-8 hours	Renal*
Cefpodoxime	200-400 mg bid	Renal*
Cefprozil	250-500 mg bid	Renal*
Ceftazidime	1-2 g q 8 hours	Renal*
Ceftibuten	400 mg daily	Renal*
Ceftriaxone	1-2 g q 24 hours	Renal/hepatobiliary
Cefuroxime IV	750-1,500 mg q 8 hours	Renal*
Cefuroxime axetil PO	250-500 mg bid	Renal*
Cephalexin	250 mg-1 g qid	Renal*

bid, twice daily; q, every; qid, 4 times daily; tid, 3 times daily.
*Modify dose for renal dysfunction.

- Third generation: cefotaxime, ceftriaxone, ceftazidime, cefpodoxime, cefixime
- Fourth generation: cefepime

Spectrum of Activity
- First generation
  - ▲ Highly active against methicillin-susceptible staphylococci, β-hemolytic streptococci, and many strains of *P. mirabilis*, *E. coli*, and *Klebsiella* spp.
  - ▲ Used commonly for methicillin-sensitive staphylococcal infections and skin and soft tissue infections
- Second generation
  - ▲ Improved gram-negative activity but slightly less gram-positive activity than first-generation agents
  - ▲ Cefuroxime and the oral agents—activity against community-acquired respiratory pathogens (*Streptococcus pneumoniae*, *H. influenzae*, *M. catarrhalis*)
  - ▲ Cefotetan and cefoxitin—gram-negative and anaerobic activity; have been used for obstetrics/gynecologic and colorectal surgical prophylaxis and treatment of community-acquired abdominal infections and pelvic inflammatory disease
- Third generation
  - ▲ Improved gram-negative activity vs. first- and second-generation agents
  - ▲ Cefotaxime and ceftriaxone—enhanced gram-negative activity compared with second-generation agents but not active against *Pseudomonas*, good activity against community-acquired respiratory, urinary, and meningeal pathogens
  - ▲ Ceftazidime—less active against staphylococci and streptococci but has activity against *P. aeruginosa*
- Fourth generation
  - ▲ Cefepime—highly active and durable gram-negative activity (including *P. aeruginosa*) and enhanced gram-positive activity (methicillin-susceptible *S. aureus* and *Streptococcus* spp)

Toxicities
- GI effects (nausea, vomiting, and diarrhea) are most common.
- Hypersensitivity reactions (cross-reactivity with penicillins, about 5%), drug fever, and *C. difficile* colitis
- Cefotetan and cefamandole (*N*-methylthiotetrazole side chain)—associated with hypoprothrombinemia (increased INR) and a disulfiram-like reaction when ethanol is consumed
- Ceftriaxone—associated with pseudocholelithiasis, cholelithiasis, and biliary colic, especially in young children

Monobactam
Agent—Aztreonam

Spectrum of Activity
- Gram-negative aerobic organisms, including most *P. aeruginosa*

Toxicities
- Similar to other β-lactams
- Because of low risk of cross-allergenicity, it can often be used in patients with penicillin or cephalosporin allergies.

Carbapenems (Table 3)
Agents—Imipenem, Meropenem, Ertapenem

Spectrum
- Very broad antibacterial activity, including gram-positives, gram-negatives, and anaerobes
- Gram-positive spectrum includes β-hemolytic streptococci, *S. pneumoniae*, and methicillin-susceptible *S. aureus*; imipenem and meropenem cover susceptible *Enterococcus* spp, but ertapenem is inactive.
- Gram-negative spectrum includes the Enterobacteriaceae (including those with extended-spectrum β-lactamase production), *H. influenzae*, and *M. catarrhalis*; meropenem and imipenem cover most *P. aeruginosa* and *Acinetobacter* spp, but, ertapenem is inactive against both.
- Anaerobic activity is excellent and includes *Bacteroides*, *Clostridium*, *Fusobacterium*, *Peptostreptococcus*, and *Prevotella*.

Table 3. Carbapenems

Drug	Usual adult dose for normal renal function	Elimination
Ertapenem	1 g q 24 hours	Renal*
Imipenem	500 mg q 6 hours	Renal*
Meropenem	1-2 g q 8 hours	Renal*

q, every.

Toxicities

- Can cause GI side effects, hypersensitivity reactions (may be cross-allergenic with penicillins), drug fever, and overgrowth of resistant organisms (yeast, *Stenotrophomonas*, *C. difficile*)
- Seizures occur rarely with these agents, but occur especially with a history of seizure disorder, renal insufficiency without proper dosage adjustment, or structural CNS defects.

Aminoglycosides (Tables 4 and 5)

Prototypic Agents

- Gentamicin, tobramycin, amikacin, streptomycin

Spectrum of Activity

- Includes most aerobic gram-negative bacilli, mycobacteria (varies by agent), *Brucella* (streptomycin), *Nocardia* (amikacin), *Francisella tularensis* (streptomycin), *Yersinia pestis* (streptomycin)
- Gentamicin and streptomycin are synergistic with certain β-lactams and vancomycin against susceptible enterococci (gentamicin, streptomycin), staphylococci, and several aerobic gram-negatives.

Toxicities

- Can cause nephrotoxicity, auditory or vestibular toxicity, and rarely neuromuscular blockade

Table 4. Aminoglycoside Dosing for Normal Renal Function*

Condition	Gentamicin/tobramycin traditional dosing	Serum level targets, µg/mL	Amikacin/strepto traditional dosing	Serum level targets, µg/mL
Pneumonia/sepsis	2-2.5 mg/kg q 8 hours	pk: 7-10 tr: <1.2	7-8 mg/kg q 8-12 hours	pk: 25-40 tr: 2.5-8
Bacteremia, SSTI, pyelonephritis	1.5-1.7 mg/kg q 8 hours	pk: 6-8 tr: <1.2	6 mg/kg q 8-12 hours	pk: 20-30 tr: 2.5-4
Lower urinary tract infection	1-1.3 mg/kg q 8 hours	pk: 4-5 tr: <1.2	5-6 mg/kg q 8-12 hours	pk: 15-20 tr: 2.5-4
Gram-positive synergy	1 mg/kg q 8 hours	pk: 3-4 tr: <1.2	--	--

pk, peak; SSTI, skin & soft tissue infection; tr, trough.
*Must adjust doses and intervals for renal dysfunction.

Table 5. Single Daily (Pulse) Dosing*

Gentamicin/tobramycin 5-7 mg/kg daily
Amikacin/streptomycin 15-20 mg/kg daily

*Adjust dosing interval for renal dysfunction.

- Nephrotoxicity—the risk is enhanced in presence of other nephrotoxins and is usually reversible; monitoring drug levels is important to minimize this.
- Ototoxicity—may be irreversible

Vancomycin
Spectrum of Activity
- Includes most aerobic and anaerobic gram-positive organisms
- Active against methicillin-resistant staphylococci, susceptible enterococci, and highly penicillin-resistant *S. pneumoniae*
- An alternative agent for infections caused by methicillin-sensitive staphylococci (less active than cefazolin, nafcillin, oxacillin), ampicillin-sensitive enterococci or streptococci in patients intolerant of β-lactam antimicrobials
- Not active against certain strains of *Lactobacillus*, *Leuconostoc*, *Actinomyces*, and vancomycin-resistant enterococci
- Use should be minimized because of emergence of vancomycin-resistant enterococci and, more recently, vancomycin-resistant staphylococci
- Oral vancomycin is not systemically absorbed and can be used for treatment of *C. difficile* colitis.

Toxicities
- Rare ototoxicity and nephrotoxicity (especially in combination with other nephrotoxins)
- Infusion-related pruritus and rash or flushing reaction involving face, neck, and upper body ("red-man" or "red-neck" syndrome—not an allergic reaction) can be minimized by prolonging the infusion and/or administering an antihistamine.

Dosing
- Usual dosing is 15-20 mg/kg every 12 hours with normal renal function.
- Dose should be decreased or interval prolonged for renal dysfunction.
- Target trough levels are 5-15 µg/mL for most infections.
- Troughs of 15-20 µg/mL may be appropriate for methicillin-resistant *S. aureus* pneumonia or meningitis.

Fluoroquinolones (Table 6)

Prototypic Agents
- Ciprofloxacin, levofloxacin, gatifloxacin, moxifloxacin, gemifloxacin

Spectrum of Activity
- Active against most aerobic gram-negative bacilli, including the Enterobacteriaceae, *H. influenzae*, and some staphylococci; gram-positive and anaerobic activity varies
- Ciprofloxacin has the best activity against *P. aeruginosa* but does not have good activity against *S. pneumoniae*, and clinical failures have been reported.
- Levofloxacin, moxifloxacin, gatifloxacin, and gemifloxacin have improved activity against *S. pneumoniae* and other gram-positive organisms; they also have good activity against atypical pneumonia pathogens such as *Chlamydia*

Table 6. **Fluoroquinolones**

Drug	Usual adult dose with normal renal function	Elimination
Ciprofloxacin IV	200-400 mg q 12 hours 400 mg q 8 hours	Renal*
Ciprofloxacin PO	250-750 mg q 12 hours	Renal*
Gatifloxacin IV/PO	400 mg daily	Renal*
Gemifloxacin PO	320 mg daily	Fecal/renal*
Levofloxacin IV/PO	250-750 mg daily	Renal*
Moxifloxacin IV/PO	400 mg daily	Hepatic/renal (minor)

q, every
*Adjust doses for renal function.

pneumoniae, *Mycoplasma pneumoniae*, and *Legionella* and thus are useful for community-acquired respiratory infections.

- Moxifloxacin, gatifloxacin, and gemifloxacin have appreciable anaerobic activity but are not drugs of choice for serious anaerobic infections.

Toxicities

- GI effects, including *C. difficile* colitis
- Rash is most frequent with gemifloxacin.
- CNS effects are rare but can include seizures in patients predisposed, especially when not dose adjusted for renal function.
- Erosions have been seen in cartilage in animals; thus, quinolones generally are not recommended in pregnant women or in patients younger than 18 years.
- Tendinitis and tendon rupture are rare complications.
- QT prolongation and rare cases of torsades de pointes have been reported.
- Gatifloxacin: hyper- and hypoglycemia have been reported
- Oral chelating agents such as aluminum, calcium, magnesium, iron, and zinc will bind fluoroquinolones and inhibit absorption. Such drugs should not be given together.

Tetracyclines and Glycylcycline (Tigecycline) (Table 7)

Prototypic Agents

- Tetracycline, doxycycline, minocycline, tigecycline

Spectrum of Activity

- Includes *Rickettsia*, *Chlamydia*, *M. pneumoniae*, *Vibrio*, *Brucella*, *B. burgdorferi* (early stages), *Helicobacter pylori*, many *S. pneumoniae*
- Minocycline is also active against methicillin-resistant staphylococci (for mild disease in patients who cannot tolerate vancomycin), *Stenotrophomonas*, and *Mycobacterium marinum*
- Tigecycline is active against several multidrug resistant organisms, including several that are tetracycline resistant.

Table 7. **Tetracyclines and Tigecycline**

Drug	Usual adult dose	Elimination
Doxycycline IV/PO	200 mg ×1, 100 mg bid	Biliary/renal
Minocycline IV/PO	250 mg ×1, 100 mg bid	Biliary/renal
Tetracycline PO	250-500 mg qid	Renal*/biliary
Tigecycline IV	100 mg ×1, 50 mg q 12 hours	Biliary-fecal/renal

bid, twice daily; q, every; qid, four times daily.
*Adjust tetracycline dose for renal function or use alternative agent.

▲ Gram-positive activity includes methicillin-sensitive and resistant staphylococci, and vancomycin-resistant enterococci

▲ Gram-negative activity is broad, including *E. coli*, *Klebsiella*, *Enterobacter*, *Citrobacter*, *Acinetobacter*, *Stenotrophomonas*, *Haemophilus*, and *Moraxella*. It does not have appreciable activity against *Proteus* or *Pseudomonas*.

▲ Good anaerobic and non-tuberculosis mycobacterial activity

Toxicities
- Include GI effects (especially prominent with tigecycline), rash, photosensitivity
- Avoid in pregnant females and children because these agents impair bone growth of the fetus and stain the teeth of children.
- Coadministration of antacids, iron, calcium, magnesium, or aluminum substantially decreases the enteric absorption of PO agents.

Macrolides and Ketolide (Telithromycin) (Table 8)
Prototypic Agents
- Erythromycin, clarithromycin, azithromycin, telithromycin

Spectrum of Activity
- Most β-hemolytic streptococci, *S. pneumoniae* (resistance is increasing), some methicillin-sensitive staphylococci, *B. pertussis*, *Campylobacter jejuni*, *Treponema pallidum*, *Ureaplasma*, *M. pneumoniae*, *L. pneumophila*, *Chlamydia* sp

Table 8. Macrolides and Telithromycin

Drug	Usual adult dose	Elimination
Azithromycin	PO: 250-500 mg daily IV: 500 mg daily	Hepatic/biliary
Clarithromycin	PO: 250-500 mg bid	Hepatic/renal*
Erythromycin	PO: 250-500 mg tid-qid IV: 500 mg-1 g qid	Hepatic/biliary
Telithromycin	PO: 800 mg daily	Biliary/hepatic/renal*

bid, twice daily; qid, 4 times daily; tid, 3 times daily
*Adjust dose for renal function.

- Azithromycin and clarithromycin have enhanced activity over erythromycin against *H. influenzae* and several nontubercular mycobacterial species.
- Telithromycin has enhanced activity for *S. pneumoniae* (including strains resistant to macrolides); it retains activity against *H. influenzae*, *M. catarrhalis*, *Mycoplasma*, *Legionella*, and *C. pneumoniae*

Toxicities
- GI side effects (more common with erythromycin and telithromycin), diplopia (telithromycin), rare reversible hearing loss with high doses
- Can prolong the QT interval, with rare reports of torsades de pointes; this may be least significant for azithromycin.
- Agents except azithromycin inhibit metabolism of other drugs through the cytochrome P-450 (CYP) 3A4 system; the potential for drug interactions should be reviewed closely.

Trimethoprim-Sulfamethoxazole (Table 9)
Spectrum of Activity
- Includes a wide variety of aerobic gram-positive cocci and gram-negative bacilli: staphylococci (moderate activity), most *S. pneumoniae*, *H. influenzae*, *M. catarrhalis*, *L. monocytogenes*, and many *Enterobacteriaceae*.

Table 9. Miscellaneous Antibacterials

Drug	Usual adult dose for normal renal function	Elimination
Clindamycin	PO: 150-450 mg qid IV: 300-900 mg q 6-8 hours	Hepatic
Daptomycin	4 mg/kg IV daily (6 mg/kg under study)	Renal*
Linezolid	600 mg bid (PO or IV)	Hepatic
Metronidazole	7.5 mg/kg (500 mg) q 6-12 hours	Hepatic
Dalfopristin-quinupristin	7.5 mg/kg IV q 8-12 hours	Hepatic
Trimethoprim-sulfamethoxazole	PO: 1 DS bid IV: 8-15 mg/kg daily in 3-4 divided doses	Renal*

bid, twice daily; DS, double strength; q, every; qid, 4 times daily.
*Adjust dose for renal function.

- Active against *Pneumocystis*, *Stenotrophomonas*, *Nocardia*, *Shigella*, and *Isospora*, but not *Pseudomonas*

Toxicities
- Hypersensitivity reactions and GI side effects are most common.
- Nephrotoxicity, myelosuppression, and hyperkalemia are less frequent but may occur, especially with high-dose therapy.
- Use with caution or avoid during the last trimester of pregnancy (to minimize risk of fetal kernicterus) and in patients with known glucose-6-phosphatase dehydrogenase deficiency.

Clindamycin (Table 9)

Spectrum of Activity
- Includes aerobic and anaerobic gram-positive organisms.
- Its anaerobic activity includes *Actinomyces* spp, *Clostridium* (except *C. difficile*), *Peptostreptococcus* and most *Bacteroides* spp, but, 10%-20% of *B. fragilis* organisms are resistant.
- Clindamycin is active against gram-positive aerobes such as many staphylococci and group A streptococci, but emergence of resistance by staphylococci can occur during treatment.

Toxicities
- Most commonly include rash and GI side effects
- Antibiotic-associated diarrhea can occur in up to 20% of patients, and *C. difficile* colitis occurs in 1%-10%.

Metronidazole (Table 9)
Spectrum of Activity
- Includes most anaerobic microorganisms, including *Bacteroides* spp.
- Exceptions include some anaerobic gram-positive organisms: *Peptostreptococcus*, *Actinomyces*, and *Propionibacterium acnes*.
- Also effective against *Entamoeba histolytica*, *Giardia*, and *Gardnerella*.

Toxicities
- Include nausea, vomiting, reversible neutropenia, metallic taste, and a disulfiram reaction when coadministered with alcohol.

Dalfopristin-quinupristin (Synercid) (Table 9)
Spectrum of Activity
- Good activity against gram-positive cocci, including vancomycin-resistant *Enterococcus faecium* and staphylococcus, including methicillin-resistant strains, but, activity against *E. faecalis* is substantially decreased.

Toxicities
- A relatively high rate of inflammation and irritation at the infusion site, arthralgias, myalgias, and hyperbilirubinemia
- Can inhibit the metabolism of other drugs metabolized via the CYP 3A4 enzyme system and close attention should be paid to possible drug interactions.

Linezolid (Table 9)
Spectrum of Activity
- Has activity against gram-positive bacteria, including methicillin-resistant staphylococci, most vancomycin-resistant enterococci, and penicillin-resistant *S. pneumoniae*

- Also has activity against *Nocardia* and some mycobacterial species

Toxicities
- The most prominent is myelosuppression, especially with prolonged use
- Headache, diarrhea, and peripheral or optic neuropathy also can occur.
- Linezolid is a weak monoamine oxidase inhibitor that can interact with some medications, such as selective serotonin reuptake inhibitors and monoamine oxidase inhibitors.

Daptomycin (Table 9)
Spectrum of Activity
- Includes *Staphylococcus* (including methicillin-resistant strains), *Streptococcus pyogenes*, *S. agalactiae*, and *Enterococcus* (including vancomycin-resistant strains)

Toxicities
- GI effects, hypersensitivity reactions, headache, insomnia, myalgias, and CK elevations.
- Manufacturer suggests stopping statins during daptomycin therapy and monitoring CK values weekly.

ANTIVIRAL AGENTS
Anti–Herpes Simplex Virus (HSV) Agents (Table 10)
Agents
- Acyclovir, valacyclovir, famciclovir

Spectrum of Activity
- Acyclovir and its prodrug, valacyclovir, have clinical activity against HSV-1 and HSV-2, are also active against varicella-zoster virus (VZV), but are not effective against cytomegalovirus (CMV).
- Famciclovir is active against HSV-1, HSV-2, and VZV.

Toxicities
- Acyclovir has been associated with neurotoxicity, nephrotoxicity (IV), and GI effects.
- Patients on high-dose IV acyclovir should be well hydrated to minimize drug precipitation in renal tubules.

Table 10. Anti-HSV Agents

Drug	Usual adult dose for normal renal function	Elimination
Acyclovir	Mucocutaneous disease: 5 mg/kg IV q 8 hours HSV encephalitis: 10 mg/kg IV q 8 hours Varicella-zoster (immunocompromised): 10-12 mg/kg IV q 8 hours Genital herpes: 400 mg PO tid or 800 mg PO bid Varicella-zoster: 600-800 mg PO 5 × per or 1,000 mg PO q 6 hours Chronic suppression for recurrent infection: 400 mg PO bid (400 mg 800 mg PO bid-tid in HIV)	Renal*
Valacyclovir	Herpes zoster: 1 g PO tid First episode genital herpes: 1 g PO bid Recurrent genital herpes: 500 mg PO bid Suppression for recurrent genital herpes: 500-1,000 mg PO daily	Renal*
Famiciclovir	Herpes zoster: 500 mg q 8 hours Recurrent genital herpes in HIV patients: 500 mg bid Recurrent genital herpes (non-HIV): 125 mg bid Suppression of recurrent genital herpes: 250 mg bid	Renal*

bid, twice daily; HSV, herpes simples virus; q, every; tid, 3 times daily.
*Adjust dose for renal function.

- Famciclovir is associated with headache, nausea, diarrhea, and rare CNS effects, specifically confusion or hallucinations; neutropenia and liver function test elevations may occur rarely.

Anti-Cytomegalovirus Agents (Table 11)
Agents
- Ganciclovir, valganciclovir, cidofovir, foscarnet

Spectrum of Activity
- Ganciclovir and its prodrug, valganciclovir, are clinically active against CMV, HSV-1 and HSV-2, VZV, and human herpesvirus (HHV)-6.
- Cidofovir and foscarnet are clinically active against CMV (including many ganciclovir-resistant strains), HSV-1 and HSV-2 (including many acyclovir-resistant strains), VZV, and HHV-6.

Toxicities
- Ganciclovir and valganciclovir are associated with myelo-suppression, generally neutropenia or thrombocytopenia.
  - ▲ Less commonly, nephrotoxicity, liver function test elevations, and fever can occur.
  - ▲ CNS effects, including headache, confusion, seizures, and coma, have been described but are rare.
- Cidofovir can cause dose-related nephrotoxicity, neutropenia, iritis, uveitis, and GI effects.
  - ▲ Saline hydration and probenecid should be used to decrease the risk of nephrotoxicity.
- Foscarnet is associated with nephrotoxicity, electrolyte disturbances, and CNS effects; fever, nausea, vomiting, and diarrhea are common.

Anti-Influenza Agents (Table 12)
Agents
- Rimantadine, amantadine, oseltamivir, zanamivir

Spectrum of Activity
- Rimantadine and amantadine are active only against influenza A; resistance is increasing.
- Oseltamivir and zanamivir are active against influenza A and B and have activity against avian influenza.

Table 11. Anti-Cytomegalovirus Agents

Drug	Usual adult dose for normal renal function	Elimination
Ganciclovir	IV induction: 5 mg/kg q 12 hours IV maintenance: 5 mg/kg q 24 hours PO: 1 g tid	Renal*
Valganciclovir	Induction: 900 mg PO bid Maintenance: 900 mg PO daily	Renal*
Cidofovir	Induction: 5 mg/kg IV weekly × 2 weeks Maintenance: 5 mg/kg IV every other week	Renal*
Foscarnet	Induction: 60 mg/kg (over 1 hour) IV q 8 hours *or* 90 mg/kg (over 1-2 hours) IV q 12 hours × 14-21 days Maintenance: 90-120 mg/kg (over 2 hours) IV q 24 hours	Renal*

bid, twice daily; q, every; tid, 3 times daily.
*Adjust dose for renal function.

Toxicities
- Rimantadine and amantadine
  - ▲ Commonly associated with GI complaints and CNS effects, including insomnia, anxiety, difficulty concentrating.
  - ▲ Neurotoxicity, including tremor, seizures, and coma, has been reported at high doses and doses unadjusted for renal function.
  - ▲ CNS effects are less pronounced with rimantadine.
  - ▲ Dose-related cardiac arrhythmias have been reported rarely.
- Zanamivir and oseltamivir
  - ▲ Generally well tolerated, with GI complaints most frequently reported
  - ▲ Zanamivir may rarely cause cough and bronchospasm and

Table 12. Anti-Influenza Agents

Drug	Usual adult dose for normal renal function	Elimination
Amantadine	Treatment or prophylaxis: 100 mg PO bid (or 100 mg PO daily for patients ≥65 years) × 5 days	Renal*
Rimantadine	Treatment or prophylaxis: 100 mg PO bid (or 100 mg PO daily for patients ≥65 years) × 5 days	Hepatic/renal*
Oseltamivir	Treatment: 75 mg PO bid × 5 days Prophylaxis: 75 mg PO daily	Hepatic/renal*
Zanamivir	Treatment: 10 mg (2 inhalations) bid × 5 days	Renal

bid, twice daily.
*Adjust dose for renal function.

is not recommended in patients with underlying chronic pulmonary disease.

Antihepatitis Agents (see Appendix 2)

Antiretroviral Agents
Prototypic Agents
- Nucleoside/nucleotide reverse transcriptase inhibitors
  - Abacavir, didanosine, emtricitabine, lamivudine, stavudine, tenofovir, zalcitabine, zidovudine
  - Combination agents—Combivir (zidovudine-lamivudine), Trizivir (zidovudine, lamivudine, abacavir), Epzicom (abacavir-lamivudine), Truvada (tenofovir-emtricitabine)
  - Non-nucleoside reverse transcriptase inhibitors—efavirenz, nevirapine, delavirdine
  - Protease inhibitors—amprenavir, atazanavir, fosamprenavir, indinavir, lopinavir-ritonavir, nelfinavir, ritonavir, saquinavir, tipranavir
  - Fusion inhibitor—enfuvirtide

Novel Adverse Effects

- Nucleoside/nucleotide reverse transcriptase inhibitors—class side effects include rare lactic acidosis, hepatic steatosis and lipoatrophy; more common with stavudine and didanosine, especially in combination.
  - ▲ Abacavir has potential for serious hypersensitivity reactions; symptoms may include fever, rash, GI (nausea, vomiting, diarrhea, or abdominal pain), constitutional (generalized malaise, fatigue, or achiness), and respiratory (dyspnea, cough, or pharyngitis).
    - • Avoid abacavir rechallenge in patients with suspected or confirmed hypersensitivity because severe and even fatal reactions can occur.
  - ▲ Didanosine, zalcitabine, and stavudine can cause peripheral neuropathy.
  - ▲ Didanosine is associated with pancreatitis.
  - ▲ Zidovudine can cause myelosuppression, especially in combination with other myelosuppressive drugs.
  - ▲ Tenofovir has been anecdotally reported to cause renal toxicity (proximal tubular dysfunction and Fanconi syndrome).
- Non-nucleoside reverse transcriptase inhibitors—class side effects include hypersensitivity reactions and hepatotoxicity
  - ▲ All can cause hepatotoxicity, especially with underlying liver disease; incidence is highest with nevirapine in women with CD4 $\geq$250 cells/mm^3 or men with CD4 $\geq$400 cells/mm^3.
  - ▲ Efavirenz can cause CNS effects such as insomnia, vivid dreams, trouble concentrating, and hallucinations; these often resolve after first 2-4 weeks.
  - ▲ Drug interactions should be reviewed closely because non-nucleoside reverse transcriptase inhibitors can induce metabolism of other drugs via the cytochrome P-450 system (efavirenz is a mixed inducer-inhibitor).
- Protease inhibitors—class side effects include hyperlipidemia (especially triglycerides), glucose intolerance, and lipodystrophy (these may be less common with atazanavir); more rarely, spontaneous bleeding has been noted in hemophiliacs.
  - ▲ GI side effects appear most frequent with lopinavir-ritonavir, high-dose ritonavir, and nelfinavir.

- ▲ Nephrolithiasis can occur with indinavir; patients should stay well hydrated to minimize this.
- ▲ Atazanavir can cause hyperbilirubinemia (usually asymptomatic)
- ▲ Drug interactions should be reviewed closely—most commonly, protease inhibitors inhibit metabolism of other drugs via CYP 3A4, and some can also be inducers of other CYP isoenzymes.
- ▪ Fusion inhibitor (enfuvirtide)—local site reactions with SQ injection are common.

For drug selection and drug dosing, see the latest guidelines from the U.S. Department of Health and Human Services: http://aidsinfo.nih.gov/guidelines/.

ANTIFUNGAL AGENTS
Azoles
Agents
- ▪ Fluconazole, itraconazole, voriconazole, posaconazole (under review by U.S. Food and Drug Administration) (Table 13)

Spectrum of Activity
- ▪ Fluconazole—active against most *Candida* spp (less activity against *C. glabrata*, inactive against *C. krusei*), *Cryptococcus*, *Coccidioides immitis*, *Histoplasma capsulatum*, *Blastomyces dermatitidis*, and *Paracoccidioides* sp
- ▪ Itraconazole
    - ▲ Active against some filamentous fungi, including *Aspergillus* spp, *Pseudallescheria* sp, *Alternaria* sp, etc.
    - ▲ Similar activity against most yeasts as fluconazole but with greater activity against *Histoplasma* and *Blastomyces* infections and active against most fluconazole-resistant *Candida* spp (but cross-resistance can occur)
- ▪ Voriconazole—active against many filamentous fungi including *Aspergillus* spp, *Pseudallescheria*/*Scedosporium* sp, *Fusarium* spp, while retaining similar anti-*Candida* activity as fluconazole and itraconazole (may be active against fluconazole and itraconazole-resistant strains, but cross-resistance can occur)
- ▪ Posaconazole—activity similar to voriconazole but possesses some activity against the Zygomycetes.

Table 13. Azole Antifungal Dosing

Drug	Usual adult dose for normal renal function	Excretion (liver/kidney)
Fluconazole (PO/IV)	200-400 mg daily	Renal*
Itraconazole PO[†]	200 mg daily-bid	Hepatic
Itraconazole IV	200 mg daily[‡]	Hepatic
Voriconazole PO	200-300 mg bid	Hepatic
Voriconazole IV	6 mg/kg q 12 hours × 2 days, then 4 mg/kg q 12 hours	Hepatic
Posaconazole[§] (PO only)	400 mg bid or 200 mg qid	Hepatic

bid, twice daily; q, every; qid, 4 times daily.

*Adjust doses for renal function.

[†]Itraconazole capsules require gastric acid (low pH) for adequate absorption, but liquid PO itraconazole does not have this requirement.

[‡]After loading dose of 200 mg IV every 12 hours × 2 days.

[§]Currently under review by U.S. Food and Drug Administration.

Toxicities

- All azoles can cause elevated liver function tests and, less commonly, hepatotoxicity.
- Itraconazole and voriconazole inhibit liver metabolism (and secondarily increase serum drug concentrations of many drugs, including cyclosporine, tacrolimus, digoxin, midazolam, and triazolam; review potential drug interactions closely).
- About 10% of patients starting voriconazole develop transient visual disturbances.
- Rash is more common with voriconazole.
- Itraconazole IV and voriconazole IV contain a cyclodextrin vehicle that can accumulate with renal dysfunction; clinical significance is unclear; use with caution in patients with renal dysfunction (assess risk/benefit).

Polyenes: Amphotericin B Products

Agents

- Amphotericin B deoxycholate and lipid formulations of amphotericin (AmBisome, Abelcet, Amphotec) (Table 14)

Table 14. Amphotericin Dosing*

Drug	Usual adult dose	Excretion (liver/kidney)
Amphotericin B deoxycholate	0.25-1.5 mg/kg daily	Intracellular degradation
AmBisome†	3-5 mg/kg daily	Intracellular degradation
Abelcet†	3-5 mg/kg daily	Intracellular degradation
Amphotec	3-5 mg/kg daily	Intracellular degradation

*Doses may be increased for invasive molds.
†Doses 5-10 mg/kg often used for treatment of Zygomycetes and other refractory invasive molds.

Spectrum of Activity

- Broadest antifungal activity, including yeasts (*Candida* spp, *Cryptococcus*, etc.), dimorphic fungi (*Histoplasma, Coccidioides, Blastomyces*), and filamentous fungi (*Aspergillus*, the Zygomycetes and dematiaceous molds).

Toxicities

- Infusion-related: fever, chills, rigors, nausea, vomiting
  - ▲ Pretreatment with diphenhydramine, acetaminophen, meperidine may lessen these reactions.
  - ▲ These are less frequent with AmBisome.
- Nephrotoxicity (usually reversible)—can be lessened by sodium crystalloid loading
- Others: hypokalemia, hypomagnesemia, anemia, phlebitis, changes in blood pressure, neurologic effects
- Lipid amphotericin agents have less nephrotoxicity than amphotericin B deoxycholate.

Echinocandins
Agents
- Caspofungin, micafungin, anidulafungin (investigational) (Table 15)

Spectrum of Activity
- Active against *Candida* spp (including azole-resistant strains) and *Aspergillus* spp

- Not active against *Cryptococcus* spp and the Zygomycetes

Toxicities (Not Common)
- Possible histamine-related effects —rash, facial swelling
- Liver function test abnormalities

ANTIMYCOBACTERIAL AGENTS
Anti-TB Agents
First-Line Agents
- Isoniazid, a rifamycin (rifampin, rifabutin, rifapentine), pyrazinamide, ethambutol (Table 16)

Toxicities
- Isoniazid—hepatitis, peripheral neuropathy, rash and other skin eruptions, rarely seizures.
- Rifampin—hepatitis (may show cholestatic pattern), orange discoloration of urine and tears (not a toxicity), rash and other skin eruptions, thrombocytopenia, anemia, flulike symptoms, nephritis, proteinuria
  - ▲ Rifampin induces hepatic CYP P-45 metabolic pathway, resulting in decreased serum concentrations of concomitantly administered drugs metabolized by this same pathway, including the following: azathioprine, azole antifungals, calcium channel blockers, corticosteroids, cyclosporine, dapsone, diazepam, digoxin, haloperidol, imidazoles, opioids/methadone, oral contraceptives, oral hypoglycemic agents, phenytoin, propranolol, protease inhibitors, quinidine, theophylline, tolbutamide, warfarin.
- Rifabutin
  - ▲ Profile similar to rifampin plus uveitis, arthritis and arthralgias, neutropenia and leukopenia, bronze skin pigmentation.
  - ▲ Less hepatic CYP P-450 induction than rifampin
- Pyrazinamide—hepatitis, arthralgias, hyperuricemia (not a toxicity), rash
- Ethambutol— optic neuritis (decreased visual acuity or red-green color discrimination)

Table 15. Echinocandins

Drug	Usual adult dose	Excretion (liver/kidney)
Caspofungin	70 mg IV load × 1, then 50 mg IV daily	Hepatic
Micafungin	50-150 mg daily	Hepatic
Anidulafungin	Investigational	Investigational

Table 16. Dosing of Anti-TB Drugs (Adult Dosing)

Drug	Usual adult dose			Excretion (liver/kidney)
Isoniazid	300 mg daily			Hepatic
	900 mg 2 or 3 times weekly			
Rifampin	600 mg daily			Hepatic
	600 mg 2 or 3 times weekly			
Rifabutin	300 mg daily			Hepatic
	300 mg 2 or 3 times weekly			
Rifapentine	600 mg once weekly			
Pyrazinamide, patient weight				Hepatic
	Daily	Twice weekly	3 times weekly	
40-55 kg	1,000 mg	1,500 mg	2,000 mg	
56-75 kg	1,500 mg	2,500 mg	3,000 mg	
76-90 kg	2,000 mg	3,000 mg	4,000 mg	
Ethambutol, patient weight				Hepatic
	Daily	Twice weekly	3 times weekly	
40-55 kg	800 mg	1,200 mg	2,000 mg	
56-75 kg	1,200 mg	2,000 mg	2,800 mg	
76-90 kg	1,600 mg	2,400 mg	4,000 mg	

Second-Line Agents

- Fluoroquinolones (moxifloxacin, levofloxacin), aminoglycosides (streptomycin, amikacin, kanamycin), capreomycin, ethionamide, cycloserine, para-aminosalicylic acid, linezolid, clofazimine

Non-TB Mycobacteria Agents

- Selection of drugs depends on specific mycobacteria species but may include macrolides (clarithromycin, azithromycin), fluoroquinolones (moxifloxacin, levofloxacin, ciprofloxacin), doxycycline, tigecycline, trimethoprim-sulfamethoxazole, amikacin, tobramycin, imipenem, linezolid, cefoxitin, clofazimine.

Acknowledgment: The authors acknowledge the specific contributions of Glenn D. Roberts, Ph.D., and Rachel M. Chambers, Pharm.D.

Appendix 1. Organism Taxonomy

Aerobic Bacteria

Gram-positive cocci

Staphylococcus spp
  S. aureus
  S. epidermidis
  S. saprophyticus
  S. lugdunensis
  Other *Staphylococcus* spp
Streptococcus spp
  S. pyogenes (group A)
  S. agalactiae (group B)
  Streptococcus groups C, F, G
  S. pneumoniae
  S. bovis
  Viridans group streptococci
    S. anginosus
    S. constellatus
    S. criceti
    S. crista
    S. downei
    S. gordonii
    S. infantis
    S. intermedius
    S. macacae
    S. mitis
    S. mutans
    S. oralis
    S. parasanguinis
    S. peroris
    S. rattus
    S. salivarus
    S. sanguis
    S. sobrinus
    S. thermophilus
    S. vestibularis
Enterococcus spp
  E. faecalis
  E. faecium
Rhodococcus equi
Micrococcus spp

Gram-positive bacilli

Bacillus anthracis
Bacillus cereus
Corynebacterium diphtheriae
Corynebacterium jeikeium
Corynebacterium spp (other)
Erysipelothrix rhusiopathiae

Gram-negative cocci

Neisseria gonorrhoeae
Neisseria meningitidis
Moraxella (Branhamella)
  catarrhalis

Gram-negative bacilli

Enterobacteriaceae
  Escherichia coli
  Klebsiella pneumoniae
  Enterobacter spp
  Citrobacter spp
  Proteus mirabilis (indole-negative)
  Proteus vulgaris (indole-positive)
  Morganella morganii
  Serratia spp
  Salmonella spp
  Shigella
  Providencia spp
  Yersinia spp
  Edwardsiella spp
  Hafnia spp
Acinetobacter spp
Stenotrophomonas maltophilia
Pseudomonas aeruginosa
Pseudomonas spp (other)
Aeromonas hydrophila
Moraxella spp
Alcaligenes spp
Flavobacterium spp
Haemophilus spp
Bartonella spp
Bordetella spp
Brucella spp
Burkholderia cepacia
Calymmatobacterium
  granulomatis
Capnocytophaga spp
Francisella tularensis
Gardnerella vaginalis
HACEK group: *Haemophilus*
  parainfluenzae, H. aphrophilus,
  H. paraphrophilus, Actino-
  bacillus actinomycetemco-
  mitans, Cardiobacterium
  hominis, Eikenella corrodens,
  Kingella kingae
Legionella spp
Providencia spp
Vibrio spp

Appendix 1 (continued)
Anaerobic Bacteria

Gram-positive cocci
  Peptostreptococcus spp

Gram-positive bacilli
  Actinomyces spp
  Bifidobacterium spp
  Clostridium botulinum
  Clostridium difficile
  Clostridium perfringens
  Clostridium tetani
  Eubacterium spp
  Lactobacillus spp
  Leptotrichia spp

Gram-positive bacilli (continued)
  Mobiluncus spp
  Propionibacterium spp
  Rothia spp

Gram-negative cocci
  Veillonella spp

Gram-negative bacilli
  Bacteroides spp
  Fusobacterium spp
  Porphyromonas spp
  Prevotella spp

Fungi*

Yeasts—grow as single cells and reproduce by budding
  Candida spp
    C. albicans
    C. tropicalis
    C. parapsilosis
    C. glabrata
    C. krusei
    C. lusitaniae
    C. guilliermondii
  Cryptococcus neoformans
  Other *Cryptococcus* spp
  Blastoschizomyces capitatus
    (formerly called *Trichosporon capitatum*)
  Malassezia spp
  Malassezia furfur
  Saccharomyces cerevisiae
  Rhodotorula spp
  Trichosporon spp includes
    T. cutaneum, asteroides, ovoides, inkin, asahii, mucoides

Dimorphic fungi—exhibit two different growth forms: outside the body, they grow as a mold, producing hyphae and asexual reproductive spores; in the body, they grow in a non-mycelial form

Dimorphic fungi (continued)
  Histoplasma capsulatum
  Blastomyces dermatitidis
  Coccidioides immitis
  Paracoccidioides brasiliensis
  Sporothrix schenckii
  Penicillium marneffei

Dermatophytes—superficial skin/hair infections
  Epidermophyton spp
  Microsporum spp
  Trichophyton spp

Filamentous fungi—reproduce principally by elongation at tips of filamentous growth forms

Hyaline hypomycetes— colorless fungi
  Aspergillus spp includes (list not complete) *A. flavus, niger, clavatus, terreus, fumigatus, glaucus* group, *nidulans, oryzae, ustus, versicolor*
  Acremonium spp
  Chrysosporium spp
  Fusarium spp
  Geotrichum spp

Hyaline hypomycetes (continued)

Paecilomyces spp
Penicillium spp
Scedosporium apiospermum (*Pseudallescheria boydii* is sexual form)
Scopulariopsis spp (sexual form is *Microascus*)
Trichoderma spp
Verticillium spp
Zygomycetes (aseptate or few septates) includes *Absidia*, *Apophysomyces*, *Basidiobolus*, *Conidiobolus*, *Cokeromyces*, *Cunninghamella*, *Mortierella*, *Mucor*, *Rhizomucor*, *Rhizopus*, *Saksenaea vasiformis*, *Syncephalastrum*

Dematiaceous Hyphomycetes

—produce dark brown or black melanin pigment in cell walls (phaeohyphomycosis)

Alternaria spp
Aureobasidium spp
Bipolaris spp
Chaetomium spp
Cladophialophora spp
Cladosporium spp
Curvularia spp
Ochroconis (*Dactylaria*) spp
Drechslera spp
Epicoccum spp
Exophiala jeanselmei
Fonsecaea spp
Lecythophora spp
Hortaea werneckii
Phialophora spp
Ramichloridium spp
Scedosporium prolificans
Ulocladium spp
Wangiella dermatidis

*Clinical and histologic groupings; not all human pathogenic fungi listed.

Viruses

DNA viruses

Pox virus group
  Vaccina virus (cowpox)
  Variola (smallpox)
  Parapoxvirus (milker's nodule)
  Molluscum contagiosum
Herpesvirus group
  Herpes simplex virus (HSV) 1 & 2
  Varicella-zoster virus (VZV)
  Cytomegalovirus (CMV)
  Epstein-Barr virus (EBV)
  Human herpesvirus 6 & 7
  Human herpesvirus 8 (Kaposi sarcoma)
  Herpes B virus
Adenovirus
Human papillomavirus (HPV)
Polyomavirus group
  JC virus
  BK virus
Hepatitis B virus (HBV)
Parvoviruses (B19 virus)

RNA viruses

Enterovirus group
  Poliovirus
  Coxsackieviruses A & B
  Echovirus
  Enterovirus
Rhinovirus
Hepatitis A virus (HAV)
Influenza virus (A, B, C)
Paramyxovirus group
  Parainfluenza virus
  Mumps virus
  Measles virus (rubeola)
  Respiratory syncytial virus (RSV)
Rabies virus
Arbovirus group
  Alphavirus group
    Eastern equine encephalitis (EEE) virus
    Western equine encephalitis (WEE) virus
    Venezuelan equine encephalitis (VEE) virus

Appendix 1 (continued)

RNA viruses (continued)
  - Chikungunya virus
  - O'nyong-nyong virus
  - Flavivirus group
    - Yellow fever virus
    - Dengue fever virus
    - St. Louis encephalitis virus
    - Japanese encephalitis virus
    - West Nile virus
    - Powassan encephalitis virus
    - Murray Valley encephalitis virus
    - Hepatitis C virus (HCV)
  - Rubella virus (German measles)
  - La Crosse encephalitis virus
  - Hantavirus
  - Retrovirus group
    - HIV 1 & 2
    - Human T-cell lymphotropic virus 1 & 2
  - Lymphocytic choriomeningitis (LCM) virus
  - Lassa virus (Lassa fever)
  - Calicivirus
  - Norwalk & Norwalk-like viruses
  - Astrovirus
  - Colorado tick fever virus (an arbovirus)
  - Ebola virus
  - Marburg virus
  - Coronavirus
  - Rotavirus
  - Hepatitis E virus

Appendix 2. Treatment of Specific Organisms

Information provided is not intended to replace clinical judgment. Patients' conditions may vary and require adjustments in therapy. An infectious disease consultation should be considered to assist in patient care.

Bacterial Organism-Specific Treatment

Organism	Preferred therapy	Alternative agents (depending on susceptibility)
Acinetobacter	Meropenem, imipenem (not ertapenem)	Tigecycline, piperacillin-tazobactam, ceftazidime, cefepime, quinolone, aminoglycoside, colistin, minocycline, tmp-smx
Actinomyces	Penicillin	Ampicillin-amoxicillin, doxycycline, cephalosporin, clindamycin, erythromycin
Aeromonas	tmp-smx, quinolone	Carbapenem,* gentamicin, 3rd-generation cephalosporin

Organism	Preferred therapy	Alternative agents (depending on susceptibility)
Bacillus anthracis (anthrax)	Ciprofloxacin, doxycycline	Amoxicillin, penicillin, levofloxacin, imipenem
Bacillus spp	Vancomycin	Clindamycin, carbapenem,* quinolone
Bacteroides fragilis	Metronidazole	Carbapenem,* β-lactam/β-lactamase inhibitor,† clindamycin, moxifloxacin, cefotetan, cefoxitin
Bartonella henselae & *B. quintana*	Macrolide,‡ doxycycline	
Bordetella pertussis	Macrolide‡	Tmp-smx
Borrelia burgdorferi (Lyme disease)	Doxycycline, amoxicillin	Penicillin, cefuroxime axetil, cefotaxime, ceftriaxone, azithromycin, clarithromycin
Brucella spp	Doxycycline plus gentamicin or streptomycin or rifampin	Tmp-smx, ciprofloxacin, chloramphenicol; each ± gentamicin/streptomycin or rifampin
Burkholderia cepacae	Often a colonizer, tmp-smx	Ceftazidime, cefepime, carbapenem,* quinolone
Campylobacter jejuni	Erythromycin, azithromycin	Doxycycline, quinolone, gentamicin, furazolidone
Capnocytophaga spp	Clindamycin, amoxicillin-clavulanate	Erythromycin, quinolone, carbapenem,* doxycycline, β-lactam/β-lactamase inhibitor†
Chlamydia pneumoniae	Doxycycline, macrolide‡	Quinolone, telithromycin
Citrobacter freundii	Carbapenem*	Quinolone, aminoglycoside, tmp-smx, 3rd or 4th-generation cephalosporin, piperacillin-tazobactam
Clostridium difficile	Metronidazole	Vancomycin (PO)

Appendix 2 (continued)

Organism	Preferred therapy	Alternative agents (depending on susceptibility)
Clostridium perfringens	Penicillin	Metronidazole, clindamycin, β-lactam/β-lactamase inhibitor,[†] carbapenem*
Clostridium tetani	Metronidazole + tetanus immune globulin & tetanus toxoid	Doxycycline, penicillin
Corynebacterium diptheriae	Erythromycin + antitoxin	Clindamycin, penicillin
Corynebacterium JK group	Vancomycin	Penicillin + gentamicin, macrolide[‡]
Coxiella burnetti (Q fever)	Acute: doxycycline Chronic (endocarditis): doxycycline + hydroxychloroquine; doxycycline + quinolone	Acute: quinolone, macrolide[‡] Chronic: doxycycline + quinolone, doxycycline + rifampin
Ehrlichia	Doxycycline	
Eikenella corrodens	Ampicillin-amoxicillin, 3rd generation cephalosporin	Doxycycline, β-lactam/β-lactamase inhibitor,[†] quinolone
Enterobacter	Carbapenem*	Quinolone, tmp-smx, cefepime, piperacillin-tazobactam, aminoglycoside
Enterococcus spp[§]		
Ampicillin-sensitive	Ampicillin-amoxicillin, penicillin	Vancomycin, β-lactam/β-lactamase inhibitor,[†] linezolid, dalfopristin-quinupristin (*E. faecium* only), tigecycline
Ampicillin-resistant, vancomycin-sensitive	Vancomycin	Linezolid, daptomycin,[//] daltopristin-quinupristin (*E. faecium* only), tigecycline
Vancomycin-resistant	Linezolid[†]	Daptomycin,[//] dalfopristin-quinupristin (*E. faecium* only), tigecycline

Organism	Preferred therapy	Alternative agents (depending on susceptibility)
Erysipelothrix rhusiopathiae	Penicillin	Cephalosporin, quinolone, clindamycin, carbapenem*
Escherichia coli	Ceftriaxone, cefotaxime, cefepime (use a carbapenem* for ESBL-producing strains)	Quinolone, aminoglycoside, other cephalosporin, β-lactam/β-lactamase inhibitor,[†] ampicillin, tmp-smx
Francisella tularensis (tularemia)	Streptomycin, gentamicin (both + doxycycline or chloramphenicol for CNS infections)	Doxycycline, quinolone, chloramphenicol
Fusobacterium	Penicillin	Metronidazole, clindamycin, β-lactam/β-lactamase inhibitor,[†] carbapenem*
Gardnerella vaginalis (bacterial vaginosis)	Metronidazole	Topical metronidazole, topical or PO clindamycin
Haemophilus influenzae	Ceftriaxone, cefotaxime	Quinolone, tmp-smx, azithromycin, clarithromycin, telithromycin, β-lactam/β-lactamase inhibitor,[†] doxycycline
Klebsiella pneumoniae	Ceftriaxone, cefotaxime, cefepime (use a carbapenem* for ESBL-producing strains)	Quinolone, aminoglycoside, tmp-smx, β-lactam/β-lactamase inhibitor,[†] carbapenem*
Leuconostoc spp	Ampicillin/amoxicillin, penicillin	Clindamycin, doxycycline, macrolide[‡]
Legionella spp	Newer quinolone,[¶] azithromycin ± rifampin	Other macrolide,[‡] doxycycline, tmp-smx; each ± rifampin
Listeria monocytogenes	Ampicillin or penicillin ± gentamicin	Tmp-smx
Moraxella catarrhalis	2nd or 3rd-generation cephalosporin	Quinolone, azithromycin, clarithromycin, telithromycin, tmp-smx, cefepime, doxycycline, β-lactam/β-lactamase inhibitor[†]

Appendix 2 (continued)

Organism	Preferred therapy	Alternative agents (depending on susceptibility)
Morganella morganii	3rd or 4th-generation cephalosporin, quinolone	tmp-smx, carbapenem,* piperacillin-tazobactam, aminoglycoside
Mycobacterium avium-intracellulare	Treatment: clarithromycin + ethambutol ± rifabutin or rifampin Prophylaxis: azithromycin, clarithromycin	As parts of combination treatment: newer quinolone,¶ amikacin
Mycobacterium chelonae	Tobramycin + imipenem + clarithromycin; Localized skin infection: clarithromycin	Amikacin, newer quinolones,¶ azithromycin, linezolid
Mycobacterium abscessus	Amikacin + cefoxitin + clarithromycin or imipenem	Newer quinolones,¶ azithromycin, linezolid
Mycobacterium fortuitum	Imipenem or cefoxitin + amikacin	Newer quinolones,¶ clarithromycin, sulfamethoxazole, doxycycline, linezolid
Mycobacterium kansasii	Isoniazid + rifampin ± ethambutol or streptomycin	Clarithromycin, azithromycin, ethionamide, cycloserine, rifabutin, quinolone
Mycobacterium leprae	Dapsone + rifampin ± clofazimine	Minocycline, clarithromycin, quinolone
Mycobacterium marinum	Clarithromycin, tmp-smx, minocycline, or rifampin + ethambutol	
Mycobacterium tuberculosis	4-drug combo: isoniazid, rifampin, ethambutol, pyrazinamide	As parts of combination treatment: newer quinolones,¶ cycloserine, capreomycin, amikacin, kanamycin, ethionamide, para-aminosalicylic acid, linezolid

Organism	Preferred therapy	Alternative agents (depending on susceptibility)
Mycoplasma pneumoniae	Macrolide[‡]	Doxycycline, quinolone, telithromycin
Neisseria gonorrhoeae	Ceftriaxone, cefixime	Cefotaxime, quinolone (variable resistance)
Neisseria meningitidis	Penicillin, ceftriaxone, cefotaxime	Ampicilln, quinolone, tmp-smx
Nocardia asteroides	Tmp-smx	Minocycline, imipenem ± amikacin, sulfonamide, ceftriaxone ± amikacin, amoxicillin-clavulanate, linezolid
Pasteurella multocida	Penicillin, ampicillin, amoxicillin	Doxycycline, 2nd/3rd-generation cephalosporin, tmp-smx, β-lactam/β-lactamase inhibitor,[‡] carbapenem[§]
Peptostrepto-coccus	Penicillin, ampicillin, amoxicillin	Clindamycin, cephalosporin, newer quinolone,[¶] carbapenem,[*] vancomycin, telithromycin, β-lactam/β-lactamase inhibitor[†]
Propionibacter-ium acnes (systemic infection)	(Common blood culture contaminant) Penicillin	Clindamycin, doxycycline, carbapenem[*]
Proteus mirabilis	Ampicillin, amoxicillin	Cephalosporin, quinolone, aminoglycoside, tmp-smx, β-lactam/β-lactamase inhibitor,[†] carbapenem[*]
Proteus vulgaris and *Providencia*	3rd or 4th-generation cephalosporin, carbapenem[*]	Quinolone, aminoglycoside, tmp-smx, piperacillin-tazobactam
Pseudomonas aeruginosa	Cefepime, ceftazidime, meropenem or imipenem (not ertapenem); consider addition of aminoglycoside or ciprofloxacin for severe infection or until susceptibilities available	Ciprofloxacin, piperacillin-tazobactam, colistin, aztreonam

Appendix 2 (continued)

Organism	Preferred therapy	Alternative agents (depending on susceptibility)
Rickettsia spp	Doxycycline	Quinolone, chloramphenicol
Salmonella spp	Treatment not indicated for uncomplicated disease; quinolone, ceftriaxone	Amoxicillin or ampicillin, chloramphenicol, tmp-smx, other 3rd/4th-generation cephalosporin
Serratia	Carbapenem*	Quinolone, aminoglycoside, 3rd/4th-generation cephalosporin, tmp-smx, piperacillin-tazobactam
Shigella	Quinolone	tmp-smx, 3rd/4th-generation cephalosporin, azithromycin
Staphylococcus#		
Penicillin-sensitive (rare)	Penicillin	Any agent below in either column
Oxacillin/ methicillin-sensitive staphylococci	Nafcillin, oxacillin, cefazolin	1st-generation cephalosporins, clindamycin, tmp-smx, minocycline Broad spectrum agents that have coverage for oxacillin-sensitive staphylococci: cefepime, β-lactam/β-lactamase inhibitor,† carbapenem,* newer quinolone¶
Oxacillin-resistant staphylococci (MRSA, MRSE)	Vancomycin, linezolid	Daptomycin,¶ tigecycline, dalfopristin-quinupristin Depending on susceptibility for mild-moderate infections or step-down therapy: tmp-smx, minocycline, newer quinolone¶

Organism	Preferred therapy	Alternative agents (depending on susceptibility)
Staphylococcus[#] (continued)		
Vancomycin-intermediate or resistant staphylococci	Notify Infection Control immediately; obtain infectious disease consultation	
Stenotrophomonas maltophilia	May be a colonizer; tmp-smx (consider adding ticarcillin-clavulanate for severe infection)	Ticarcillin-clavulanate, tigecycline, quinolone, minocycline
Streptococcus pneumoniae		
Penicillin-susceptible (MIC <0.1)	Penicillin, ampicillin	Cephalosporin, a macrolide,[‡] tmp-smx, clindamycin, doxycycline, newer quinolone,[¶] or any of agents below in either column
Penicillin-intermediate (MIC 0.1- ≤2)	Ceftriaxone, cefotaxime, newer quinolone,[¶] high-dose penicillin or ampicillin, amoxicilln (non-meningeal infection)	Cefepime, vancomycin, linezolid, dalfopristin-quinupristin, telithromycin, carbapenem* Variable resistance with macrolides,[‡] tmp-smx, or clindamycin
Penicillin-high-level resistance (MIC >2)	Meningitis: vancomycin + ceftriaxone, cefotaxime ± rifampin Other infections: newer quinolone,[¶] vancomycin ± cefotaxime/ ceftriaxone	Linezolid, dalfopristin-quinupristin

Appendix 2 (continued)

Organism	Preferred therapy	Alternative agents (depending on susceptibility)
Streptococcus group A, B, C, or G	Penicillin	Cephalosporin, other penicillin class drug, macrolides‡ or clindamycin (variable resistance), vancomycin, linezolid, daptomycin
Streptococcus viridans group	Penicillin For endocarditis, base treatment on susceptibility testing (see Circulation. 2005;111:e394-c434)	Cephalosporin, vancomycin, newer quinolone¶
Treponema pallidum (syphilis)	Penicillin	Doxycycline, ceftriaxone
Ureaplasma	Macrolide,‡ doxycycline	
Vibrio cholerae	Doxycyclne	Quinolone, tmp-smx
Vibrio vulnificus	Doxycyclnc	Ceftriaxone, cefotaxime, ciprofloxacin
Yersinia enterocolitica	Quinolone, gentamicin, tmp-smx, doxycycline	Chloramphenicol, ceftriaxone, cefotaxime
Yersinia pestis (plague)	Streptomycin	Tmp-smx, gentamicin, doxycycline, chloramphenicol, ciprofloxacin

CNS, central nervous system; ESBL, extended spectrum β-lactamase; MIC, mean inhibitory concentration; MRSA, methicillin-resistant *Staphylococcus aureus*; MRSE, methicillin-resistant *Staphylococcus epidermidis*; tmp-smx, trimethoprim-sulfamethoxazole.

*Carbapenems: meropenem, imipenem, ertapenem (ertapenem is not active against *Pseudomonas* or *Acinetobacter*).

†β-Lactam–β-lactamase inhibitors: piperacillin-tazobactam (Zosyn), ampicillin-sulbactam (Unasyn), amoxicillin-clavulanate. Ticarcillin-clavulanate (Timentin) is an agent and does not have good enterococcal coverage.

‡Macrolides: erythromycin, clarithromycin, azithromycin.

Appendix 2 (continued)

Footnotes (continued)

§Gentamicin or streptomycin is added when cidal activity is required (e.g., endocarditis) and agents are susceptible for synergy.

//Daptomycin: insufficient data for serious enterococcal infections. Do not use for pneumonia (high failure rates).

¶Newer (respiratory) quinolones: moxifloxacin, levofloxacin, gatifloxacin.

#Rifampin may be added for deep-seated staphylococcal infections (e.g., endocarditis) that are not responding well or in the presence of prosthetic material. Coagulase-negative staphylococci are common contaminants but can also cause serious infection.

Fungal Organism-Specific Treatment

Organism	Preferred therapy	Alternative agents (depending on susceptibility)
Aspergillus	Voriconazole	Amphotericin product,* itraconazole, caspofungin, posaconazole (investigational)
Blastomyces	Amphotericin product* (life-threatening or CNS disease) Itraconazole (for mild-moderate disease)	Voriconazole, fluconazole
Systemic infection		
Candida unspeciated†	Fluconazole (stable patient), caspofungin (in life-threatening/unstable patient)	Voriconazole, amphotericin product,* itraconazole, micafungin
C. albicans *C. tropicalis* or *C. parapsilosis*	Fluconazole, caspofungin‡ (in life-threatening/unstable patient)	Amphotericin product,* voriconazole, itraconazole, micafungin
C. glabrata	Caspofungin, voriconazole, higher dose fluconazole§	Amphotericin product,*, // itraconazole,§ micafungin
C. krusei	Caspofungin, voriconazole	Amphotericin product,*, // micafungin
C. lusitaniae or *C. guilliermondii*	Voriconazole, fluconazole	Caspofungin,‡ amphotericin product,*, // micafungin

Appendix 2 (continued)

Organism	Preferred therapy	Alternative agents (depending on susceptibility)
Systemic infection (continued)		
Oropharyngeal/ thrush	Topical nystatin, clotrimazole, fluconazole	Voriconazole, amphotericin (PO liquid), itraconazole, caspofungin, micafungin
Esophagitis¶	Fluconazole	Voriconazole, amphotericin product,* itraconazole, caspofungin, micafungin
Urinary tract infection	Fluconazole	Amphotericin product*
Vulvovaginal infection	Intravaginal azole, fluconazole	Itraconazole, intravaginal boric acid (refractory cases)
Coccidioides	Fluconazole, itraconazole, amphotericin product* (initial therapy for diffuse/ disseminated diseases)	Voriconazole
Cryptococcus	Fluconazole, amphotericin product* (often with flucytosine for induction therapy for CNS disease)	Itraconazole, voriconazole
Fusarium	Voriconazole, amphotericin product*	
Histoplasma	Itraconazole, amphotericin product*	Fluconazole (after amphotericin induction for CNS disease), voriconazole

Organism	Preferred therapy	Alternative agents (depending on susceptibility)
Paracoccidioides	Itraconazole	Voriconazole, sulfonamide, amphotericin product* (with maintenance sulfonamide or azole), ketoconazole, terbinafine
Scedosporium (*Pseudallescheria*)	Voriconazole	Itraconazole, terbinafine (in combo with azole)
Sporothrix	Itraconazole, amphotericin product*	
Zygomycetes (*Mucor*)	Amphotericin product*, //	Posaconazole (investigational)

CNS, central nervous system; MIC, mean inhibitory concentration.

*Amphotericin products include amphotericin B deoxycholate, liposomal amphotericin (Ambisome), and amphotericin B lipid complex (Abelcet is nonformulary).

†Speciation and susceptibility testing for serious infections is recommended.

‡Caspofungin may display higher MICs for *C. parapsilosis* and *C. guilliermondii*; clinical implication is unclear.

§Fluconazole and itraconazole MICs for *C. glabrata* are often in the susceptible but dose-dependent category. If used, higher than usual doses are suggested. If susceptibility results show susceptible isolate (MIC ≤8 for fluconazole or <0.125 for itraconazole), usual doses can be used.

//May exhibit higher MICs to amphotericin; consider use of higher-than-usual doses.

¶Do not use topical therapy (e.g., nystatin, clotrimazole, amphotericin PO suspension) for esophageal disease. Systemic therapy is needed.

Appendix 2 (continued)

Viral Organism-Specific Treatment (non-HIV Infections)

Organism	Preferred therapy	Alternative agents
Cytomegalovirus (CMV)	Ganciclovir, valganciclovir	Foscarnet, cidofovir, ganciclovir implant* (Vitrasert), fomivirsen* (Vitravene implant)
Herpes simplex virus (HSV)	Acyclovir,[†] famciclovir, valacyclovir	Foscarnet (acyclovir-resistant strains), trifluridine eye drops (for keratoconjunctivitis), ganciclovir,[‡] valganciclovir[‡]
Hepatitis B virus[§]	Pegylated interferon	Entecavir, lamivudine,[//] adefovir, tenofovir,[¶] emtricitabine,[#] interferon alpha
Hepatitis C virus	Pegylated interferon + ribavirin	
Influenza virus (treatment or prophylaxis)	Rimantadine (infl A), amantadine (infl A), oseltamivir (infl A or B)	Zanamivir (infl A or B)
Varicella-zoster virus (VZV)	Acyclovir,[†] famciclovir, valacyclovir	Foscarnet (acyclovir-resistant strains)

Infl, influenza.

*Ocular inserts for CMV retinitis should generally be used in combination with systemic therapy to prevent spread to contralateral eye and other organs.

[†]IV acyclovir should be used for HSV central nervous system disease and for sight-threatening or severe VZV disease in immunocompromised patients.

[‡]Active against acyclovir-susceptible strains for HSV but not preferred agents because of toxicity and cost.

[§]Hepatitis B vaccine should be administered as preventive strategy to those at risk (including health care workers).

[//]Lamivudine is approved by U.S. Food and Drug Administration for hepatitis B and is also a good option to include in an HIV treatment regimen for patients infected with hepatitis B.

[¶]Not approved for hepatitis B but may be reasonable option to include an antiretroviral regimen in HIV-infected patients.

Appendix 3. Novel Bacterial Drug Resistance Mechanisms

Selected Bacterial Resistance Issues*

Pertinent organisms	Resistance issue*	Treatment
	Extended spectrum β-lactamase–producing (ESBL) gram-negative bacilli	
E. coli, Klebsiella, Serratia	Generally resistant to penicillins and cephalosporins[†] May appear susceptible to piperacillin-tazobactam, but data from case series and observational reports indicate a potentially higher failure rate than with carbapenem therapy	**Preferred**: a carbapenem (meropenem, imipenem), but some regions have seen carbapenem resistance in *Klebsiella* **Alternatives**: a fluoroquinolone, but there is less clinical experience
	Inducible AmpC-mediated resistance in gram-negative bacilli	
Enterobacter & Citrobacter (less commonly, *Morganella* spp, *Providencia* spp, *Serratia*)	3rd-generation cephalosporins (e.g., ceftazidime, cefotaxime, ceftriaxone) should generally be avoided even if they are reported as susceptible There is potential for induction or selection of ampC-mediated β-lactamase (de-repressed β-lactamase production) which can lead to development of resistance while on therapy	**Preferred**: a carbapenem (meropenem, imipenem, or ertapenem) **Alternatives**: depending on susceptibility testing: quinolones, tmp-smx, piperacillin-tazobactam, aminoglycosides, cefepime (better activity than 3rd-generation cephalosporins[‡]) If inducible resistance occurs, carbapenems are typically the only active β-lactams

Appendix 3 (continued)

Pertinent organisms	Resistance issue*	Treatment
Methicillin-resistant *Staphylococcus aureus*		
S. aureus	Oxacillin (methicillin)-resistant staphylococci are resistant to all β-lactam antibiotics Both nosocomial & community-acquired strains are seen Community-acquired MRSA isolates tend to be more susceptible to non-β-lactams (e.g., tmp-smx, clindamycin, quinolones) than nosocomial isolates	**Preferred:** vancomycin, linezolid **Alternatives** (depending on susceptibility): minocycline, tmp-smx, clindamycin (need to test for inducible resistance), daptomycin,§ & dalfopristin-quinupristin, tigecycline, newer quinolone//
Vancomycin intermediate or vancomycin-resistant staphylococci		
S. aureus with vancomycin MIC >4	Organisms with reduced susceptibility or complete resistance to vancomycin have been reported	Contact Infection Control immediately and obtain an infectious disease consultation Reportable to State Dept. of Health
Vancomycin-resistant enterococci		
Enterococcus	Enterococci with resistance to vancomycin Can cause invasive infection but can also be a colonizer Colonizers (e.g., positive stool cultures) do not require treatment	**Preferred:** linezolid **Alternatives:** daptomycin,§ dalfopristin-quinupristin (for *E. faecium* only), tigecycline; can use penicillin/ampicillin if susceptible

807

Appendix 3 (continued)

Pertinent organisms	Resistance issue*	Treatment
	Stenotrophomonas	
Stenotrophomonas maltophilia	Can cause invasive disease but is a frequent colonizer Colonizers do not typically require treatment If treatment required, this organism is typically multi-drug resistant and treatment should be guided by susceptibility testing	**Preferred**: tmp-smx, ticarcillin-clavulanate, tigecycline **Alternatives** (depending on susceptibility): quinolones, minocycline

MIC, mean inhibitory concentration; tmp-smx, trimethoprim-sulfamethoxazole.

*See also institutional policies and procedures on microorganisms requiring isolation or contact an Infection Control officer.

[†]May show in vivo susceptibility to cephamycins (cefotetan, cefoxitin), but failures have been reported and other mechanisms can confer resistance.

[‡]Cefepime is less likely to induce resistance than 3rd-generation agents, but resistance has been reported. If inducible β-lactamase production occurs, organisms should be considered resistant to penicillins and β-lactams.

[§]Daptomycin should not be used for pneumonia because of lack of penetration and higher failure rates. It has in vitro activity against enterococci, but studies are very limited for serious enterococcal infections.

[‖]Newer quinolones: moxifloxacin, levofloxacin, gatifloxacin, gemifloxacin. Staphylococcal resistance to quinolones has been reported to develop while patient is receiving therapy.

CARDIAC ARREST

Joseph G. Murphy, M.D.
Gillian C. Nesbitt, M.D.
R. Scott Wright, M.D.

- Patient survival is critically dependent on first responders and actions taken in the first few minutes after cardiac arrest.
- Most adult patients with sudden cardiac arrest have unstable ventricular tachycardia (VT) or ventricular fibrillation (VF), more rarely asystole or pulseless electrical activity (PEA) (formerly called electromechanical dissociation).
- Immediate cardiopulmonary resuscitation (CPR) is the best treatment for cardiac arrest until defibrillation and advanced cardiac life support (ACLS) can be instituted.
- Early effective CPR improves patient survival in cardiac arrest by delaying rhythm degeneration from VF into asystole, preventing acidosis, and reducing anoxic brain damage.
- Early defibrillation is the most important determinant of survival after cardiac arrest
- Survival following VF decreases by about 8% for each minute without defibrillation.
- Survival after VF for >15 minutes is <5%
- Cardiac arrest victims with hypothermia, usually associated with drowning or cold weather exposure, are partially protected and may be successfully resuscitated after longer periods of time.

BASIC LIFE SUPPORT FOR ADULTS
- Check responsiveness.
- Activate emergency response system.
- Check airway.

Special abbreviations used in this chapter: ACLS, advanced cardiac life support; CPR, cardiopulmonary resuscitation; PEA, pulseless electrical activity; VF, ventricular fibrillation; VT, ventricular tachycardia.

- Check breathing.
- Give two effective breaths.
- Check circulation.
- Compress chest if no signs of circulation are detected.
- An unresponsive patient who is breathing and has adequate circulation should be placed in the lateral position to prevent airway obstruction.
- A patient with absent respiration requires rescue breathing provided at 10-12 inhalations per minute. Significantly faster rates of rescue breathing are less beneficial.
- Assess circulation by palpation of the carotid artery. If in doubt about the status of the carotid pulse in an unconscious patient, start chest compressions.

CHEST COMPRESSIONS
- Rhythmic pressure over the lower half of the sternum
- Compression rate of 100/minute
- Ratio of 15 compressions to 2 ventilations
- Compress sternum approximately 2 inches and assess adequacy of compression by palpating carotid or femoral pulse.
- Effective chest compression produces a systolic blood pressure of about 70 mm Hg and a cardiac output about one-third of normal.
- Do not interrupt CPR for more than 10 seconds except to defibrillate.
- After each compression, chest pressure must be completely released.
- The most effective cerebral and coronary perfusion is achieved when 50% chest compression phase and 50% chest relaxation phase.

COMPLICATIONS OF CPR
- Inadequate chest compression
- Gastric inflation resulting from excessive ventilation
- Regurgitation of gastric contents and lung aspiration
- Rib fractures, sternum fracture, separation of ribs from sternum
- Pneumothorax, hemothorax
- Lung contusions, laceration of liver and spleen
- Defibrillation burns
- Dental injury from traumatic intubation

ACLS

DEFIBRILLATOR
- Defibrillate up to three times for VF/VT, using energies of 200 J, 300 J, and 360 J for monophasic defibrillators or a nonescalating energy of 150-170 J for biphasic defibrillators (preferred option).
- After three shocks, CPR should be resumed for at least 1 minute; after this period, the rhythm should be reassessed and repeat shock delivered if appropriate.
- Defibrillation should be attempted after each medication is administered or after each minute of CPR.

DRUG THERAPY OF CARDIAC ARREST
- Drug therapy is second-line therapy for cardiac arrest.
- Epinephrine can be administered at 1 mg IV every 3-5 minutes for PEA, asystole, or refractory VF/VT not responding to defibrillation.

DEFIBRILLATION-REFRACTORY VT/VF
- Amiodarone—300 mg IV push. If VF or pulseless VT recurs, a second 150-mg dose can be administered.
- Lidocaine—1 mg/kg IV push. This dose can be repeated every 3-5 minutes up to a maximum dose of 3 mg/kg.
- Magnesium sulfate—1-2 g IV is recommended for treatment of polymorphic VT (torsades de pointes) and suspected low magnesium.
- Sodium bicarbonate—1 mEq/kg IV is indicated for hyperkalemia, metabolic acidosis, or aspirin or tricyclic antidepressant drug overdose.
- Not routinely used for acute lactic acidosis associated with CPR, but may be given to correct acidosis with shock refractory VF/VT

PEA (ELECTROMECHANICAL DISSOCIATION)
- Cardiac rhythm other than VT or VF in absence of a detectable pulse

- Pulmonary embolism
- Cardiac tamponade
- Hypovolemic shock
- Septic shock
- Hypokalemia and hyperkalemia
- Hypothermia
- Acidosis or hypoxia
- Drug overdoses

Cardiac Medication Used in PEA
- Epinephrine—1-mg IV push every 3-5 minutes may be tried for PEA.
- Atropine—1 mg every 3-5 minutes for PEA

ASYSTOLE
- Asystole as the primary cause of cardiac arrest or following VF/VT has a very poor prognosis.

PATIENTS FACTORS USED IN THE DECISION-MAKING PROCESS FOR TERMINATION OF CPR
- Duration of CPR >30 minutes
- Initial ECG rhythm was asystole or asystole has now replaced earlier VF/VT
- Prolonged interval (>10-15 minutes) between estimated time of arrest and initiation of CPR
- Severity of comorbid disease
- Absence of brainstem reflexes
- Absence of hypothermia
- Availability of living will or patient's relatives to indicate patient's wishes in the event of cardiac arrest

INSULIN THERAPY FOR HOSPITALIZED PATIENTS

Cacia V. Soares-Welch, M.D.
William C. Mundell, M.D.

CLASSIFICATION

- SQ insulin is classified into rapid-, intermediate-, and long-acting agents (Table 1).
- IV insulin—rapid-acting (the only insulin used IV)
- Insulin pump—uses rapid-acting insulin

INDICATIONS FOR INSULIN

- Hyperglycemia
  - ▲ Diabetic patient on usual diet
  - ▲ Diabetic patient who is NPO
  - ▲ Steroid-induced hyperglycemia
  - ▲ Parenteral nutrition-induced hyperglycemia
- Diabetic ketoacidosis
- Nonketotic hyperosmolar syndrome
- Acute hyperkalemia

MONITORING INSULIN THERAPY

- Monitoring insulin therapy in various medical conditions is described in Table 2.
- If fingerstick glucose is <60 mg/dL or >400 mg/dL, check a confirmatory serum glucose to determine exact glucose value.

PRESCRIBING INSULIN

- The time and type of insulin prescribed are listed in Table 3.
- A patient whose blood glucose level is well controlled at home may become hypoglycemic when given the usual insulin dose in the hospital on an American Diabetes Association diet, which may be more restrictive than the home "diabetic diet."
- Make sure that the meal is not delayed or missed when patients receive insulin.

Table 1. Onset, Peak Action, and Duration of SQ Insulin

SQ insulin	Onset, hours	Peak action, hours*	Duration, hours
Rapid-acting			
Lispro	0.25	1-3	3-6
Aspart	0.25	1-3	3-6
Regular	0.5-1	2-6	4-12
Semilente	0.5-1	3-10	8-16
Intermediate-acting			
NPH	2-4	6-16	14-28
Lente	3-4	6-16	14-28
Long-acting			
Ultralente (human or bovine)	3-8	4-20	10-40
Protamine zinc	3-8	14-26	24-40
Glargine	3-8	4-24	11 to >24

*Peak effect varies from person to person and depends on dose.

Hyperglycemia
- Goal—restore normal glucose
- Stable diabetic patient on usual diet
  - ▲ Continue usual insulin therapy and use insulin supplementation as needed.
- Critically ill diabetic patient
  - ▲ Continue usual insulin therapy and use insulin supplementation to achieve appropriate glucose control.
  - ▲ Do not withhold insulin, otherwise patient will be driven into diabetic ketoacidosis!
- Diabetic patient NPO for procedure
  - ▲ Withhold oral antihyperglycemic agent before the procedure.
  - ▲ Give one-half the usual dose of intermediate-acting insulin (NPH or Lente).
  - ▲ If fasting glucose is <100 mg/dL, add glucose to IV fluid (5% dextrose in 0.45% normal saline at 100 mL/hour = 5 g of glucose/hour).
  - ▲ If fasting glucose is >200 mg/dL, give only supplemental insulin (do not add to usual rapid-acting insulin dose).
  - ▲ After the procedure, resume the oral agent when patient is able to eat.

Table 2. Monitoring Insulin Therapy in Various Medical Conditions

Medical condition	Frequency of RMG	Also monitor	End point
Stable	1-2 times/day		RMG = 100-150 mg/dL
Critically ill	4-5 times/day		RMG = 100-120 mg/dL
Perioperative period	In recovery room (pre- and postoperative)		RMG = 100-180 mg/dL
Steroid-induced hyperglycemia	2-4 times/day		RMG = 100-150 mg/dL
Parenteral nutrition	2-4 times/day	Electrolytes daily	RMG = 100-150 mg/dL
Diabetic ketoacidosis	Every 30-60 minutes	Electrolytes every 1 hour; Urine output	Resolution of acidosis
NKHS	Every 30-60 minutes	Electrolytes every 1 hour	RMG = 100-150 mg/dL
Acute hyperkalemia	30-60 minutes after insulin administration	Potassium every 1 hour	Stabilization of hyperkalemia

NKHS, nonketotic hyperosmolar syndrome; RMG, reflectance meter glucose.

Table 3. Time and Type of Insulin Prescribed

Time and type of insulin	Glucose value affected
AM Rapid acting	Lunch glucose
AM NPH or Lente	Supper glucose
PM Rapid acting	Bedtime glucose
PM NPH or Lente	Breakfast glucose

- Perioperative period (coordinate with the anesthesiologist)
  - ▲ Goal blood glucose = 120-200 mg/dL
- Measure preoperative and postoperative (recovery room) blood glucose level.
- Patients usually on diet or oral agent control (type 2)
  - ▲ Withhold oral antihyperglycemic agent before the procedure.
  - ▲ If preoperative glucose is >200 mg/dL, add 5-10 U regular insulin per 50 g glucose (1 L of 5% dextrose) in IV *or* give 5-10 U of short-acting insulin SQ.
  - ▲ If postoperative glucose is >200 mg/dL, continue adding 5-10 U regular insulin per 50 g glucose in IV and give short-acting insulin SQ every 4-6 hours.
- Patients usually on insulin control
  - ▲ If preoperative glucose is >200 mg/dL, add 5-10 U regular insulin per 50 g glucose in IV (e.g., 5% dextrose in 0.45% normal saline with 20 mEq KCl/L at 100 mL/hour = 5 g glucose/hour).
  - ▲ Give 1/2 the total AM intermediate insulin dose preoperatively.
  - ▲ Use rapid-acting insulin supplement for the first day postoperatively.
- Steroid-induced hyperglycemia
  - ▲ Goal—fasting blood glucose <150 mg/dL
  - ▲ Use supplemental regular insulin for the first day.
  - ▲ On the second day, add the amount of insulin used the first day and divide the total amount into 2/3 in the morning and 1/3 at supper.
  - ▲ Continue to adjust the dosages daily based on amount of supplemental insulin needed and steroid doses.
- Parenteral nutrition-induced hyperglycemia

- ▲ Add 0.1 U regular insulin per 1 g glucose in total parenteral nutrition (e.g., 20 U/L; dextrose 20% is 200 g/L).
- ▲ Add SQ insulin if reflectance meter glucose is >150 mg/dL on full total parenteral nutrition insulin coverage.
- ■ An algorithm for calculating the amount of supplemental insulin is given in Figure 1.
- ■ Another way to calculate the amount of supplemental insulin is the "1,500 rule":
  - ▲ Divide 1,500 by the total daily insulin usually required by the patient.
  - ▲ This is the amount the blood glucose will decrease when 1 U of rapid-acting insulin is given SQ.
  - ▲ For example, total daily insulin = 50 U
    - • 1,500/50 = 30
    - • 1 U of rapid-acting insulin will decrease blood glucose by 30 mg/dL.

Diabetic Ketoacidosis
- ■ Goal—resolve acidosis
- ■ Initial dose—10-15 U (or 0.15 U/kg) rapid-acting insulin IV bolus
- ■ Continuous dose—10 U/hour (or 0.1 U/kg per hour) IV or IM rapid-acting insulin
- ■ Rate of glucose decrease should *not* exceed 80-100 mg/dL per hour.
  - ▲ If glucose decreases >100 mg/dL per hour, continue insulin infusion and add 5% dextrose to IV fluids.
  - ▲ As glucose approaches 250-300 mg/dL, add 5% dextrose to IV fluids.
  - ▲ Maintain blood glucose at 200-300 mg/dL.
- ■ Increase insulin dose by 50%-100% per hour if insulin resistance is suspected.
- ■ When serum bicarbonate >15 mEq/L, change insulin to 1-2 U/hour.
- ■ Maintenance dose for diabetic patients
  - ▲ Start usual insulin regimen when acidosis has resolved (ketones are no longer present in serum), and discontinue insulin drip 1 hour after SQ insulin is given.

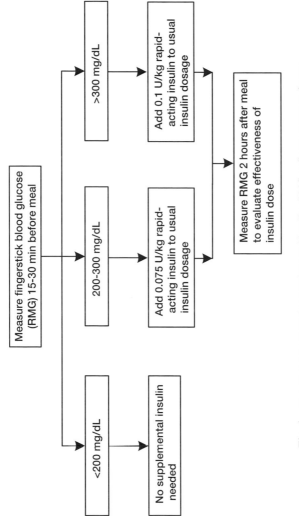

Fig. 1. Algorithm for calculating supplemental insulin. RMG, reflectance meter glucose.

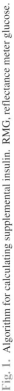

- Maintenance dose for newly diagnosed diabetic patients
  - ▲ First 24 hours—0.1-0.25 U/kg rapid-acting insulin every 6-8 hours to determine a daily insulin requirement
  - ▲ Second 24 hours
    - 1/2 the previous day's total dose in the morning (1/3 rapid-acting, 2/3 intermediate-acting) and
    - 1/2 the previous day's total dose in the evening (1/2 rapid-acting, 1/2 intermediate-acting)

      or
    - The previous day's total dose divided as 1/4 rapid-acting at breakfast, 1/4 rapid-acting at lunch, 1/4 rapid-acting in the evening, and 1/4 intermediate-acting at bedtime

Nonketotic Hyperosmolar Syndrome
- Goal—restore normal glucose
- Initial dose—5-10 U IV regular insulin bolus if glucose is >600 mg/dL
- Continuous dose—5-10 U/hour IV or IM to lower glucose to ~200 mg/dL
- Maintenance dose—SQ insulin
- Fluid repletion is the most important aspect of treatment.

COMPLICATIONS OF INSULIN THERAPY
Hypoglycemia
- Symptoms and signs—diaphoresis, tremors, tachycardia, confusion, seizure, stupor, coma, etc.
- Diagnosis
  - ▲ Stat measurement of plasma glucose
  - ▲ Plasma glucose <70 mg/dL
- Treatment
  - ▲ 15 g of fast-acting oral carbohydrate (1 cup of milk or juice, cheese and crackers) if patient is alert

    or
  - ▲ IV dextrose (25-50 mL 50% dextrose) if patient is NPO or unable to swallow. Then infusion of 5% dextrose in water

    or
  - ▲ Glucagon 1 mg IM or SQ

- Monitoring
  - ▲ Retest reflectance meter glucose 15 minutes after treatment.
  - ▲ If <70 mg/dL, repeat above treatment.
  - ▲ If >70 mg/dL and >30 minutes to meal or snack, give 15 g of carbohydrate + protein.
  - ▲ If >70 mg/dL and <30 minutes to meal or snack, proceed with meal or snack.

Allergic Reaction

- Symptoms and signs
  - ▲ Local—erythema, induration, and pruritus at injection site
  - ▲ Systemic—urticaria, angioneurotic edema, and anaphylaxis
- Diagnosis—clinical exam
- Treatment
  - ▲ Local—antihistamine
    - • Switch to biosynthetic human insulin if animal insulin was used originally.
    - • Desensitization may be needed.
  - ▲ Systemic—supportive care, antihistamine, epinephrine and/or corticosteroids if needed
    - • Insulin desensitization is mandatory.

Hypokalemia

- Make sure the serum potassium level is normal before insulin administration and measure the serum potassium level frequently.
- Correct potassium as needed.

LIPID MANAGEMENT

R. Scott Wright, M.D.
Gillian C. Nesbitt, M.D.
Joseph G. Murphy, M.D.

- Atherosclerosis—diffuse inflammatory-proliferative arterial reaction initiated by endothelial injury
- Atherosclerotic lesions that appear focal and limited on coronary angiography are pathologic, widespread within the arterial tree.
- Risk factor modification, especially low-density lipoprotein (LDL), high-density lipoprotein (HDL), and triglyceride optimization, is mandatory for all patients with atherosclerosis irrespective of presentation syndrome.

CLASSIFICATION OF DYSLIPIDEMIA

- Dyslipidemia—a heterogeneous disorder with multiple causes.
- In Western societies, most dyslipidemia is secondary to lifestyle and poor dietary habits.
- Physiologic LDL is probably in the range of 50-70 mg/mL, as determined by findings in non-westernized societies where atherosclerosis is unknown.
- Most patients have mixed dyslipidemia: frequently elevated LDL cholesterol in combination with low HDL cholesterol and/or elevated serum triglyceride.
- Many patients with dyslipidemia have multiple confounding medical issues such as diabetes or metabolic syndrome, obesity, hypertension, and occasionally, obstructive sleep apnea, all of which necessitate treatment.
- Dietary reductions in saturated fat and total caloric content typically reduce LDL cholesterol values 10%-15% and plasma triglycerides can fall 20%-40%.

Special abbreviations used in this chapter: HDL, high-density lipoprotein; LDL, low-density lipoprotein.

- Regular, vigorous exercise can raise HDL cholesterol values by 10%-15%, comparable to changes induced by pharmacologic therapy.
- Diet therapy, undoubtedly effective in a highly motivated person, fails to achieve goal LDL levels in most patients.

PHARMACOLOGIC TREATMENT OF DYSLIPIDEMIA
- Goal-directed therapy for dyslipidemia is outlined in Table 1.

Statins
- Statin agents work through at least two mechanisms in patients with dyslipidemia.
- Statins inhibit the enzyme responsible for the rate limiting step of cholesterol biosynthesis and HMG coenzyme A reductase and thus directly inhibit cholesterol biosynthesis.
- Statins promote LDL receptor upregulation on hepatocytes and thus promote biologic clearance of LDL-cholesterol.
- Statins typically lower LDL-cholesterol 25%-55%
- Statins lower total cholesterol similarly in magnitude to that observed with LDL-cholesterol.
- Statins also increase HDL-cholesterol by 5%-15%.
- Potent statins may reduce plasma triglycerides 15%-45%.
- Statins are associated with elevation of liver enzymes and rarely rhabdomyolysis.

Niacin
- Niacin—currently the most potent U.S. Food and Drug Administration–approved HDL-cholesterol raising drug available.
- Treatment with niacin increases HDL-cholesterol 20%-30% in most patients and decreases plasma triglycerides 30%-40%.
- Niacin also reduces plasma LDL-cholesterol an additional 20%-30%.
- Niacin is generally well tolerated if started at lower doses and gradually increased over time.
- Aspirin pretreatment reduces flushing and headache frequently seen with niacin.
- Niacin can be used safely in combination with statins, fibrates, and ezetimibe.

Table 1. Goal-Directed Therapy for Dyslipidemia*†‡§

| Patients | Goals | | Therapy |
	LDL, mg/dL	HDL, mg/dL	
With established CAD	≤70	≥40	Statin *or* Statin + ezetimibe
With diabetes mellitus or hypertension but not CAD events	70-100	≥40	Statin *or* Statin + ezetimibe *or* Statin + fibrate
With diabetes mellitus or hypertension + known CAD	≤70	≤40	Statin *or* Statin + ezetimibe *or* Statin + fibrate
Populations with multiple cardio-vascular risk factors or family history of severe, premature CAD	≤100	≥40	Statin *or* Statin + niacin or fibrate

CAD, coronary artery disease; HDL, high-density lipoprotein; LDL, low-density lipoprotein.

*All patients should be educated about and adhere to AHA Step 2 Diet.

†All patients should reduce body weight to body mass index ≤25

‡All patients should exercise 4-5 times per week for at least 30 minutes per session.

§All patients should stop using any tobacco products.

Fibrates

- Fibrates
  - ▲ Gemfibrozil and fenofibrate are potent triglyceride-lowering agents.
  - ▲ They reduce plasma triglycerides 40%-60% when utilized with dietary modification.
- Fibrates also increase HDL-cholesterol by additional 10%-20% but are generally less effective than niacin for this situation.

▲ Rare but serious cases of rhabdomyolysis have been reported with combination statins and fibrates.

Ezetimibe
- Directly inhibits cholesterol absorption in small intestine and lowers plasma LDL-cholesterol additional 15%-20% when used with a statin

Resin-Binding Agents
- Cholestyramine and colestipol decrease total cholesterol and LDL-cholesterol by binding bile acids in intestine to interrupt enterohepatic circulation of bile acids. This action stimulates a secondary increase in hepatic LDL receptors, which in turn remove LDL-cholesterol from the circulation.
- Resins have no important effect on HDL but increase plasma triglycerides.
- Major side effects of resins: gastrointestinal intolerance with gas, bloating, constipation, nausea, and esophageal reflux
- Resins inhibit absorption of vitamin K, digoxin, warfarin, thyroxine, and diuretics

MECHANICAL AND NONINVASIVE POSITIVE PRESSURE VENTILATION

Kirby D. Slifer, D.O.
Steve G. Peters, M.D.

MECHANICAL VENTILATION

■ The initiation of intubation and mechanical ventilation is an attempt to accomplish one, or all, of the following:
  ▲ Protect the airway or overcome airway obstruction
  ▲ Support or maintain pulmonary gas exchange
  ▲ Increase lung volume
  ▲ Reduce the work of breathing

Indications

■ Acute respiratory failure
  ▲ Respiratory activity is insufficient to maintain adequate oxygenation or ventilation (carbon dioxide clearance)
  ▲ Develops over a short period
  ▲ Hypercapneic (hypercarbic) respiratory failure—a reflection of inadequate ventilation, e.g., alveolar hypoventilation
    • When acute, a rapid rise in $PaCO_2$, with an accompanying drop in arterial pH (assuming no metabolic component), is observed.
    • Clinical signs include recruitment of accessory respiratory muscles, mental status changes, agitation, tachypnea and, eventually, unresponsiveness.
    • Causes include three general groups of disorders:
      - Central nervous system disorders
      - Neuromuscular disorders
      - Disorders resulting in increased work of breathing or characterized by increased alveolar dead space (in

---

Special abbreviations used in this chapter: FIO_2, fraction of inspired oxygen; I:E, inspiratory-to-expiratory timing; NPPV, noninvasive positive pressure ventilation; PEEP, positive end-expiratory pressure; SIMV, synchronized intermittent mandatory ventilation.

which total minute ventilation might seem adequate but alveolar ventilation is reduced)

▲ Hypoxemic respiratory failure—the inability to maintain adequate arterial oxygenation
  • This can occur despite adequate ventilation as reflected by a normal or low P_{CO_2}.
  • Clinical signs include tachypnea, dyspnea, cyanosis, mental status changes, hypertension, and peripheral vasoconstriction.

▪ General anesthesia
▪ Intentional hyperventilation (increased intracranial pressure, although adaptive mechanisms render this treatment modality ineffective after 24-36 hours)
▪ Common causes of hypercapneic and hypoxemic respiratory failure are listed in Table 1.

Ventilator Settings

▪ The following parameters are typically set by the physician on initiation of mechanical ventilation:
  ▲ Tidal volume
    • This parameter is set directly by the physician or is determined by the ventilator after the minute volume and respiratory rate are set.

Table 1. Common Causes of Acute Respiratory Failure

Hypercapneic	Hypoxemic
Cerebrovascular accident	Ventilation-perfusion mismatch
Head trauma	ARDS
Drug effect	Pneumonia
General anesthetics,	Acute lung injury
barbiturates	Pulmonary edema
Paralytic agents	Diffusion defects
Aminoglycoside antibiotics	Right-to-left shunts
Corticosteroids	Aging
Chest wall deformity	Hypoventilation
Amyotrophic lateral sclerosis	Inadequate F_{IO_2}
Pulmonary fibrosis	
Morbid obesity	
Guillain-Barré syndrome	
Poliomyelitis	

ARDS, acute respiratory distress syndrome; F_{IO_2}, fraction of inspired oxygen.

- Tidal volume cannot be set in pressure control ventilation; it is determined by the amount of pressure given, the lung and chest wall compliance, and the inspiratory effort.
- Generally, 10-12 mL/kg ideal body weight is used for mechanically ventilated patients.
- Low tidal volumes set at 6 mL/kg ideal body weight improve survival in acute lung injury and acute respiratory distress syndrome.

▲ Fraction of inspired oxygen (FIO_2)
  - Generally, this should be set for 100% for most patients initiated on mechanical ventilation.
  - Further adjustments are guided by arterial blood gas measurements and pulse oximetry.
  - To avoid oxygen toxicity, it is prudent to reduce FIO_2 to ≤0.6.

▲ Respiratory rate
  - This is set once the physician has considered inspiratory-to-expiratory ratio (I:E) and the patient's own respiratory rate.
  - Ventilator backup rate should be close to the patient's actual respiratory rate.

▲ Inspiratory flow rate
  - After patient-ventilator interactions have been observed, this is generally set to minimize patient-ventilator asynchrony.
  - In pressure-cycled modes, this is not a set variable.

▲ Inflation pressure setting
  - Inflation pressure is a dependent function of volume with volume-cycled ventilation and is preset with pressure-preset modes.
  - Generally, keep inflation pressures <35 cm H_2O to decrease risk of barotrauma.
  - Coughing and sneezing can cause random increases in inflation pressure.

▲ Positive end-expiratory pressure (PEEP)
  - This refers to application of a positive pressure at the end of passive expiration.

- When PEEP is not selected, airway pressure returns to ambient atmospheric pressure.
- PEEP is used to recruit atelectatic and flooded alveoli to participate in gas exchange and improve oxygenation.
- It can be used in any ventilator mode.
- Intrinsic PEEP (auto-PEEP, "breath stacking," dynamic hyperinflation)
  - Phenomenon of increased airway pressure at end of exhalation without intentional selection of PEEP on the ventilator
  - Detect intrinsic PEEP by occluding the exhaust port of the ventilator at end-expiration just before the next inspiration, observing the airway pressure.
  - Many ventilators have a feature that allows the ventilator to evaluate intrinsic PEEP with the push of a button.
  - The main adverse effects of PEEP are decreased cardiac output (by decreasing preload), hypotension, and barotrauma, including pneumothorax.
  - If intrinsic PEEP is present above the intentional application of PEEP, these effects may be severe. PEEP is usually titrated to the lowest level necessary to achieve adequate oxygenation (arterial saturations $\geq 90\%$ or Po_2 ≥ 60 mm Hg with Fio_2 <0.6).

Modes of Mechanical Ventilation
- When discussing mechanical ventilation, some terms must be defined to facilitate understanding of ventilator function.
  - ▲ Triggered
    - Refers to the initiation of the breath delivered by the ventilator
    - Can be set by time, flow, motion (pediatric ventilators), or pressure and can be initiated by the patient or the ventilator
    - Ventilators can be triggered manually, usually by a push button.
  - ▲ Cycled
    - Refers to the termination of the mechanical inspiratory breath and the beginning of exhalation
    - This is predetermined and is set, most commonly, as a function of time (most ventilators measure how much

time it takes to deliver a preset volume at a preset flow rate and, thus, are actually time-cycled).

▲ Limited
  • Refers to a preset variable being reached before the end of inspiration
  • A limit can be set as a function of flow, pressure, or volume.

■ Mechanical ventilation is a form of positive pressure ventilation, which is either volume-cycled or pressure-preset.

  ▲ Volume-cycled ventilation
    • Provides a constant volume with each delivered breath
    • Airway pressure varies as a function of volume; thus, if compliance of the lungs or chest wall decreases (increased stiffness), airway pressure will increase because a set volume is guaranteed.

  ▲ Pressure-preset ventilation
    • Delivers a breath to a preset pressure that is limited
    • If a pressure-preset mode is used for the example above, the volume will vary as a function of pressure. If compliance decreases, then volume will decrease because the preset pressure is reached earlier during inspiration (limited).

■ The usual modes of mechanical ventilation are listed below with a brief description.

  ▲ Assist/control ventilation
    • Preselected tidal volume, minimum respiratory rate and inspiratory flow rate
    • Time- or patient-triggered
    • It is set to detect the patient's inspiratory effort. Once detected, this mode provides an assisted mechanical breath until the preset tidal volume is delivered.
    • If no inspiratory effort is detected in a predetermined amount of time (as determined by the minimum respiratory rate), the ventilator automatically delivers a mechanical breath.
    • If the patient's respiratory rate exceeds the preset minimum respiratory rate, all breaths will be assisted. If apnea occurs, the patient receives the ventilator's set minimum respiratory rate.

- Assist/control is indicated when it is desired that the ventilator assume most or all the work of breathing, e.g., neuromuscular weakness, paralysis, or respiratory muscle fatigue.
- Some patients may develop respiratory alkalosis.
  - Alkalosis can be severe if the patient had preexisting hypercapneic respiratory failure with compensatory increase in bicarbonate.
  - Also, the assist/control mode poses the greatest risk of air-trapping and dynamic hyperinflation for patients with airflow obstruction.
▲ Controlled mechanical ventilation
  - All parameters (tidal volume, inspiratory flow rate, I:E, and respiratory rate), are determined entirely by the operator and are machine set.
  - The only indication for this mode is to provide mechanical ventilation to a patient experiencing apnea.
  - Sedation and paralysis are usually required.
▲ Synchronized intermittent mandatory ventilation (SIMV)
  - Preselected tidal volume or pressure and minimum respiratory rate
  - Time- or patient-triggered
  - Spontaneous breaths can be pressure-supported.
  - Sensitized to detect the patient's inspiratory effort, but unlike the assist/control mode, only assists the patient's effort at the minimum respiratory rate preset on the ventilator (e.g., if this rate is 8 and the patient is making 22 inspiratory efforts per minute, only 8 of these efforts will be assisted. Any full breaths over the rate of 8 are breaths that the patient achieves alone. If the patient becomes apneic, the ventilator will deliver 8 breaths per minute)
  - The breaths are "synchronized" with the patient's inspiratory efforts to avoid a double breath.
  - Allows for spontaneous breathing between ventilator-assisted breaths
  - Between ventilator-assisted breaths, the ventilator provides warm, humidified air with a predetermined FIO_2.
  - SIMV was developed initially as a "weaning" mode; the minimum respiratory rate could be gradually reduced.
    - The most useful functions of this mode may be when a patient needs substantial respiratory support and

has a very high respiratory rate or when it is desirable for the patient to assume some of the work of breathing to preserve respiratory muscle function.

▲ Pressure control ventilation
- Preselected pressure, minimum respiratory rate, and duration of inspiration
- Time- or patient-triggered, pressure-limited, and time-cycled
- Can be used with assist/control ventilation or SIMV
- Ventilator raises airway pressure (detected at the endotracheal tube) to a level preselected by the physician.
- If patient becomes apneic, the ventilator cycles at the minimum respiratory rate and tidal volume will depend entirely on the incremental increase in airway pressure in addition to the compliance of the lungs and chest wall.
- If the patient makes inspiratory efforts, tidal volume will be a function of the intensity of the patient's inspiratory effort as well as the incremental increase in airway pressure and the compliance of the lungs and chest wall.
- Patient has little control over tidal volume and pattern of breathing (inspiratory time is preset), so generally the patient must be sedated and paralyzed.
- Useful when further lung injury by high pressures needs to be avoided, as in acute lung injury and acute respiratory distress syndrome
  - In these situations, lung injury may be increased by overdistension of lung tissues (barotrauma or volutrauma).

▲ Pressure support ventilation
- Preselected pressure to help achieve desired tidal volume with each spontaneously triggered breath thus decreasing the work of breathing
- The patient must be breathing spontaneously to use this mode (always patient-triggered).
- During exhalation, airway pressure returns to zero or the preselected PEEP.
- Patient has more control over inspiratory time, tidal volume, and flow.

- This may be a more comfortable mode of breathing for patients.
- It is frequently a "weaning" mode. The level of pressure support is reduced gradually, allowing the patient to assume more of the work of breathing.

Mechanical Ventilation Strategies

- Commonly encountered clinical situations and typical ventilator strategies for which mechanical ventilation is used are listed in Table 2.
  - ▲ Keep in mind that *initial* ventilator settings are suggested.
  - ▲ The clinical situation and arterial blood gas determinations should guide further ventilator adjustments.

Weaning

- After the precipitating cause of acute respiratory failure has resolved, fully 80%-90% of patients on mechanical ventilation can be weaned and extubated without difficulty.
  - ▲ Some patients can be extubated without a weaning process.
  - ▲ However, for a small group of mechanically ventilated patients, the weaning process can be long and difficult.
- Several weaning strategies have been used, the most common being the following:
  - ▲ "T-piece trials," in which periods of spontaneous breathing are alternated with partial, or full, ventilatory support
  - ▲ SIMV, in which the number of mandatory breaths is decreased over hours to days
  - ▲ Pressure support ventilation, in which the amount of pressure support is decreased over hours to days and the patient gradually assumes more of the work of breathing
- Two studies have shown conflicting results with weaning methods.
  - ▲ One study—Pressure support ventilation is superior to SIMV and T-piece trials.
  - ▲ Other study—T-piece trials are superior to the others.
  - ▲ Both studies—SIMV is inferior to other two methods.
- Weaning trials should be attempted only when the patient is hemodynamically stable, improving, awake and alert, cooperative, and informed that the weaning process is to take place.
  - ▲ A recent study showed that daily interruption of sedative

Table 2. Mechanical Ventilation Strategies

Scenario	Modes	Initial settings	Goals/comments
Head injury/trauma	A/C, SIMV	V_T 10-12 mL/kg f 20-25 breaths/minute (intentional hyperventilation) PEEP 0-5 cm H_2O Fio_2 1.0 initially	Avoid high intrathoracic pressure which impedes venous return from the brain (ICP monitored and <10) Increase Fio_2 rather than PEEP for hypoxemia If ICP not elevated, intentional hyperventilation not indicated Volume or pressure ventilation may be used
Asthma	A/C, PCV	V_T 6-8 mL/kg f 12-16 breaths/minute Q 60-100 L/minute Fio_2 1.0 initially P_{PLAT} <35 cm H_2O	Permissive hypercapnia? If used, keep pH 7.1-7.2 If intrinsic PEEP observed, increase expiratory time
COPD	A/C, SIMV, PCV	V_T 8-10 mL/kg f 6-8 breaths/minute P_{PLAT} <35 cm H_2O Q 60 L/minute Pao_2 60-70 mm Hg PEEP 2.5-5 cm H_2O	Maintain CO_2 at patient's baseline Prone to intrinsic PEEP

Table 2 (continued)

Scenario	Modes	Initial settings	Goals/comments
ARDS	PCV, A/C	V_T 5-8 mL/kg (volume-cycled) PIP <40 cm H_2O (pressure preset) f 20-30 breaths/minute PEEP no upper limit	May need sedation and/or paralysis Permissive hypercapnia? Proning? If sedated/paralyzed, use lower respiratory rates Keep O_2 saturation ≥90% at FiO_2 <0.6
CHF/pulmonary edema	A/C, SIMV (? NPPV)	V_T 8-12 mL/kg f 8-12 breaths/minute Q ≥60 L/minute FiO_2 1.0 initially PEEP 5-10 cm H_2O	PEEP applied to recruit flooded & collapsed lung units Volume or pressure ventilation may be used
ARF	A/C, SIMV, PCV	V_T 8-10 mL/kg (volume-cycled) PIP 10-15 cm H_2O (pressure preset) PEEP 5-10 cm H_2O FiO_2 1.0	Restore adequate ventilation & oxygenation Monitor for intrinsic PEEP

A/C, assist/control; ARDS, acute respiratory distress syndrome; CHF, congestive heart failure; f, frequency; FiO_2, fraction of inspired oxygen; ICP, intracranial pressure; NPPV, noninvasive positive pressure ventilation; PCV, pressure control ventilation; PIP, peak inspiratory pressure; P_{PLAT}, plateau pressure; Q, flow rate; SIMV, synchronized intermittent mandatory ventilation; V_T, tidal volume.

infusions shortened the time of mechanical ventilation and length of stay in the ICU.

▲ Physiologic parameters that help determine a patient's readiness for weaning are listed in Table 3.

▲ The index of rapid shallow breathing (f/VT) is the most sensitive and specific single predictor of weaning success.

■ Factors to be considered in the weaning process are as follows:

▲ Prepare the patient.
  • The patient must be reassured that ventilatory backup is immediately available in the event of a failure.
  • Communicate to the patient that the weaning process is gradual and progressive.
  • Encourage and support the patient.

▲ Address nonrespiratory factors that may contribute to weaning failure, e.g., cardiac status, acid-base and metabolic status, drugs (sedatives, narcotics, etc.), nutrition, and psychologic dependency.

▲ Therapist-driven protocols have been found to shorten the time of mechanical ventilatory support and to reduce hospital costs.

▲ The patient's pain level (recent thoracic or abdominal surgery)

■ After a weaning trial is under way, signs of clinical deterioration, which may indicate the need for reinstitution of ventilatory support, include

Table 3. Weaning Parameters

Patient alert, cooperative, improving
FIO_2 requirement <0.50
Maximum inspiratory pressure < −10 to −20 cm H_2O
PEEP requirement <5 cm H_2O
f/VT <100 (VT measured in liters)
Respiratory rate <25 breaths/minute
Minute ventilation <10-20 L/minute

FIO_2, fraction of inspired oxygen; f/VT, respiratory rate/tidal volume (index of rapid shallow breathing); PEEP, positive end-expiratory pressure.

- ▲ Subjective dyspnea, rated 5/10 by the patient
- ▲ Heart rate >30 beats/minute above baseline
- ▲ Ventricular ectopy, supraventricular tachyarrhythmias
- ▲ Arterial oxygen saturation <90%
- ▲ Respiratory rate >35 breaths/minute for at least 5 minutes
- ▪ Clinical judgment must be used when interpreting these signs, which are not absolute.
- ▪ It is important not to terminate a weaning trial prematurely, because this can prolong the weaning process.

Complications
- ▪ Many complications can occur and vigilance must be constant when caring for patients on mechanical ventilation.
- ▪ Complications include, but are not limited to, the following:
  - ▲ Barotrauma (volutrauma)—pneumothorax (with and without tension), pneumomediastinum, pneumoperitoneum, pneumoretroperitoneum, SQ emphysema
  - ▲ Machine failure, alarm failure, ventilator asynchrony, bacterial contamination
  - ▲ Endotracheal tube migration or rupture, vocal cord granuloma, self-extubation, cuff rupture
  - ▲ Nasotracheal intubation associated with nasal necrosis and sinusitis
  - ▲ Hyperventilation, alveolar hypoventilation, ventilator-associated pneumonia, tracheoesophageal fistula, hypotension and decreased cardiac output associated with PEEP and intrinsic PEEP resulting in vascular insufficiency

Other Modes of Mechanical Ventilation
- ▪ High-frequency ventilation
  - ▲ The two most common variations are "high-frequency jet ventilation" and "high-frequency oscillation."
  - ▲ Both use an extremely small tidal volume (50%-100% of dead space volume).
  - ▲ High-frequency oscillation is used in the pediatric population.
  - ▲ Neither variation depends on bulk gas transport for oxygenation or ventilation.
- ▪ Partial liquid ventilation
  - ▲ Uses perfluorocarbons, which dissolve very large amounts of oxygen, but readily release it

▲ May replace absent surfactant and is attractive strategy for acute respiratory distress syndrome, but is experimental (trials are under way)

■ Inverse ratio ventilation

▲ Reverses I:E time in an attempt to improve oxygenation by increasing mean airway pressure.

▲ Normal inspiratory time is one-half to one-third of expiratory time, so with inverse ratio ventilation, this is reversed.

▲ Can be used with volume-control ventilation, however, pressure-control ventilation used most often

▲ Very uncomfortable, requires sedation or paralysis

■ Proportional-assist ventilation

▲ Pressure, inspiratory flow rate, and tidal volume are delivered proportional to the patient's spontaneous inspiratory effort.

▲ Only provides for assisted ventilation

NONINVASIVE POSITIVE PRESSURE VENTILATION

■ Noninvasive positive pressure ventilation (NPPV) refers to positive pressure ventilation delivered without the use of an endotracheal tube.

▲ The most obvious advantage is that it avoids many of the complications that occur during intubation or with the use of a ventilator.

■ The most common delivery methods include the following:

▲ Positive pressure ventilators, which provide ventilatory support through a tight-fitting facemask or other interface, such as a nasal mask.

• Type depends on fit and patient preference.

• With this type of delivery, a preset airway pressure or tidal volume is delivered, either with full support or by assisting spontaneous patient inspiratory efforts.

• Exhalation is passive to a preset PEEP or to atmospheric pressure.

• In patients with a nasogastric tube, the facemask may be "leaky," but some ventilators, in a pressure-limited mode, are able to quantitate the amount of leak and compensate for the amount lost during inspiration. If a volume-limited mode is used, no compensation can be made for leak, but an increase in tidal volume will allow for compensation.

▲ Continuous positive airway pressure provides for a *constant* positive pressure (relative to atmospheric pressure) to be delivered to the airway during the entire respiratory cycle.

- It does not provide for an inspiratory assist; however, it does reduce the work of breathing by keeping small airways open (avoiding intrinsic PEEP).
- It is commonly used in the treatment of obstructive sleep apnea.

Indications

■ Before using NPPV, consideration must be given to the patient's status.
  ▲ Cooperative
  ▲ Minimal secretions
  ▲ Hemodynamically stable
  ▲ Able to protect airway
  ▲ Impending endotracheal intubation
  ▲ Evidence of acute respiratory failure

■ Indications for this modality are continuing to expand as physicians become more familiar with the use and capabilities of NPPV. The following list is not exhaustive:
  ▲ Exacerbations of COPD
  ▲ Exacerbations of asthma
  ▲ Pulmonary edema
  ▲ "Do not intubate"
  ▲ Restrictive lung disease
  ▲ Obesity hypoventilation syndrome
  ▲ Neuromuscular disease
  ▲ Acute lung injury

Initial Settings

■ Virtually any ventilator can be used for NPPV; however, units designed strictly for NPPV have extremely rapid cycling times, minimizing patient-ventilator asynchrony.

■ Generally an inspiratory pressure of 8-10 cm H_2O and an expiratory pressure, or PEEP, of 2-5 cm H_2O are reasonable initial settings.

- Further adjustments are guided by patient tolerance and arterial blood gas measurements.
- When using bilevel positive pressure ventilators, which are pressure-limited and time- or flow-cycled, the variable settings are referred to as inspiratory positive airway pressure and expiratory positive airway pressure. Inspiratory positive airway pressure can be patient- or time-triggered.

Weaning

- When clinical improvement is observed, NPPV can be discontinued abruptly or reduced gradually, as with pressure-support ventilation, with the patient being monitored closely for signs of respiratory decompensation and distress, in which case NPPV is reinstituted.
- Patients may remove the mask for eating and conversation and generally can replace it when feeling dyspneic.

Complications

- When NPPV is used in appropriately selected patients, complications generally are minor.
- Complications include the following:
  - ▲ Nasal bridge necrosis
  - ▲ Nasal dryness
  - ▲ Corneal irritation or ulceration
  - ▲ Gastric insufflation
  - ▲ Skin rash at points of skin contact with the mask
  - ▲ A small proportion of patients cannot tolerate the mask because of discomfort or, less commonly, claustrophobia.
  - ▲ Explaining the role of the mask, giving patient encouragement, and selecting different interfaces may obviate the need for endotracheal intubation.

NUTRITION SUPPORT IN HOSPITALIZED PATIENTS

Kurt A. Kennel, M.D.
M. Molly McMahon, M.D.

CLINICAL ASSESSMENT OF NUTRITIONAL STATUS

Malnutrition

- Depletion of body protein stores from starvation and/or severe illness
- Assessment combines history, exam, and lab tests to identify malnourished patients or patients at risk for malnutrition
- History—recent dietary habits (usual diet, supplements, herbs, and fad diets), presence of anorexia, nausea, vomiting, dysphagia, or diarrhea, medical illness, surgical procedure, medications, alcohol, and unintentional weight loss (see below)
- Exam—muscle wasting (temporalis muscle, interosseous muscles, thin extremities), subcutaneous fat loss, dehydration, and symptoms and signs of vitamin deficiencies
- Lab tests
  - ▲ Albumin and prealbumin are negative acute phase proteins that are altered by stress and are not sensitive markers of nutritional status.
  - ▲ Lab assessment should be individualized but usually includes electrolytes, glucose, CBC, and kidney and liver function tests. These also are not nutritional markers but can easily be altered by disease coupled with poor nutrition.

Risk Factors

- Unintentional weight loss >5%-10% of usual weight over 3-6 months (use chart or nursing home weights)
  - ▲ Consider weight in relation to fluid status.
- Inadequate (<50% of estimated needs) nutrition over previous 2-4 weeks

Special abbreviations used in this chapter: BEE, basal energy expenditure; BMI, body mass index; HB, Harris-Benedict (equation).

- Body mass index (BMI) <18.5, wasted appearance, chronic disease, alcohol abuse, eating disorders, elderly or institutionalized patients
- Dysphagia—If suspected, keep patient NPO until swallowing is evaluated

ORAL SUPPLEMENTATION

Indications
- Able to safely eat but intake inadequate to meet needs

Prescribing
- Ask dietitian to clarify food preferences and to initiate calorie and protein record. Involve patient, dietitian, and nurse in assessment and implementation.
- Many varieties of solid and liquid supplements are available. Consult your formulary.
- Specialty products are available for certain disease states, e.g., renal failure.
- Consider small frequent meals; liberalize diet.
- Add daily multivitamin.

Monitoring
- Review intake and output and weight trends and compare calorie/protein intake with estimated requirements.
- Frequent reassessment—Is nutrition support needed?

INDICATIONS FOR NUTRITION SUPPORT (TUBE FEEDING OR PARENTERAL NUTRITION)
- Moderate or severe illness
  and
- >7-10 days of past or anticipated inadequate intake (<50% of requirements)
- Goals of nutrition support
  - ▲ Enhance immune function, organ function, and wound healing
  - ▲ Improve net protein balance
  - ▲ Prevent sequelae of malnutrition by providing substrates, electrolytes, vitamins, and minerals
- If patient requires nutrition support, first determine route (enteral or parenteral) and then estimate nutrition and fluid requirements.

ESTIMATION OF NUTRITION AND FLUID REQUIREMENTS

■ Estimation for hospitalized patients is described in Table 1.
■ Hamwi estimation of lean body weight (useful when feeding obese patients)
  ▲ Men: 106 lb for 5 ft + 6 lb per additional inch
  ▲ Women: 100 lb for 5 ft + 5 lb per additional inch

Estimated Daily Fluid Requirements

■ Euvolemic patient with normal heart and kidney function and no unusual losses needs ~30 mL/kg daily.
■ If high kidney or gastrointestinal tract losses (nasogastric, diarrhea, drains, fistulas, ostomy), required daily fluid equals losses + urine output + 500 mL for insensible losses.
  ▲ Nondextrose crystalloid solutions, rather than parenteral or enteral nutrition, should be used to replace unusual gastrointestinal tract or kidney losses that may vary in amount from day to day.

Table 1.   Estimation of Daily Calorie, Protein, and Fat Requirements in Hospitalized Patients

	ICU patient	Non-ICU patient
Total calories*	Basal calories using the Harris-Benedict (HB) equation†	HB to HB plus 20%
Protein‡	1.5 g/kg of body weight	1.0-1.5 g/kg of body weight
Fat	20%-30% of total calories	20%-30% of total calories

*If patient's body mass index is 25 to <30, limit calories to basal estimate; if it is ≥30, provide 75% of basal caloric needs (based on the obese weight).
†Harris-Benedict (HB) equation for estimating basal energy expenditure (BEE)
  Males: BEE (kcal/day) = 66.5 + 13.8 (weight in kg) + 5 (height in cm) − 6.8 (age in years)
  Females: BEE (kcal/day) = 655 + 9.6 (weight in kg) + 1.8 (height in cm) − 4.7 (age in years)
  (Weight is current or "dry weight")
‡The guidelines for protein assume normal liver and kidney function. The estimated lean body weight is often used in obese patients to estimate protein needs of 1.5 g/kg.

- Maximally concentrated enteral and parenteral nutrition formulas are advised for critically ill patients (often receiving extra fluid and blood products) or fluid overloaded patients.

TUBE FEEDING

Indications

- If nutrition support is indicated and patient is not able to safely meet nutritional needs by mouth and gastrointestinal tract is functioning
- Examples—stroke and dysphagia; amyotrophic lateral sclerosis and dysphagia

Prescribing

Tubes

- For short-term use (<30 days), nasoenteric tubes with tip in stomach, duodenum, or jejunum are recommended; 12F diameter tubes are preferred.
  - ▲ Flexible, small diameter feeding tube with a weighted tip is preferred.
  - ▲ Semirigid nasogastric tube initially placed for decompression is suitable only for short-term use.
  - ▲ Gastrostomy or jejunostomy tube (endoscopic, surgical, or radiologic)
    - If anticipated need >4 weeks and
    - If ethical and acceptable by patient or guardian
  - ▲ Placement of nasoenteric tubes
    - Bedside or with fluoroscopic or endoscopic assistance
    - Position of tip must be confirmed radiographically before use.
    - Reconfirm position if any question of tube migration.

Prepyloric vs. Postpyloric Tubes

- Prepyloric (preferred) allows intermittent feeding (more physiologic), does not require a pump, and there is more information about drug absorption with gastric delivery.
- Postpyloric feedings should be considered if tube-feeding–related aspiration, elevation of head of bed >30° is contraindicated, or gastrointestinal dysmotility intolerant of gastric feeding. All postpyloric tubes must use continuous feeding program.

Baseline Lab Tests
- Glucose, sodium, potassium, chloride, bicarbonate, BUN/creatinine, AST, albumin, calcium, magnesium, and phosphorus
- Other tests individualized to patient

Formulas
- Determine estimated need for calories, protein, and fluid.
- We include protein in caloric estimate because amino acids are oxidized and provide energy.
- Standard formulas (appropriate for most patients) contain about 1 kcal/mL, 40 g/L protein, 40 mEq/L sodium, 40 mEq/L potassium, and 300 mOsm/kg water (isosmolar).
  - ▲ Typically, 1,200-1,500 mL formula provides 100% of recommended daily intake of vitamins and minerals.
  - ▲ If feeding <1,500 mL, check formula label and add daily multivitamin if necessary.
- One can of formula ~250 mL
- Isotonic feedings are generally administered full-strength. The exception is infusion of hypertonic (>400 mOsm/L) feeding into small bowel.

Intermittent (Gravity) vs. Continuous (Pump-Controlled)
- Standard progression for continuous tube feeding
  - ▲ Begin with 20 mL/hour and increase by 10-20–mL/hour increments every 12-24 hours to the goal rate.
- For intermittent (gravity) feeding
  - ▲ Start 1/2 can over 60-90 minutes with each feeding the first day of feeding and increase each feeding daily by 1/2 can increment until goal is reached (maximum 2 cans at any feeding).
- Tube patency requires flushing the tube with at least 30 mL water every 6 hours (more if necessary to meet fluid requirements, see below).

Medications and Tube Feeding
- Medications in liquid form are preferred.
- Opened capsules and crushed or ground tablets are mixed with 10-15 mL water and flushed through tube.

- ▲ Extended release and enteric-coated medications should not be used.
- ▪ Multiple medications should not be mixed together.
- ▪ Water is flushed through the tube before and after the administration of medications.
- ▪ Generally, medications should not be added to the tube feeding formula.
- ▪ Be aware of
  - ▲ Drugs with high osmolality or sorbitol content, such as potassium chloride, acetaminophen, and theophylline
  - ▲ Drugs that clog tubes, such as psyllium, ciprofloxacin suspension, sevelamer, and potassium chloride (do not use potassium chloride tablets, use liquid or powder form)
  - ▲ Drugs whose absorption is interfered with by tube feeds, such as phenytoin
- ▪ Consult with a pharmacist about tube feeding and medication issues.
- ▪ Consult nutrition team or dietitian for use of specialty formulas or if patient will be dismissed home on tube feedings for assistance with nutrition program, supplies, insurance, and follow-up.

Example
- ▪ A 66-year-old man unable to eat because of dysphagia after a stroke. Gastrointestinal tract is functioning. He is not in ICU. Height is 168 cm, weight is 60 kg, and BMI is 21.
- ▪ HB (male) = 66.5 + 13.7 (60) + 5 (168) − 6.8 (66), so BEE = 1,280 kcal/day
- ▪ Calorie goal—HB plus 20% is ~1,500 kcal/day.
- ▪ Protein goal—1 g/kg daily = 60 g/day
- ▪ Estimated fluid requirement—30 mL/kg daily × 60 mg = 1,800 mL/day
- ▪ Therefore, standard formula with 1.0 kcal/mL and 44 g protein/L would require 1,500 mL/day to provide 1,500 kcal/day (HB + 20%), 66 g protein (1.1 g/kg daily), and adequate vitamins
  - ▲ 1,800 mL − 1,500 mL in tube feeding formula = 300 mL/day fluid still required

Continuous Feeding Program (Requires Pump)
- ▪ 1,800 mL/24 hours = 75 mL/hour

- 300 mL fluid still needed divided 4× per day = 75 mL of water tube flush every 6 hours

Intermittent Feeding (Gravity) Program
- One can standard formula is ~250 mL, so ~250 kcal/can.
- Two cans (AM), 2 cans (midday), 2 cans (early evening) = 1,500 kcal/day and 1,500 mL/day fluid
- 300 mL fluid is still needed because six flushes (before and after each feeding) = 50 mL per flush

Monitoring
- Check residuals of feeding tube.
  - ▲ For prepyloric feeding, the residual fluid should be <100 mL, otherwise hold feeding for 1 hour and recheck.
  - ▲ If residual remains increased, check for abdominal distension and tube placement.
  - ▲ For postpyloric feeding, the residual fluid should be monitored to rule out tip migration back into the stomach.
- Is patient tolerating feeding? Check for abdominal distension or pain, diarrhea, or constipation.
- Intake and output, daily weights, lab tests (see below), increase >0.25 kg/day should be attributed to fluid gain
- 1-1.5 L of urine output is generally adequate.
- Frequent reassessment—Is more or less nutrition support needed? Is fluid still appropriate?

Complications
- Diarrhea—common problem but might not be caused by tube feeding
  - ▲ Review medications for sorbitol (in liquid medicines), magnesium, and osmolality.
  - ▲ Consider an infectious cause (especially *Clostridium difficile*).
  - ▲ Rule out infusion of full-strength hyperosmolar formula or medications into jejunum.
  - ▲ Can try fiber-containing formula and, if no infection, loperamide or tincture of opium.
- Abdominal distension or pain

- ▲ Assess for ileus, obstruction, or other abdominal lesion.
- ▲ Stop the tube feeding until problem has been resolved, then restart slowly.
- ■ Constipation
  - ▲ Be certain fluid (including water program) is adequate.
  - ▲ Fiber-containing formula can be used.
- ■ Aspiration
  - ▲ Elevate the head of the bed 30°- 45° during feeding.
  - ▲ Check residual volumes every 6 hours if continuous program or before feeding if intermittent program.
  - ▲ Consider postpyloric placement (see above).
  - ▲ Recheck tube placement by X-ray after placement or manipulation.
- ■ Metabolic abnormalities
  - ▲ Hypernatremia—Ensure adequate volume.
  - ▲ Hyperglycemia—Monitor glucose and treat as appropriate.
- ■ Tube-related—sinusitis, clogged tube, and tract infection
- ■ "Refeeding syndrome" (see below)

PARENTERAL NUTRITION—DEXTROSE, PROTEIN, FAT, ELECTROLYTES, VITAMINS, AND MINERALS

Indications
- ■ If nutrition support is indicated and gut cannot be used (i.e., ileus, distal bowel obstruction, short-gut syndrome/malabsorption, or severe dysmotility—if tube feeding is not tolerated)

Prescribing
- ■ Determine estimated need for daily calories (carbohydrate, protein, fat) and fluid.
- ■ We include protein in caloric estimate because amino acids are oxidized and provide energy.
- ■ Recall that a 10% solution = 10 g/dL = 100 g/L, i.e., 10% dextrose = 100 g/L (3.4 kcal/g dextrose), 5% amino acid = 50 g/L (4 kcal/g protein), 10% fat emulsion = 1.1 kcal/mL, and 20% fat emulsion = 2 kcal/mL.
- ■ Central access, central parenteral nutrition—Confirm catheter tip is in superior vena cava by chest X-ray before initiating parenteral nutrition.
- ■ Peripheral access; peripheral parenteral nutrition
  - ▲ Peripheral parenteral nutrition may be used if the patient

is mildly to moderately stressed and requires short-term parenteral nutrition.

▲ Infrequently used because 1 L provides few calories and large volumes are required to meet nutrition needs

▲ Osmolarity should be <900 mOsm/L and is estimated as follows:

- % amino acids × 100 + % dextrose × 50 + Na (mEq/L) × 2 + K (mEq/L) × 2 + 25

■ Baseline lab values—glucose, sodium, potassium, chloride, bicarbonate, BUN/creatinine, AST, albumin, calcium, magnesium, and phosphorus

▲ Other tests individualized to the patient

■ Check triglycerides if patient has pancreatitis, is taking propofol, has a history of hypertriglyceridemia or poorly controlled diabetes.

▲ If >400 mg/dL, stop or reduce fat emulsion.

■ Parenteral nutrition can help correct chronic metabolic abnormalities but should not be used as the sole treatment for acute metabolic abnormalities, e.g., electrolyte, mineral, or acid-base disorders.

■ Some drugs can be added to parenteral nutrition, especially if fluid restriction is needed (ask pharmacist).

■ If patient will be dismissed home on parenteral nutrition, consult nutrition team for assistance with patient selection, catheter selection and placement, outpatient nutrition program, monitoring, reimbursement, and insurance issues.

Example

■ A 54-year-old woman is unable to eat because of ileus due to abdominal abscess and sepsis. Features: 15% recent weight loss, is in ICU, is euvolemic, height is 172 cm, weight is 53 kg, estimated lean weight is 53 kg, and BMI 18.

■ HB (female) = 655 + 9.6 (53) + 1.8 (172) − 4.7 (54), so BEE = 1,220 kcal/day

■ Caloric goal—HB = 1,228 kcal/day

■ Protein goal—1.5 g/kg daily = 1.5 g × 53 kg = 80 g protein/day

■ Fat goal—20%-30% calories from fat

- Estimated fluid requirement—30 mL × 53 kg = 1,590 mL/day
- Distributing the calories among macronutrients
  - Protein—80 g × 4 kcal/g = 320 kcal
  - Fat—250 mL of 10% fat emulsion = 275 kcal (22% of total kcal)
  - Dextrose—need additional 633 kcal from dextrose to meet BEE requirement
    - 633 kcal/3.4 kcal/g of dextrose = 186 g dextrose
- Nonfluid-restricted formula
  - 1,590 mL/day total − 250 mL of fat = 1,340 mL for amino acids and dextrose
  - 80 g amino acids in 1,340 mL requires 80 g/13.4 dL = 6% amino acid solution
  - 186 g dextrose in 1,340 mL requires 186 g/13.4 dL = 14% dextrose solution
  - Therefore, formula would be 1,340 mL of 14% dextrose and 6% amino acid + 250 mL of 10% fat emulsion to provide 1,228 kcal (HB), 80 g protein (1.5 g/kg daily), and 22% of kcal from fat. Infuse over 24 hours, so 1,340 mL/24 = 56 mL/hour.
- Fluid-restricted (maximally concentrated) formula
  - 80 g protein from 10% amino acid source (100 g amino acid/L) requires 800 mL
  - 186 g dextrose from 70% dextrose (D70, 700 g dextrose/L) requires 266 mL
  - Thus, 1,066 mL is minimal fluid needed for dextrose and amino acids.
  - Therefore, formula would be 1,066 mL of 17% dextrose and 7.5% amino acid + 250 mL of 20% fat emulsion to provide 1,228 kcal (HB), 80 g protein (1.5 g/kg daily), and 22% kcal from fat.
  - 1,066 mL/24 hours = 45 mL/hour

Monitoring

- Chest X-ray to confirm position of catheter tip
- Daily intake and output and weight—Increase in excess of 0.25 kg/day should be attributed to fluid gain.
- Daily heart and lung exam, assessment of fluid status
- Catheter site for infection—always suspect if fever
- Glucose after initiation of parenteral nutrition
  - Aim for 80-120 mg/dL in critically ill patients with

hyperglycemia. Given that there is limited information
for glucose goals for stable patients on wards and tight
glucose control is difficult to achieve safely with SQ insulin
programs in hospitalized patients, a goal range of 100-
150 mg/dL is reasonable for patients on wards.

▲ If above is the goal, regular insulin can be added to
parenteral nutrition starting with 0.1 U per gram dextrose
and increasing up to 0.2 U per gram dextrose in parenteral
nutrition.

▲ Some patients will also require SQ insulin or graded insulin
infusion.

■ Check sodium, potassium, and glucose daily to start, other
tests and frequency should be individualized.

■ Check for added calories such as dextrose or propofol (for-
mulated in 10% fat emulsion, provides 1.1 kcal/mL). Fat
emulsion may need to be reduced or discontinued if patient
takes propofol.

■ Frequent reassessment—Is more or less nutrition support
needed? Is volume still appropriate? Can program be converted to tube feeding?

Complications

■ Central line-related—malposition, pneumothorax, infection,
thrombosis, and bleeding

■ Overfeeding can cause hyperglycemia, abnormal liver tests,
and increased carbon dioxide production.

■ Metabolic abnormalities—acid-base and electrolytes, hyperglycemia

■ "Refeeding syndrome" can occur when severely malnourished patients are aggressively refed. Complications
typically occur within first 5 days of feeding and include
hypokalemia, hypophosphatemia, fluid overload, and cardiac
arrhythmias.

▲ Check and replace potassium, phosphorus, and magnesium in patients at risk before initiating nutrition support.

▲ Avoid overfeeding. Begin with basal (using current, not
ideal, weight) calorie requirement, watch fluid balance,
monitor and replace electrolytes, and give thiamine.

OXYGEN THERAPY

Apoor S. Gami, M.D.
Jeffrey T. Rabatin, M.D.

CLASSIFICATION

Delivery Devices

- Oxygen delivery devices are described in Table 1.
- Oxygen flow and expected fraction of inspired oxygen (FIO_2) for different delivery devices are listed in Table 2.

Indications

- Indications for low-flow and high-flow devices are listed in Table 3.
- Acute myocardial infarction and congestive heart failure
  - ▲ For hypoxemia due to left ventricular failure, pulmonary edema, ventilation perfusion mismatch
  - ▲ Does not increase oxygen delivery if patient is not hypoxemic
  - ▲ May increase systemic vascular resistance and decrease cardiac output slightly.
  - ▲ Can be omitted if PaO_2 is normal
  - ▲ No effect on complications or survival
- Acute cor pulmonale
  - ▲ Rapid and dramatic improvement of pulmonary hemodynamics
  - ▲ Decreases right ventricular afterload with pulmonary infarction, infection, COPD
- Chronic cor pulmonale
  - ▲ Criteria for chronic oxygen therapy
    - • PaO_2 <55 mm Hg or SaO_2 ≤88%
    - • Or in the presence of cor pulmonale, heart failure, or erythrocytosis (hematocrit >55%), PaO_2 56-59 mm Hg or SaO_2 ≤89%

Special abbreviations used in this chapter: A-a, alveolar-arterial; ABG, arterial blood gas; FIO_2, fraction of inspired oxygen; SaO_2, arterial oxygen saturation.

Table 1. Oxygen Delivery Devices

Type	Delilvery device	Notes
Low-flow	Nasal cannula	FIO_2 variable dependent on:
	Simple face mask	Minute volume (RR ×
	Partial rebreather mask (reservoir)	tidal volume)
		Inspiratory flow rate
	Others—nasal catheter, transtracheal catheter	
High-flow	Non-rebreather mask (reservoir + 1-way valve)	FIO_2 more precise
		Oxygen delivery >4 × patient's minute volume
	Venturi mask	Larger oxygen reservoir
	Down's Flow Generator*	

FIO_2, fraction of inspired oxygen; RR, respiratory rate.
*Vital Signs, Inc., Totowa, New Jersey.

- Or in the presence of lung disease or other clinical needs, PaO_2 ≤60 mm Hg or SaO_2 ≤90%
  - ▲ Oxygen therapy should be prescribed for daytime and nighttime (and appropriately titrated) if these criteria are met during the day
  - ▲ Oxygen therapy should be prescribed for exercise or sleep if these criteria are met during that activity
  - ▲ Order sufficient oxygen to achieve PaO_2 >60 mm Hg.
  - ▲ Note: Oxygen therapy is the only treatment that improves survival in COPD.
  - ▲ Air travel
    - Patients who require oxygen therapy at sea level will require it when traveling by airplane.
    - Patients are not allowed to carry their own oxygen supply aboard a commercial airplane. Patients must notify the airline of their oxygen need, and they must carry a detailed oxygen prescription. Airlines usually require 48 hours to arrange for in-flight oxygen.
- ■ Hypoxemia
  - ▲ Is due to many conditions—interstitial lung disease, pulmonary fibrosis, acute respiratory distress syndrome, asthma, pulmonary embolism, pneumonia, pneumothorax, laryngeal infections, sickle cell crisis, anaphylaxis, circulatory shock

Table 2. **Delivery Devices, Oxygen Flow, and Expected FIO₂**

Device	100% O₂ flow, L/minute	FIO₂, %
Nasal cannula	1	24
	2	28
	3	32
	4	36
	5	40
	6	44
	7	48
	8	52
Simple face mask	5-7	40-50
	8-10	50-60
Partial rebreather	6	50
	7	65
	8-15	80
Non-rebreather	15-flush ($\approx$ 60)	90+
Venturi mask	Usually >40	Up to 50
Down's Flow Generator*	80-100	Room air-100

FIO₂, fraction of inspired oxygen.
*Vital Signs, Inc., Totowa, New Jersey.

▲ Goal
  • Maintain PaO₂ >60 mm Hg or SaO₂ >90%
  • PaO₂ levels >80 mm Hg are rarely necessary.
■ Carbon monoxide poisoning
  ▲ Oxygen is the definitive treatment.
  ▲ Hyperbaric oxygen treatments may reduce long-term complications, but there is no consensus about the best dose and schedule. Administration of 3 treatments within 24 hours showed benefit in one trial.
  ▲ Order 100% FIO₂ by a non-rebreather mask at 10 L/minute until carbon monoxide levels are <10% and all symptoms and any cardiovascular or central nervous system instability resolve.
  ▲ Infants and pregnant women require treatment hours after symptoms resolve because of predominance of fetal hemoglobin, which has a higher affinity for carbon monoxide.

Table 3. Indications for Low-Flow and High-Flow Devices

Device	Indications
Low-flow	Short-term therapy (e.g., postoperatively)
	Long-term therapy (e.g., chronic hypoxemia)
	Temporizing measure
High-flow	Temporizing measure before assisted ventilation becomes necessary

- Cluster headaches
  - ▲ Oxygen is the most effective treatment for an acute attack.
  - ▲ Order 100% F_{IO_2} for 15 minutes.
- Gas gangrene—Hyperbaric oxygen therapy is controversial.
- Obstructive sleep apnea—Nocturnal oxygen alone is not effective.
- Important points
  - ▲ Cyanosis is not an accurate indicator of Pa_{O_2} (many false-positive and false-negative results).
  - ▲ Compromised brain function at Pa_{O_2} 55 mm Hg
  - ▲ Loss of consciousness at Pa_{O_2} 30 mm Hg

Monitoring

- Arterial blood gas (ABG) measurements
  - ▲ Routine ABG monitoring is misleading because of poor precision.
  - ▲ Inconsistent with repeated measurements: variation = 13 ± 18 mm Hg.
  - ▲ A Pa_{O_2} change on a "routine ABG" is not necessarily abnormal if the patient's clinical status has not changed.
  - ▲ Advantage
    - Wealth of other information about clinical status
    - Useful when clinical status deteriorates and pulse oximetry waveform is unreliable.
- Important points
  - ▲ The alveolar-arterial (A-a) P_{O_2} gradient is affected by oxygen therapy—The normal A-a P_{O_2} gradient increases 5-7 mm Hg for every 10% increase in F_{IO_2} (because of loss of regional hypoxic vasoconstriction in poorly ventilated lung regions).
- Pulse oximetry

- ▲ Advantages
  - Excellent accuracy, superior precision
  - High sensitivity for detection of hypoxic episodes
  - Inexpensive, noninvasive, and free of complications
- ▲ Limitations
  - Accuracy within $\pm$ 3% (when SaO_2 >70%)
  - Overestimates
    - Elevated methemoglobin (high-dose nitroglycerin)
    - Elevated carboxyhemoglobin (smoke inhalation)
  - Underestimates
    - Hypotension—accurate down to blood pressure of 30 mm Hg
    - Anemia—accurate down to hemoglobin 3 g/dL
    - Nail polish
    - Jaundice and skin pigmentation
    - Hypothermia, motion artifact
- ■ Important points
  - ▲ Ear probes have faster response times than finger probes.
  - ▲ Check pulse oximetry or ABG $\geq$20 minutes after changing patient's FIO_2.
  - ▲ Continuous pulse oximetry typically is only for ICU or unstable patients.
  - ▲ Always check different sites and waveforms before making therapeutic decisions.

Prescribing
- ■ Low-flow devices
  - ▲ FIO_2 depends on the patient's minute volume and inspiratory flow rate.
  - ▲ If large tidal volumes or tachypnea, FIO_2 is lower than estimates in Table 2.
  - ▲ Good initial choice for patient who is hemodynamically stable but mildly hypoxemic
- ■ High-flow devices
  - ▲ They provide the total inspiratory volume at predictable FIO_2 levels.
  - ▲ Prescribe for those who need consistent FIO_2 and have varying tidal volumes and respiratory rates.

- Important points
  - With nasal cannula, F_{IO_2} generally does not vary with mouth vs. nose breathing.
  - Order therapy early because it may take time to obtain the next needed device.
- COPD
  - Problem—Ventilatory drive is PaO_2-dependent in a small percentage of patients with COPD.
    - If patient is hypoxic, aggressive oxygen therapy can decrease the respiratory rate, leading to progressive hypoxemia and respiratory acidosis.
    - Goal—maintain adequate PaO_2 while limiting hypercapnia
    - *Withholding oxygen therapy may be harmful.*
  - If oxygenation is inadequate and/or patient has progressive hypercapnia, initiate assisted ventilation (i.e., Ambu-bag, noninvasive mechanical ventilation, intubation and mechanical ventilation).
  - Important point
    - Pediatric flow meters accurately measure oxygen flow from 0.25 to 3.0 L/minute. If these are available, titrate flow in 0.25-L/minute increments in patients with COPD.

Complications
- Nasal cannula
  - Mucosal irritation, drying, and bleeding
  - Especially with flow rates >4 L/minute and nonhumidified oxygen
- Masks
  - Aspiration, "emesis traps"
  - Because of difficulty eating and drinking, there is risk of acute hypoxemia with noncompliance.
  - Venturi one-way valve may stick because of moisture.
- Important points
  - Order a humidifier or nebulizer to increase the water content of inspired gases.
  - Order the lowest flow rate necessary to achieve the goals of therapy.
- Complications
  - Progressive symptoms of oxygen toxicity include

- Substernal discomfort or pain
- Cough
- Deeper breathing, worsening cough and pain
- Decreased vital capacity

▲ Complications of toxic oxygen therapy are listed in Table 4.

▲ Reasonable limits of toxic FIO_2 therapy are listed in Table 5.

▲ Important points
  - The shunt fraction determines the effect of FIO_2 on PaO_2.
  - When shunt fraction is >50%, PaO_2 is essentially independent of changes in FIO_2.
  - Thus, with high shunt fractions (acute respiratory distress syndrome), FIO_2 can be lowered to nontoxic levels.

Table 4. Clinical Complications of Toxic Oxygen Therapy

Time breathing toxic FIO_2	Clinical complications
12 hours to days	Tracheobronchitis
	Decreased vital capacity
Days to 1 week	Interstitial pulmonary edema
>1 week	Pulmonary fibrosis

FIO_2, fraction of inspired oxygen.

Table 5. Reasonable Limits of Toxic FIO_2 Therapy

FIO_2, %	Time, hours
100	12
80	24
60	36
50	Unlimited*

FIO_2, fraction of inspired oxygen.

*Even "nontoxic" levels of FIO_2 have potential to cause complications listed in Table 4, especially in more debilitated patients. Some have advocated supplementing antioxidants (e.g., selenium) for these patients to prevent complications of oxygen therapy, but no evidence supports this.

PAIN MANAGEMENT

K. L. Venkatachalam, M.D.
Paul E. Carns, M.D.

PAIN CONTROL

- Three approaches to controlling pain are as follows:
  - ▲ Modify the source of pain.
  - ▲ Alter the central perception and spinal cord modification of pain.
  - ▲ Block the transmission of pain to the central nervous system.
- Treat pain aggressively and quickly to provide the patient sustained relief.

DEFINITIONS

- Tolerance—condition in which a larger dose of opioid analgesic is required to maintain the original effect (a common occurrence in chronic users)
- Dependence—physical condition in which the abrupt discontinuation of an opioid (after chronic use) or the administration of an opioid antagonist produces an abstinence syndrome (anxiety, irritability, chills, hot flashes, salivation, lacrimation, rhinorrhea)
- Addiction—psychologic condition defined as a pattern of compulsive drug use characterized by a continued craving for an opioid and the need to use opioids for effects other than pain relief
- Pseudoaddiction—iatrogenic condition resembling addiction due to opioid doses that are too low or spaced too far apart to relieve pain

INDICATIONS

- Obtain a thorough pain history.
  - ▲ Use the mnemonic OLD CARTS—onset, location,

Special abbreviation used in this chapter: PCA, patient-controlled analgesia.

duration, characteristic, aggravating factors, relieving factors, treatments, and severity.

▲ Ascertain and verify pain intensity frequently from the patient by using a reliable verbal or numerical scale.
  • Mild pain—1-4
  • Moderate pain—5-6
  • Severe pain—7-10

■ Perform a thorough physical exam, probing for tender points of inflammation or muscle spasm.
  ▲ It is important to arrive at the correct diagnosis.
  ▲ Treat pain during the diagnostic work-up, but do not miss treatable underlying causes, e.g., pulmonary embolism, acute abdomen, radiculopathic pain with progressive neurologic deficit.

■ The World Health Organization recommends the use of a "Three-Step Analgesic Ladder" to guide therapy:
  ▲ Treat mild-moderate pain with nonopioid analgesics (step 1).
  ▲ Maximize the dose of the nonopioid analgesic, and add a step 2 opioid analgesic if the pain is mild-moderate despite the use of nonopioid analgesics. Increase the dose for patients with moderate-severe pain despite step 2 opioids.
  ▲ If this is not feasible, use a step 3 opioid.

CLASSIFICATION OF THERAPY

■ The various classes of therapy and the corresponding medications and indications are outlined in Table 1.
■ Note that all prescribing information is based on adult dosages.
■ If possible, start with PO analgesics because they are the preferred form.
  ▲ Avoid IM injections.
  ▲ When administering IV medication, patient-controlled analgesia (PCA) is the preferred mode of delivery.

THE GIST OF PCA

■ The following adjustments may be made to a PCA machine (Table 2):
  ▲ IV drug bolus dose per patient request
  ▲ Lockout interval—time following bolus dose during which the PCA machine will not dispense any medication despite patient requests

Table 1. Classes of Therapy, Representative Medications, and General Indications

Class of therapy	Representative medications	General indications
Nonopioid analgesics	Acetaminophen Aspirin Choline magnesium trisalicylate NSAIDs (many classes) Tramadol (both opioid & nonopioid)	Good baseline control of mild-moderate pain
Opioid analgesics	Codeine Dihydrocodeine Hydrocodone Oxycodone Morphine Hydromorphone Fentanyl	Step 2 opioids for moderate pain despite nonopioids Step 3 opioids for severe pain despite step 2 opioids
Analgesic adjuvants	Tricyclic antidepressants Benzodiazepines Caffeine Corticosteroids Anticonvulsants	Used to enhance effects of analgesics or counteract their side effects

▲ Maximum dose—set so that the patient may receive medication only ≈ 10 times per 4 hours.
  • Patients can request it as much as they want but will be locked out.
▲ Baseline infusion—not always required but useful if patient is trying to sleep or is unable to operate PCA machine
■ Equianalgesic opioid conversion factors (Table 3)
■ Equianalgesic dose of transdermal fentanyl to morphine (Table 4)
■ Conversion of IV morphine to sustained-release morphine
  ▲ Total the daily requirement of immediate-release morphine (IV and PCA) and convert to PO dosage. Next, convert to the nearest equivalent of sustained-release morphine,

Table 2. Patient-Controlled Analgesia Dosage

Drug concentration	Bolus dose	Lockout interval, minutes	Maximum dose, per 4 hours	Baseline infusion, per hour
Morphine (MSIR) (1 mg/mL)	1-5 mg	5-20	10-50 mg	1-10 mg
Fentanyl (10 µg/mL)	15-50 µg	3-10	150-500 µg	20-100 µg
Hydromorphone (0.2 mg/mL)	0.1-0.5 mg	5-15	1-5 mg	0.2-0.5 mg

Data from Mayo Clinic Anesthesia Department Inpatient Pain Service Guidelines.

Table 3. Equianalgesic Opioid Conversion Factors*

Opioid	IM/IV	PO, mg
Codeine	--	200
Fentanyl	100 µg	--
Hydrocodone	--	5-10
Hydromorphone	1.5 mg	7.5
Meperidine	75 mg	300
Morphine	10 mg	30
Oxycodone		20

*Note that these are not recommended doses but only conversion factors.

Table 4. Transdermal Fentanyl to Morphine Conversion

Transdermal fentanyl, µg/hour	Morphine PO, mg/24 hours	Morphine IV, mg/24 hours
25	30-90	10-30
50	91-150	31-50
75	151-210	51-70
100	211-270	71-90

Modified from Donner B, Zenz M, Tryba M, Strumpf M. Direct conversion from oral morphine to transdermal fentanyl: a multicenter study in patients with cancer pain. Pain. 1996;64:527-34. Used with permission.

e.g., PCA—2 mg/bolus dose, 10-minute lockout, 30 mg maximum per 4 hours. Actual 24-hour usage found to be 60 mg IV. (*Check PCA machine for specific daily usage.*)
▲ Convert to PO dosage using the equianalgesic opioid conversion factors chart (Table 3).
  • 60 mg IV morphine = 180 mg PO morphine (1:3 conversion)
▲ Use long-acting morphine sulfate 90 mg PO every 12 hours *or* 60 mg PO every 8 hours (180 mg/day) plus 15-30 mg MSIR PO every 4 hours as needed for breakthrough pain.

PAIN PEARLS AND PITFALLS
▪ Always believe the patient.
▪ Be mindful of the patient's baseline analgesic use, because

he or she may have developed tolerance. Adjust dosages accordingly.

- Patients may need initial boluses of opioid before IV PCA is started.
- Acetaminophen and ibuprofen can provide excellent baseline control of pain as long as they are used on a scheduled basis (Tables 5 and 6).
- Always provide constipation prophylaxis when using opioid (Table 7).
- If the duration of analgesia is insufficient or decreases with time, increase the magnitude of each dose, not the dosing frequency.
- Morphine can provide pain relief without interfering with the patient's ability to give consent or the physician's ability to make a diagnosis (Table 5).
- The incidence of addiction in patients with pain is low and not affected by opioid administration by health care providers.
- Administer analgesics regularly (not just as needed) if pain is present most of the time.
- With the elderly, start low and go slow. Initial doses should be 25%-50% lower than for young adults.
- Do not use placebos to assess pain.

Table 5. Symptom-Oriented Prescribing Information and Adult Dosages for Acute Pain

Condition	Treatment
Headache (severe tension or migraine)	Ibuprofen 600 mg PO tid
	Add acetaminophen 1 g PO qid
	If refractory, ketorolac 30 mg IV or 60 mg IM
Unresponsive migraine	Sumatriptan 25 mg PO/6 mg SQ: increase PO dose to 50 mg every 2 hours (300 mg max/day); repeat SQ dose in 1 hour (12 mg max/day)
	Rizatriptan (Maxalt, Maxalt MLT) 5-10 mg PO, may repeat in 2 hours tmax dose, 30 mg/24 hours); Maxalt MLT tablets dissolve under tongue
	Adjunctive therapy with metoclopramide 10 mg IV or prochlorperazine 10 mg IV/25 mg PR
	Caffeine 100 mg PO every 4-6 hours
	Dihydroergotamine (DHE, migranal) 1 mg IV, IM, or SQ: may repeat once
Trigeminal neuralgia	Gabapentin started at 300 mg PO at bedtime, increasing by 300 mg every 3 days to a goal of 600 mg tid over 15 days; this may be increased further depending on patient response to a max of 3,600 mg/day
	Carbamazepine 200-400 mg PO qid
Odynophagia (from oral infections or irradiation)	Haddad's solution (2% viscous lidocaine 10 mL, Maalox 10 mL, diphenhydramine elixir 10 mL) swished & swallowed every 6 hours

Table 5 (continued)

Condition	Treatment
Costochondritis	Ibuprofen 600 mg PO tid
	If ulcer history or gastrointestinal distress, rofecoxib 25 mg PO daily (short term use only)
	Add acetaminophen 1 g PO qid
Dyspepsia	Ketorolac 30 mg IV/IM for immediate relief
	"GI cocktail" (Maalox or Mylanta 30 mL, 2% viscous lidocaine 10 mL, and Donnatal 10 mL) PO; repeat once in 2-4 hours
	For long-term relief, pantoprazole 40 mg PO daily or lansoprazole 30 mg PO daily
Angina pectoris	For stable angina, nitroglycerin 0.4-mg tablets SL or 1 spray under tongue every 5 minutes to max of 3 doses; for prophylaxis, isosorbide dinitrate 40-80 mg PO bid
Unstable angina	Nitroglycerin IV bolus 12.5-25 µg, then 10-20 µg/minute; titrate to effect
	If refractory and patient agitated, morphine sulfate 1-3 mg slow IV every 10 minutes
Abdominal pain	If severe enough to merit analgesics, morphine sulfate 2-4 mg IV every 15 minutes (will not interfere with patient's ability to give informed consent or physician's ability to make diagnosis)
	Alternatively, morphine sulfate PCA—2-4 mg/dose, 10-minute lockout, 20-40 mg max every 4 hours
Pelvic pain	Ibuprofen 600 mg PO tid
	Add acetaminophen 1 g PO qid

Table 5 (continued)

Condition	Treatment
Pelvic pain (continued)	For breakthrough pain, acetaminophen with codeine (300 mg/30 mg) 1-2 tablets every 4 hours (*do not exceed 4 g/day total of acetaminophen*)
	Oxycodone 5-10 mg PO every 6 hours
	Tramadol 50-100 mg PO every 4-6 hours to 400 mg max/day
	Meperidine 50-100 mg PO every 4-6 hours (do not use for more than 48 hours)
Renal colic	Ketorolac 15-30 mg IM/IV or indomethacin 100 mg PR initially
	If refractory morphine sulfate PCA—2-4 mg/dose, 10-minute lockout, 20-40 mg max every 4 hours
Vaso-occlusive crisis	Aggressive control required; morphine sulfate IV or PCA—baseline infusion 1-10 mg/hour, 2-4 mg/dose, 10-minute lockout, 40-80 mg max every 4 hours

bid, twice daily; PCA, patient-controlled analgesia; PR, per rectum; qid, 4 times daily; SL, sublingual; tid, 3 times daily.

Table 6. Symptom-Oriented Prescribing Information and Adult Doses for Chronic Pain

Condition	Treatment
Cancer pain (may be somatic, visceral, or neuropathic pain)	For mild-moderate pain, ibuprofen 600 mg PO tid with acetaminophen 1 g PO qid If intolerant of ibuprofen, replace with rofecoxib up to 50 mg PO daily (short term use only) For continued pain, oxycodone 5-10 mg PO every 6 hours prn or 30-60 mg of codeine every 4-6 hours prn If refractory, add morphine sulfate, immediate release (MSIR) 15-30 mg PO every 4 hours & determine effective daily dose; replace with equivalent dose of sustained-release morphine bid (see Table 3) with MSIR for breakthrough pain *(the maximum dose of morphine under these conditions is determined only by the degree of pain control & side effects)*
Cancer pain with dysphagia	Morphine elixir or rectal suppositories (except for patients with bone marrow suppression) in equivalent doses; alternatively, transdermal fentanyl (see Table 4); replace transdermal fentanyl every 72 hours; slightly higher serum levels may be achieved by replacing fentanyl every 48 hours; continue other pain medications for at least 24 hours until transdermal fentanyl takes effect; fentanyl transmucosal lozenges in equivalent doses may also be used Morphine PCA—2-4 mg/dose, 10-minute lockout, 20-40 mg max every 4 hours Fentanyl PCA—baseline infusion 20-100 µg/hour, 15-50 µg/dose, 3-10-minute lockout, 150-500 µg/4 hours

Table 6 (continued)

Condition	Treatment
Adjuvant therapy for neural plexus malignancy	Dexamethasone 16 mg/day
Metastatic bone pain	Pamidronate IV 90 mg over 2 hours every 4 weeks
Joint pain	Acetaminophen 1 g PO qid & ibuprofen 600 mg PO tid
	For ibuprofen intolerance, rofecoxib 25 mg PO daily
	Codeine/acetaminophen (30 mg/300 mg) every 4-6 hours for moderate-severe pain
Bursitis	Betamethasone + 1% lidocaine (specific volumes for each bursa) intrabursal injection

PCA, patient-controlled analgesia; prn, as needed; qid, 4 times daily; tid, 3 times daily.

Table 7. Drug Complications and Contraindications

Medication	Complications and contraindications
NSAIDs	Dyspepsia, ulcers, gastrointestinal tract perforation, colitis, renal insufficiency, prolonged PT & bleeding
Acetaminophen	Over-anticoagulation with warfarin; severe hepatotoxicity in alcoholics & patients with liver disease Do not use more than 4 g/day in nonalcoholics with normal liver function
Aspirin	Gastritis, gastric bleeding; associated with Reye syndrome in children <12 years Aspirin hypersensitivity with rhinitis or asthma or more serious combination of angioedema, hypotension & urticaria may occur
Carbamazepine	Aplastic anemia & liver function abnormalities; monitor serial CBCs & liver function tests for prolonged use
Gabapentin	Sedation, ataxia, nystagmus, SIADH Sedation, ataxia, & nystagmus Dose reduction needed in renal failure
Haddad's solution	Marked reduction in gag reflex (do not give near meal times)
GI cocktail	Avoid in renal failure
Nitroglycerin	Contraindicated with hypotension, severe bradycardia or tachycardia, right ventricular infarction, & sildenafil use within 24 hours
Morphine	Respiratory depression, constipation, hypotension, sedation, nausea, vomiting; change dose or route of drug, aiming for more constant levels; add medication to counteract side effect For sedation, caffeine 60–200 mg PO daily For constipation, prophylaxis with docusate sodium, 100 mg PO bid with senna 2-6 tablets PO bid (goal of 1-2 soft bowel movements/day); lactulose, laxative suppositories, & magnesium citrate to relieve constipation

Table 7 (continued)

Medication	Complications and contraindications
Morphine (continued)	For mild nausea, prochlorperazine 10 mg IV every 6-8 hours
	For severe nausea, ondansetron 4 mg IV every 3 hours
	For respiratory depression that needs reversal, use dilute solution of naloxone (0.4 mg in 10 mL normal saline administered as 0.5 mL IV push every 2 minutes); watch for profound withdrawal, seizures, & severe pain
	Morphine-6-glucuronide is active metabolite with decreased elimination in renal failure, resulting in enhanced potency & prolonged duration of action
Tramadol	Avoid in opioid-dependent patient
	Lowers seizure threshold (avoid in patients with history of seizures or taking antidepressants)
	Dose reduction needed in renal insufficiency
Meperidine	Normeperidine, a metabolite produces anxiety, tremors, myoclonus, & generalized seizures with repetitive dosing
	Avoid in renal insufficiency
	Limit use to 48 hours
	Do not use for chronic pain
Sumatriptan	Nausea, vomiting, malaise, vertigo, warmth

bid, twice daily; SIADH, syndrome of inappropriate antidiuretic hormone

PROCEDURES

Matthew W. Martinez, M.D.
Adam J. Locketz, M.D.
Jon O. Ebbert, M.D., M.Sc.

DOCUMENTATION

- Obtain informed consent before the procedure.
  - ▲ The patient or person making medical decisions for the patient should be clearly informed of the following:
    - Purpose of the procedure (diagnosis and/or therapy)
    - Risks of the procedure (bleeding and infection)
    - Alternative interventions
    - General procedural technique
    - Patients, guardians, or power of attorney should be allowed to ask questions.
- Procedural note
  - ▲ "Discussed risks, benefits, and alternatives of (insert procedure here) with the patient (and/or guardian/power of attorney). Patient expressed an understanding of risks, benefits, and alternatives and asked appropriate questions, which were answered. Patient agreed to proceed."
  - ▲ Include the following:
    - Date
    - Name
    - Pager
    - Supervised by (if indicated)
    - Indication
    - Brief description of the procedure, including
      - Amount of anesthetic used
      - Estimated blood loss
      - Fluid removed (if any)
      - Testing performed
      - Notable hemodynamics (if any monitored)
      - Complications (if any)

ARTHROCENTESIS

- All joint procedures require "Indications," "Contra-indications," "Suggested Equipment for Joint Aspiration," and "Preparation and Anesthesia" (see below).
- Specific joints are outlined beginning with "Specific Joints."

Indications

- Diagnostic indications of arthrocentesis include evaluating the cause of a joint effusion (including crystal-induced, traumatic, infectious, or inflammatory or degenerative processes).
  - ▲ *It is particularly important to rule out a septic joint, which is perhaps the only rheumatologic emergency.*
- Therapeutic indications include removing pus from a septic joint, pain relief from removal of fluid, injection of local anesthetic, corticosteroid, or visco-supplementation.

Contraindications

- Severe coagulopathy
- Broken skin or cellulitis over intended entry site
- Joint prosthesis—should always be performed by an orthopedic surgeon
- Bacteremia or sepsis syndrome—This seems counterintuitive to many residents. You *can* tap a joint if it is suspected to be infected but the patient is without diagnosed bacteremia or sepsis.
- Note—Arthrocentesis can be performed safely with normal anticoagulation (INR 2-3).

Suggested Equipment for Joint Aspiration

- Most hospitals have a prepared "Aspiration Tray" that can be ordered.
- Bottle of povidone-iodine solution
- Alcohol swab
- Needles—1-inch 25 gauge and a 1.5-inch 25, 20, 18, or 15 gauge (depending on joint injection)
- Syringes—two 6 mL, 35 mL (for large knee volumes)
- Lidocaine 1% 30 mL
- Drape
- Sterile gloves
- Tubes for culture, Gram stain, cell count, crystal analysis
- Disposable pad for placing under the joint

- Bandage for covering injection site when completed
- If you suspect an anaerobic infection, obtain a special anaerobic culture vial.
- *Therapeutic*
  - ▲ For therapeutic injections, you also need to obtain 1 bottle of 0.25% preservative-free bupivacaine (or equivalent) and 1 bottle of methylprednisolone acetate 40 mg/mL or equivalent.
  - ▲ Explain to the patient that the joint may be painful for up to 24 hours after the injection.
  - ▲ The full benefit from a corticosteroid injection may take several days.
  - ▲ The joint should also be rested for 1-2 days.

Preparation and Anesthesia

- Confirm that you have all the required materials.
- Stamp several labels with the patient's name.
- Complete the appropriate microbiology card.
- Labels should be applied to all clinical specimens (or the lab will not accept them).
- Review the patient's current CBC (platelets), aPTT, and INR if available.
- In the outpatient setting, coagulation studies typically are not ordered before arthrocentesis.
  - ▲ Instead, the patient is asked if he or she is taking warfarin or other blood thinners.
- *Make sure there is not an artificial joint.*
- Review relevant X-rays of the joint if available.
- It may be useful to have a nurse or fellow resident in the room to assist you.
- Position the patient, and mark the insertion site (after careful review of the appropriate anatomic landmarks).
- *Confirm that the patient does not have a history of allergy to lidocaine or iodine.*
  - ▲ Also ask about drug allergies in general.
- Place a disposable pad under the joint.
- Open the kit on a bedside table.
- Pour iodine into the iodine cup.
- Change into sterile gloves.

- Prepare the skin using gauze dipped into the iodine solution.
  - ▲ Remember to allow 5 minutes to dry or there is little bacteriocidal effect.
- Drape the fenestrated drape over the insertion site.
- Wipe the area with a sterile alcohol swab.
- Optional—Raise a skin wheal with lidocaine by using a 25-gauge 1-inch needle attached to a 6-cc syringe.
- Optional—Infiltrate anesthetic into SQ tissue in the direction that the arthrocentesis will occur, aspirating as you go, so as not to inject anesthetic directly into a blood vessel.
- Remove the anesthetic needle and syringe and place them back on the tray.

Specific Joints—Shoulder, Elbow, Wrist, Knee, Ankle
Shoulder Joint
- To aspirate the glenohumeral joint, use either a posterior or anterior approach.
- For the posterior approach, rotate the shoulder internally across the chest, which opens the joint space.
- Identify the sulcus between the head of the humerus and the acromion.
- Mark the insertion site with skin indentation 1 cm inferior and 1 cm medial to the lateral edge of the acromion process.
- Note—Avoid going too far inferiorly with this approach because you may enter the quadrangular space and risk hitting the axillary artery.
- Prepare the joint, and anesthetize the insertion site as described under "**Preparation and Anesthesia**."
- Connect the 18-gauge 1.5-inch needle to the 6-cc syringe.
  - ▲ A longer needle may be needed depending on body habitus; consider this for all the injections.
- Advance the needle through the skin wheal, perpendicular to the skin aiming for the coracoid process anteriorly.
- Aspirate as much fluid as can be easily obtained.
- *Therapeutic*—If a therapeutic injection is to be performed, attach a 25-gauge 1.5-inch needle to another 6-mL syringe and inject a mixture of 2 mL 0.25% preservative-free bupivacaine or equivalent and 1 mL 40 mg/mL of methylprednisolone acetate or equivalent.
- The solution should go in smoothly if the needle is within the joint space.

▪ Remove the needles, and place a bandage over the site.

Elbow Joint

▪ Flex the elbow to 90°.
▪ Have the patient rest the ulnar side of the hand on a table, allowing the thumb to point upward.
▪ Identify a triangle involving the lateral epicondyle of the humerus, the olecranon process, and the head of the radius.
▪ The radial head is identified by having the patient supinate and pronate the forearm while you palpate for movement in the area.
▪ The needle will be directed in the space just inferior to the lateral epicondyle and superior to the olecranon process of the ulna and proximal to the head of the radius.
▪ Mark the site with a skin indentation.
▪ Prepare the joint and anesthetize the insertion site as described under "Preparation and Anesthesia."
▪ Connect a 20-gauge 1.5-inch needle to a 6-mL syringe.
▪ Introduce the needle perpendicular to the surface of the skin.
▪ Advance the needle through the skin wheal.
▪ Aspirate as much fluid as can be easily obtained.
▪ *Therapeutic*—If a therapeutic injection is to be performed, attach a 25-gauge 1-inch needle to another 6-mL syringe and inject a mixture of 1 mL 0.25% preservative-free bupivacaine or equivalent and 1 mL of 40 mg/mL methylprednisolone acetate or equivalent.
▪ The solution should go in smoothly if the needle is within the joint space.
▪ Remove the needles, and place a bandage over the site.

Wrist Joint

▪ Place a rolled towel under the wrist, which opens the joint space.
▪ The needle should be directed at a site on the dorsal wrist lateral to the extensor digitorum communis tendon, proximal to the indentation of the capitate bone.
▪ A concave space can be palpated here as the wrist is flexed

and extended; this space indicates the correct position for needle placement.

- *Avoid the dorsal metacarpal* vein, "intern's vein," when using this approach.
- Mark the site of insertion with a skin indentation.
- Prepare the joint and anesthetize the insertion site as described under "Preparation and Anesthesia."
- Connect a 20-gauge 1.5-inch needle to the 6-mL syringe.
- Advance the needle through the skin wheal, perpendicular to the skin.
- Aspirate as much fluid as can be easily obtained.
- *Therapeutic*—If a therapeutic injection is to be performed, attach a 25-gauge 1-inch needle to another 6-mL syringe and inject a mixture of 0.5-1 mL 0.25% preservative-free bupivacaine or equivalent and 1 mL of 40 mg/mL of methyl-prednisolone acetate or equivalent.
- The solution should go in smoothly if the needle is within the joint space.
- Remove the needles, and place a bandage over the site.

Knee Joint

- Confirm the effusion.
- Position the patient lying down on the bed, and slightly flex the knee with a towel placed under the knee.
- A lateral, medial, or inferior approach may be used. The medial approach is discussed here.
- The site of entry medially is just below the middle point for the patella.
- Introduce the needle parallel to the ground toward the intra-condylar notch of the femur.
- With this approach, there is no major artery nearby, but an infrapatellar branch of the saphenous nerve is nearby.
- Mark the site of insertion with a skin indentation.
- Prepare the joint and anesthetize the insertion site as described under "Preparation and Anesthesia."
- Connect the 18-gauge 1.5-inch needle to a 6-mL syringe (a 35-mL syringe may be used if a large volume of fluid is anticipated).
- Advance the needle through the skin wheal, parallel to the ground, proceeding under the patella at a 20°-40° incline from parallel.

- You may hit the ostium of the undersurface of the patella. This is painful for the patient. If this occurs, withdraw the needle slightly, reposition, and aim more inferiorly.
- You will often feel a "pop" or lessening of resistance as the needle enters the joint space.
- As the fluid is aspirated, it can be "milked down" by controlled pressure with one hand placed over the suprapatellar pouch.
- *Therapeutic*—If a therapeutic injection is to be performed, attach a 25-gauge 1.5-inch needle to another 6-mL syringe and inject a mixture of 3-4 mL 0.25% preservative-free bupivacaine and 1 mL of 40 mg/mL of methylprednisolone.
- The solution should go in smoothly if the needle is within the joint space.
- Remove the needles, hold pressure for 5 minutes (to reduce any hematoma or ecchymosis), and place a bandage over the site.

Ankle Joint

- The ankle joint is composed of the tibiotalar joint, subtalar joint, and talonavicular joint.
- The tibiotalar joint is aspirated or injected.
- The patient should be lying down, with the ankle in neutral position.
- Identify the tibialis anterior tendon and the extensor hallucis longus tendon by having the patient dorsiflex the foot.
- Identify the hollow medial or lateral to these two tendons at the articulation of the tibia and the talus.
  - ▲ You should inject medially or laterally to these tendons to avoid the dorsalis pedis artery.
- Mark the site of insertion with a skin indentation.
- Prepare the joint, and anesthetize the insertion site as described under "Preparation and Anesthesia."
- Connect the 20-gauge 1.5-inch needle to the 6-mL syringe.
- Direct the needle medially or laterally to the extensor hallucis longus tendon and the anterior tibialis tendon.

- Direct the needle tangentially to the curve of the talus and slightly laterally.
  - ▲ It must be inserted approximately 3 cm before fluid will be obtained.
- Advance the needle through the skin wheal, aspirating as you go.
- Aspirate as much fluid as can be easily obtained.
- *Therapeutic*—If a therapeutic injection is to be performed, attach a 25-gauge 1.5-inch needle to another 6-mL syringe and inject a mixture of 1-2 mL 0.25% preservative-free bupivacaine or equivalent and 1 mL of 40 mg/mL or equivalent of methylprednisolone.
- The solution should go in smoothly if the needle is within the joint space.
- Remove the needles, and place a bandage over the site.

Synovial Fluid Analysis
- Features of synovial fluid characteristic of various conditions are listed in Table 1.

LUMBAR PUNCTURE
Indications
- For internists, lumbar puncture is performed primarily for the diagnosis of
  - ▲ Central nervous system infection (meningitis, encephalitis, neurosyphilis)
    - • If suspicion is high, begin antibiotics or antivirals before procedure.
  - ▲ Subarachnoid hemorrhage
  - ▲ Demyelinating conditions (Guillain-Barré syndrome, multiple sclerosis)
  - ▲ Other (pseudotumor cerebri, malignancy)

Contraindications
- Local lumbar skin infection over puncture area
- Suspicion of empyema
- Increased intracranial pressure from a mass lesion
- Uncooperative or combative patients (relative contraindication)
- Severe bleeding diathesis (relative contraindication)
- Platelet count $<50 \times 10^9$/L (relative contraindication)

Table 1. Synovial Fluid Analysis

Condition	Appearance	WBCs/μL	% PMNs	Glucose % serum level	Crystals under polarized light
Normal	Clear	<200	<25	95-100	None
Noninflammatory (e.g., DJD)	Clear	<2,000	<25	95-100	None
Acute gout	Turbid	2,000-5,000	>75	80-100	Negative birefringence, needle-like crystals
Inflammatory (e.g., rheumatoid arthritis)	Turbid	2,000-10,000	50-75	~75	None
Pseudogout	Turbid	5,000-50,000	>75	80-100	Positive birefringence, rhomboid crystals
Septic arthritis	Purulent/turbid	>50,000*	>75	<50	None

DJD, degenerative joint disease.

*Higher with untreated or virulent organisms.

Data from www.uptodate.com [cited 2005 May 2] and Cush JJ, Lipsky PE. Disorders of the joints. In: Fauci AS, Martin JB, Braunwald E, Kasper DL, Isselbacher KJ, Hauser SL et al, editors. Harrison's principles of internal medicine. Vol 2. 14th ed. New York: McGraw-Hill; 1998. p. 1931.

Equipment

- Kits are available that contain the following:
  - ▲ Skin needle (25 gauge with 3-mL syringe)
  - ▲ Infiltration needle (22-gauge 1.5-inch needle)
  - ▲ Spinal needle with stylet
  - ▲ Lidocaine HCl, 1%
  - ▲ Sterile gloves
  - ▲ Three-way stopcock
  - ▲ Manometer
  - ▲ Extension tube, 5 inches
  - ▲ Prelabeled specimen vials with caps, 10 mL
  - ▲ Gauze pads
  - ▲ Sterilization swab sticks
  - ▲ Fenestrated drape
  - ▲ Bandage

Procedure

- Perform an ophthalmoscopic exam to assess for papilledema or retinal hemorrhage.
- Perform CT of the head, check platelets and aPTT, PT, and INR as indicated.
- Position the patient in the lateral decubitus or sitting position.
  - ▲ Proper positioning with frequent assessment will ensure successful and safe placement of the lumbar needle.
- Have the patient flex the spine anteriorly with his or her chin on the chest.
- Ensure that the patient keeps the shoulders and hips perpendicular to the bed.
- Arch the patient's back to open the vertebral spaces to allow easier entrance of the spinal needle into the subarachnoid space.
- Identify the L3-4 interspace at the level of the iliac crests.
- Mark the space over the midline with a skin indentation.
- Prepare the skin over the preselected interspace, as well as one above and below, with antiseptic solution.
- Prepare equipment on an adjacent table using sterile technique.
- Change into sterile gloves.
- Verify that all the necessary items are present and working properly.
- Assemble the manometer and attach the three-way stopcock.
- Align the specimen tubes in order in an upright position on the tray.

- Drape the area with sterile draping, and remove excess iodine from the marked insertion site.
- Use a skin wheal to anesthetize the skin.
- With the infiltration needle, anesthetize deeper into the posterior spinous region after superficial analgesia is adequate.
- Select the spinal needle with stylet in place, and verify that superficial anesthesia is still adequate.
- Instruct the patient that he or she may feel pressure.
- If sharp pain is felt, the anesthesia is not adequate.
- Also, the patient should inform the operator if he or she feels pain down either leg at any time during the procedure.
- With the bevel up, direct the needle in the midsagittal plane cephalad toward the umbilicus.
  - If immediate resistance is felt, the needle should be withdrawn slightly and redirected.
  - The subarachnoid space is often deeper than expected, and you may feel a "pop" upon penetrating the ligamentum flavum and dura mater.
- Check for CSF return frequently by withdrawing the stylet to look for fluid return.
- After CSF has been obtained, measure the opening pressure with the three-way stopcock and manometer.
  - After asking the patient to straighten his or her legs, measure the CSF meniscus in the manometer tube.
- Empty the fluid from the manometer into the first tube and fill each subsequent tube with approximately 2-3 mL.
- *Reinsert the stylet*, alert the patient that you are about to remove the needle, and withdraw the needle.
- Place the bandage over the insertion site.
- Perform blood tests if needed (i.e., glucose).

Complications
- Headaches occur in up to 30% of patients.
  - This complication can be minimized by using a 20-gauge or smaller needle and by reinserting the stylet before withdrawing the needle.
- Nerve root herniation—avoid by retracting the needle with a well-fitting stylet in place

- Transient cranial nerve VI palsy—caused by traction on the cranial nerve from removal of large amounts of CSF

CSF Analysis
- CSF features associated with various conditions are listed in Table 2.

PARACENTESIS

Indications
- Evaluation of new ascites
- Evaluation of established ascites for infection
- Relief of respiratory compromise
- Relief of gastrointestinal complaints
- Impending peritoneal rupture

Contraindications
- Uncooperative or agitated patient
- Pregnancy
- Bowel obstruction
- Suspected adhesion of bowel to abdominal wall
- Adjacent infection
- Abdominal wall cellulitis
- Infraumbilical surgical scar (excludes a midline approach)
- Hematoma

Equipment
- Kits are available that contain the following:
  - A catheter device such as an 8F catheter over 18-gauge introducer needle with stopcock
  - Lidocaine
  - Povidone-iodine swab sticks
  - Needles (25 and 22 gauge)
  - Two syringes
  - Scalpel blade with handle
  - Evacuated fluid collection bottles
  - Drainage tubes with and without needles
  - Specimen vials
  - Sterile gloves
  - Bandage
  - IV albumin if the projected volume removed will exceed 4 L of ascitic fluid

Table 2. CSF Findings in Various Conditions

Condition	Pressure, mm H_2O	Cell count, mm³, & differential	Glucose, mg/dL	Protein, mg/dL
Normal	100-180	0-5 WBC (no PMNs) Traumatic tap may have 1 WBC per 700 RBCs	50-175 (alternative = CSF/blood ratio of 0.67)	15-45
Bacterial meningitis	200-300	>100 WBCs (mostly PMNs)	<40	100-1,000 (rapid antigen test)
Viral meningitis	90-200	100-300 monocytes	Normal (decreases slightly with mumps)	50-100
Herpes encephalitis	90-400	50-500 lymphocytes (RBCs present in 80%, PMNs may be present early)	Normal (small % of patients <40 years)	50-100 (PCR for antigen)
Subarachnoid hemorrhage	>200	>1,000 RBCs	Normal	>45 (for each 1,000 RBCs, protein increases by 1 mg/dL)

PCR, polymerase chain reaction.

- One recommendation is to give 25 g of albumin for more than 4 L removed.

Procedure

- Have the patient lie in the horizontal dorsal decubitus position.
- Raise the bed to a comfortable level for the operator.
- Reexamine for location of the ascitic fluid, and mark an insertion site with an indentation.
- A midline insertion should be placed 2 cm inferior to the umbilicus. A lateral approach is placed 5 cm cephalad and medial to the anterior superior iliac crest, typically on the left side (to avoid the cecum).
- Prepare the skin with the povidone-iodine solution.
- Prepare equipment on an adjacent table using sterile technique.
- Change into sterile gloves.
- Examine the kit to verify that all the necessary items are present and working properly.
- Remove excess iodine from the marked insertion site.
- Drape the area with sterile draping.
- Use a skin wheal to anesthetize the skin.
  - ▲ After superficial analgesia is adequate, infiltrate deeper to anesthetize to the peritoneum.
- Use a small scalpel to make a small superficial incision at the marked site (~3 mm long).
  - ▲ Take care not to puncture the peritoneum in patients with abdominal wall atrophy.
- Insert the catheter device into the incision site approximately perpendicular to the abdominal wall.
- Create a Z tract to reduce subsequent oozing in two different ways:
  - ▲ Use the free hand to stretch the skin near the entry site until the catheter is inserted and fluid is obtained.
  - ▲ Make a Z tract by using a zigzagging approach on entry by varying the catheter angle on insertion to produce a self-sealing site.
- While using a twisting motion with the catheter, draw back slowly on the syringe until ascitic fluid is visualized.
- Once ascitic fluid is visualized, remove the introduced needle while advancing the catheter into the peritoneal cavity.
- Attach the plastic tubing to the catheter via the three-way stopcock, and verify catheter placement by withdrawing

ascitic fluid into a large syringe.

- If the procedure is for diagnostic purposes only, this fluid can be sent for the desired testing.
- If the procedure is performed for therapeutic benefit, attach one end of plastic tubing to the stopcock and the other end to a needle.
- Place the needle in the evacuated container.
  - ▲ On opening the stopcock to the tubing, ascitic fluid return should be seen immediately.
- If the flow of fluid is inadequate or stops during the procedure, the catheter can be repositioned gently with a twisting motion or slightly withdrawn until fluid flow improves.
- When desired amounts of fluids are obtained or flow of fluid stops despite catheter repositioning, withdraw the catheter.
- Dress the site with a bandage.
- After paracentesis is completed and the patient stabilized, any necessary blood tests can be performed (e.g., albumin).

Complications
- Common complication—local hematoma
- Bowel entry
- Hemoperitoneum
- Infection
- Ascites leak

Testing
- Fluid testing usually includes
  - ▲ CBC and differential
  - ▲ Gram stain and bacterial cultures
  - ▲ Albumin
    - • SAAG = [serum albumin (SA)] – [ascites albumin (AG)] (Table 3)
  - ▲ Total protein
- Additional testing may include
  - ▲ Amylase
  - ▲ Glucose
  - ▲ LDH
  - ▲ Bilirubin

- ▲ Triglycerides
- ▲ Cytology
- ▲ Acid-fast bacilli and mycobacterial cultures
- Indicate to store remaining fluid
- Abnormal test values and their clinical importance are listed in Table 4.

THORACENTESIS

Indications

- Diagnostic evaluation of pleural effusions of unknown etiology
- Therapeutic indication for symptomatic pleural effusions

Contraindications

- Uncooperative or agitated patient
- Small loculated effusions (diagnosed by chest X-ray)
- Insufficient amount of pleural fluid (<10 mm on lateral decubitus film)
- Bleeding diathesis or excess anticoagulation (platelets $<25 \times 10^9$/L)
- Marginal respiratory reserve or unstable medical condition
- Positive end-expiratory pressure
- Adjacent infection (cellulitis) that may be introduced into the pleural space

Equipment

- Kits are available that contain the following:

Table 3. **Ascitic Fluid Analysis**

		SAAG, g/dL	
		≥1.1	<1.1
Serum total protein, g/dL	<2.5	Cirrhosis Portal hypertension	Malnutrition Nephrotic syndrome
	>2.5	Congestive heart failure Pulmonary hypertension Right-sided heart failure Budd-Chiari syndrome	Peritoneal carcinomatosis TB

Table 4. Abnormal Values and Clinical Importance of Additional Tests

Additional test	Abnormal value	Clinical importance
Amylase	>100 g/dL	Pancreatic source, intestinal rupture
Triglycerides	>200 mg/dL	Ruptured lymphatic system
PMNs	>250 cells/mm^3	Bacterial peritonitis
Glucose	<50 mg/dL	Spontaneous bacterial peritonitis or gut perforation
Bilirubin	>6 mg/dL	Gallbladder or upper gut perforation

▲ A catheter device such as an 8F catheter over an 18-gauge introducer needle with stopcock
▲ Lidocaine
▲ Povidone-iodine swab sticks
▲ Needles (25 and 22 gauge)
▲ Two syringes (large and small)
▲ Scalpel blade with handle
▲ Evacuated fluid collection bottles
▲ Drainage tubes with and without a needle
▲ Specimen vials
▲ Sterile gloves
▲ Arterial blood gas (ABG) (heparinized) syringe in a bag of ice (for pH analysis)
▲ Mask
▲ Bandage

Procedure
■ Check platelets aPTT, PT, INR as indicated, and view the chest X-ray to verify the side of the effusion.
  ▲ Verify the side of the effusion again.
  ▲ Bringing the film into the room with you will help you avoid tapping the wrong side.
■ Have the patient sit comfortably on the edge of a chair or bed with arms crossed in front.

- Select the insertion site for fluid removal ~1 to 2 interspaces below the fluid level and in line with the posterior scapular line.
  - ▲ Do not go below the 10th intercostal interspace.
- Mark the insertion site with a skin indentation.
- Prepare the equipment on an adjacent table using sterile technique.
- Prepare the skin with povidone-iodine solution.
- Change into sterile gloves.
- Examine the kit to verify that all the necessary items are present and working properly.
- Remove excess povidone-iodine from the marked insertion site, and drape the area with sterile draping.
- Use a skin wheal to anesthetize the skin.
- Use the 22-gauge needle to infiltrate the anesthetic into the rib and pleura.
- Continue to aspirate and inject as you advance by guiding the needle over the *superior* margin of the rib until the parietal pleura is entered.
- Use the scalpel to make a small horizontal incision over the rib.
- Insert the catheter device in the same tract as the anesthesia needle, drawing slowly on the syringe until pleural fluid is seen.
- Once pleural fluid is seen, slowly remove the needle while advancing the catheter.
  - ▲ Verify catheter placement by withdrawing pleural fluid into a large syringe.
- If the procedure is for diagnostic purposes only, this fluid can be sent for the desired testing.
- If the procedure is performed for therapeutic benefit, attach one end of plastic tubing to the stopcock and the other end to a needle.
- Place the needle in the evacuated container.
  - ▲ On opening the stopcock to the tubing, pleural fluid return should be seen immediately.
- If the flow of fluid is inadequate or stops during the procedure, the catheter can be repositioned gently with a twisting motion or slightly withdrawn until fluid flow improves.
  - ▲ Do not replace the needle!
- Once the desired amount of fluid is obtained or fluid flow stops despite catheter repositioning, withdraw the catheter.
- Dress the site with a bandage.

- After thoracentesis has been completed and the patient stabilized, the necessary blood tests can be performed (i.e., serum protein and LDH).
- Obtain a chest X-ray to assess for pneumothorax, and personally view the film.

Complications
- Pain in up to 20% of patients
- Pneumothorax in up to 10% of patients
- Dry tap
- Bleeding
- Empyema
- Visceral trauma (spleen, heart, liver)
- Reexpansion pulmonary edema

Testing
- Fluid testing may include
  - Gram stain and bacterial cultures
  - LDH
  - Protein
  - Cytology
  - pH using a heparinized ABG syringe that is kept on ice
  - Amylase
  - Glucose
  - Triglycerides
  - Acid-fast bacilli and fungal evaluations
  - Anaerobic culture
- Transudate and exudate fluids are compared in Table 5.
- Additional features of exudate are listed in Table 6.
- Pleural fluid tests and their clinical importance are listed in Table 7.

Table 5. Comparison of Transudate and Exudate Fluid Analysis

Feature	Fluid	
	Transudate	Exudate
Appearance	Straw-colored	Turbid
Protein ratio (pleural/serum)*	<0.5	>0.5
LDH ratio (pleural/serum)*	<0.6	>0.6
Total LDH*		>200

*Meeting 1 of the above criteria has a sensitivity of 70%, 2 criteria have 97%, and 3 have a 99% sensitivity (Light criteria [Light RW, MacGregor I, Luchsinger PC, Ball WC Jr. Pleural effusions: the diagnostic separation of transudates and exudates. Ann Intern Med. 1972;77:507-13]).

Table 6. Additional Features of Exudates

Feature	Value
Pleural fluid protein*	>2.9 g/dL
Pleural fluid cholesterol*	>45 mg/dL
Pleural fluid LDH*	>45% of normal serum value

*In one study, the use of the values in this table was as successful in differentiating transduate from exudate as the use of 2 or 3 of the Light criteria in Table 5.

Table 7. Pleural Fluid Tests

Test	Clinical importance
Glucose <60 mg/dL	Suggests rheumatoid pleurisy, empyema, malignancy, TB
pH	<7.3 indicates an increased need for pleural space drainage in parapneumonic effusions
Amylase (> normal serum amylase or ratio >1.0)	Acute pancreatitis, esophageal rupture, malignancy
Total pleural fluid LDH	>1,000 suggests empyema, rheumatoid arthritis
Triglycerides >115 mg/dL	Chylothorax

RENAL REPLACEMENT THERAPIES

Steven J. Younger, M.D.
John W. Graves, M.D.

INDICATIONS FOR DIALYSIS (AEIOU)

Remember

- **A** is for refractory **a**cidosis, i.e., pH is <7.0 and not improving.
- **E** is for refractory **e**lectrolyte disturbance, i.e., potassium is >6.0 with or without ECG changes despite medical management.
- **I** is for **i**ntoxicants, i.e., overdose of dialyzable substances (Table 1).
- **O** is for refractory fluid **o**verload (failure to respond to escalating doses of diuretics).
- **U** is for **u**remia, i.e., pericarditis, neuropathy, or decline in mental status not otherwise explained.

DEFINITIONS

Dialysis

- A transport process by which a solute diffuses through a concentration gradient from one compartment to another
- Typically, hemodialysis maintains water but
  - ▲ Removes potassium, creatinine, and BUN
  - ▲ Replaces bicarbonate and calcium

Filtration

- The process by which water and middle-sized molecules (>5,000 daltons) move across a membrane, not because of a concentration gradient but by hydrostatic pressure and a mechanism called "solvent drag"
- This process removes solutes such as potassium and urea *in the same concentration* as plasma.

Special abbreviations used in this chapter: AV, arteriovenous; VV, venovenus.

Table 1. Common Agents for Which Hemodialysis Enhances Elimination

Barbiturates
Bromides
Chloralhydrate
Alcohols
    Ethanol
    Isopropanol
    Acetone
    Methanol
    Ethylene glycol
Lithium
Procainamide
Theophylline
Salicylates
Heavy metals (possible)
Trichloroethanol
Atenolol
Sotalol

- Substitution fluid with lower concentrations of electrolytes is often needed to prevent hypovolemia while reducing plasma concentrations of solutes.

Diafiltration
- Combination of dialysis and filtration

Arteriovenous (AV)
- A single-lumen catheter uses the blood pressure gradient to deliver arterial blood into the extracorporeal circuit returning the treated blood to the venous system.

Venovenous (VV)
- The use of a double-lumen catheter (more common) or two different catheters placed within the venous system that requires an external pump to push the blood into the extracorporeal circuit

INTERMITTENT RENAL REPLACEMENT THERAPIES
Hemodialysis
- Standard modality for hemodynamically stable patients

- Advantage
  - ▲ Most effective means of renal replacement therapy
- Disadvantages
  - ▲ Inconvenience
  - ▲ Difficulty with vascular access (thrombosis and infections)
  - ▲ Severe dietary and fluid restrictions
- Acute hemodialysis
  - ▲ Performed through a temporarily placed dual-lumen catheter (e.g., Mahukar or Quinton) either in a femoral or jugular vein
  - ▲ Subclavian access is not recommended because of possible subclavian stenosis interfering with fistula placement in that arm.
- Chronic hemodialysis
  - ▲ Performed through
    - Brescio-Cimino AV fistula—either a connection between the radial or brachial vascular systems; best long-term access
    - Gore-Tex synthetic graft—the best alternative if Brescio-Cimino AV fistula is not technically possible
      - – Disadvantage, a foreign body and more likely to be infected
    - Tunneled catheter—can also be used for long-term access but has the most potential for infection
- Initiating hemodialysis
  - ▲ Patients in acute renal failure new to dialysis should have runs of 1-2 hours for 2 consecutive days.
  - ▲ This is to avoid disequilibrium syndrome—Aggressive dialysis markedly decreases plasma concentration of urea. Because intracellular urea cannot move out into the plasma quickly enough, there is disequilibrium between the intracellular and extracellular urea concentrations. This syndrome may cause mild (headache, cramping, nausea) to severe (seizures, cerebral herniation, and death) symptoms.
  - ▲ After patients are stabilized and chronic dialysis is needed, the runs are typically for 4-6 hours 3 days a week.

Peritoneal Dialysis

- Advantages
  - ▲ Patient controls own treatment.
  - ▲ May be done at home
  - ▲ Less severe fluid and dietary restrictions than for hemodialysis
  - ▲ Diabetic patients can place insulin into dialysate to avoid SQ injections.
- Disadvantages
  - ▲ Weight must be <80 kg (otherwise must do more than 5 exchanges/day)
  - ▲ Mental and physical dexterity required to change the dialysate fluid regularly.
  - ▲ Risk of peritonitis is the major disadvantage (scarring, pain, and sepsis).
- Peritoneal dialysis uses the patient's abdominal lining as the semipermeable membrane (the surface area of the abdominal lining is 1 m^2, which is almost the same as the surface area of the renal glomeruli).
  - ▲ Fluid (dialysate) is placed in the abdomen through a plastic catheter.
  - ▲ The fluid is allowed to sit ("dwell") in the abdomen for 30 minutes to 4 hours.
  - ▲ BUN, potassium, and other molecules diffuse through the peritoneal lining and accumulate in the fluid.
  - ▲ Water is pulled into the peritoneal dialysate by having a very high glucose concentration (1.5%-4.25%), which makes glucose osmotically active and draws water from the plasma into the dialysate.
  - ▲ The fluid is then drained from the peritoneal cavity and the cycle repeated with fresh dialysate.

CONTINUOUS RENAL REPLACEMENT THERAPIES

- These are used only in acute renal failure for those who are not hemodynamically stable.
- In choosing which form of continuous therapy to use, consider the following:
  - ▲ Goals of therapy
  - ▲ Which forms of therapy are available
  - ▲ Which forms of continuous therapy the nephrologist and staff are comfortable with using

- For several reasons, intermittent acute hemodialysis causes more hemodynamic problems than the continuous therapies:
  - ▲ Excess plasma volume is removed and can decrease blood pressure
  - ▲ Dialysis can cause major shifts of solutes, whereas hemofiltration removes solute at the same concentration as in the plasma. The shifts of solute out of the plasma mean that the intracellular osmolality is higher than in plasma and water then shifts out of the vascular space into the intracellular space.
  - ▲ Dialysis membranes used in intermittent hemodialysis are not as porous as the membranes used in hemofiltration and the middle- to large-sized molecules are thought to have more vasodilatory or cardiodepressant effects.
- Continuous AV hemofiltration
  - ▲ This modality of renal replacement is best for hemodynamically unstable patients in whom refractory fluid overload is the major problem (filtration does remove very small amounts of solutes as well).
  - ▲ Disadvantage—Arterial access is needed.
- Continuous VV hemofiltration
  - ▲ Similar to continuous AV hemofiltration except arterial access is not needed.
  - ▲ Best for fluid removal
- Continuous AV hemodialysis
  - ▲ Uses a dialysate to run countercurrently, but set to remove fluid at a low rate
  - ▲ Use if solute removal is more important than fluid balance and patient is hypotensive
- Continuous VV hemodialysis
  - ▲ Very similar to continuous AV hemodialysis but different access
- Continuous AV hemodiafiltration
  - ▲ Similar to continuous AV hemodialysis except the ultrafiltration rate is allowed to be higher than needed to establish euvolemia and replacement fluid is then placed back into the plasma
  - ▲ Use for hemodynamically unstable patients who need

large amounts of solute removed and who have arterial access
- Continuous VV hemodiafiltration
  - ▲ Same as continuous AV hemodiafiltration except arterial stick is not needed

RENAL TRANSPLANTATION
- The treatment of choice for chronic renal failure
- Advantages—better quality of life and decreased mortality compared with chronic hemodialysis and peritoneal dialysis methods
- Contraindications
  - ▲ HIV or other active infection
  - ▲ Malignancy with expected short life span
  - ▲ Poorly controlled psychosis
  - ▲ Active substance abuse
  - ▲ Any illness likely to end life within a year
- Disadvantages—Availability of organs is the usual disadvantage to transplantation, but with increasing use of living related and unrelated donors (some centers are even trying cross-match positive kidneys), renal transplantation should be considered for nearly all patients with chronic renal failure.

STEROID THERAPY

Stanley I. Martin, M.D.
William F. Young, Jr., M.D.

INDICATIONS

- The indications for steroid therapy by medical specialty are listed in Table 1.

CLASSIFICATION

- Potency and duration of action of steroids are listed in Table 2.

MONITORING

- Monitoring response to steroids varies widely and depends on the disease being treated.
- Side effects of steroids that should be monitored universally include
  - ▲ Bone mineral density—measured annually
  - ▲ Intraocular pressure—checked at least every 6 months
  - ▲ Blood glucose—monthly for outpatients, daily for inpatients
  - ▲ Blood pressure—monthly for outpatients, daily for inpatients
- Consider *Pneumocystis carinu* prophylaxis if long-term therapy.
- Consider gastrointestinal tract protection with a proton pump blocker, especially if patient is concurrently taking an NSAID.

PRESCRIBING

- Oral steroids are absorbed almost 100% within about 30 minutes.
- Topical steroid absorption depends on the area of the body to which agent is applied, e.g., intertriginous folds have a higher rate of absorption than the forearm.
- Salicylic acid and occlusive dressings enhance cutaneous absorption.
- Alternate-day dosing was devised to alleviate undesirable

side effects of long-term high-dose therapy with less suppression of hypothalamic-pituitary-adrenal axis.

- ▲ Begin use within 3 weeks after starting treatment.
- ▲ Prescribe approximately twice the usual daily dose of steroids every other day and use a shorter-acting agent.

COMPLICATIONS

Withdrawal

- The most frequent complication from steroid withdrawal is flare-up of underlying disease for which the patient was being treated.
- Withdrawal can also lead to adrenocortical insufficiency from suppression of hypothalamic-pituitary-adrenal axis.
  - ▲ Symptoms may include myalgias, fever, hypotension, nausea and vomiting, and confusion.
  - ▲ Pseudotumor cerebri is a rare effect of acute withdrawal.

Supraphysiologic Doses

- Side effects at supraphysiologic doses are listed in Table 3.

Table 1. Indications for Steroid Therapy by Medical Specialty

Medical specialty	Indications
Allergy & immunology	**Allergic rhinitis**
	Triamcinolone & fluticasone are used 2 sprays/nostril daily
	Flunisolide, budesonide, & beclomethasone are used 2 sprays/nostril twice daily
	Beclomethasone also comes in 84 μg preparation which is applied 4 sprays/nostril daily
Dermatology	**Inflammatory disorders of skin**
	1% Hydrocortisone cream topically twice daily
	Oral glucocorticoids such as 40-120 mg of prednisone daily are used for severe disease (e.g., Stevens-Johnson syndrome) or exacerbations of chronic disorders
Endocrinology	**Exogenous glucocorticoid replacement**
	Hydrocortisone 15 mg each AM & 5-10 mg each PM (first choice) *or* prednisone 3 7.5 mg daily *or* dexamethasone 0.25 mg daily closely mimic the body's normal supply
	Mineralocorticoids are needed only in primary adrenal insufficiency
	Stress dosing
	In mild illnesses, double or triple steroid dose
	For severe trauma or surgical stress, hydrocortisone 50 mg IV every 6 hours or 100 mg IV every 8 hours is recommended

Table 1 (continued)

Medical specialty	Indications
Gastroenterology	**Ulcerative colitis or Crohn disease— acute exacerbations** 　　Prednisone 10-120 mg PO daily depending on severity **Autoimmune hepatitis** 　　80% of patients have biopsy-proven remission with prednisone 40-60 mg daily until transaminases decrease, then taper to 7.5-10 mg as tolerated
Hematology & oncology	**Autoimmune hemolytic anemia (Coombs-positive)** 　　Prednisone 1 mg/kg daily can be tried; higher doses in severe hemolysis; may require small maintenance doses for long periods **ITP** 　　Prednisone 1-1.5 mg/kg daily is usual treatment; refractory disease may respond to pulsed, higher-dose glucocorticoids **Chemotherapy** 　　Used in combination with various agents in leukemias, lymphomas, multiple myeloma, amyloidosis, etc.
Nephrology	**Minimal change glomerulonephritis** 　　Start prednisone 1-2 mg/kg for 6 weeks, then taper over 6-8 weeks; 90% will have remission in 3 months **Membranous & membranoproliferative glomerulonephritis with focal sclerosis** 　　Conflicting data on efficacy of steroid therapy; many nephrologists recommend 120 mg prednisone qod for 8-10 weeks, with a 1-2 month taper; response must be monitored **Rapidly progressive glomerulonephritis (lupus nephritis WHO type III and IV)** 　　IV steroid pulse 1 g daily × 3 days

Table 1 (continued)

Medical specialty	Indications
Neurology	**Spinal cord injuries within 8 hours** Methylprednisolone up to 30 mg/kg initially, followed by 5.4 mg/kg every hour for 23 hours causes pronounced decrease in neurologic deficits **Primary or metastatic CNS neoplasms with intracranial hypertension or cord compression** Dexamethasone 4-6 mg PO or IV every 6 hours (controlled clinical trials do not support steroid use for traumatic injuries of the brain or for stroke) **Multiple sclerosis** Relapses can be treated with steroids; efficacy is controversial; methyl-prednisolone for 5 days can be used; no consensus about optimal dosages or duration of therapy **Myasthenia gravis** Prednisone 60-100 mg PO daily until improvement is sustained for about 2 weeks, then gradually taper to 5-15 mg PO daily over several months Dexamethasone high-dose administration has been highly successful when used in a 10-day course & then repeated (e.g., 20 mg PO daily) Also, low-dose alternate-day therapy with prednisone 25 mg PO daily & then increasing by 12.5 mg PO qod until 100 mg PO qod is achieved. This should be done for at least 3 months because improvement may not occur for up to 7 weeks. Taper doses as allowed **CNS vasculitides** Methylprednisolone pulse 1 g IV for 3 days

Table 1 (continued)

Medical specialty	Indications
Ophthalmology	**Inflammation of the outer eye & anterior segment**
	Topicals, such as 0.1% dexamethasone sodium phosphate solution applied 2 drops to the conjunctiva every 4 hours while awake, can be beneficial in noninfectious conjunctivitis. *Do not use* for bacterial, viral, or fungal conjunctivitis
	Inflammation of the posterior segment
	Systemic steroids
Pulmonology	**Severe asthma or COPD exacerbations**
	Methylprednisolone 60-125 mg every 6-12 hours
	As the attack resolves, switch to prednisone 40-60 mg PO daily; attempt to taper over 5-14 days, then stop altogether
	For less severe exacerbations of asthma, prednisone 40-60 mg daily for 5-7 days
	Acute respiratory distress syndrome
	Results of studies have not shown any benefit in treatment, at least in early stages of disease. Steroids are commonly used at high doses, usually with IV methylprednisolone, similar to acute asthma or COPD exacerbations
	***Pneumocystis carinii* pneumonia**
	If PaO_2 <70 or A-a gradient >35, prednisone 40-60 mg PO bid for 5 days, 20 mg bid on days 6-10, & 20 mg daily on days 11-21

Table 1 (continued)

Medical specialty	Indications
Rheumatology	**SLE, sarcoidosis, rheumatoid arthritis, & vasculitides such as polyarteritis nodosa, Wegener granulomatosis, temporal arteritis** Specific doses depend on disease, organ involvement, severity, & other factors **Gout** Prednisone 40-60 mg PO daily for patients with contraindications to NSAIDs (e.g., renal failure) **Tendinitis, bursitis, & arthritis** Intra-articular injections for inflammatory, crystal, and osteoarthritis. Dose depends on joint size. Use 5-20 mg of triamcinolone acetonide or equivalent. Give injections sparingly with at least 3 months between each dose
Transplantation	**At time of operation** Prednisone 50-100 mg usually given in conjunction with other immunosuppressive agents; the patient's doses are tapered to lower maintenance regimen as effects of organ rejection are monitored

A-a, alveolar-arterial; bid, twice daily; CNS, central nervous system; ITP, idiopathic thrombocytopenic purpura; qod, every other day; SLE, systemic lupus erythematosus.

Table 2. Glucocorticoid Preparations

	Potency	Duration of activity	Equivalent doses, mg	Aldosterone activity
Cortisol	1	Short	20	1
Cortisone	0.8	Short	25	0.8
Fludrocortisone	10	Short	NA	125
Prednisone	4	Intermediate	5	0.8
Prednisolone	4	Intermediate	5	0.8
Methylprednisolone	5	Intermediate	4	0.5
Triamcinolone	5	Intermediate	4	0
Betamethasone	25	Long	0.75	0
Dexamethasone	25	Long	0.75	0

NA, not applicable.

Table 3. Side Effects at Supraphysiologic Doses

Cardiovascular
  Hypertension
  Atherosclerosis
  Coronary artery disease
Dermatologic
  Hirsutism, skin atrophy, striae, and purpura
Endocrine
  Hyperglycemia—4× increase in risk of diabetes mellitus with
    long-term use
  Truncal obesity
  Hyperlipidemia
  Growth suppression in pediatric patients
  Sodium & fluid retention
  Hypokalemia
Gastrointestinal tract
  No peptic ulcer disease (unless concurrent use of NSAIDs or
    alcohol)
  Acute pancreatitis—rare
  Steroids can mask symptoms of life-threatening gastrointestinal
    tract perforation & peritonitis, particularly worrisome in
    patients with inflammatory bowel disease
Hematologic
  Acutely, steroids lead to leukocytosis with neutrophilia &
    lymphopenia, but usually with no left shift
  Eosinophils & basophils tend to be suppressed
Infectious
  Increased risk for infections with >10 mg of prednisone or
    equivalent daily
  PCP may develop in patients taking steroids equivalent to 30 mg
    of prednisone daily for >2 months; in such cases, some
    recommend TMP-SMX prophylactically
  Beware of using steroids in vasculitides in which underlying
    infection may have a role such as polyarteritis nodosa with
    hepatitis B infection, steroids may exacerbate the infection
Musculoskeletal
  Myopathy occurs in up to half of patients with long-term steroid
    therapy; muscle enzymes are usually normal, but urine
    creatinine level is often increased

Table 3 (continued)

Musculoskeletal (continued)

    Osteoporosis—rapid loss of bone density in first 6 months of
        therapy, then at slower pace; a net reduction in calcium
        absorption and enhanced urinary excretion stimulates
        increased parathyroid hormone levels; trabecular bone (femoral
        neck, distal radius, vertebral bodies) affected more than
        cortical bone

    Avascular necrosis—increased risk with SLE, renal transplan-
        tation, antiphospholipid syndrome, trauma, & alcoholism
        (femoral head most at risk, distal femur, talus, humeral head,
        proximal tibia, navicular, and scaphoid bones)

Ophthalmic

    Posterior subcapsular cataracts

    Glaucoma—topical applications of ocular steroids can lead to
        increased intraocular pressure; monitor if topical steroids are
        used >2 weeks

Psychiatric

    Acutely—steroids may cause minor confusion to severe
        psychosis

    Long-term—anxiety & depression are common, as are
        irritability, insomnia, & decreased libido

PCP, *Pneumocystis carinii* pneumonia; SLE, systemic lupus erythematosus.

TRANSFUSION THERAPY

Grace K. Dy, M.D.
Dennis A. Gastineau, M.D.

INDICATIONS
- Indications for transfusion of cellular components are listed in Table 1 at end of chapter.
- Indications for transfusion of plasma derivatives are listed in Table 2 at end of chapter.
- Indications for special coagulation factor products are listed in Table 3 at end of chapter.

SPECIAL MONITORING PARAMETERS
- Platelet transfusion
  - ▲ When the next AM count is no higher than pretransfusion level, measure 1-hour posttransfusion count.
  - ▲ If no or insignificant increase, consider platelet refractoriness from alloimmunization, sepsis, effect of antibiotics, or hypersplenism.
- Frozen lymphocyte antibody panel to look for HLA alloimmunization

COMPLICATIONS OF TRANSFUSION THERAPY
- Febrile nonhemolytic reaction
  - ▲ Increase in temperature of 1°C without hemolysis
  - ▲ Alloantibodies in recipient against donor leukocyte or platelet antigens
  - ▲ Usually seen in multiply transfused patients
  - ▲ Cannot distinguish from hemolytic reaction clinically, evaluation for transfusion reaction required
- Hemolytic transfusion reaction
  - ▲ Minor symptoms—fever, chills, back pain
  - ▲ Major symptoms or signs—dyspnea, chest pain, hemoglobinuria, oliguria, shock, intravascular coagulation and

fibrinolysis (formerly called "disseminated intravascular coagulation")

- ▲ Stop transfusion, hydration, alkalization of urine.
- ▲ Investigate—Check for clerical error, repeat ABO/Rh typing, antibody screen on pre- and posttransfusion samples.
- ■ Anaphylactoid reaction
  - ▲ Nausea, abdominal cramping, diarrhea
  - ▲ Use washed product.
- ■ Allergic reactions
  - ▲ Urticaria
    - • Circulating antibody against foreign donor serum proteins
    - • Treat with antihistamines.
    - • Blood may be restarted if urticaria is sole reaction and episode has resolved.
- ■ Transmission of microorganisms
  - ▲ Bacterial contamination—symptoms similar to those of hemolytic reaction, highest risk with platelet concentrates
  - ▲ Use of leukocyte-reduced products reduces but does not eradicate risk of transmission of viral infection.
- ■ Volume overload
  - ▲ Bacterial contamination—symptoms similar to those of hemolytic reaction, highest risk with platelet concentrates
  - ▲ Use of leukocyte-reduced products reduces but does not eradicate risk of transmission of viral infection.
- ■ Volume overload
  - ▲ Dyspnea, exacerbation of congestive heart failure, cardiogenic pulmonary edema
  - ▲ Use lowest rate of administration allowable in nonurgent situations (1-2 mL/kg per hour in high-risk patients).
  - ▲ Use factor-specific concentrates.
  - ▲ Diuresis ± morphine (for severe pulmonary edema)
- ■ Hypotension
  - ▲ Patients taking angiotensin-converting enzyme inhibitors receiving leukocyte-reduced products through bedside filters
  - ▲ Use prestorage leukocyte-reduced products (bradykinin is degraded in minutes).
- ■ Hypocalcemia, hyperkalemia
  - ▲ Seen in massive transfusion, defined loosely as >10 units of whole blood or equivalent to one blood volume

- Hemostasis and coagulation defects
  - ▲ Coagulopathy, dilutional thrombocytopenia during massive transfusions
  - ▲ Posttransfusion purpura 5-10 days after transfusion of RBCs containing fragments of PlA1 platelet antigen
    - Frequently associated with severe bleeding—treat with IV immunoglobulin; plasma exchange for nonresponse to IV immnoglobulin
    - Seen mostly in multiparous women, previously transfused patients
  - ▲ Drug-induced thrombosis with desmopressin (DDAVP) in patients with atherosclerotic vascular disease
  - ▲ Prolonged factor IX or XI concentrate infusion may be associated with thromboembolic events (deep venous thrombosis, pulmonary embolism, intravascular coagulation and fibrinolysis, rarely myocardial infarction).
- Iron overload—transfusion hemosiderosis
  - ▲ Seen in persons who received 60-200 units of RBCs
  - ▲ Prophylactic iron chelation (deferoxamine) in patients with thalassemia
- Immunological
  - ▲ Alloimmunization
    - Causes refractoriness to random-donor platelet products
    - Use leukocyte-reduced products when multiple transfusions are anticipated with ongoing therapy (e.g., acute myelogenous leukemia).
    - Use cross-match negative single-donor apheresis product or HLA-matched product if alloimmunized.
  - ▲ Transfusion-associated lung injury
    - Rare; most often associated with transfusion of whole blood, packed RBCs, and fresh frozen plasma
    - Result of donor leukoagglutinins causing recipient-WBC aggregation, capillary leak, and acute respiratory distress syndrome
    - Usually resolves
    - No special selection of products is appropriate—a donor implicated in a transfusion-associated lung injury reaction is eliminated from the donor pool.

- ▲ Transfusion-associated graft-versus-host disease
  - • Nearly always fatal, results in multiorgan system failure in susceptible patients
  - • Prevented by using gamma-irradiation of products
- ▲ Immunomodulation
  - • Controversial issues and analyses of results equivocal
  - • May be reduced by using leukocyte-reduced products
    - – Postoperative infections—increased incidence among patients receiving transfusion who underwent surgery
    - – Cancer recurrence—colorectal cancer studied most

Table 1. Transfusion of Cellular Components

Component	Types	Characteristics/unit	Indications
RBCs	Packed RBCs	Hematocrit 70%–75% ~350 mL/unit Infused at 2–4 mL/kg per hour 3% Hematocrit or 1 g/dL Hb increment 225–250 mg iron (1 mg/cm³ of RBC volume)	Symptomatic anemia (e.g., angina, dyspnea, postural hypotension, etc.) Hb ≤7.0 g/dL Hb <10 g/dL with acute myocardial infarction, unstable angina Ongoing hemorrhage—used alone if estimated blood loss is 20%–50% total blood volume
	Special RBC products Washed	Hematocrit 80% ~180 mL/unit Saline washes (machine) remove 90% of WBCs, most platelets, & 98% of plasma proteins	Above indications plus any of the following: Anaphylactoid reactions IgA or IgA subclass deficiency (presence of anti-IgA antibodies) Paroxysmal nocturnal hemoglobinuria
	Frozen	Hematocrit 65% (ultra-washed) ~180 mL/unit High glycerol solution (40% w/v) for storage 95% of WBCs, platelets, & plasma proteins removed	Rare RBC types (McLeod phenotype, etc.) Store autologous blood >42 days Indications for washed RBCs (but more expensive)

Table 1 (continued)

Component	Types	Characteristics/unit	Indications
RBCs (continued)	Leukocyte-reduced	In US, <5 × 10⁶ (by filtration) In Europe, <1 × 10⁶ (by filtration) ~350 mL/unit	Nonhemolytic febrile transfusion reaction unresponsive to acetaminophen Avoid HLA alloimmunization in nonsensitized patients Avoid transmission of new variant CJD prion (speculative) Prevent transmission of leukocyte-associated viruses (CMV, HHV-8, EBV, HTLV) Cross-match incompatibility
	CMV-negative	Seronegative for CMV	CMV-negative, immunodeficient hosts (bone marrow, organ transplant recipients); leukocyte-reduced is considered equivalent
	Irradiated	Higher potassium content Gamma radiation, 25 Gy	Prevent transfusion-associated GVHD in Immunodeficient patients (congenital immunodeficiencies, purine analogue-treated, *not* HIV, or standard chemotherapy-treated malignancies) Bone marrow, organ transplant recipients Related donor or HLA-selected component transfusion

Table 1 (continued)

Component	Types	Characteristics/unit	Indications
WBCs	Granulocytes	1×10^{10}/L, irradiated Collected by apheresis 0.1-0.3 $\times 10^9$/L increment Contains 3×10^{11}/L platelets	Immunodeficient hosts with overwhelming bacterial/fungal sepsis refractory to antimicrobials & recombinant granulocyte colony-stimulating factor *and* Severe neutropenia <0.5 $\times 10^9$/L *and* Prolonged marrow recovery anticipated (>7-10 days) Serious infection in patients with granulocyte dysfunction, e.g., CGD
	Lymphocytes		Induce remission in CML patients with molecular or cytogenetic relapse after bone marrow transplant
Platelets	Random-donor pooled platelet concentrates	5.5-7.5 $\times 10^{10}$/unit (60%-70% of whole blood unit platelets) ~50 mL dose—1 U/10 kg body weight (standard dose, 6 U)	Therapeutic transfusion in acute hemorrhage in patients with thrombocytopenia $\leq$50 $\times 10^9$/L Prevent coagulopathy in massive transfusions (150% of blood volume)

Table 1 (continued)

Component	Types	Characteristics/unit	Indications

Platelets (continued)			Prophylactic transfusion in:
			  Treatment of acute leukemia patients with platelet count $\leq 10 \times 10^9$/L[*]
			  Chemotherapy of solid tumor patients with platelet count $\leq 10 \times 10^9$/L, except those with bladder & necrotic tumors (threshold, $\leq 20 \times 10^9$/L)
			  Febrile or anticoagulated patients with platelet count $< 20 \times 10^9$/L
			  Dental extraction, many invasive procedures, & major operations if platelet count $\leq 50 \times 10^9$/L)[‡‡]
			Reserve for serious bleeding in ITP; avoid in TTP, heparin-associated thrombocytopenia unless bleeding is life-threatening

Table 1 (continued)

Component	Types	Characteristics/unit	Indications
Platelets (continued)	Irradiated	Gamma radiation, 25 Gy	Indications for random-donor platelet concentrates plus the following: Prevent transfusion-associated GVHD in: Bone marrow, organ transplant recipients Severely immunodeficient or immunosuppressed patients Related-donor or HLA-selected component transfusion Histocompatible platelet transfusion for alloimmunized patients with active hemorrhage
	Single-donor (apheresis)	$>3 \times 10^{11}$ ~200 mL $10\text{-}50 \times 10^9/L$ increment	Indications for random-donor platelet concentrates plus either of the following: Avoid HLA alloimmunization in patients anticipated to have multiple transfusions (e.g., AML at diagnosis) during therapy to prevent refractoriness to random-donor platelets *or* Nonhemolytic febrile transfusion reaction unresponsive to acetaminophen
	Leukocyte-reduced		

Table 1 (continued)

AML, acute myelogenous leukemia; CGD, chronic granulomatous disease; CJD, Creutzfeldt-Jakob disease; CML, chronic myelogenous leukemia; CMV, cytomegalovirus; EBV, Epstein-Barr virus; GVHD, graft-versus-host disease; HHV, human herpesvirus; HTLV, human T-lymphotropic virus; ITP, idiopathic thrombocytopenic purpura; TTP, thrombotic throbocytopenic purpura.

*Transfusion at higher levels may be necessary in patients with hemorrhage, high fever, hyperleukocytosis, rapid fall of platelet count, or coagulation abnormalities (e.g., acute promyelocytic leukemia), and in those undergoing invasive procedures or in situations in which platelet transfusions may not be readily available in case of emergencies.

†Bone marrow aspirations and biopsies can be performed safely at counts <20 × 10⁹/L.

‡Central nervous system operation may require >100 × 10⁹/L.

Table 2. Transfusion of Plasma Derivatives

Derivative	Factors	Characteristics/unit	Indications
FFP	All factors (fibrinogen, factors II, V, VII, VIII, IX, X, XI, XIII, proteins C & S, AT III)	No RBCs, essentially no platelets ~220 mL/unit Dose: 10-20 mL/kg (except warfarin reversal = 5-8 mL/kg)	Hemorrhage in multiple coagulation factor deficiency (e.g., liver disease) Coagulopathy in factor XI, AT III, protein C, protein S deficiency Urgent reversal of warfarin therapy Correction of known coagulation factor deficiencies for which specific products are not available Coagulopathy in massive blood transfusion (hemorrhage, PT & aPTT ≥1.5× control) Used in TTP for plasma exchange when cryo-poor plasma is not available
Cryoprecipitate	vWF, factor VIII, fibrinogen, factor XIII, fibronectin	~25 mL/unit 80-120 U factor VIII 150-200 mg fibrinogen Infused at ≥200 mL/hour Not virally inactivated	Transient reversal of platelet dysfunction in uremic patients Dysfibrinogenemia, hypofibrinogenemia Replacement of factors when specific products are not available
Cryo-poor plasma	FFP factors except vWF	Supernatant of cryo-precipitate	Used in TTP apheresis (avoids transfusion of vWF)

AT, antithrombin; FFP, fresh frozen plasma; TTP, thrombotic thrombocytopenic purpura; vWF, von Willebrand factor.

Table 3. Special Coagulation Factor Products

Condition	Product	Administration/indications

Hemophilia A	Recombinant factor VIII (Recombinate, Kogenate, Bioclate, Helixate FS, Refacto) Monoclonal antibody purified (Monoclate-P, Hemofil M, Monarc-M)	1 U/kg increases level by 2% ($t_{1/2}$ = 8-12 hours) Target activity level
		  Dental extraction prophylaxis: 50%-100%
		  Mild hemorrhage: 20%
		  Moderate hemorrhage: 30%-50%
		  Severe hemorrhage, surgery: 100%
		Bolus before procedure
		Continuous infusion during surgery, active hemorrhage (4 U/kg per hour)

	DDAVP (1-desamino-8-d-arginine vasopressin, desmopressin)	0.3 µg/kg IV (median increment of 62% in factor VIII activity) Use for mild bleeding episodes Intranasal: <50 kg-150 µg, >50 kg-300 µg
Hemophilia B	Recombinant factor IX (Benefix) Monoclonal antibody purified (Mononine, Alphanine SD)	1.2 U/kg increases level by 1% ($t_{1/2}$ = 24 hours) 1 U/kg increases level by 1% ($t_{1/2}$ = 24 hours)
Factor inhibitors	Activated prothrombin complex concentrate (Feiba [factor VIII inhibitor bypassing activity], Autoplex T), NovoSeven recombinant factor VIIa	50-100 U/kg every 8-12 hours (not to exceed 200 U/kg daily) Hemophilia A or B patients with factor inhibitors
	Porcine factor VIII (Hyate C)	100-150 U/kg (product ineffective if inhibitor level is >10 Bethesda U/mL)

Table 3 (continued)

Condition	Product	Administration/indications
von Willebrand disease	DDAVP	See above For mild type 1 vWD vWD types 2 and 3 respond poorly or variably Contraindicated for vWD type 2B
	Certain factor VIII products (e.g., Humate-P, Koate-DVI or HP, Alphanate)	Hemorrhage for which desmopressin is inade-quate or inappropriate Dose: 40-80 IU vWF:ristocetin cofactor (RCoF)/kg every 8-12 hours; goal of vWF:RCoF activity >50% (2-3 IU vWF/IU factor VIII)
AT III deficiency	AT III	1 U/kg increases level by 1%-2.1% ($t_{1/2}$ = 2-4 days) Dose: [Desired – actual AT III % level] × weight/1% Desired level: 80%-120% Replacement in congenital deficiency: During major surgery, prolonged immobilization Thrombosis during pregnancy (facilitate heparin) Acute DVT or PE Replacement in acquired deficiency: Severe liver failure to prevent or control ICF

Table 3 (continued)

Condition	Product	Administration/indications
AT III deficiency (continued)		Hemorrhage in cirrhosis (prevent thrombosis or ICF when factor IX is given)
		Acute DVT or PE when AT III <70%
		Surgery in those with disease associated with increased AT III loss (e.g., nephrotic syndrome)

AT, antithrombin; DVT, deep venous thrombosis; ICF, intravascular coagulation and fibrinolysis (formerly termed "DIC" [disseminated intravascular coagulation]); PE, pulmorary embolism; vWD, von Willebrand disease; vWF, von Willebrand factor.

EMERGENCY RESPONSE TEAM RESPONSIBILITIES AND GUIDELINES

Rendell W. Ashton, M.D.
T. Jared Bunch, M.D.
Edwin G. Wells III, M.D.
Nicola E. Schiebel, M.D.

EMERGENCY RESPONSE TEAM

- Most medical centers have a team of physicians and other professionals designated to respond to medical emergencies, such as cardiac arrest, in the hospital or outpatient clinics.
  - ▲ This team is the "emergency response team" or the "code team."
  - ▲ The assumption is that having a well-trained and prepared team ready to respond to emergencies will improve the outcomes of these situations.
  - ▲ For this goal to be realized, the team members must know their respective roles and the protocols recommended for handling medical emergencies so they can work together to provide timely and appropriate care for patients in distress.

ERT LEADER RESPONSIBILITIES

- Overall conduct of emergency situation ("code"); maintaining focus on medical priorities
  - ▲ Rhythm interpretation
  - ▲ Defibrillation– *early defibrillation is highest priority when indicated!*
  - ▲ Pharmacologic therapy
- Overseeing other team members' performance
  - ▲ Basic life support (adequate cardiopulmonary resuscitation, etc.)
  - ▲ Proper airway management (endotracheal tube placement, etc.)

Special abbreviations used in this chapter: AHA, American Heart Association; DNR, do not resuscitate.

- Managing the scene of the emergency
  - ▲ Managing the many people who respond to codes is a major challenge.
  - ▲ Anyone who does not have a defined role should be asked to leave.
  - ▲ Look for someone to delegate this responsibility (e.g., nursing supervisor, charge nurse).
- Managing patient transfer after resuscitation
- Documenting the emergency and management in the medical record
- Assisting the primary service in communicating with the family
- Special concerns
  - ▲ Over-response with loss of control at scene
  - ▲ Inadequate infection control precautions
  - ▲ Misunderstanding of do not resuscitate (DNR) policies
  - ▲ Poor documentation
  - ▲ Quality improvement issues
  - ▲ Family presence at scene—Data suggest that this may be acceptable, and even preferable, but only with adequate attention from medical personnel.

MAYO DNR POLICY—CONSULT INSTITUTIONAL GUIDELINES

The following excerpt is quoted directly from the Mayo 2005 pocket calendar and the institutional procedural guidelines (emphasis added):

1. **A Do Not Resuscitate (DNR) order implements a decision to withhold resuscitation in event of cardiac arrest. It is an order to withhold treatment when and only when the unresponsive patient has become clinically pulseless.**
2. DNR refers to the withholding of the following treatments in event of cardiac arrest:
   1) endotracheal intubation and initiation of ventilatory support,
   2) chest compression,
   3) electrical countershock,
   4) external cardiac pacing, and
   5) bolus administration of inotropes, vasopressors, or antiarrhythmics.

   Except in exceptional circumstances, these five therapies

should be withheld together or potentially provided together. Orders to provide some but not all potential therapies for cardiac arrest are strongly discouraged.

3. **A DNR order may be compatible with maximum therapy.** The patient may be receiving vigorous support in all other therapeutic modalities and justifiably have a DNR order. Some components of resuscitation (endotracheal intubation, pacemaker placement, inotropic or vasopressor infusions, antiarrhythmic therapy) may be given to a patient with a DNR order who has not suffered cardiac arrest. **Decisions to withhold such treatments in nonarrest circumstances are often appropriate but must be made consensually with the patient or surrogate and are not encompassed by the DNR order.**

4. A DNR order may be written by a physician involved in the care of the patient:
   - after consultation with the patient or the appropriate surrogate decision maker
   - and when, in the opinion of the patient or surrogate, the burdens of the potential resuscitation outweigh the anticipated benefits

5. The individuals involved in decision-making discussions for implementation of a DNR order will vary depending on the decision-making capacity of the patient:
   - For the patient with decision-making capacity, the decision shall be reached consensually by the patient and the physician.
   - For the patient lacking decision-making capacity, and who has been declared legally incompetent by the courts, the decision shall be reached consensually by the court-appointed guardian and the physician.
   - For the patient lacking decision-making capacity who has, by means of an Advance Directive, designated a surrogate decision maker, the decision shall be reached consensually by the designated surrogate and the physician.
   - For the patient lacking decision-making capacity without a designated surrogate decision maker, the decision shall

be reached consensually by the most appropriate surrogate decision maker and the physician. Typically, the most appropriate surrogate decision maker will be a family member, or a consensus opinion of family members.

- For the patient lacking decision-making capacity who has an Advance Directive specifying a DNR status, a DNR order will be written unless specifically rescinded by an appropriate surrogate.
- In all circumstances, the decision should be consistent with the patient's values and desires.

6. A DNR order should not be implemented if the patient or appropriate surrogate decision maker does not consent to the order.

7. Parental/guardian approval is required for a DNR order for a minor. The primary staff physician should talk with the parents/guardians of the child and provide support to the minor and parents/guardians in arriving at a decision.

8. A DNR order may be rescinded by the patient or appropriate surrogate at any time.

9. To the extent possible, a DNR order should be reviewed with all involved parties when:

- there is a change of physicians on the primary service or another service assumes primary care of the patient.
- the patient is taken from the patient care unit to a diagnostic or therapeutic procedure.
- the patient is transferred to another patient care unit (e.g., ICU to general care unit).
- the patient undergoes a surgical operation or a procedure requiring sedation. In the event a DNR order was rescinded for surgery by the patient or appropriate surrogate, the perioperative resuscitation status and the postoperative resuscitation status should both be clearly and distinctly documented in the medical record. The surgical episode includes the anesthetic, operation, and recovery time in postanesthetic care unit. The surgical episode ends when the patient is admitted to a monitored or general care bed unless otherwise specified in the medical record. It may be appropriate for a DNR order to stand during operation and anesthesia. A nonrescinded "do not intubate" order is not appropriate for the patient undergoing general anesthesia.

- there is a significant change in the patient's clinical condition.

10. The primary (or co-primary) staff physician is responsible for discussions with the patient or appropriate surrogate regarding a DNR order. The staff physician may personally conduct these discussions or delegate this responsibility to a resident physician in training involved in the care of the patient. However, other health team members involved in the care of the patient (e.g., nurse, chaplain, social worker) may participate in the discussions and decision-making process.

11. Careful considerations must be given to a patient's Advance Directives. Clarification should be sought from the patient or appropriate surrogate regarding any ambiguity introduced by such a document, and the physicians should document the clarification in the chart.

12. Conflicts may arise in arriving at a DNR order. In such an event, institutional resources available to assist in identifying the underlying issues creating the conflict and to facilitate the decision-making process include the Hospital Ethics Consultation Service, Resuscitation Committee, Mayo Clinical Ethics Council, and Legal Department.

EMERGENCY RESPONSE ALGORITHMS

- The following algorithms (Fig. 1-9) are based on the 2000 American Heart Association (AHA) guidelines for advanced cardiac life support. Every effort has been made to ensure accuracy; however, these adaptations have not been officially reviewed by the AHA, and no guarantee can be inferred that they reflect the intent of the AHA or any subsequent revisions to the official guidelines.

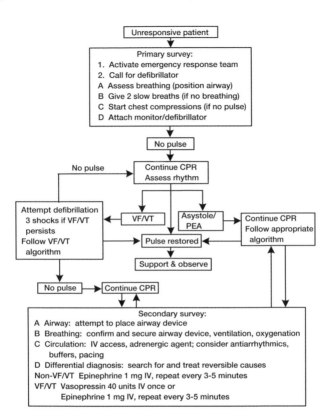

Fig. 1. Comprehensive emergency care algorithm. CPR, cardiopulmonary resuscitation; PEA, pulseless electrical activity; VF, ventricular fibrillation; VT, ventricular tachycardia.

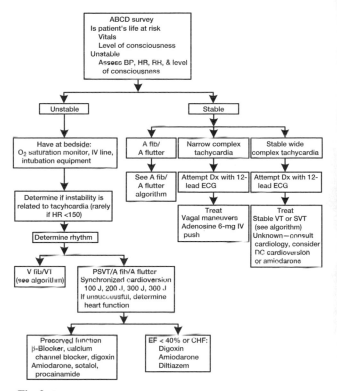

Fig. 2. Tachycardia algorithm. A, atrial; BP, blood pressure; CHF, congestive heart failure; Dx, diagnosis; EF, ejection fraction; fib, fibrillation; HR, heart rate; PSVT, paroxysmal supraventricular tachycardia; RR, respiratory rate; SVT, supraventricular tachycardia; VT, ventricular tachycardia.

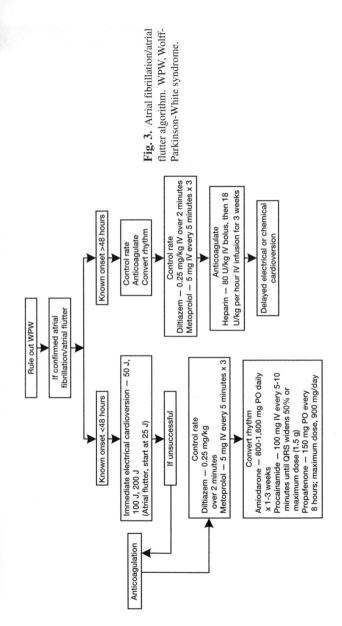

Fig. 3. Atrial fibrillation/atrial flutter algorithm. WPW, Wolff-Parkinson-White syndrome.

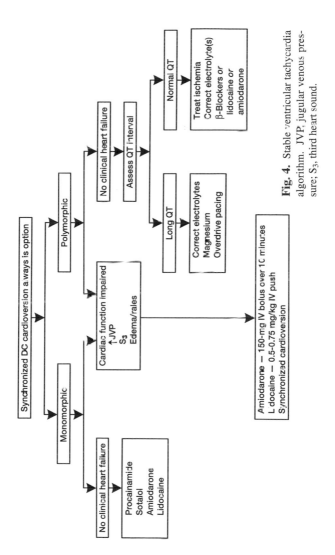

Fig. 4. Stable ventricular tachycardia algorithm. JVP, jugular venous pressure; S_3, third heart sound.

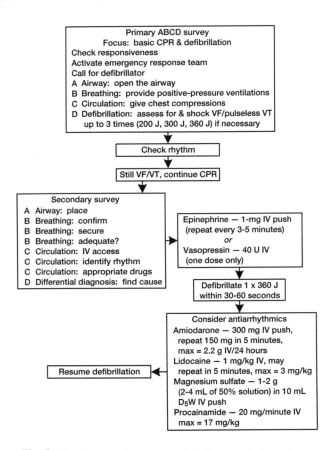

Fig. 5. Ventricular fibrillation (VF)/pulseless ventricular tachycardia (VT) algorithm. CPR, cardiopulmonary resuscitation; D5W, 5% dextrose in water; max, maximum dose.

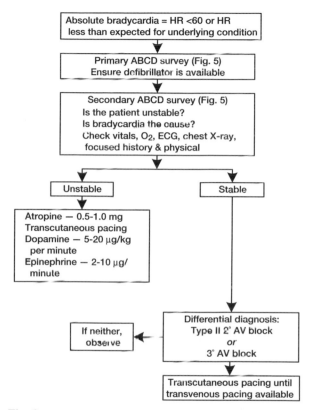

Fig. 6. Bradycardia algorithm. AV, atrioventricular; HR, heart rate.

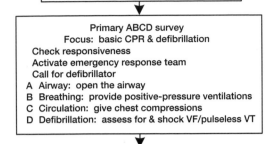

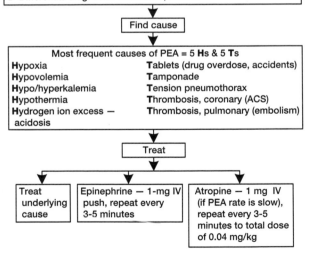

Fig. 7. Pulseless electrical activity (PEA) algorithm. ACS, acute coronary syndrome; CPR, cardiopulmonary resuscitation; VF, ventricular fibrillation; VT, ventricular tachycardia.

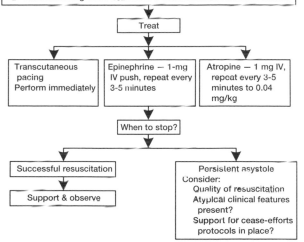

Primary ABCD survey
Focus: basic CPR & defibrillation
Check responsiveness
Activate emergency response team
Call for defibrillator
A Airway: open the airway
B Breathing: provide positive-pressure ventilations
C Circulation: give chest compressions
C Circulation: confirm true asystole
D Defibrillation: assess for & shock VF/pulseless VT
Rapid scene survey: is there any evidence that personnel should not attempt resuscitation (e.g., DNR order, signs of death)?

Secondary ABCD survey
Focus: more advanced assessments & treatments
A Airway: place airway device as soon as possible
B Breathing: confirm airway device placement by exam plus confirmation device
B Breathing: confirm effective oxygenation & ventilation
C Circulation: confirm true asystole
C Circulation: establish IV access
C Circulation: identify rhythm → monitor
C Circulation: give medications appropriate for rhythm & condition
D Differential diagnosis: search for & treat identified reversible causes

Treat

| Transcutaneous pacing Perform immediately | Epinephrine — 1-mg IV push, repeat every 3-5 minutes | Atropine — 1 mg IV, repeat every 3-5 minutes to 0.04 mg/kg |

When to stop?

Successful resuscitation

Support & observe

Persistent asystole
Consider:
Quality of resuscitation
Atypical clinical features present?
Support for cease-efforts protocols in place?

Fig. 8. Asystole algorithm. CPR, cardiopulmonary resuscitation; DNR, do not resuscitate; VF, ventricular fibrillation; VT, ventricular tachycardia.

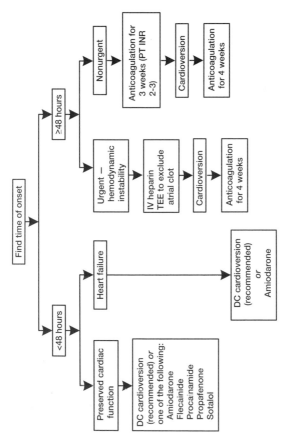

Fig. 9. Atrial fibrillation/flutter with Wolff-Parkinson-White syndrome algorithm.

END OF LIFE

Anna M. Georgiopoulos, M.D.
Casey R. Caldwell, M.D.

GOALS OF PALLIATIVE CARE

- Palliative care involves shifting efforts from an attempt to cure disease to relief of symptoms and improvement of quality of life. Hospice care is a multidisciplinary approach to palliative care of the dying patient and family. Palliative and hospice care may be provided at home or in a hospital, a nursing home, or a dedicated hospice facility.
- Many losses can accompany terminal illness. Patients' social and financial status, their relationships with friends and family, and their ability to independently perform activities of daily living often change as illness progresses. Symptoms causing distress for patients with advanced disease include pain, dyspnea, weakness and fatigue, insomnia, loss of alertness or confusion, depression and anxiety, anorexia and cachexia, nausea and vomiting, and constipation.
- Multiple effective therapies are available to manage patients' physical and mental suffering at the end of life. In the time leading up to death, patients may draw hope from deepening their relationships and spirituality, bringing a sense of closure to their lives, and finding meaning in their achievements and legacies.

MEDICAL DECISION MAKING

- To consent to a proposed course of care, a patient must be able to demonstrate understanding of the risks, benefits, and alternatives of the plan and to reasonably evaluate this information and communicate his or her decision. A health proxy is someone appointed by a patient to make health care decisions when the patient is no longer able to do so. The most useful advance directives designate a health proxy who knows the patient well and has talked to the patient about his or her goals and values. Long lists of acceptable and unacceptable medical interventions may unnecessarily constrain care, and vague statements ("no heroic measures") may be difficult to interpret when tough decisions need to be made. Find out what the laws are in your state for surrogate decision making when a patient does not have advance directives appointing a health proxy.

- Conflicts between medical personnel and family members over medical futility and withdrawal of support often come down to issues of communication and trust. It may help for both the family and medical team to appoint one person as the primary contact and to schedule regular communications. The types of questions patients and families have and the level of detail they desire to know may vary. Remember that the goals of care are set by the patient or the patient's proxy, but that rational decision making about the best way to pursue those goals is more likely to occur when the medical team provides appropriate information in an empathetic manner.

SYMPTOM CONTROL
Pain Management
- Medications for specific pain syndromes are listed in Table 1.
- Opioids are the mainstay of care for severe pain at the end of life. As long as there is informed consent, it is ethically and legally acceptable to use doses of opioids necessary to control a patient's suffering, even if this may unintentionally hasten his or her death. This is known as the "principle of double effect."
  - ▲ There is no upper dose limit for opioids, but be careful with adjuvants such as acetaminophen or NSAIDs. You may want to separate the opiate from the adjuvant.
  - ▲ For example, rather than risk acetaminophen overdose in patients with moderate pain by using Percocet, prescribe Tylenol 1,000 mg every 6 hours on a scheduled basis, sustained release oxycodone (OxyContin), 10 mg every 12 hours, and rapid release oxycodone, 5-10 mg every 4 hours, for breakthrough pain.
- Balance alertness and pain control in accordance with patient and family values and goals. An exhausted patient sleeps a lot but is alert between naps, whereas a sedated patient cannot be fully awakened.

Table 1. Medications for Specific Pain Syndromes

Burning, tingling neuropathic pain	Shooting, stabbing, electrical neuropathic pain	Bone pain	Bowel obstruction (inoperable)
Gabapentin—100 mg PO tid, escalate every 1-2 days by 100 mg PO tid, up to 3,600 mg/day or more		Opioids NSAIDs	
Desipramine—10-25 mg PO qhs, increase every 4-7 days	Carbamazepine—100 mg PO bid-tid, increase by 100-200 mg every 5-7 days	Dexamethasone—2-20 mg daily (also for capsular liver pain)	Scopolamine—0.1-0.4 mg SQ/IV every 4 hours or transdermal patches 1-3 every 3 days or 10-80 µg/hour IV/SQ infusion
	Valproic acid—250 mg PO qhs, increase 250 mg every 7 days in divided doses	Pamidronate—90-120 mg IV every 4-6 weeks Calcitonin—200 IU or nasally daily-bid Radiation Orthopedic interventions, braces	Octreotide—100 µg SQ every 8-12 hours or 10 µg/hour IV

bid, twice daily; qhs, at bedtime; tid, 3 times daily.

▲ If the patient has opiate-induced delirium or respiratory depression (<6 breaths/minute), opiates may be reversed with naloxone, 0.1-0.2 mg IV every 1-2 minutes until alert. Monitor and repeat as needed. This should rarely be necessary.

- If the patient requires increasing doses of pain medications, disease progression is a more likely explanation than drug tolerance.
- Dying patients with a history of substance abuse still deserve adequate pain control.
- Urticaria and pruritis occurring with opioids are usually due to mast cell destabilization, not true drug allergy. Try fexofenadine 60 mg PO twice daily or doxepin 10-30 mg PO at bedtime.
- Treat drug-associated nausea, vomiting, and constipation aggressively rather than compromise pain control. Consider a psychostimulant to combat sedation.
- All opioids that can be given IV can also be given SQ, even in continuous infusion. This may be preferable to IM dosing, which is painful. Do not forget liquid preparations or administration to buccal mucosa (oral morphine elixir).
  ▲ Also consider rectal administration, transdermal patches, or insertion of a feeding tube to deliver pain medications.
- Consider nonpharmacologic approaches such as transcutaneous electrical nerve stimulation, acupuncture, heat, cold, relaxation therapy, music, or massage.
- Refer to specialists for persistent pain or consideration of nerve blocks or other procedures if acceptable to patient.

Depression and Anxiety
- Medications for depression or anxiety are listed in Table 2.
- Major depression and hopelessness are not normal or inevitable consequences of serious illness; they increase patients' suffering and may shorten life.
  ▲ If you feel depressed around the patient, consider that the patient may be depressed.
- Physical symptoms such as altered sleep, appetite, and energy are less useful for the diagnosis of depression in patients at the end of life.
  ▲ Simply asking, "Are you depressed?" is a quick, accurate way to screen for depression in this population.

Table 2. Medications for Depression or Anxiety

Class of agent	Comments	Examples
Psychostimulant	Drugs of choice for depression: quick response, often in 24 hours May stimulate appetite Increase dose if tolerance develops Can precipitate delirium	Methylphenidate—start 2.5-5 mg bid (8 AM & noon), titrate daily, up to 20 mg bid; extended-release available Dextroamphetamine—start 2.5-5 mg PO bid, up to 20 mg bid; extended-release available Pemoline—18.75-37.5 mg PO every AM, up to 75 mg bid; chewable SL form available
SSRIs	Treat both depression & anxiety Response in 2-4 weeks	Fluoxetine—2.5-5 mg PO qhs, increase weekly up to 80 mg/day Paroxetine—10-60 mg PO qhs Sertraline—25-200 mg PO daily Citalopram—20-40 mg PO daily
Tricyclic antidepressant	Only if also needed for pain control, insomnia, appetite stimulation Some effect on anxiety	Nortriptyline—10-125 mg PO daily Desipramine—12.5-150 mg PO daily

Table 2 (continued)

Class of agent	Comments	Examples
Other	Mixed depression & anxiety	Mirtazapine—start 7.5 mg PO qhs, up to 15-60 mg qhs (sedating, stimulates appetite) Nefazodone—100-300 mg PO bid (sedating) Venlafaxine—18.75 mg PO bid, up to 187.5 mg bid
Benzodiazepine	Anxiety	Diazepam—2-10 mg qhs-tid Clonazepam—0.25-2 mg daily-bid Lorazepam—0.25-2 mg PO/SL tid-qid

bid, twice daily; qhs, at bedtime; qid, 4 times daily; SL, sublingual; SSRI, seleceive serotonin reuptake inhibitor; tid, 3 times daily.

   ▲ Anhedonia, irritability, helplessness, hopelessness, worthlessness, excessive guilt, intractable pain, and suicidal ideation are also suggestive of depression.

- Asking about suicidal ideation does not increase the risk of suicide.
- A combination of counseling/psychotherapy and medications is optimal for severe mood disorders.
- Benzodiazepines may worsen memory or precipitate confusion. Consider antipsychotics for these patients.
- Look for medications that may worsen depression (β-blockers) or anxiety (albuterol nebulizer, caffeine).

Delirium
- Neuroleptics are listed in Table 3.
- Look for underlying reversible cause; decide how far to look in accordance with goals.
- Day-night reversal may be first sign of delirium in patients nearing death.
- Consider antipsychotic medications and benzodiazepines.
- Severely agitated, delirious patients nearing death may benefit from high-dose infusion of benzodiazepines, propofol, or barbiturates.

Dyspnea
- Many effective therapies are available for managing dyspnea at the end of life (Table 4).

Table 3. Neuroleptics

Agent	Dose
Haloperidol	0.5-1 mg PO, IV, SQ every 1 hour as needed, then every 6-12 hours to maintain (1-20 or more mg/day)
Risperidone (fewer extrapyramidal effects)	0.5-1 mg every 12 hours & titrate
Olanzapine (fewer extrapyramidal effects)	2.5-7.5 mg PO every 12 hours

- Empiric management of dyspnea is outlined in Table 5.

Nausea
- Medications for nausea are listed in Tables 6 and 7.

Constipation
- Medications for constipation are listed in Table 8.
- Prescribe stimulant laxatives prophylactically for patients taking opioids.
  - ▲ Stool softeners or dietary changes alone are unlikely to be effective.

Table 4. Specific Management of Dyspnea

Cause	Therapy
Bronchospasm	Nebulized albuterol 2.5-5 mg and/or ipratropium 0.125 mg every 4 hours
	Dexamethasone—2-20 mg PO, IV, SQ daily
Thick secretions	
Good cough	Nebulized saline
	Guaifenesin
Poor cough	Scopolamine—0.1-0.4 mg SQ/IV every 4 hours *or* 1-3 transdermal patches every 3 days *or* continuous IV/SQ infusion
	Glycopyrrolate—0.4-1 mg daily SQ infusion *or* 0.2 mg SQ/IV every 4-6 hours as needed
	Hyoscyamine—0.125 mg PO/SL every 8 hours
Anemia	Transfuse to >10 g/dL hemoglobin, repeat if provides symptomatic relief
	Erythropoetin (epoetin alfa)—10,000 IU SQ 3 times weekly if life expectancy is several months, increase as needed
Aspiration	Thicken foods
Airway obstruction	Nebulized racemic epinephrine
	Dexamethasone—2-20 mg PO, IV, SQ daily
	Oxygen-helium mixture
	Surgery, radiation if in accordance with patient goals

SL, sublingual.

Table 5. Empiric Management of Dyspnea

Oxygen	Opioids	Dopamine blockers	Anxiolytics
Follow subjective breathlessness, not arterial blood gases or oxygen saturation	Mild dyspnea—acetaminophen 325 mg/codeine 30 mg PO every 4 hours plus breakthrough dose 30 mg codeine every 2 hours Severe dyspnea—morphine 5-15 mg PO every 4 hours, titrate	Chlorpromazine or promethazine has had anecdotal success when used in conjunction with opioids Use in same doses as for nausea (Table 6)	Lorazepam—0.5-2 mg PO, SL, IV hourly as needed, then every 4-6 hours to maintain Clonazepam—0.25-2 mg PO every 12 hours

SL, sublingual.

Table 6. Medications for Nausea

Class of medication	Try in these conditions	Examples
Dopamine antagonists	Cerebral/liver metastases Opioid or other medication side effect Chemotherapy Metabolic—hypercalcemia, hyponatremia, liver/kidney failure CHF/ischemia	Haloperidol—0.5-2 mg PO, IV, SQ every 6 hours, then titrate (less sedating) Metoclopramide—10-20 mg PO every 6 hours Droperidol—2.5-5 mg IV every 6 hours
Antihistamines	Opioid or other medication side effect Metabolic—hypercalcemia, hyponatremia, liver/kidney failure CHF/ischemia	Diphenhydramine—25-50 mg PO every 6 hours Meclizine—25-50 mg PO every 6 hours Hydroxyzine—25-50 mg PO every 6 hours
Anticholinergics	Movement-induced nausea Bowel obstruction Failure of other agents (expensive)	Scopolamine—0.1-0.4 mg SQ/IV every 4 hours *or* 1-3 transdermal patches every 3 days
Serotonin antagonists	Chemotherapy	Ondansetron—8 mg PO tid Granisetron—1 mg PO daily-bid
Corticosteroids	Cerebral/liver metastases Meningeal irritation Chemotherapy Metabolic—hypercalcemia, hyponatremia, liver/kidney failure	Dexamethasone—6-20 mg daily PO, IV, or IM

bid, twice daily; CHF, congestive heart failure; tid, 3 times daily.

Table 7. Additional Antinausea Agents

Class of agent	Try in these conditions	Example
Prokinetic	Opioid side effect Ileus	Metoclopramide—10-20 mg PO every 6 hours
Antacids	Hyperacidity GERD	Maalox—2 Tb every 2 hours as needed
		Famotidine—20 mg PO/IV or other H_2 blocker
		Omeprazole—20 mg PO daily-bid or other proton pump inhibitor
Cytoprotective	Gastric irritation from NSAIDs	Misoprostol—200 µg bid-qid
		Omeprazole—20 mg PO daily-bid or other proton pump inhibitor
Anxiolytic	Nausea associated with anxiety	Lorazepam—0.5-2 mg PO every 4-6 hours
		Tetrahydrocannabinol—2.5-5 mg PO tid

bid, twice daily; GERD, gastroesophageal reflux disease; qid, 4 times daily; Tb, tablespoon; tid, 3 times daily.

- Bulking agents such as psyllium can exacerbate constipation in patients with poor fluid intake and immobility.
- Use a maximum dose before deciding that an agent is ineffective.
- Look for medications that may be contributing (calcium channel blockers, tricyclic antidepressants), and look for causes such as dehydration.

Diarrhea
- Medications for diarrhea are listed in Table 9.
- Consider dietary modifications.
- Look for easily treatable causes.
- Monitor for perianal skin breakdown.

Table 8. Medications for Constipation

Peristaltic stimulants	Osmotic agents	Stool softeners	Prokinetic agents	Lubricants/irritants
Prune juice—120-240 mL PO daily-bid	Lactulose—30 mL PO every 4-6 hours, titrate	Docusate sodium—50-100 mg PO bid	Metoclopramide—10-20 mg PO every 6 hours	Glycerin suppositories
Senna—1-2 tablets PO qd-bid (or cascara sagrada 4-12 mL qhs)	Sorbitol—30 mL 70% every 2 hours until results	Fleet enema—as needed		Mineral oil
Bisacodyl—5 mg PO/PR qhs, titrate	Milk of magnesia—1-2 tablets daily-tid	Warm soapy enema (also induces peristalsis)		
	Magnesium citrate—1-2 bottles as needed			

bid, twice daily; PR, rectally; qd, daily; qhs, at bedtime.

Anorexia and Weight Loss

- Appetite stimulants are listed in Table 10.
- Family and friends may be more distressed than patient is about poor appetite and cachexia.
- Discontinue dietary restrictions. Experiment with different foods.
- Patients typically stop oral intake in the last days to hours of life.
- Dehydration and ketosis may stimulate endorphin production and often are not uncomfortable for patients at the end of life.
  - ▲ Dry mouth can be combated by good oral care and is not likely to improve with IV fluids.
- In some cases, delirium may respond to IV hydration; this is unlikely in terminal delirium.
- Feeding tubes are associated with risk of infection and aspiration, discomfort, and occasional need for restraints.
- IV fluids and total parenteral nutrition may worsen ascites, peripheral edema, and pulmonary edema and may not prolong life in a terminal setting.

Table 9. Medications for Diarrhea

| | Diarrhea | |
Mild/transient	Moderate	Severe
Attapulgite—30 mL or 2 tablets as needed Bismuth salts— 15-30 mL bid-qid	Loperamide—2-4 mg PO every 6 hours or more Diphenoxylate-atropine—2.5-5 mg PO every 6 hours or more Tincture of opium—0.7 mL PO every 4 hours or more (may cause delirium)	Octreotide—50 µg SQ every 8-12 hours, up to 500 µg SQ every 8 hours or more, or continuous SQ/IV infusion 10-80 µg/hour IV fluid support if in accordance with patient goals

bid, twice daily; qid, 4 times daily.

Table 10. Appetite Stimulants

Drug	Comments
Dexamethasone—2-20 mg PO every AM	Side effects less of concern in patients with short life expectancy Other steroids may be used
Megestrol acetate—200 mg PO every 6-8 hours, titrate to effect	
Tetrahydrocannabinol	
Psychostimulants—methyl-phenidate, dextroampheta-mine, pemoline	Reduce appetite in healthy popula-tion but may increase it at end of life See Table 2 for dosing
Androgens—oxandrolone, nandrolone	

Fatigue and Weakness
- Consider corticosteroids and psychostimulants.
- Good hygiene, frequent turning, hydrocolloid dressings, and air mattresses may help prevent skin breakdown and pressure ulcers.
- Active or passive range of motion and massage on intact skin may also help.

Insomnia
- Medications for insomnia are listed in Table 11.
- Use extended-release medications for pain control overnight.
- Use good sleep hygiene—have patient maintain a regular schedule; avoid alcohol, caffeine, and nicotine; and stay out of bed when awake.
- Consider the contribution of medications such as bron-chodilators or corticosteroids to insomnia.

Table 11. Medications for Insomnia

Class of drug	Example	Comments
Antihistamines	Diphenhydramine– 25-50 mg PO qhs	Tolerance is common Anticholinergic effects
Benzodiazepines	Lorazepam—0.5-2 mg PO qhs	May worsen or precipitate dementia or delirium
Sedating neuroleptics	Chlorpromazine— 10-25 mg qhs	May help day-night reversal or delirium
Other options	Trazodone—25-200 mg PO qhs	Less daytime sedation
	Zolpidem—5-10 mg PO qhs	Fewer side effects

qhs, at bedtime.

EPONYMS IN INTERNAL MEDICINE

Guilherme H. M. Oliveira, M.D.
John B. Bundrick, M.D.

A

Abadie sign—spasm of the levator palpebrae superioris in thyrotoxicosis.

Addison disease—autoimmune chronic adrenal insufficiency.

Adie pupil—one pupil larger than the other; both show slow or no reaction to light and accommodation (also called tonic pupil).

Adson maneuver—palpation of the radial pulse with elevation of the chin and rotation of the head to the side contralateral to the pulse palpated demonstrates decrease in amplitude of the pulse and indicates thoracic outlet syndrome.

Albright syndrome—hereditary osteodystrophy-pseudohypoparathyroidism.

Allen test—test of arterial supply to the hand, observing color change with sequential compression of the radial and ulnar arteries.

Alport syndrome—autosomal dominant hereditary nephritis and neural hearing loss.

Alzheimer disease—slowly progressive degenerative cortical dementia.

Anton syndrome—blindness, denial of blindness, and confabulation

Argyll Robertson pupil—pupil accommodates but does not react to light; seen with syphilis, Wernicke encephalopathy, and diabetes mellitus.

Arnold-Chiari malformation—congenital occipital bone and proximal spine malformation causing displacement of cerebellar tonsils into cervical canal, resulting in hydrocephalus, papilledema, cranial nerve palsies, and cerebellar ataxia. Often associated with spina bifida and meningocele.

Aschoff bodies—endocardial granuloma pathognomonic for rheumatic fever.

Auer bodies—rod-shaped inclusions seen at microscopy in acute myeloid leukemia.

Austin Flint murmur—functional late diastolic murmur simulating mitral stenosis in severe aortic regurgitation.

Austrian syndrome—pneumococcal pneumonia, endocarditis, and meningitis.

B

Babinski sign—hyperextension of the big toe after lateral plantar stimulation; indicative of upper motor neuron disease.

Bainbridge reflex—increased heart rate due to increased right atrial pressure.

Baker cyst—posterior enlargement and herniation of the popliteal bursa.

Banti disease—portal hypertension with congestive splenomegaly, hypersplenism, and anemia.

Barlow syndrome—mitral valve prolapse murmur and chest pain.

Barrett esophagus—columnar metaplasia of distal esophagus secondary to long-standing reflux.

Bartholin cyst—inflammation of Bartholin gland near the introitus of the vagina.

Bartter syndrome—hypokalemic alkalosis, hyperaldosteronism, and normal blood pressure.

Basedow (Graves) disease—thyrotoxicosis.

Batista procedure—left ventricular myomectomy with mitral valvuloplasty in patients with end-stage dilated cardiomyopathy in an attempt to restore ventricular geometry, Frank-Starling curve, and function.

Battle sign—retroauricular ecchymosis indicating fracture of the base of the skull.

Bazex syndrome—paraneoplastic acrokeratosis affecting ears, nose, hands, and feet and associated with laryngeal and esophageal cancer.

Beau lines—transverse lines in fingernails resulting from nail growth interruption as a result of severe systemic illness.

Beck triad—hypotension, increased jugular venous pressure, and absence of apex beat, with pericardial tamponade.

Behçet syndrome—oral and genital ulcers, pyoderma, uveitis.

Bekhterev disease—ankylosing spondylitis.

Bell palsy—unilateral lower motor neuron paralysis of cranial nerve VII (facial nerve).

Bence Jones protein —monoclonal light chains of IgG seen in urine of patients with multiple myeloma.

Berger disease—IgA nephropathy.

Bernard-Soulier syndrome—thrombocytopenia, congenital giant platelets, bleeding diathesis, and platelet dysfunction due to lack of glycoprotein Ib.

Bernheim syndrome—bulging of the interventricular septum into the right ventricle as a result of increased left-sided pressures, causing right ventricular failure.

Bezold reflex—vagal reflex causing bradycardia, hypotension, syncope, and nausea after inferior wall infarction.

Bezold-Jarisch reflex—vagal hyperstimulation usually following an inferior myocardial infarction, with hypotension and bradycardia.

Billroth operation—I, removal of distal stomach with end-to-end anastomosis with duodenum; II, gastroduodenal anastomosis with duodenal closure.

Binswanger disease—premature atherosclerotic vascular dementia characterized by memory loss, paranoia, and emotional lability.

Blackfan-Diamond syndrome—rare, progressive, hematologic disorder that presents in early childhood as a normocytic and normochromic aplastic or hypoplastic anemia and results from defective erythropoiesis and lack of nucleated erythrocytes in the bone marrow.

Blumberg sign—rebound tenderness indicating peritoneal inflammation.

Blumer shelf—metastatic gastric cancer to the pelvic floor palpable on rectal examination.

Boerhaave syndrome—esophageal rupture as a result of repetitive vomiting.

Bouchard nodes—hard nodular deformity of the proximal interphalangeal joints, pathognomonic for osteoarthritis.

Bourneville disease—tuberous sclerosis, characterized by adenoma sebaceum, seizures, and mental retardation.

Bouveret syndrome—giant gallstone erodes into the duodenum and causes intestinal obstruction and gastrointestinal tract bleeding.

Bowen disease—intraepidermal epithelioma, with 15%-30% incidence of malignancy.

Bradbury-Eggleston syndrome—idiopathic orthostatic hypotension, primary autonomic failure.

Branham sign—bradycardia caused by compression of hemodynamically important arteriovenous fistula.

Bright disease—chronic nephritis.

Broadbent sign—systolic retraction of the ictus cordis as a result of constrictive pericarditis.

Broca aphasia—motor aphasia (i.e., person understands but cannot produce words).

Brown-Séquard syndrome—ipsilateral flaccid paralysis and impairment of touch, position, and vibration sense, with contralateral loss of pain and temperature from a lesion affecting one-half of the spinal cord.

Brudzinski sign—flexion of neck results in flexion of hip and knee, indicates meningeal inflammation.

Brugada syndrome—hereditary disorder characterized by right bundle branch block, ST-segment elevation, and sudden death.

Budd-Chiari syndrome—suprahepatic vein thrombosis, with jaundice, ascites, and portal hypertension.

Buerger disease—thromboangiitis obliterans.

Burkitt lymphoma—most rapidly progressive human tumor, a rare type of non-Hodgkin lymphoma.

C

Caplan syndrome—pneumoconiosis (typically silicosis) with rheumatoid arthritis.

Carey Coombs murmur—mid-diastolic murmur heard during acute rheumatic fever and indicative of carditis.

Carney complex or syndrome—autosomal dominant condition characterized by spotty pigmented skin lesions with atrial myxomas, psammomatous melanotic schwannoma, and Cushing syndrome.

Caroli disease—congenital biliary tree ectasia with biliary cyst formation.

Carvallo sign—increase in tricuspid regurgitation murmur with deep inspiration.

Castleman disease—angiofollicular lymph node hyperplasia, a lymphoma variant.

Chaddock reflex—noxic stimulus of lateral malleolus produces extension of great toe, equivalent of a Babinski sign.

Chagas disease—systemic disease caused by *Trypanosoma cruzi* that preferentially affects the myocardium and smooth muscle, causing dilated cardiomyopathy, megacolon, and achalasia.

Charcot joint—deformed joint caused by repetitive trauma as a result of diabetic neuropathy, syphilis, leprosy, or syringomyelia.

Charcot-Leyden crystals—colorless needle-shaped crystals found in sputum of patients with asthma and stools of patients with ulcerative colitis and amebiasis.

Charcot-Marie-Tooth disease—peroneal nerve atrophy.

Charcot triad (gastroenterologic)—abdominal pain, fever, and jaundice; indicates ascending cholangitis.

Charcot triad (neurologic)—intention tremor, nystagmus, and scanning speech seen in multiple sclerosis with brainstem involvement.

Chédiak-Higashi syndrome—autosomal recessive neutrophil and eosinophil disorder characterized by oculocutaneous albinism, photophobia, nystagmus, and recurrent pyogenic infections.

Cheyne-Stokes respiration—recurrent pattern of hyperpnea followed by transient apnea; seen in patients with cerebrovascular and cardiovascular disease.

Chilaiditi syndrome—loops of bowel between liver and diaphragm causing loss of liver dullness; associated with abdominal distension, pain, and vomiting.

Christmas disease—hemophilia B, factor IX deficiency.

Churg-Strauss syndrome—allergic granulomatous angiitis; small-vessel vasculitis of skin, kidneys, and lungs associated with eosinophilia and asthma.

Chvostek sign—percussion of facial nerve in front of the tragus of the ear causes ipsilateral muscular spasm; seen in severe hypocalcemia.

Cogan syndrome—nonsyphilitic interstitial keratitis with vestibuloauditory symptoms; associated with systemic vasculitis and aortic valvulitis.

Conn syndrome—primary hyperaldosteronism, hypertension, and hypokalemic alkalosis.

Cooley anemia—thalassemia major.

Corrigan pulse—water-hammer pulse of chronic aortic regurgitation, also seen in hyperdynamic states.

Courvoisier sign—painless, hard, palpable gallbladder caused by ampullary cancer, most commonly carcinoma of the head of the pancreas.

Cowden disease—autosomal dominant inheritance with virginal hypertrophy of breasts, fibrocystic disease, carcinoma of breasts, bird-like facies, pectus excavatum, and multiple hamartomas of colon and cerebellum.

Creutzfeldt-Jakob disease—progressive degenerative disease of the central nervous system caused by proteinaceous infectious particles devoid of nucleic acid (prions); typically presents with dementia and myoclonus, and usually causes death within 1 year after onset.

Crigler-Najjar syndrome—hereditary defect in bilirubin conjugation causing high (type I) to intermediate (type II) degrees of elevation in serum indirect bilirubin and normal liver histology.

Crohn disease—granulomatous enterocolitis.

Cruveilhier-Baumgarten syndrome—recanalization of the umbilical vein secondary to high portal pressures, leading to caput medusae and a venous bruit over the umbilicus.

Cullen sign—abdominal wall periumbilical ecchymosis indicative of retroperitoneal hemorrhage; first described with acute pancreatitis.

Curling ulcer—gastric ulcer caused by severe systemic stress; originally associated with large burns.

Cushing disease—primary adrenocorticotrophic hypersecretion from pituitary, causing cortical adrenal tumor with hypersecretion of systemic steroids

Cushing phenomenon—hypertension and bradycardia indicative of increased intracranial pressure.

Cushing syndrome—phenotype created by long-term exposure to endogenous or exogenous corticosteroid excess.

Cushing ulcer—gastric, duodenal, or esophageal ulcer associated with increased intracranial pressure; presumably due to gastric acid hypersecretion.

D

Darier sign—stroking of the skin results in edema and erythema in systemic mastocytosis.

De Musset sign—head bobbing synchronous with heart beat in severe chronic aortic insufficiency.

De Quervain tenosynovitix—chronic tenosynovitis due to a narrowing process in the tendon sheaths around abductor pollicis longus and extensor pollicis brevis muscles.

De Quervain thyroiditis—subacute nonbacterial thyroiditis.

Devic disease—neuromyelitis optica, acute attacks of optic neuritis, and transverse myelitis.

Dieulafoy lesion—eroded aberrant gastric submucosal artery that causes catastrophic upper gastrointestinal tract bleeding.

DiGeorge syndrome—cardiac abnormality and abnormal facies, T-cell deficit due to thymic hypoplasia, cleft palate, hypocalcemia due to hypoparathyroidism resulting from 22q11 deletion (*CATCH22* is a helpful mnemonic for this syndrome).

Down syndrome—trisomy of chromosome 21.

Dressler syndrome—inflammatory pleuropericarditis usually occurring in the second week after myocardial infarction.

Dubin-Johnson syndrome—inherited benign disorder of bilirubin metabolism characterized by low-grade direct hyperbilirubinemia and classic "black liver" due to accumulation of a dark, granular pigment in the lysosomes of centrilobular hepatocytes.

Duchenne muscular dystrophy—X linked muscular dystrophy characterized by weakness and hypertrophy of affected muscles.

Duncan syndrome—also known as "X-linked lymphoproliferative syndrome," a recessive disorder of young boys who die of fulminant infectious mononucleosis or develop malignant B-cell lymphomas after infection with Epstein-Barr virus.

Dupuytren contracture—contracture of palmar fascia causing the ring and little fingers to bend into the palm so they cannot be extended.

Duroziez sign—systolic and diastolic two-phase murmur that can be heard over the femoral artery in severe aortic regurgitation when it is compressed with the bell of the stethoscope.

E

Eales disease—retinal vasculitis with acute sudden loss of vision.

Eaton-Lambert syndrome—peripheral motor-sensory polyneuropathy associated with non–small cell lung cancer.

Ebstein anomaly—congenital noncyanotic heart disease with ventricularization of the right atrium secondary to downward displacement of the tricuspid valve from the annulus fibrosus.

Ehlers-Danlos syndrome—inherited disorder of collagen characterized by hyperelasticity of the skin, hypermobility of the joints because of extremely lax ligaments and tendons, and poor wound healing.

Eisenmenger syndrome—cyanotic heart defect characterized by ventricular septal defect, dextroposition of the aorta, pulmonary hypertension with pulmonary artery enlargement, and hypertrophy of the right ventricle as well as a left-to-right shunt (ventricular, occasionally also atrial) reverted to right-to-left by pulmonary hypertension.

Ewart sign—localized area of dullness to percussion, increased fremitus, and bronchial breathing in lungs of patients with large pericardial effusions, likely caused by compressive atelectasis.

Ewing tumor—malignant sarcoma of shafts of long bones.

Evans syndrome—hemolytic anemia of warm antibodies and immune thrombocytopenia.

F

Fabry disease—X-linked hereditary disorder of α-galactosidase A deficiency, characterized by skin telangiectasias in abdominal and pelvic regions, with paresthesias and exertional fevers.

Fallot tetralogy—cyanotic heart disease characterized by pulmonic stenosis, ventricular septal defect, dextraposition of the aorta, and right ventricular hypertrophy.

Fanconi syndrome—pancytopenia with mental retardation, absence of a radius, and deformity of long bones; autosomal recessive disorder.

Felty syndrome—atypical form of rheumatoid arthritis with fever, splenomegaly, and leukopenia and, in some cases, anemia and thrombocytopenia.

Finkelstein test—bend thumb into palm and grasp thumb with remaining fingers; pain caused by bending wrist away from thumb, hyperextending the abductor pollicis longus, indicates a positive finding and is suggestive of De Quervain tenosynovitis.

Fitz-Hugh-Curtis syndrome—gonococcal perihepatitis.

Forschheimer spots—petechial enanthema of the soft palate associated with acute viral syndromes, initially thought to be pathognomonic for rubella (German measles).

Fournier gangrene—necrotizing fasciitis of the scrotum and perineal region, usually in diabetics.

Frank sign—oblique fissure of the ear lobe associated with coronary artery disease, hypertension, and diabetes mellitus.

Friedreich ataxia—autosomal recessive inherited progressive degenerative disease with spinal cord atrophy and sclerosis of the dorsal and lateral columns of the spinal cord that presents before age 25; characterized by ataxia, dysarthria, and cardiac manifestations.

G

Gaisböck syndrome—relative erythrocytosis due to decreased plasma volume.

Gallavardin phenomenon—midsystolic murmur of aortic stenosis becomes more audible, less harsh, and higher pitched at the apex rather than the base of the heart.

Gardner syndrome—polyposis coli associated with soft tissue tumors, bony tumors, and ampullary cancer.

Gaucher disease—autosomal recessive disorder that results from defective activity of acid β-glucosidase and infiltration of lipid-laden macrophages (Gaucher cells) in viscera, bones, and central nervous system; may present as hepatosplenomegaly, bone disease, or progressive disease of the central nervous system.

Gerstmann syndrome—combination of acalculia, dysgraphia, finger anomia, and right-left disorientation; points to damage in inferior parietal lobule (angular gyrus) of the left cerebral hemisphere.

Gibson murmur—continuous machinery murmur of patent ductus arteriosus; best heard over the left second intercostal space.

Gilbert syndrome—hereditary defect of bilirubin metabolism that causes mild, benign increase in indirect bilirubinemia.

Gilles de la Tourette syndrome—autosomal dominant hereditary disorder characterized by motor and phonic tics, with coprolalia, echolalia, and palinphrasia.

Gitelman syndrome—inherited autosomal recessive mineralocorticoid deficiency syndrome characterized by renal salt wasting, activation of the renin-aldosterone system, with low blood pressure, low serum levels of potassium and magnesium, high serum levels of bicarbonate, and decreased urinary calcium excretion.

Glanzmann thrombasthenia—autosomal recessive disorder due to deficiency of the glycoprotein IIb-IIIa complex, thus unable to bind fibrinogen; characterized by normal-sized platelets that adhere but do not aggregate, causing impaired hemostasis and severe spontaneous mucosal bleeding.

Gohn focus—calcified nodule seen on chest X-ray; due to healed primary TB.

Goodpasture syndrome—antiglomerular basement membrane nephritis with lung hemorrhage.

Gottron sign—erythema of the knuckles, with a raised, violaceous, scaly eruption characteristic of dermatomyositis.

Gowers sign—patients with muscular dystrophy use arms to push themselves erect by moving their hands up their thighs to compensate for weakness of leg and hip flexors.

Graham Steell murmur—high-pitched, diastolic, decrescendo, blowing murmur of pulmonary regurgitation heard along the left sternal border; result of dilatation of the pulmonic valve ring from severe pulmonary hypertension.

Graves disease—thyrotoxicosis caused by thyroid-stimulating immunoglobulins directed against thyroid-stimulating hormone receptor, resulting in the classic clinical state of hyperthyroidism with goiter, ophthalmopathy, and dermopathy.

Guillain-Barré syndrome—rapidly evolving, ascending, autoimmune, symmetric areflexic motor paralysis with or without sensory involvement.

H

Hageman factor—factor XII.

Hallervorden-Spatz disease—neurodegeneration with brain iron accumulation type 1; is either sporadic or autosomal recessive progressive disease, with onset in late childhood; characterized by extrapyramidal signs, spasticity, dystonia, dysarthria with dementia, and emotional disturbances.

Hamman-Rich syndrome— more commonly known as "acute interstitial pneumonia," a fulminant type of interstitial lung disease characterized by diffuse, bilateral airspace opacification on chest X-ray and diffuse alveolar damage on lung biopsy.

Hamman sign—auscultatory crunching sound synchronous with the heartbeat; heard in pneumomediastinum.

Hampton hump—radiographic wedge-shaped density above the diaphragm seen in pulmonary embolism and thought to reflect a peripheral area of lung infarction.

Ham test—outdated laboratory demonstration of lysis of RBCs after complement activation by acid; diagnostic of paroxysmal nocturnal hemoglobinuria.

Hand-Schüller-Christian disease—diabetes insipidus, exophthalmos, and punched-out bone lesions; caused by histiocytosis X.

Hansen disease—leprosy.

Hashimoto thyroiditis—autoimmune lymphocytic infiltration of the thyroid gland causing hypothyroidism.

Heberden nodes—hard nodules that develop around the distal interphalangeal joints; pathognomonic of osteoarthritis.

Heerfordt syndrome—one of two acute sarcoidosis syndromes; characterized by fever, parotid enlargement, anterior uveitis, and facial nerve palsy.

Hecht pneumonia—primary giant cell pneumonia in rubeola.

Heinz bodies—small deep purple granular inclusions in RBCs of patients with certain hemolytic anemias, especially thalassemia.

Henoch-Schönlein purpura—small-vessel vasculitis characterized by palpable purpura in buttocks and thighs, abdominal pain, arthralgias, and IgA glomerulonephritis.

Heimlich maneuver—sudden and forceful application of sub diaphragmatic pressure to the chest in an attempt to expel a foreign body from the trachea or pharynx, where it is causing danger of suffocation.

Hill sign—blood pressure in the arm >30 mm Hg when compared with blood pressure in the leg; seen in severe aortic regurgitation.

Hodgkin disease—malignant lymphoma characterized by diffuse, symmetric lymphadenopathy.

Hoffmann sign—thumb flexion caused by flicking the nail of either the second, third, or, fourth finger, in hyperreflexia states, including upper motor neuron disease.

Hollenhorst plaque—cholesterol embolus seen in branching of retinal arterioles of patients with amaurosis fugax.

Holt-Oram syndrome—autosomal dominant disorder with upper limb dysplasia, atrial septal defects, and conduction disturbances in the atrioventricular node.

Homan sign—calf pain caused by dorsiflexion of the foot in patients with deep venous thrombosis of the lower extremities.

Hoover sign—inspiratory retraction of lower rib margins in patients with COPD.

Horner syndrome—unilateral ptosis, miosis, and anhidrosis; can be associated with lung cancer impinging on the sympathetic chain, carotid dissection, or brainstem stroke.

Howell-Jolly bodies—globular nuclear fragments in RBCs of patients who have been splenectomized or have megaloblastic anemia.

Hunner ulcer—chronic vesical ulcer at the vertex of the bladder suggestive of interstitial cystitis.

Huntington disease—inherited autosomal dominant degenerative brain disorder characterized by chorea and behavioral abnormalities.

Hurler syndrome—autosomal recessive mucopolysaccharidosis, resulting from alpha-L-iduronidase deficiency; characterized by coarse (gargoyle) facial features, hunchback, mental retardation, hepatosplenomegaly, and cardiac defects.

Hutchinson triad—cranial nerve VIII deafness, notched teeth, and interstitial keratitis; seen in congenital syphilis.

J

Jaccoud arthritis—progressive, deforming arthropathy of hands and feet of young patients with recurrent rheumatic fever or systemic lupus erythematosus.

Jacksonian seizure—seizure activity that starts in a localized part of the body, such as the hand or arm, and spreads, becoming generalized; indicative of a focal lesion in the contralateral motor cortex.

Jacod triad—optic atrophy, total ophthalmoplegia, and trigeminal neuralgia usually due to nasopharyngeal tumor.

Janeway lesion—a painless hemorrhagic macule on the palms or soles thought to be a vasculitic process in infectious endocarditis.

Jarisch-Herxheimer reaction—generalized rash, fever, and malaise during the first days of antibiotic treatment of leptospirosis, Lyme disease, or syphilis.

Jatene operation—operation to correct transposition of the great vessels.

Jendrassik maneuver—used to facilitate testing of the knee jerk by asking patients to hook their fingers together and then pull strongly in abduction.

Jod-Basedow phenomenon—hyperthyroidism induced by exogenous iodine.

K

Kaposi sarcoma—multicentric neoplasm consisting of multiple vascular nodules and strongly associated with human herpesvirus type 8 (HHV-8); occurs in skin, mucous membranes, and viscera and is seen most frequently in patients with AIDS.

Karnofsky performance scale—an index of clinical estimate of a patient's physical state, performance, and prognosis to help evaluate his or her suitability for a therapeutic procedure; most commonly used in oncology before chemotherapy and surgery.

Kartagener syndrome—subgroup of immotile cilia syndrome, autosomal recessive; characterized by situs inversus, chronic sinusitis, and bronchiectasis.

Kasabach-Merritt syndrome—extensive and progressively enlarging vascular malformation that causes stagnant blood flow and disseminated intravascular coagulation, with thrombocytopenia and purpura.

Kawasaki disease—mucocutaneous lymph node syndrome; acute febrile multisystem disease of children that may be associated to coronary aneurysms in 25% of patients and may cause acute myocardial infarction in children.

Kayser-Fleischer ring—gray-green or brownish pigmented ring, 1-3 mm broad, in the deep epithelial layers at the outer border of the cornea and pathognomonic for copper deposition in Wilson disease.

Kearns-Sayre syndrome—sporadic noninherited mitochondrial DNA disorder characterized by the triad of progressive external ophthalmoplegia, pigmentary degeneration of the retina, and heart block.

Kehr sign—radiated pain and hyperesthesia of the left shoulder in splenic rupture or subdiaphragmatic abscess.

Kernig sign—an attempt to extend the knee when the thighs are flexed over the hips causes pain in patients with meningeal irritation.

Kikuchi disease—benign cervical necrotizing lymphadenitis in young women.

Kimmelstiel-Wilson lesion—nodular diabetic glomerulosclerosis.

Klatskin tumor—bile duct carcinoma localized at the bifurcation of the hepatic ducts.

Klinefelter syndrome—XXY syndrome with hypogonadism, hypogenitalism, and mental retardation.

Klippel-Trénaunay syndrome—sporadic syndrome with vascular malformation of the limbs, gross limb hypertrophy, and arteriovenous fistulas.

Klüver-Bucy syndrome—bilateral lesions of the amygdala and temporal cortex produce visual agnosia, hyperphagia, emotional apathy, and hypersexual behavior.

Koebner phenomenon—also called "isomorphic response," refers to formation of skin lesions along a site of injury; seen with lichen planus, psoriasis, and systemic juvenile rheumatoid arthritis.

Koplik spots—bright red spots on the inside of the cheek and pathognomonic for rubeola.

Korotkoff sounds—pulse-synchronous circulatory sounds heard through the stethoscope in auscultation of blood pressure using a sphygmomanometer when pressure over the artery is reduced below systolic arterial pressure.

Krukenberg tumor—gastric carcinoma metastases to the ovary, usually bilateral.

Kussmaul respiration—rhythmic, gasping, and very deep type of respiration with normal or reduced frequency; associated with severe diabetic or renal acidosis or coma.

Kussmaul sign—jugular venous pulse increases with deep inspiration (when it normally would decrease because of increased venous return to the right atrium), indicating limited expansion of the right ventricle, as found in restrictive pericarditis.

Kveim-Stilzbach test—formation of a granuloma after injection of Kveim antigen in patients with sarcoidosis.

L

Laënnec cirrhosis—macronodular cirrhosis caused by alcohol consumption.

Lasègue signs—when a patient is supine with the hip flexed, dorsiflexion of the ankle causes pain or muscle spasm in the posterior thigh and back; seen in irritation of lumbar root or sciatic nerve.

Legg-Calvé-Perthes disease—autosomal dominant disorder causing unilateral or bilateral aseptic vascular necrosis of the femoral head.

Lemierre syndrome—suppurative thrombophlebitis of the internal jugular vein with sepsis and septic metastasis to the lung, brain, and kidneys, usually caused by fusobacteria.

Lenègre disease—primary sclerodegenerative disease of the conducting system of the heart causing heart block with no other cardiac abnormalities.

Leriche syndrome—atheromatous involvement or occlusion of the abdominal aorta just above its bifurcation, causing inability to maintain penile erection, fatigue in the lower limbs, cramps in the calf area, ischemic pain of intermittent bilateral gluteal claudication, absent or diminished femoral pulse, pallor, and coldness of the feet and legs.

Lesch-Nyhan syndrome—X-linked complete deficiency of hypoxanthine phosphoribosyltransferase causing hyperuricemia, self-mutilating behavior, choreoathetosis, spasticity, and mental retardation.

Lev disease—calcification of the fibrous cardiac skeleton, which frequently involves the aortic and mitral valves, the fibrous skeleton, and the apical ventricular septum, causing atrioventricular and bundle branch block.

Levine sign—a gesture of clenching the fist over the sternum used by patients when describing anginal chest pain; it is highly specific for a coronary origin of the pain.

Lewy body disease—dementia caused by diffuse cortical infiltration of Lewy bodies (intraneuronal cytoplasmic inclusions).

Lhermitte sign—sensation of an electric shock down the spine caused by neck flexion or coughing in patients with multiple sclerosis or other spinal cord disease.

Libman-Sacks endocarditis—noninfectious thrombotic endocarditis in patients with systemic lupus erythematosus or malignancies.

Löffler endocarditis—endocardial and myocardial infiltration by eosinophils in hypereosinophilic syndrome, with formation of large ventricular mural thrombi.

Löffler syndrome—benign acute eosinophilic syndrome characterized by migrating pulmonary infiltrates and mild clinical symptoms.

Löfgren syndrome—one of two acute sarcoidosis syndromes characterized by erythema nodosum with bilateral hilar adenopathy seen on chest X-ray and polyarthritis.

Lou Gehrig disease—amyotrophic lateral sclerosis.

Ludwig angina—Periodontal infection, usually arising around the third molar, which causes submandibular cellulitis, trismus, and neck swelling with respiratory distress.

Lutembacher syndrome—congenital or acquired heart disease in which atrial septal defect is combined with mitral stenosis.

Lyme disease—infectious tick-borne disease caused by *Borrelia burgdorferi*, begins with a characteristic skin rash (erythema migrans) but may become systemic.

Lynch syndrome—hereditary nonpolyposis colon cancer.

M

MacCallum patch—vegetations found along the mural surface of a cardiac chamber.

Machado-Guerreiro test—a complement-fixation test for *Trypanosoma cruzi* infection (Chagas disease).

Machado-Joseph disease—spinocerebellar ataxia type 3; rare, progressive hereditary ataxia initially described in Portuguese descendants; features are similar to those of Parkinson disease.

Mallory-Weiss tears—vertical tears in the esophagus caused by severe repetitive vomiting.

Marfan syndrome—Autosomal dominant hereditary disorder of connective tissue affecting primarily the musculoskeletal system, cardiovascular system, and eye; characterized by tall stature, long extremities, arachnodactyly, arm span greater than height, poorly developed musculature, laxity of the joints and ligaments, thoracic cage abnormalities, kyphosis, dorsal scoliosis, flat feet, hammer toes, dislocation of the lens, aortic insufficiency, and ascending aortic aneurysms (not all these features need to be present).

Means-Lerman scratch—scratchy systolic ejection murmur due to hyperthyroidism.

Meckel diverticulum—diverticulum of the ileum, a vestige of the yolk stalk, about 6-10 cm long, shaped like a glove's finger, found approximately 2 ft from the ileocecal valve.

Mees lines—white transverse lines in fingernails associated with chronic arsenic intoxication.

Meige syndrome—chronic familial lymphedema of the limbs, which manifests with pittings and brawny edema of the ankles and shins; often associated with inflammation and various defects, including distichiasis, extradural cysts, vertebral anomalies, cerebrovascular malformations, yellow nails, and sensorineural hearing loss.

Meigs syndrome—characterized by a solid ovarian tumor, usually a fibroma, accompanied by ascites and hydrothorax.

Meleney ulcer—gradually expanding ulcer developing at the site of trauma or surgery; caused by synergistic infection, including anaerobic streptococci.

Mendelson syndrome—chemical aspiration pneumonitis caused by regurgitation and aspiration of gastric contents.

Ménétrier disease—caused by large tortuous gastric mucosal folds resulting in epigastric pain and protein-losing gastropathy.

Meniere disease—progressive sensorineural hearing loss and vertigo; frequently accompanied by nausea and vomiting, ringing in the ears, a sensation of fullness or pressure in the ears, and sometimes nystagmus.

Milroy disease—congenital lymphedema, same as Meige disease.

Mitsuda reaction—a local immune response to SQ injection of *Mycobacterium leprae* used to measure delayed-type hypersensitivity to the pathogen.

Mondor disease—rare entity characterized by sclerosing thrombophlebitis of the veins in the anterior chest wall, usually a result of direct trauma.

Morton neuroma—a painful, benign fibroinflammatory tumor developing around the plantar digital nerve, most commonly between the third and fourth interdigital spaces, caused by entrapment neuropathy, most often in women.

Moyamoya disease—occlusive disease involving large intracranial arteries with development of rich collateral circulation, which is prone to bleeding, around the occluded artery, producing the diagnostic arteriographic appearance of "puff of smoke" (Japanese "moyamoya").

Müller sign—systolic pulsations of the uvula in aortic insufficiency.

Munchausen syndrome—somatiform disorder characterized by severe, chronic, dramatic factitious illness, particularly seizures, asthma, hematuria, or chronic diarrhea.

Murphy sign—interrupted inspiration by palpation of a tender, enlarged gallbladder in acute cholecystitis.

N

Negri bodies—pathognomonic cytoplasmic inclusions in neurons of patients with rabies.

Nelson syndrome—hyperpigmentation and high ACTH levels despite adequate corticosteroid replacement, caused by residual pituitary tumor after bilateral adrenalectomy in patients with pituitary Cushing disease.

Nikolsky sign—separation of epidermis of patients with pemphigus vulgaris by manual compression of the skin.

Niemann-Pick disease—inherited autosomal recessive lysosomal storage disorder of early infancy characterized by failure to thrive, hepatosplenomegaly, and rapidly progressive neurodegeneration.

Noonan syndrome—a complex multisystem syndrome similar to Turner syndrome but can occur in both sexes and has no karyotype abnormality; features include unusual facies (i.e., hypertelorism, down-slanting eyes), webbed neck, congenital heart disease, short stature, chest deformity, and mental retardation.

O

Ogilvie syndrome—acute metabolic colonic pseudo-obstruction.

Oliver-Cardarelli sign—pulsation of the larynx synchronous with ventricular systole; elicited when the larynx is grasped between the thumb and index finger while the patient is in the erect position. It is indicative of an aneurysm of the aortic arch, mediastinal tumors, and COPD.

Ondine curse—observed in primary alveolar hypoventilation, in which patients have frequent episodes of central apnea when asleep.

Oppenheim reflex—(a Babinski equivalent) firm stroke or other irritation along the medial side of the tibia causes dorsiflexion of the great toe of patients with upper motor neuron disease.

Ortner syndrome—hoarseness caused by compression of recurrent laryngeal nerve by enlarged left atrium in patients with mitral stenosis.

Osborne wave—an electrocardiographic wave that distorts the QRS-ST junction in patients with hypothermia.

Osgood-Schlatter disease—osteochondrosis of the tibial tuberosity.

Osler maneuver—easily palpable and rigid radial artery despite obliteration of the radial pulse by a sphygmomanometer; indicating unreliability (and likely overestimation) of cuff measurement of blood pressure because of severe arteriosclerosis of the artery.

Osler nodes—small, erythematous, exquisitely painful nodes at the tips of fingers and toes, thought to be embolic phenomena from infective endocarditis.

Osler-Weber-Rendu syndrome—hereditary telangiectasia syndrome.

P

Page kidney—renal subcapsular hematoma that causes parenchymal compression with secondary hypertension.

Paget disease—osteitis deformans, caused by generalized excessive resorption of bone by osteoclasts; causes bone pain, bone deformity, and widespread intraosseous fistulas that may result in high-output heart failure.

Palla sign—radiologic enlargement of the right descending pulmonary artery seen in pulmonary embolism.

Pancoast syndrome—usually a squamous cell carcinoma at the apex of the lungs compresses the sympathetic plexus and erodes into the rib cage, causing back and arm pain and Horner syndrome.

Parinaud syndrome—dorsal midbrain syndrome characterized by supranuclear palsy of vertical conjugate movement, most often upwards, and caused by lesions near the aqueduct of Sylvius

Parkinson disease—progressive degenerative central nervous system disease characterized by destruction of neurons in the pigmented substantia nigra (pars compacta), locus ceruleus, globus pallidus, and putamen, resulting in loss of dopaminergic cells and depletion of striatal dopamine; clinically characterized by rest tremor, rigidity, bradykinesia, and gait instability.

Pastia lines—petechiae in body folds of patients with scarlet fever.

Paterson-Kelly syndrome—esophageal web in association with glossitis and iron deficiency anemia. (Better known as Plummer-Vinson syndrome.)

Pel-Ebstein fever—fever that persists for days to weeks, disappears and then recurs; seen in Hodgkin disease.

Pemberton sign—face plethora and syncope caused by compression of neck vasculature by large retrosternal goiter.

Peutz-Jeghers syndrome—autosomal dominant inherited disorder characterized by intestinal hamartomatous polyps in association with mucocutaneous melanocytic macules; has a high predisposition to cancer of the gastrointestinal tract.

Peyronie disease—induration of the corpora cavernosa of the penis, causing distortion and pronounced curvature of the penis, with erectile dysfunction.

Phalen test—paresthesia in the median nerve distribution by pressing the extensor surfaces of the two flexed wrists against each other, in carpal tunnel syndrome.

Pick disease—slowly progressive neurodegenerative disorder similar to Alzheimer disease; diagnosis requires autopsy confirmation with the pathologic finding of Pick bodies.

Pickwickian syndrome—obesity-hypoventilation syndrome, with daytime hypersomnolence, hypercapnea, polycythemia, pulmonary hypertension, and right-sided heart failure.

Plummer nails—separation of the nail from the nailbed (onycholysis) in Graves disease

Plummer-Vinson syndrome—same as Paterson Kelly syndrome.

Pott disease—tuberculous osteomyelitis of the spine.

Prinzmetal angina—vasospastic angina.

Purtscher retinopathy—hemorrhagic and vaso-occlusive vasculopathy characterized by multiple white retinal patches and retinal hemorrhages with acute blindness; associated with severe head and chest trauma and acute pancreatitis.

Q

Quincke sign—systolic plethora and diastolic blanching in the nail bed with slight compression; observed in aortic insufficiency.

R

Ramsay Hunt syndrome—varicella-zoster virus infection involving the geniculate ganglion of the sensory branch of cranial nerve VII (facial nerve) and resulting in pain and vesicles in the auditory canal, loss of taste sensation in the anterior two-thirds of the tongue, and ipsilateral facial palsy.

Rasmussen aneurysm—dilated vessel that ruptures into a tuberculous pulmonary cavity and causes hemoptysis.

Raynaud disease—occurrence of Raynaud phenomenon in the absence of its known secondary causes.

Raynaud phenomenon—episodic digital ischemia manifested by sequential blanching, cyanosis, and rubor of the fingers following cold exposure.

Reed-Sternberg cell—giant connective tissue cells with one or two large nuclei (mirror image nuclei) characteristic of the lesions of Hodgkin disease.

Reiter syndrome—nongonococcal urethritis, uveitis, and reactive arthritis.

Reye syndrome—acute childhood illness associated with the combination of viral illness and drugs (especially salicylates), causing cerebral edema and renal and hepatic insufficiency.

Reynolds pentad—fever, abdominal pain, jaundice, hypotension, and confusion in septic acute cholangitis.

Richter syndrome—transformation of chronic lymphocytic leukemia or small lymphocytic lymphoma into aggressive diffuse large B-cell lymphoma.

Riedel thyroiditis—chronic fibrosing, painless thyroiditis.

Riley-Day syndrome—familial dysautonomia.

Ritter disease—staphylococcal toxic epidermal necrolysis in newborns.

Romaña sign—unilateral painless edema of the palpebrae in acute Chagas disease.

Romberg sign—the patient cannot maintain body balance when standing with feet together and eyes closed; the sign is present if the patient sways and falls when the eyes are closed; falling is often to the same side and indicates posterior column disease.

Roth spots—retinal red spots with white center seen in infective endocarditis and some leukemias.

Rovsing sign—pressure over the descending colon causes pain in the right lower quadrant of the abdomen of patients with acute appendicitis.

S

Saint Vitus dance—Sydenham chorea of rheumatoid fever.

Schatzki ring—a thin weblike constriction at the squamocolumnar junction or near the border of the lower esophageal sphincter.

Schmidt syndrome—autoimmune polyglandular failure.

Schober test—test that measures flexion of the lumbar spine in patients with ankylosing spondylitis who have impaired flexion.

Sézary syndrome—cutaneous T-cell lymphoma (mycosis fungoides) with peripheral blood involvement.

Sheehan syndrome—postpartum pituitary infarction in the setting of hemorrhage and systemic hypotension.

Shy-Drager syndrome—a form of multiple system atrophy characterized by autonomic dysfunction and parkinsonian features.

Sipple syndrome—multiple endocrine neoplasia type IIA; characterized by medullary thyroid carcinoma, hyperparathyroidism, and pheochromocytoma.

Sister Mary Joseph nodule—periumbilical metastases from gastrointestinal tract malignancies.

Sjögren syndrome—chronic autoimmune lymphocytic infiltration of exocrine glands causing xerostomia, dry eyes, and systemic manifestations.

Somogyi phenomenon—rebound hyperglycemia after an episode of hypoglycemia.

Starling law—the force of contraction of the cardiac muscle is proportional to its initial length.

Stauffer syndrome—paraneoplastic nonmetastatic liver dysfunction in patients with renal cell carcinoma.

Stevens-Johnson syndrome—drug-induced severe erythema multiforme-like eruption of the skin, lesions of the oral, genital, and anal mucosae, and hemorrhagic crusting on the lips; associated with fever, headache, and arthralgia.

Still disease—adult juvenile rheumatoid arthritis.

Stokes-Adams syndrome– intermittent high-degree atrioventricular block with syncope.

Strachan syndrome—also known as "Jamaican neuritis" and characterized by amblyopia, optic neuritis, painful peripheral neuropathy, and urogenital dermatitis; occurs in undernourished populations of tropical countries.

Sturge-Weber syndrome—neurocutaneous syndrome characterized by unilateral facial port-wine nevus, cerebral atrophy, and oculomeningeal capillary hemangiomata.

Sydenham chorea—chorea associated with acute rheumatic fever.

Symmers fibrosis—periportal liver fibrosis associated with schistosomiasis.

Sweet syndrome—acute febrile neutrophilic dermatosis characterized by sudden onset of fever, leukocytosis, and tender, erythematous, well-demarcated papules and plaques showing dense neutrophilic infiltrates on histologic examination. Although Sweet syndrome may occur in the absence of other known disease, it is often associated with hematologic disease (including leukemia) and immunologic disease (rheumatoid arthritis, inflammatory bowel disease).

T

Takayasu arteritis—inflammatory and stenotic disease of medium- and large-sized arteries, especially the aortic arch and its branches.

Tako-tsubo syndrome—transient ballooning of the cardiac apex associated with severe acute illness in the absence of coronary disease.

Tietze syndrome—painful, swollen, and red costochondrial joint.

Tinel sign—paresthesia in the distribution of median nerve produced by tapping the volar aspect of the wrist.

Todd paralysis—transient limb paralysis after generalized seizures.

Tolosa-Hunt syndrome—recurrent, sharp unilateral retro-orbital pain with extraocular palsies, usually involving cranial nerves III, IV, V, and VI; other features include proptosis and sensory loss over the forehead, sluggish pupil reaction to light, and diminished corneal sensitivity with blurred vision up to complete blindness.

Troisier sign—metastatic enlargement of left supraclavicular lymph nodes from an obscurely located primary cancer, usually in the gastrointestinal tract or lungs.

Trousseau syndrome—paraneoplastic migratory thrombophlebitis; usually associated with pancreatic cancer.

Turcot syndrome—polyposis coli associated with malignant tumors of the central nervous system.

Turner sign—blue-purple discoloration of the costovertebral angles that occurs in hemoperitoneum caused by acute pancreatitis.

Turner syndrome—gonadal dysgenesis in women caused by genetic defects of the X chromosome; characterized by primary amenorrhea, sexual infantilism, short stature, and multiple congenital defects.

V

Valsalva maneuver—the patient maintains a constant expiratory pressure for at least 15 seconds while changes in blood pressure and heart rate are observed.

Verner-Morrison syndrome—watery diarrhea, hypokalemia, and renal failure in association with pancreatic islet cell tumors (VIPomas) that secrete large quantities of vasoactive intestinal peptide (VIP).

Vincent angina—acute necrotizing ulcerative gingivitis caused by *Treponema vincentii* and *Fusobacterium nucleatum*.

Virchow node—supraclavicular adenopathy associated with malignancy of the gastrointestinal tract.

Virchow triad—three functional causes of thrombosis: epithelial changes, changes in blood flow, and changes in blood viscosity.

Vogt-Koyanagi-Harada syndrome—uveomeningeal syndrome characterized by anterior uveitis associated with poliosis, vitiligo, auditory disturbances, and meningeal irritation.

von Hippel-Lindau syndrome—association of central nervous system tumor, renal cell carcinoma, pheochromocytoma, and islet cell neoplasm.

von Recklinghausen disease—neurofibromatosis type I, multiple skin neurofibromas, café au lait spots, and pheochromocytomas.

von Willebrand disease—autosomal dominant disease characterized by bleeding disorder resulting from deficiency of von Willebrand factor.

W

Waldenström macroglobulinemia—hematologic malignancy of lymphoplasmacytoid cells that secrete IgM; similar to multiple myeloma except it has a more benign course.

Wallenberg syndrome—occlusion of the posterior inferior cerebellar artery supplying the dorsolateral medulla and posteroinferior cerebellum results in pain and impaired sensation in the ipsilateral half of the face, ataxia of limbs and falling toward the side of the lesion, nystagmus, diplopia, Horner syndrome, dysphagia, hoarseness, and impaired pain and temperature on contralateral side of the body.

Waterhouse-Friderichsen syndrome—bilateral hemorrhagic necrosis of the adrenal glands in severe meningococcal disease.

Wegener granulomatosis—an antineutrophil cytoplasmic antibody (ANCA)-associated systemic necrotizing granulomatous vasculitis of small arteries and veins of the upper and lower respiratory tracts, kidneys, and other organ systems.

Weil syndrome—hemorrhagic form of leptospirosis causing acute renal failure, shock, and disseminated intravascular coagulation.

Wermer syndrome—multiple endocrine neoplasia type I, characterized by neoplasia of the parathyroid, pituitary, and pancreatic islet cells.

Werner syndrome—adult progeria; hereditary multisystem disorder characterized by premature aging, dwarfism, premature graying of the hair (canities), alopecia, scleroderma-like skin changes, trophic leg ulcers, cataracts, hypogonadism, diabetes mellitus, calcification of blood vessels, and osteoporosis.

Wernicke aphasia—inability to comprehend written and spoken language.

Wernicke encephalopathy—metabolic encephalopathy caused by thiamine deficiency, usually in the setting of alcoholism, and characterized by the clinical triad of ophthalmoplegia, ataxia, and global confusion.

Westermark sign—focal oligemia on chest X-ray in pulmonary embolism.

Whipple disease—systemic indolent infection caused by *Tropheryma whippelii* and manifested by arthralgia, abdominal pain, chronic diarrhea, progressive weight loss, low-grade fever, skin hyperpigmentation, and peripheral lymphadenopathy.

Whipple triad—symptoms of hypoglycemia, documentation of hypoglycemia, and relief of symptoms with administration of glucose; originally described in association with insulinomas.

Williams syndrome—idiopathic hypercalcemia of infancy; characterized by elfin facies, mental retardation, and supravalvular aortic stenosis in association with hypercalcemia secondary to increased sensitivity to vitamin D.

Wilms tumor—the most common renal tumor in children; it arises from the primitive embryonal renal tissue and contains epithelial, stromal, and blastemal elements; it presents as an abdominal mass and has a 90% rate of cure.

Wilson disease—autosomal recessive defect of biliary copper excretion that may lead to liver disease and neuropsychiatric manifestations.

Wiskott-Aldrich syndrome—X-linked recessive disorder with a defect in both T- and B-cell function and characterized by the triad of eczema, profound thrombocytopenia, and frequent infections.

Wolff-Parkinson-White syndrome—cardiac preexcitation syndrome in which atrioventricular conduction may occur through an accessory pathway, most commonly the bundle of Kent; it is characterized by episodes of supraventricular tachycardia, short PR interval, and the presence of a delta wave on the ECG.

Y

Young syndrome—triad of bronchiectasis, obstructive azoospermia with reduced fertility, and chronic rhinosinusitis infections.

Z

Zenker diverticulum—outpouching of the esophageal wall in the posterior hypopharyngeal wall.

Zollinger-Ellison syndrome—excessive gastrin production by a gastrinoma, clinically manifested by numerous gastrointestinal ulcers and recurrent gastrointestinal tract bleeding.

EVIDENCE-BASED PRACTICE

Guilherme H. M. Oliveira, M.D.
Victor M. Montori, M.D., M.Sc.

PROBLEM

- The interview and examination represent the first diagnostic test.
- How do you select lab tests?
- What treatments do you start?
- How do you explain the risks and benefits of your diagnostic and therapeutic strategies to the patient, the one who takes those risks and suffers the harms and benefits?

GENERAL APPROACH

Patient-Centered Approach

- The patient's best interest is the only interest to be considered.

Evidence-Based Approach

- Do not be evidence-centered—research reports alone never tell you what to do.
- Do not ignore evidence—patients suffered to produce it.
- Do not ignore the advice of local experts, but be critical.
- Do not believe all you read, be very critical.

Explicit and Mindful

- If you make a decision, know why you are making it and be ready to defend it.
- In all decisions, be aware of the patient's preferences and values—only the patient knows these and they could be different from yours.
- Be aware of the limits set by the care environment on the options you can consider.
- Be aware of the reactions and emotions you experience and explore them—they influence your judgment.

How to Make a Problem Familiar
- Read. Acquire knowledge. Know patterns. See patients. Recognize patterns. Problems become familiar with experience. Be ready to learn from every patient.

How to Structure Solutions to Problems
Analyze the Problem
- For each case, determine the differential diagnosis.
- To determine your approach, stratify the differential diagnosis according to the following (Table 1):
  - ▲ Plan your diagnostic strategy; know the test characteristics.
  - ▲ Choose a sensitive test to rule out disease.
  - ▲ Choose a specific test to rule in disease.

Formulate the Clinical Question
- Fill in the following blanks:
  - ▲ Your patient:_____
  - ▲ Test: _____
  - ▲ Reference standard: _____
  - ▲ Diagnosis:_____
- Search for evidence to formulate a diagnostic strategy.
- Critically appraise the data.
  - ▲ Was the study prospective, with a spectrum of patients similar to those in whom the test will be applied (was there diagnostic uncertainty)?
  - ▲ Were the assessment of the reference standard and the test independent and blind to each other? Did everyone receive the same reference standard?

Results
- Look for sensitivity, specificity, or likelihood ratios.
- The likelihood ratio is the proportion of people with disease and the test result divided by the proportion of people without disease and the test result (Fig. 1).
- Calculation of posttest probability is shown in Figure 2.

Plan the Therapeutic Strategy
- Know the risks and benefits of treating. Value observation (over the need to act).
- Treatment goals need to be negotiated with the patient.
- Monitor the treatment.

Table 1. Diagnostic Strategy

Strategy	Reason	Example
Treat probable disease	Disease probability is high and/or disease is severe Treatment can be started without test results	Sublingual nitroglycerin & aspirin for a smoker with coronary artery disease who has chest pain
Diagnostic tests	Disease probability is intermediate Wait for test results to start treatment	Ferritin level in a middle-aged man with anemia to diagnose iron-deficiency anemia
Rule out	Disease probability is low *but* risk of late/missed diagnosis is not acceptable	Serial ECG and cardiac enzymes in patient with atypical chest pain to rule out myocardial infarction
Keep in mind	Disease probability is extremely low *or* Risk of late/missed diagnosis is acceptable	Metanephrines in urine to diagnose pheochromocytoma in patient with recurrent headaches

▲ What are the measures to judge effectiveness, harm, side effects?

Validity Criteria
- Was the assignment to treatment randomized?
- Was the allocation concealed? (Were the persons who decided about participant inclusion separated from those who allocated patients to the experimental arms?)
- Were the groups similar at the beginning of the trial? Were all subjects followed to its completion?
- Were all groups (patients, healthcare providers, data collectors, data analysts, judicial assessors of outcomes, authors) in the study blinded?
- Were patients analyzed in the groups to which they were randomly assigned (intention to treat)?

$$LR+ \atop \text{(of a positive test)} = \frac{+ \text{ test/disease}}{+ \text{ test/no disease}} = \frac{\text{sensitivity}}{1\text{-specificity}}$$

$$LR- \atop \text{(of a negative test)} = \frac{- \text{ test/disease}}{- \text{ test/no disease}} = \frac{1\text{-sensitivity}}{\text{specificity}}$$

Fig. 1. Likelihood ratio (LR).

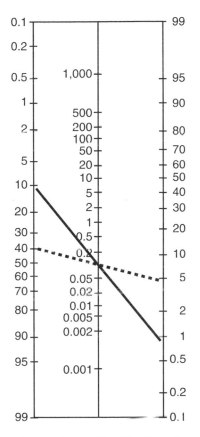

Fig. 2. Plug in the pretest probability of the disease (prevalence of the disease in your practice setting, your best guess). Next, use a straight angle through the likelihood ratio to calculate the posttest probability. (From Fagan TJ. Nomogram for Bayes's theorem [letter]. N Engl J Med. 1975;293:257. Used with permission)

Results

- Look for the risks of both groups.
  - ▲ The risk difference is the absolute risk reduction.
  - ▲ The inverse is the number needed-to-treat.
- Look for the risks of harm in both groups.
  - ▲ Follow the same steps, and calculate the number needed-to-harm.
- It is easier to trust a body of literature (or a systematic review of several trials) than a single trial.
- The evidence alone does not tell you what to do.
- Lack of evidence of effectiveness does not mean lack of effectiveness.
- Before you use these results, ask if your patient and setting is so different from the average patient and setting in the study that the results are likely to be different in your patient and setting.
- Once you are familiar with the evidence and with your patient's preferences and values, try to identify the following:
  - ▲ What are the limits imposed by my reality on the range of options I am considering?
  - ▲ What are the local standards for the treatment and diagnostic options considered?
- After this extensive evaluation, you are more likely to feel comfortable with the diagnostic and therapeutic answers to your patient problem.
- With more experience, you will be able to recognize this problem, be familiar with it, and have a structured answer to apply to its solution.

EVIDENCE SOURCES

- The ACP Journal Club: www.acpjc.org
  - ▲ Summaries of important research of high methodologic validity. Valuable for remaining updated.
- The Cochrane Collaboration (systematic reviews of therapy trials): www.cochranelibrary.com
  - ▲ High-quality systematic review of therapeutic trials.
- MEDLINE: www.pubmed.gov
  - ▲ Massive database of biomedical research.

HOW TO BE A GOOD INTERN

Jason Persoff, M.D.

GENERAL ADVICE

- All interns feel overwhelmed by the awesome "step-up" in responsibility and accountability that marks the transition from being a student to being a physician.
- Cornerstones for a successful transition and more meaningful learning experience depend on the following:
  - ▲ Organization
    - Have a system that you use consistently to track patients—a system detailing everything from a patient's birthday to medical history (use notecards, sheets of paper, or a personal digital assistant).
    - Record and keep accessible your patients' medical histories and pertinent lab and other data (you never know when a clinical situation or an attending physician will insist that you know this information).
  - ▲ Attention to detail
    - Be able to explain every abnormal clinical finding, abnormal lab result, or abnormal test result.
    - Be the first one who finds out these results.
  - ▲ Time management
    - Patient care comes first, but always find a way to complete everything before attending rounds or conferences. Note: conferences and rounds will provide the fundamental knowledge base you will need to gain confidence and independence.
    - If you are consistently behind in your work in the mornings, you need to learn ways to be more efficient—

Special abbreviation used in this chapter: PRN, as needed; q, every; qid, 4 times daily; tid, 3 times daily.

you should not sacrifice your education (i.e., missing conferences) to complete your morning rounding.
- Be mindful of work hour rules and do not violate them.

ROUNDS AND NOTES
Prerounds
- Before meeting with the senior resident each morning, it is critical that the successful first year resident preround on all of his or her patients.
  - ▲ This means
    - Finishing all progress notes on each patient
    - Personally reviewing all the patients' radiology studies
    - Reviewing and interpreting all the patients' lab values
    - Writing all initial daytime orders
- The senior resident is an invaluable resource who will be eager to help you organize your thoughts, to interpret the data, and to teach you the mechanics of residency—take advantage of his or her experience.
- You are at a point in your career where the team will base management decisions largely on your daily subjective and objective evaluation of the patient.
  - ▲ Be thorough and accurate and have a low threshold to ask for help if you do not understand an issue.
- Because patient care is primarily the intern's responsibility—and patient care is the primary method of learning and becoming a well-rounded and efficient physician—consistently relying on the senior resident to help you "catch up" limits your growth and suggests the need for you to find innovative ways that improve your efficiency and foster patient care.
  - ▲ The occasional use of the senior resident to round on unseen patients because of unforeseen complications is acceptable and appropriate.
- Each patient should be seen before you attend rounds.

Afternoon Rounds and Addendums
- Round on the patients in the afternoon to follow up on lab results and to discuss with the patients and their families the new data or the plans that have been delineated.
- Because the chart is a communications tool, it is generally suggested that a very brief addendum note be left every afternoon updating the patient's clinical course.

- Remember that your colleagues (who are less familiar with your patients) may need to review the chart on cross-over to deal with an important issue that occurs overnight.
- Therefore, it is imperative to leave an addendum note whenever
  ▲ Lab data return that require interpretation or explanation— e.g., was the thoracentesis specimen consistent with a transudate or exudate? Was the patient's decrease in hemoglobin an anticipated response to volume resuscitation?
  ▲ Lab or other data return that will alter the treatment plan— e.g., CT confirmed the presence of a large pseudocyst that requires drainage
  ▲ Discussions occur with the patient or family about prognosis, code status, etc.
  ▲ Any important change in the patient's clinical status that changes the clinical plan from the morning note, e.g., new-onset atrial fibrillation with rapid ventricular rate requiring moving the patient to a monitored bed

Progress Note Etiquette
- Progress notes are meant as a tool to communicate your evaluation, treatment plan, and rationale behind the work-up and treatment.
- Progress notes are *not* a place to document grievances or complaints.
  ▲ It is inappropriate to leave notes in the chart that document disapproval or irritation with other members of the care team (nurses, consultants, the patient, etc.).
  ▲ Always maintain a professional and neutral demeanor in your writing—a demeanor that reflects scientific thought and consideration rather than personal feelings about others.

ADMISSIONS AND ORDERS
Multiple Admissions at the Same Time
- Frequently, multiple admissions arrive on the floor simultaneously.
- Always see the sickest patients as a priority, and initially take a very brief history and perform a targeted physical.

- Enter initial orders in the chart so that treatment can begin, and then see the next patient.
- Your write-ups should be done only after every patient has been seen and has orders on the chart.
- Patient care is primary, with documentation secondary.
- The senior resident can help you "divide and conquer" when several patients arrive at the same time; however, you are ultimately responsible for the admission orders and treatment plan for all your admissions.

Orders
- No standardized format exists for admission orders, but most residents prefer to use ADDCC-VAN-DISMAL as standard, as follows:
  - ▲ **A**ssign as (inpatient/outpatient observation) status to ____ team (details about appropriate inpatient vs. outpatient assignment are in the next section).
    - Include the service name, the attending's name, and then your name and pager number
    - You must also decide on the bed type—does the patient require a monitored bed (telemetry), regular medical bed, surgical bed, oncology bed, orthopedic bed, ICU bed, etc.?
  - ▲ **D**iagnosis—The patient's preliminary diagnosis; this does not have to be exact but should offer nursing and other staff a working idea of the patient's main diagnosis.
  - ▲ **D**eep venous thrombosis prophylaxis—one of the most important, avoidable, hospital-acquired complications is deep venous thrombosis or venous thromboembolism. Discuss with your senior resident if the patient is a candidate for pharmacologic therapy (such as low-molecular-weight heparin) or mechanical prophylaxis (antiembolic hose or alternating compression devices).
  - ▲ **C**ondition—Fair, stable, unstable, critical, etc.
  - ▲ **C**ode status—Every patient should have a code status notation (in some states, this is considered the law).
    - If a patient opts for any condition other than full code, a notation must be made in the chart (see the section on DNR orders below).
  - ▲ **V**ital signs
    - If you order vital signs hourly, you should also check on

the patient that frequently.

- Also consider the patient's comfort—do you actually need the patient's vital signs at 2:00 AM?
- Standard frequencies vary from every (q) 4 to 8 hours, but you can also add "WA" to signify that you want vital signs obtained only while the patient is awake.
- There is a difference between "tid" and "q 8 hours" and between "qid" (4 times daily) and "q 6 hours," etc.; anytime you specify "q x hours," the lab, medication, glucose check, and so forth, will occur precisely separated by x hours. The other times, e.g., tid, are performed at standardized times (e.g., 0700, 1300, 1800 hours).

▲ Allergies
- Distinguish between allergies and untoward side effects.
- For example, hives are allergies, and a little dyspepsia is probably a side effect.
- Be sure to list the type of reaction the patient has to the drug in question (e.g., penicillin causes rash) because this can guide other physicians' drug choices.

▲ Nursing—Requests such as aspiration precautions, fall precautions, and seizure precautions should be listed here.

▲ Diet—This will be the first thing you will be called on for most patients (see Diets section below).

▲ Ins/outs
- Requests for strict accounting of the patient's ins/outs are made here.
- You can also specify IV fluids and flow rates as well as the need for catheters here.
- Avoid giving IV fluids without an indication and avoid fluids that are running at "To Keep Open" rates because this essentially attaches the patient to an IV pole, usually with a beeping flow regulator that is sure to disgruntle the patient.
- You can request that an IV be "capped," i.e., IV access is present but drips are not.

▲ Special—Other miscellany can be ordered in this section, such as ambulating pulse oximetry. Consider physical, occupational, and speech therapy as warranted.

- ▲ Medications
  - • Medications preferably should be listed by generic name.
  - • Be sure to include PRN ("as needed") medications to cover possible contingencies as warranted (e.g., sleeping medications, laxatives).
  - • Order only medications you think can be given safely to the patient.
  - • A good mental exercise and practice is to check for drug-drug interactions if you intend to prescribe more than three medications.
  - • Most personal digital assistant programs and online programs such as Micromedex offer an engine that checks for pertinent reactions given a set of medications.
- ▲ Activity
  - • All patients should have an order "encourage ambulating tid" while in the hospital unless you can think of a contraindication (acute myocardial infarction, new-onset seizures, mental status change, etc.). Patients who cannot ambulate should be "up to a chair tid." This helps decrease the risk of deep venous thrombosis developing and maintains or improves the patient's conditioning.
- ▲ Labs/radiology
  - • Order only tests needed to confirm or to rule out a diagnosis.
  - • Avoid ordering "shotgun" daily labs, which can markedly increase the costs of hospitalization and can lead to the need for a secondary work-up to explain an unexpected abnormality.

Outpatient vs. Inpatient Status
What it Means
- ■ The guidelines for what constitutes "outpatient status" or "admit status" are beyond the scope of this handbook (especially because they are a continually moving target and vary by diagnosis), but some general notes are included below.
- ■ Assignment of the appropriate status is not trivial.
  - ▲ Improper patient status assignment costs hospitals billions of dollars annually and results in very large hospital bills—not covered by insurance.

- ▲ Take "assignment" seriously, and do not merely "guess."
- ▲ Ideally, if there is some issue about which status is the better one, discuss the case with a case manager; the senior resident may also be able to help guide you with making this difficult and frequently nebulous decision.
- In general, "outpatient status" is reserved for
  - ▲ Semiurgent work-up requiring low-level but constant nursing care for a low-risk diagnostic group
  - ▲ Hospitalization of no more than 48 hours
- Patient status should be upgraded from "outpatient" to "inpatient" if the work-up intensifies, the diagnosis becomes higher acuity, or hospitalization will be longer than 48 hours.
- In general, "inpatient status" is reserved for
  - ▲ Urgent or unstable patient work-up requiring intensive nursing care or monitoring and considerable medical intervention for a high-risk diagnostic group
  - ▲ Hospitalization of any length of time, even <24 hours
- Patients cannot be reclassified to "outpatient status" if the inpatient criteria are not met.

The Details

- "Outpatient status" generally is used to complete a semiurgent work-up or treatment that requires low-level, but constant, nursing care (e.g., atypical chest pain for a low-risk patient with active bleeding of lower gastrointestinal tract).
- Outpatient status expires after 2 hospital days (i.e., 48 hours from the time of the admission order).
- After the end of 48 hours, patient status should be changed from "outpatient" to "inpatient;" otherwise, the test or the hospitalization may not be covered by Medicare or insurance.
- Any patient who requires major medical intervention (myocardial infarction, stroke, diabetic ketoacidosis, etc.), intensive nursing care, or specialized monitoring should be admitted formally on an "inpatient status."
  - ▲ Patients also should be on an inpatient status if they are admitted with any kind of IV drip (heparin, insulin, nitroglycerin, etc.) except for routine fluids or if they require ICU monitoring.

- All hospital-to-hospital transfers are considered inpatient status.
- Direct admissions (admissions to the floor that bypass the emergency department by physician order) tend to be inpatient status.
- Although outpatient status can later be changed to inpatient status, once a patient is assigned inpatient status, he or she can never be switched to outpatient status.
  - ▲ Many physicians (residents and staff) opt for outpatient status as default because it offers "flexibility."
    - However, if used incorrectly, the hospitalization may not be covered by insurance or Medicare and this can adversely affect both the hospital and patient financially.
- In summary, assigning proper admission status is complicated and a constant challenge for physicians, case managers, and patients.
  - ▲ Take this part of your orders seriously, and consult with the case manager or senior resident whenever you are in doubt.

Diets
- As soon as the patient gets to the floor, the nurses invariably will contact you for a diet order regardless of how sick the patient is. Use your judgment carefully.
- Some choices for diet include the following:
  - ▲ Strict NPO
    - This unnecessarily severe order is needed only for obtunded patients or for patients in whom any PO intake may worsen their care (such as acute dysphagia or recent throat surgery).
    - Use it sparingly.
  - ▲ NPO except for medications, sips, and ice chips
    - This is an ideal option, allowing patients to have sips of water, ice chips, and their medications.
    - Even patients scheduled for esophagogastroduodenoscopy, surgery, etc., can generally have this diet.
    - Use this order when you are not sure whether the patient should eat.
  - ▲ xxxx kcal American Diabetes Association diet:
    - The diet for diabetics
    - You should calculate the patient's caloric needs.

- ▲ Renal diet—a low phosphate, low potassium, low residue diet for patients with renal failure
- ▲ Cardiac diet
  - • A low sodium, low fat diet
  - • You can specify "no sodium" or "2 g sodium daily" options.
- ▲ Clears—basically only water-based, thin liquids such as broths, Jello, and tea
- ▲ Soft diet
  - • A diet that is easily digested and contains more calories and substance than a clear diet
  - • Includes apple sauce, thicker soups, etc.
  - • A good choice as a transition diet for patient who is starting to eat after a long time of NPO, etc.
- ▲ Thickened liquid or pureed
  - • This diet usually consists of pureed food.
  - • It is ordered for patients who tend to aspirate or cough when they eat.
  - • Although usually ordered by speech therapy, it is a reasonable choice if you believe the patient is at high risk for aspiration on basis of history.
- ■ Be creative
  - ▲ Combinations of diets (renal + cardiac) can be ordered.
  - ▲ Remember that the more limitations you place on a patient's diet, the more likely the food is to taste bland, and the more likely the patient is to protest.
  - ▲ Make sure your choice of diet is medically necessary, and discuss with the patient why you may be limiting his or her dietary choices.

Notify the Patient's Primary Care and Other Outside Physicians

- ■ This is a critical aspect of admitting the patient.
  - ▲ Primary care physicians are often able to provide historical details a patient does not remember about previous work-ups or diagnoses.
  - ▲ Furthermore, patients frequently need reassurance that their physicians are involved in their care.

▲ Regular updates and notification before discharge are essential parts of patient care.

Writing Up the History and Physical
■ Write-ups may vary by institution.
■ An approach is suggested below:
  ▲ Chief complaint—Use the patient's words.
  ▲ Reason for admission—one line stating the physician's assessment why the patient needed to be admitted to the hospital
  ▲ History of present illness
   • Thorough but concise summary
   • Can include lab data, previous work-up, etc., if it is critical part of patient's history
   • A history of present illness should guide the reader or listener toward the diagnosis. Do not withhold data for dramatic effect; think of the history of present illness as a preemptive argument defending your ultimate conclusions (that you will detail in your diagnosis).
  ▲ Past medical history
   • A chronologic summary is best.
   • Include pertinent supporting details that help provide a contextual idea of disease severity.
   • For example, if the patient has a history of heart failure, the date of the last echocardiogram, with the ejection fraction and wall motion abnormalities, is helpful. For diabetes, you should include the last hemoglobin A_1C and evidence of end-organ damage (retinopathy, last creatinine, neuropathy, history of diabetic ketoacidosis, etc.).
   • For patients with a history of malignancy, it is essential to outline the dates and types of chemotherapy and radiotherapy, surgery, and adverse events.
   • This exercise also educates you about the patient and allows you to be more prepared for rounds and decisions on treatment plans.
  ▲ Past surgical history
   • A chronologic summary is best.
   • Try to include dates, institution where the operation was performed, indication, and complications.
  ▲ Allergies

- Write the generic name of the medication and the type of reaction the patient had.
- This will ensure the delineation between allergy (e.g., urticaria, wheezing) and side effect (e.g., nausea, diarrhea).
- A side effect should not be recorded as "allergy" but as "medication intolerance."

▲ Medication intolerances (see above)

▲ Medications
- List all the patient's medications (try to use generic names because they offer more clarity and less commercial bias).
- Be sure to inquire about and include over-the-counter medications, eye medications, and herbal supplements, which patients may not consider medications.

▲ Family history
- List only pertinent history, e.g., if the patient's father died at age 99 of "old age," this is probably superfluous.
- List histories of early cardiac disease, diabetes, bleeding history, familial disease, and cancer history.
- Use judgment, e.g., an 88-year-old being admitted for unstable angina has outlived his or her familial cardiac risk.
- "Noncontributory" can be used for these and similar circumstances.
- Do not mark the family history as "negative" without specifying for what it is negative (e.g., family history is negative for diabetes or malignancy).

▲ Social history—Include marital status, smoking history, drug history, ethanol use (including response to CAGE questions), travel history, pet or animal exposures, and occupational exposures.

▲ Review of systems
- By necessity, be *brief.*
- List items that are pertinent but not listed in the "history of present illness" (such as fevers, chills, night sweats, weight changes).

▲ Physical exam

- Include vital signs.
- Document only what you examined.
- Include negative findings when pertinent.
▲ Lab data
  - Limit to pertinent results
  - Circle all abnormal values.
▲ Radiographic data
  - List your impressions of the radiographic studies.
  - Avoid relying solely on the radiologist's report.
▲ Miscellaneous—Include ECG interpretation, etc.
▲ Assessment and plan
  - Make a problem list that includes all the abnormalities you have found.
  - This important exercise is necessary for an intern.
  - Avoid early closure such as listing a problem as "cardiac ischemia" if the patient has chest pain because "cardiac ischemia" infers a purely cardiac etiology.
  - Be as general as possible and list the likely differential diagnosis for each problem.
  - Justify your reasoning on the basis of the data you have.
■ You do not need to make a diagnosis on admission.
  ▲ A problem list allows you to consider items in the differential which would otherwise be missed.
  ▲ Furthermore, problem lists, rather than stabs at diagnosis, facilitate learning.
■ One approach is to divide each problem into the following:
  ▲ Differential diagnosis
    - Most likely cause of the problem
    - Other potentially lethal causes that need to be excluded
    - Rare and unlikely diagnoses that will be considered if the initial work-up is negative
  ▲ Diagnostic plan
    - Your plan needs to justify every test you are planning to order, accentuating the clinical importance of the data you hope to obtain.
    - This ensures that other physicians (consultants or cross-covering residents) will know what your overall plan is, e.g., "Will order CT of abdomen (rule out diverticulitis vs. neoplasm) that may prompt invasive evaluation (such as a flexible sigmoidoscopy) depending on these results."
  ▲ Treatment plan

- What medicines and other treatments you intend to use in the meantime

CHECKOUT

- Nothing can be more challenging on a call night than providing cross-over for other residents' patients about whom you know little.
  - ▲ Although some programs have night-float systems, many programs continue to have on-call residents provide nighttime cross-over.
  - ▲ To improve your call nights, and those of your colleagues, you should commit to the following "golden rules":

Leave No Work Unfinished

- You should avoid checking out work to the cross-over team, because the team will be busy with admissions and will not be sufficiently familiar with your patients to provide routine care.
- If you order labs or radiology studies late in the day, make sure the on-call team knows what tests they are and how you would manage the results.
- You are ultimately responsible for your patients and their care.
- Be efficient but mindful of work hours. You should never violate your program's work hour rules. Develop plans to make you efficient at care while you are scheduled to work in order to improve patient care and to decrease the on-call workload of colleagues.

Try to Avoid Writing "Call M.D./House Officer If..." Orders

- Frequently, physicians will write orders for nurses to call the on-call M.D. It is best to limit writing these orders unless you also have thought of what the on-call M.D. should do with these data. If you think you need to place an indication for calling the M.D. (sometimes it is essential, e.g., for a hemoglobin <8.0 g/dL in a patient with gastrointestinal tract bleeding), indicate in your progress notes or history and physical what you are monitoring and why. This is extraordinarily helpful for cross-over.

- Your goal is to minimize your colleague's distress in the middle of the night by anticipating what should be done with these results.
- You may either point out your plan of action during check-out or you may write orders to handle these potential eventualities (such as a PRN sliding scale of insulin for high levels of blood glucose).
- This does not mean the on-call team should not be disturbed at all; matters of patient care are paramount.
  - ▲ Your job is to try to limit unnecessary telephone calls (especially those that could interfere with sleep) by restricting "notify" orders to necessary or pertinent concerns only.

Talk With the Patient's Nurse and Family
- Before leaving for the day, talk with the patient's nurse to make sure no issues of concern remain (there will frequently be minor questions the nurse would like to ask or clarify, and if the nurse does not get to ask you, she or he may have to call the on-call team who do not know your patients well enough to answer most questions).
- It is especially important to discuss the current work-up information and subsequent treatment plan with the patient and the patient's family before you leave for the day.

PRN Orders
- Be sure to have PRN orders written for constipation, diarrhea, dyspepsia, insomnia, and pain, as you deem reasonable.
  - ▲ Nothing is more disruptive than answering a call at 3 AM because a patient needs a sleeping pill.
  - ▲ However, if you have concern about ordering a sleeping pill (e.g., a patient with hypoxia who hypoventilates), relay this to the nurse, write an order explaining that you wish to avoid sleeping pills for the patient, and document it in your progress notes.
  - ▲ Remember, if you are trying to avoid giving a PRN order for a certain problem, you should also communicate that at checkout.

Checking Out
- When you transfer care to the on-call team, be sure to include

code status and active problems for which the on-call team may be notified.

- It is helpful to know what antibiotics a patient is taking and what you would like the on-call physician to do if a fever develops.
- You should provide the on-call team with an updated patient list; be sure to update the patient's problems to accurately reflect current issues.
- Once the on-call physician feels comfortable, you can leave and you should turn off your pager.

CONSULTS

Curbside Consults

- If you have a brief, general question you think can be answered without a consultant actually seeing a patient (e.g., "What is the best treatment for ACE-inhibitor–induced coughs?"), contact an on-call physician for a curbside consult.
- Curbside consults should be brief, general, and require minimal knowledge of the patient by the consultant.
- Do *not* write the curbside consultant's name in the chart ("Discussed case with Dr. Smith who said...") because the consultant has not seen the patient and provided only general information.
  - ▲ Putting the name of the consultant in the chart unfairly increases his or her liability especially since he or she has not had an opportunity to interview or examine the patient.

Formal Consults

- Always discuss obtaining a formal consult with your senior resident and/or attending before requesting one.
- Before requesting a consult
  - ▲ You and the senior resident should formulate a specific issue the consultant is asked to evaluate.
  - ▲ You should have begun or completed a basic work-up before calling the consultant so that you will be able to provide him or her critical data (and potentially to answer the question yourself, avoiding the need for a consult).

- ▲ You need to ascertain if the consult must be done with the patient in the hospital or if it can be safely deferred until the patient is discharged.
    - • Remember, just because the patient is in the hospital does not mean that all his or her medical issues and consults need to be completed before discharge.
- ▲ As part of the daily progress note about the patient or as an addendum, you must make a clear notation in the chart about the specific information you want from the consulting service.
- ■ Consults should be requested as early in the day as possible, particularly on weekends.
- ■ Avoid calling for consults during the middle of the night unless an emergency exists.
- ■ Proper use of consultants will result in an environment conducive to learning and teaching.
    - ▲ Example of an improper consult—"The patient is short of breath and we do not know why. Could you look at the patient and tell us?"
    - ▲ Example of a proper consult—"The patient is short of breath and hypoxemic. His alveolar-arterial gradient is widened, but a ventilation-perfusion scan was normal. He continues to worsen. Attempts at improving oxygenation have failed, and he now is requiring a 50% Venturi mask. We would appreciate your help with diagnostic and treatment suggestions about his hypoxemia."

PROCEDURES
Informed Consent Forms
- ■ Obtaining informed consent means educating the patient about the benefits and risks of having a procedure performed before he or she authorizes you to perform the procedure.
- ■ All procedures more invasive than a simple IV require that an informed consent form be signed by the patient or the patient's proxy.
- ■ It is important to have the patient repeat to you the potential risks and benefits before signing the form.
    - ▲ It is also important to know that this form means only that the patient is aware of potential risks, not that he or she is relieving you of any liability if an unforeseen complication occurs.

Procedure Notes
- After completing a procedure, you need to document the procedure in the progress notes or to dictate the procedure, depending on your hospital's protocol.
- A suggested format follows:
  - ▲ Procedure performed—self-explanatory
  - ▲ Indication—Summarize in one or two words.
  - ▲ Consent
    - "The patient (or proxy) signed an informed consent form after the potential risks (bleeding, hemorrhage, etc. [list them]) and benefits (definitive diagnosis and treatment, etc.) were discussed at length and the patient was able to verbally repeat these to me. All questions about the procedure were answered to the patient's satisfaction."
  - ▲ Operators—List yourself and whoever is supervising or assisting you.
  - ▲ Technique—"The patient was prepped and draped in the usual sterile fashion. Using aseptic technique..."
    - Give a cursory summary of the procedure, such as "...a TLC was advanced over the wire using aseptic Seldinger technique into the right IJ."
    - This does not need to be particularly detailed unless there were complications.
    - Assuming there were no complications, close with, "There were no immediate complications, and the patient tolerated the procedure well."
  - ▲ Estimated blood loss—Guess the amount, but always list some value (often, the author lists <5 mL if the blood loss was not appreciable).
  - ▲ Disposition –Note here if you checked a chest X-ray, if the patient's pulse was present distally, if the patient's ports flushed easily, etc.

Complications
- Rarely, complications occur.
  - ▲ Be sure to document them neutrally and factually in the chart and what was done about them.

▲ The senior resident and attending must be informed promptly and will help guide how the complications will be presented to the patient and family.

CHANGE OF SERVICE
Off-Service and Transfer Notes

- Whenever a patient is transferred from one service to another or whenever you are leaving a service (e.g., at the end of a rotation), it is an act of courtesy for you to provide a detailed note.
  - ▲ These notes should be handwritten because of the delay between dictation availability and the time the accepting service needs to access the information.
- A recommended format is as follows:
  - ▲ Date of admission
  - ▲ Reason for admission—general problem that led to admission
  - ▲ Primary care provider(s)—This helps the accepting resident know with whom he or she needs to coordinate discharges or changes in condition.
  - ▲ Hospital course
    - Briefly describe the patient's hospital course, summarizing all studies (radiology, echocardiography, etc.) that were performed and why they were performed.
    - Detail the reason behind the addition or subtraction of any medications.
    - Summarize surgical procedures and their findings or complications.
    - *Try to include* specific diagnoses and treatments, responses to therapies, and adverse outcomes.
    - *Try to avoid* restating procedures and findings previously noted in the summary, rehashing the patient's hospital course day by day, and including insignificant (e.g., transient constipation) or too much data.
    - Remember, clinicians can review the chart if more detailed information is needed.
  - ▲ Pertinent physical findings—Summarize key abnormalities.
  - ▲ Consulting services—Indicate which services have been consulted and which are still following the patient.
  - ▲ Current medications
    - List all current medications.
    - When listing antibiotics, list the antibiotic day number.

▲ Active problem list—Outline the patient's current problem list and goals before discharge (if appropriate).
▲ Code status

Acceptance Notes

■ The point of writing an acceptance note is not to rehash verbatim your colleague's off-service or transfer note but to document your own physical exam and create your own problem list.
■ A recommended format is as follows:
  ▲ "Above transfer note/off-service note by Dr. _____ reviewed and discussed with the patient and his/her family."
  ▲ Current physical exam—Perform a complete exam as you would normally.
  ▲ Current problem list—Formulate your own assessment and plan.
  ▲ Code status

DISCHARGES

On Admission

■ Begin discharge planning on the day of admission.
■ Try to anticipate special needs the patient may have on discharge because some needs may take several days to coordinate.
  ▲ Will the patient need a home health nurse?
  ▲ Will the patient need physical therapy after discharge?
  ▲ Will the patient require dietary education (new onset diabetes)?
  ▲ Will the patient need home physical and occupational therapy?
■ Request that a nurse case manager assist you in discharge planning.
  ▲ The case manager is a critical aspect of the patient's care; he or she will help find placement for the patient and will also handle all insurance matters relating to the hospitalization.
  ▲ The case manager will arrange for health care, hospice, and nursing home.

▲ Including case managers as early as possible in the hospitalization improves disposition planning considerably.

Days Before Discharge
- Be proactive in discussing matters of follow-up with the primary care physician before discharge.
- The patient's primary care physician may have very specific instructions for follow-up arrangements (such as tests, consults, and appointment dates).
  - ▲ It is your responsibility, not the patient's, to make these arrangements.

Discharging Patients Home
- To discharge a patient to home, you need to complete four things:
  - ▲ Prescriptions
  - ▲ An interdisciplinary discharge instruction sheet
  - ▲ Scheduled follow-up with the primary care physician
  - ▲ A discharge order

Prescriptions
- Give patients prescriptions for medications that have been changed or added during the hospitalization.
- You may give a 30-day supply with one refill—additional refills must be through the patient's primary care physician.

Interdisciplinary Discharge Instructions
- The format of this sheet varies by institution, but it usually contains the following information:
  - ▲ Follow-up—Specify the physicians with whom the patient is to follow up and the dates and times.
  - ▲ Diet—Leave specific recommendations ("low salt and low fat" instead of "cardiac").
  - ▲ Activity—Fill in restrictions ("no driving until cleared by your primary doctor") or encourage a resumption of normal exercise.
    - • Studies have shown that a written exercise prescription increases patient's adherence to exercise.
  - ▲ Medications
    - • Write down all the patient's medications (even if they have

not been changed), and be sure to write both the generic and brand names along with the pill dosage and frequency.

- This sheet goes home with the patient, and many patients refer to this for their pill schedule; therefore, directions for taking the medications and their frequency must be written in plain English.
- *Do not write*, "Furosemide 120 mg PO every AM, 60 mg PO every PM."
- *Do write*, "Furosemide (Lasix) 40 mg 3 pills every morning and 1 1/2 pills at night."

Scheduled Follow-up With the Patient's Primary Care Physician

- Continuity of patient care is essential when transitioning a patient to the outpatient environment.
- Although most patients probably are responsible enough to schedule a follow-up visit with their primary care physician, some may not know that this is important.
- Failure to schedule appropriate follow-up may expose you to considerable liability if anything adverse occurs to the patient.

Discharge Order

- As intuitive as it may seem, you need to write a discharge order before a patient can be discharged.

Home Health Care Orders

- Patients going home with home health care will need orders documenting specific things they are requested to do.
- It is paramount that you name the attending physician who will be responsible for telephone calls from the home health nurse and for all the paperwork regarding the home health visits.
- A recommended format is as follows:
  - ▲ Home health orders
    - Attending for home health will be Dr. _____. This should be a physician who will be responsible for the patient's outpatient care (e.g., a primary care physician) and *not* your attending on an inpatient service.

- This doctor's office telephone number is _____.
▲ Medication orders
  - List all medications and dosages.
▲ Miscellaneous—includes some or all the following:
  - Home physical therapy, occupational therapy, speech therapy
  - Home safety evaluation
  - Medication administration
  - Vital signs assessments
  - Social worker evaluation
  - Insulin teaching and monitoring
  - Administration of IV medication
  - Central line care and dressing changes
  - Wound care and dressing changes
  - Hospital beds, bedside commodes, etc.

Notification of the Primary Care Physician
- You should call the primary care physician on the next business day to discuss the care rendered and the patient's disposition issues.

Discharge Summaries
- Primary care physicians rely on discharge summaries for understanding what happened to the patient during the hospitalization.
- These should be completed on the day of discharge.
- Brevity is the key to an effective summary; almost all the important information should appear on the first page.
- Requirements vary by institution; the following template is recommended:
  ▲ Date of admission
  ▲ Date of discharge
  ▲ Discharge diagnoses
    - Include only the important diagnoses and comorbidities
    - Always number them from most to least important, if possible.
  ▲ Procedures performed
    - List all procedures.
    - If the procedure was for diagnostic purposes, include the pertinent data found (e.g., "Lumbar puncture—CSF was normal except for a high protein at 58").

▲ Other pertinent findings
  • List other grossly abnormal physical or lab findings.
▲ Treatment rendered and hospital course
  • Give a very brief synopsis of the hospital course.
  • *Try to include* specific diagnoses and treatments, responses to therapies, and adverse outcomes.
  • *Try to avoid* restating procedures and findings previously noted in the summary, rehashing the patient's hospital course day by day, and including insignificant (e.g., transient constipation) or too much data.
  • Remember, clinicians can review the chart if more detailed information is needed.
▲ Disposition—State where the patient is going: to home, to hospice, to nursing home, etc.
▲ Discharge medications
  • This is critical.
  • Include doses and frequency.
  • Do not forget that oxygen is a medication.
▲ Diet—List fluid restrictions or specific dietary restrictions that are not immediately obvious.
▲ Activity—Specify if the patient has specific restrictions (driving restriction, lifting restrictions, etc.)
▲ Follow-up—List with whom patient has follow-up and the dates and times.
▲ Carbon copies
  • Include all physicians who care for the patient outside the hospital.
  • For out-of-town physicians, be considerate of the transcriptionist and include the office address, telephone number, and fax number of the clinician.
  • Patients cannot receive copies without going to medical records and specifically requesting them.

HOSPITAL DEATHS
Pronouncing a Patient
■ There is no standardized format for doing this. However, you should feel no palpable pulse, you should not be able to auscultate breath or heart sounds, you should note no response

to deep pain, and you should note no pupil response to light.
- When the patient meets the criteria of death, you should notify the nurse of the time of death (which is the time the patient is pronounced) and make a notation in the chart.
- Be compassionate and professional, especially when the patient's family is present.
  - ▲ It is important to tell the family that the patient has "died" rather than using euphemisms such as "expired" or "passed away."

Who to Contact
- The nursing supervisor will be notified of all deaths by the nurses and will handle all the paperwork and details (such as mortician transfer and organ donation).
- You should discuss the death with the family if any are present.
- If the family is not present, the decision about how to inform them should be made by the senior resident or attending.
- Generally, it is always better for the family to be told in person.
- A chaplain usually is available 24 hours a day and is trained in dealing with most religious persuasions.
- Ask the unit secretary to page the on-call chaplain if the family desires religious help.
- Allow the family as much time with the body as needed and be available for questions until the family leaves.
- Avoid speculating on the cause of death except in general terms, and if you are unsure of the cause, be honest and say so.

Autopsy Requests
- Patients who die in the hospital may have an autopsy performed with the family's permission.
- For learning or determining the possible pathologic basis for death, it is nearly always important to ask the family for an autopsy.
- Autopsies can be partial (such as a limited brain autopsy) and can be coordinated with the morticians.
- Most teaching institutions do not charge for an autopsy performed on patients who die in the hospital.
- It may help to tell the patient's family that this is a nonmutilating, precise surgical procedure to explore why the patient may have died.

- You may also suggest that findings from an autopsy may be the "ultimate gift" and an unparalleled opportunity to educate physicians, improve subsequent patient care, and provide possible diagnoses that were not clinically apparent before death.
- It is important to reassure the family that an autopsy will not preclude an open casket funeral and generally will not delay burial.
- Understand that the patient's family may have objections, and do not push too hard.
- You should attend autopsies on your patients if possible.

Organ Donation

- Laws vary by state on whether physicians may approach families to request organ donation.
  - ▲ Check with your nursing supervisor or hospital attorney about the law in your area.
- Frequently, highly qualified persons with an organ procurement team are best able to approach the patient's family about this topic.
- Deceased patients can still be organ donors for corneas, ligaments, and bone.

Body for Science

- Patients and families may wish to donate the patient's body to science.
  - ▲ This may range from an extended autopsy for educational reasons to cadaveric donation.
- Ask the on-call nursing supervisor or case manager to arrange for this generous act.

Your Own Emotions

- After a patient dies, you will often be confronted with your own doubts about treatment or will be saddened by the loss of someone about whom and for whom you cared.
- You are encouraged to discuss these feelings with your colleagues, attending, or program director.
- All in-hospital deaths on academic services will be addressed at a monthly morbidity and mortality conference aimed at

learning what, if anything, may have been done differently to improve patient outcomes.

▲ This conference is a supportive atmosphere to discuss your own concerns about management and to grow as a clinician.

Death Summary
- Date of admission
- Date of death—The date the patient was pronounced.
- Reason for hospitalization—List the medical reason the patient was hospitalized.
- Treatment rendered and events leading up to death
  - ▲ Give a very brief synopsis of the hospital course.
  - ▲ There is no need to give extensive detail because the death summary will not be used by other physicians.
  - ▲ Try to include only major pertinent observations in a chronologic order ending with the patient's death.

PREOPERATIVE MEDICAL EVALUATION

Ripudamanjit Singh, M.D.
Charanjit S. Rihal, M.D.

GENERAL GOALS

- To identify unrecognized comorbid disease and risk factors for medical complications of surgery
- To optimize preoperative medical condition
- To foresee, prevent, and treat potential complications

PRINCIPLES OF CONSULTATION

- Restrict advice to the internist's unique areas of expertise, e.g., advise on perioperative insulin management but leave anesthetic technique to the anesthesiologist.
- Keep number of recommendations to a minimum.
  - ▲ Adherence to recommendations diminishes for consults with more than 5 recommendations.
  - ▲ Follow patients through the postoperative period because many perioperative complications occur during this time.
- Correct documentation.
  - ▲ The preoperative patient is not being "cleared." This may incorrectly imply there is no risk; rather, the evaluation may determine that the patient is "at average risk for the proposed procedure," which should be documented in your note (if no factors are found which increase perioperative risk).
- Modern anesthesia is extremely safe.
  - ▲ Patient and surgical factors are more important risk predictors than anesthetic considerations.
  - ▲ The American Society of Anesthesiology classification is a powerful predictor of overall perioperative mortality; it also predicts cardiac and pulmonary morbidity (Table 1).

Special abbreviations used in this chapter: CABG, coronary artery bypass graft; MET, metabolic equivalent; PTCA, percutaneous transluminal coronary angioplasty.

Table 1. American Society of Anesthesiology Classification

Class	Systemic disturbance	Mortality, %
1	Healthy patient with no disease outside the surgical process	<0.03
2	Mild-to-moderate systemic disease caused by the surgical condition or other pathologic processes	0.2
3	Severe disease process that limits activity but is not incapacitating	1.2
4	Severe incapacitating disease process that is a constant threat to life	8
5	Moribund patient not expected to survive 24 hours with or without an operation	34
E	Suffix to indicate emergency surgery for any class	Increased

PREOPERATIVE EVALUATION OF HEALTHY PERSONS
- Perioperative risk is very low for healthy persons.
  - ▲ Estimated at ≤0.03%
- Additional evaluation will have a low yield and high likelihood of false-positive results.
- History is the most important factor in evaluation of healthy persons.
- For patients <40 years with normal history and physical exam findings, no additional testing is needed.
- Good exercise capacity generally predicts a low cardiac and pulmonary risk for surgery.

SPECIFIC TESTS
CBC
- Anemia is present in 1% of asymptomatic patients.
- Blood loss is common during major operations.
- Baseline value may be helpful before major operations.

Electrolytes
- Incidence of unexpected abnormalities is <1%.
- *Not routinely recommended*

Renal Function
- Renal insufficiency increases with age.

- Its presence may require adjustment of the medication dose.
- Recommend renal function testing for patients >50 years and if hypotension or nephrotoxic medications are likely.

Glucose
- No definite relation between asymptomatic hyperglycemia and perioperative morbidity.
- *Not routinely recommended*

Liver Function Tests
- Asymptomatic mildly abnormal liver function tests are not associated with perioperative morbidity.
- Clinical liver disease may pose a risk; these patients are identified without screening.
- *Not routinely recommended*

Tests of Hemostasis
- Incidence of surgically important abnormalities in patients without a clinical history of bleeding tendency is extremely low.
- Reserve these tests for patients with a known bleeding diathesis or an illness associated with bleeding tendency.
- *Not routinely recommended*

Urinalysis
- No evidence for asymptomatic pyuria increasing the risk of surgical site infections
- Renal dysfunction is better detected with serum creatinine level.
- *Not recommended*

ECG
- Goal—detection of previous silent myocardial infarction or unsuspected arrhythmia that would increase cardiac risk
- Recommended for
  - Men >40 years and women >55 years
  - Clinical evaluation suggesting heart disease
  - Patients at risk for electrolyte abnormalities

▲ Systemic disease associated with possible unrecognized heart disease

Chest X-Ray
- In one study, incidence of surgically important abnormalities was 0.3%, with no risk factors for cardiac or pulmonary disease.
- Obtain it for patients >60 years (if not done within past 6 months).

Pregnancy Test
- If any suspicion of pregnancy

CARDIAC DISEASE
- Most important cause of perioperative morbidity and mortality
- Guidelines for perioperative cardiovascular evaluation for noncardiac surgery from American College of Cardiology and American Heart Association (Fig. 1)
- Overriding theme of these guidelines—Intervention is rarely necessary to lower the risk of surgery.

Clinical Predictors
Major
- Unstable coronary syndromes such as recent myocardial infarction with evidence of important ischemic risk and unstable or severe angina
- Decompensated congestive heart failure
- Significant arrhythmias—high-grade atrioventricular block, symptomatic arrhythmias in the presence of underlying heart disease, supraventricular arrhythmias with uncontrolled ventricular rate
- Severe valvular disease

Intermediate
- Stable angina pectoris
- Previous myocardial infarction
- Compensated or previous congestive heart failure
- Diabetes mellitus

Minor
- Advanced age

Start at step 1 Fig. 1

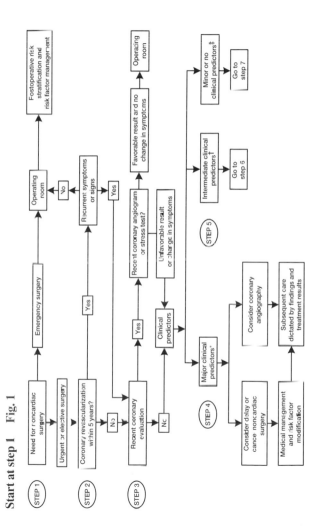

For intermediate clinical predictors, go to step 6   Fig. 1 (continued)

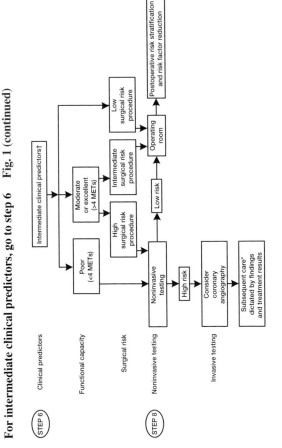

Fig. 1. Algorithm for preoperative cardiac evaluation. MET, metabolic equivalent. *Major clinical predictors: unstable coronary syndrome, decompensated congestive heart failure, significant arrhythmias, severe valvular disease. †Intermediate clinical predictors: mild angina pectoris, prior myocardial infarction, compensated or prior congestive heart failure, diabetes mellitus. ‡Minor clinical predictors: advanced age, abnormal ECG, rhythm other than sinus, low functional capacity, history of stroke, uncontrolled systemic hypertension. (From Report of the American College of Cardiology/American Heart Association Task Force on Practice Guidelines [Committee on Perioperative Cardiovascular

For minor or no clinical predictors, go to step 7 Fig. 1 (continued)

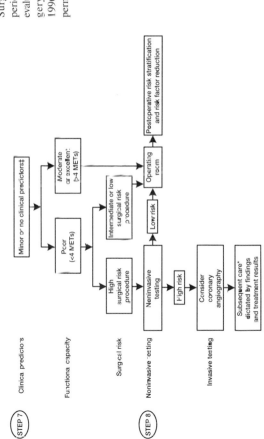

Evaluation for Noncardiac Surgery]. Guidelines for perioperative cardiovascular evaluation for noncardiac surgery. J Am Coll Cardiol. 1996;27:910-48. Used with permission.)

- Abnormal ECG
- Rhythm other than sinus
- Low functional capacity
- History of stroke
- Uncontrolled systemic hypertension

Functional Capacity
- Expressed in metabolic equivalent (MET) levels
- Perioperative cardiac and long-term risk is increased in patients unable to meet a 4-MET demand during most normal daily activities.

Duke Activity Status Index
- Eating, dressing, walking around the house, and dishwashing can range from 1 to 4 METs.
- Climbing a flight of stairs, walking on level ground at 6.4 km/hour, running a short distance, scrubbing floors, or playing a game of golf equals 4 to 10 METs.
- Strenuous sports such as swimming, singles tennis, and football exceed 10 METs.

Type of Surgery
- Surgery-specific risk for noncardiac operations can be stratified as high, intermediate, and low (Table 2).

Indications for Angiography
- High-risk results during noninvasive testing
- Angina pectoris unresponsive to medical therapy
- In most patients, unstable angina pectoris
- Nondiagnostic or equivocal noninvasive test in a high-risk patient undergoing a high-risk procedure

Indications for Coronary Artery Bypass Graft (CABG) Surgery and Percutaneous Transluminal Coronary Angioplasty (PTCA)
- Indications for CABG before noncardiac surgery are identical to those in general.
- CABG is rarely indicated to simply "get a patient through" the operation.
- Similarly, indications for PTCA in the perioperative setting are the same as those for PTCA in general.

Table 2. Cardiac Risk Level for Noncardiac Surgical Procedures

Low risk	Intermediate risk	High risk
Breast surgery	Carotid endarterectomy	Major emergency surgery, particularly in elderly
Superficial procedures	Head & neck surgery	Aortic & other major vascular surgery
Endoscopic surgery	Intraperitoneal surgery	Involving large fluid shifts and/or blood loss & prolonged procedures
Cataract surgery	Intrathoracic surgery	Peripheral vascular surgery
	Orthopedic surgery	
	Prostate surgery	

PULMONARY DISEASE

- Postoperative pulmonary complications are a major source of morbidity and mortality.
  - ▲ They are at least as frequent as clinically important cardiac complications and contribute to prolonged hospital stay and expense.

Risk Factors Associated With Increased Pulmonary Complications
COPD

- A 3- to 5-fold increase in pulmonary complications
- In one study, decreased breath sounds, prolonged expiration, rales, wheezes, and rhonchi on physical examination predicted a 5-fold increase in pulmonary complications.

Smoking

- A 2- to 6-fold increase in risk, even for patients without apparent COPD.
- Risk is highest for current smokers and those who have smoked within the past 1-2 months.
- The risk is higher for smokers who stop or decrease the number of cigarettes within 1 month than for those who continue to smoke!

- Therefore, advise smokers to stop smoking for a full 8 weeks before elective surgery

Obesity
- Most studies show no increase in pulmonary complications, even for morbid obesity.

Respiratory Infection
- Bronchitis or pneumonia is a risk factor.
- Delay the operation if any change in the character or amount of sputum.

Surgical Site
- This is the strongest overall risk factor for pulmonary complications.
- Upper abdominal and thoracic operations are greatest risk (20%-50%) because of splinting, diaphragmatic dysfunction from pain.
- Lower abdominal operations have a lower risk (0-5%).

Duration of Surgery
- Operations >3 hours increase the risk of pulmonary complications.

Preoperative Assessment of Patients At Increased Risk for Pulmonary Complications
- History and physical exam are most important.
  - ▲ Evaluate for exercise capacity, exertional dyspnea, cough, and presence of above risk factors.
- American College of Physicians position statement on preoperative pulmonary function tests is the standard. These tests are needed in all patients undergoing the following:
  - ▲ Coronary artery bypass or upper abdominal operation if patient has a history of tobacco use or dyspnea
  - ▲ Lower abdominal operation if patient has uncharacterized pulmonary disease and a prolonged or extensive operation is anticipated
  - ▲ Head and neck or orthopedic operation if patient has uncharacterized pulmonary disease
  - ▲ Lung resection

Risk Reduction Strategies
- Preoperative
  - ▲ Cigarette cessation for at least 8 weeks
  - ▲ Optimize COPD or asthma.
    - • Bronchodilators for symptomatic patients
    - • Theophylline only if used long-term
    - • Liberal use of inhaled corticosteroids to optimize pulmonary function
    - • Goal peak flow of 80% of personal best or predicted for asthmatic patients
  - ▲ Antibiotics only if change in character of sputum suggests infection, not warranted routinely
  - ▲ Begin patient education on lung expansion maneuvers.
- Postoperative
  - ▲ Lung expansion maneuvers
    - • Deep breathing exercises (chest physical therapy) or incentive spirometry is preferred.
    - • Both of above maneuvers reduce risk of pulmonary complications by half.
    - • Continuous positive airway pressure is equally effective but more expensive and labor intensive.
      - – Reserve for patients unable to cooperate with deep breathing or incentive spirometry.
    - • Adequate postoperative pain control greatly reduces pulmonary complications, especially in patients who had upper abdominal, thoracic, or aortic operations.

CORTICOSTEROID SUPPRESSION
- Suspect pituitary-adrenal axis suppression in
  - ▲ Any patient receiving long-term corticosteroid therapy
  - ▲ Any patient who has had 1 week of suppressive doses (i.e., prednisone >7.5 mg daily) within past 12 months
  - ▲ ACTH (corticotropin) stimulation test is usually unnecessary.

DIABETES MELLITUS
- Risks include altered wound healing, presence or development of electrolyte abnormalities, susceptibility to infection, risk of ketoacidosis, and hyperosmolar nonketotic coma.

- Focus on end-organ complications, especially cardiac disease because it is the most common cause of perioperative mortality.
- Lab tests
  - Routine ECG, given potential for silent myocardial infarction
  - Electrolytes, renal function, glucose
  - Urinalysis (exclude occult urinary tract infection)

THROMBOEMBOLISM PROPHYLAXIS

- Stratify the risk of thromboembolism on the basis of patient factors and type of operation (Table 3).

Very High Risk

- Major operation
- Age >40 years plus one of the following:
  - Previous venous thromboembolism
  - Hypercoagulable state
  - Malignant disease
  - Major orthopedic operation on lower extremity
  - Hip fracture
  - Stroke
  - Multiple trauma
  - Spinal cord injury

High Risk

- Major operation
- Age >60 years
- None of the following clinical risk factors:
  - Obesity
  - Immobilization
  - Malignancy
  - Varicose veins
  - Estrogen use
  - Paralysis
  - Congestive heart failure
  - Myocardial infarction
  - Stroke
  - Indwelling femoral vein catheter
  - Inflammatory bowel disease
  - Nephrotic syndrome
  - Hypercoagulable state

Table 3. Thromboembolism Prophylaxis According to Type of Operation*

Type of operation	Prophylaxis	
	Preferred	Alternative
Low-risk general surgery, <40 years old, minor operation	None	
Moderate-risk general surgery, ≥40 years old, major operation, no additional risk factors	Low-dose unadjusted heparin *or* LMWH *or* Intermittent pneumatic compression *or* Elastic stockings	Intermittent pneumatic compression if prone to hematoma or wound infection
High-risk general surgery, >40 years old, major operation, additional risk factors	Low-dose unadjusted heparin *or* Higher dose regimen of LMWH	Warfarin to INR 2-3
Highest risk general surgery, multiple additional risk factors	Low-dose unadjusted heparin *plus* LMWH *plus* Intermittent pneumatic compression	Low-dose unadjusted heparin *or* LMWH
Intracranial neurosurgery	Intermittent pneumatic compression ± Elastic stockings	
Hip replacement	Warfarin *or* LMWH *or* Adjusted-dose heparin	
Hip fracture	Warfarin *or* LMWH	

Table 3 (continued)

Type of operation	Prophylaxis	
	Preferred	Alternative
Knee replacement	LMWH *or* Warfarin *or* Intermittent pneumatic compression	

LMWH, low-molecular-weight heparin.

*Aspirin is not recommended as prophylaxis for surgical patients because other measures are more efficacious.

▲ Previous venous thromboembolism

or

- Major operation
- Age 40-60 years
- Clinical risk factors (listed above)

or

- Patients with myocardial infarction

or

- Medical patients with clinical risk factors (listed above)

Moderate Risk
- Any operation for patients 40-60 years old
- Major operation for patients <40 years
- No clinical risk factors (listed above)

or

- Minor operation
- Clinical risk factors (listed above)

Low risk
- Minor operation
- Age <40 years
- No clinical risk factors (listed above)

ENDOCARDITIS PROPHYLAXIS
- High-risk category—prophylaxis recommended
  - ▲ Prosthetic valves (metallic and bioprostheses)
  - ▲ Previous endocarditis
  - ▲ Complex cyanotic congenital heart disease
  - ▲ Surgical systemic pulmonary shunts or conduits
- Moderate-risk category—prophylaxis recommended
  - ▲ Most other congenital malformations
  - ▲ Acquired valvular dysfunction (i.e., rheumatic heart disease)
  - ▲ Hypertrophic cardiomyopathy
  - ▲ Mitral valve prolapse with regurgitation and/or thickened leaflets
- Negligible risk category—no prophylaxis recommended
  - ▲ Isolated secundum atrial septal defect
  - ▲ Surgical repair of atrial septal defect, ventricular septal

defect, patent ductus arteriosus
- ▲ Previous CABG
- ▲ Mitral valve prolapse without regurgitation
- ▲ Physiologic, innocent, or functional murmurs
- ▲ Previous Kawasaki disease or rheumatic fever without valvular dysfunction
- ▲ Pacemakers
- ■ Dental procedures for which prophylaxis is recommended
  - ▲ Dental extractions
  - ▲ Periodontal procedures, including surgery, scaling, planing, probing
  - ▲ Dental implant placement
  - ▲ Endodontic root canal instrumentation
  - ▲ Subgingival placement of antibiotic fibers or strips
  - ▲ Initial placement of orthodontic bands
  - ▲ Intraligamentary local anesthetic injections
  - ▲ Prophylactic cleaning if bleeding is anticipated
- ■ Other procedure for which prophylaxis is recommended
  - ▲ Respiratory tract
    - • Tonsillectomy
    - • Surgical operations of respiratory mucosa
    - • Rigid bronchoscopy
  - ▲ Gastrointestinal tract
    - • Sclerotherapy of esophageal varices
    - • Esophageal stricture dilatation
    - • Endoscopic retrograde cholangiopancreatography with biliary obstruction
    - • Biliary tract surgery
    - • Surgical operations involving intestinal mucosa
  - ▲ Genitourinary tract
    - • Prostate surgery
    - • Cystoscopy
    - • Urethral dilatation
- ■ Prophylactic regimens for dental, oral, esophageal, and respiratory procedures
  - ▲ Standard
    - • Amoxicilln 2 g 1 hour before procedure (no post procedure dose) *or*
    - • Ampicillin 2 g IV or IM 30 minutes before procedure
  - ▲ Allergic to penicillin
    - • Clindamycin 600 mg PO 1 hour before procedure *or*

- Cephalexin or cefadroxil 2 g PO 1 hour before procedure (not if immediate type hypersensitivity reaction to penicillin) *or*
- Azithromycin or clarithromycin 500 mg 1 hour before procedure
  - ▲ Allergic to penicillin and unable to take medication PO
    - Clindamycin 600 mg IV 30 minutes before procedure *or*
    - Cefazolin 1 g IV or IM 30 minutes before procedure.
- ■ Prophylactic regimens for genitourinary or gastrointestinal tract procedures
  - ▲ High-risk patients
    - Ampicillin 2 g IM or IV plus gentamicin 1.5 mg/kg IV or IM (not to exceed 120 mg) 30 minutes before procedure *and*
    - Ampicillin 1 g IV or IM or amoxicillin 1 g PO 6 hours afterward
  - ▲ High-risk patients allergic to penicillin
    - Vancomycin 1 g IV over 1-2 hours plus gentamicin 1.5 mg/kg IV or IM (not to exceed 120 mg).
    - Complete injection within 30 minutes before starting procedure.
  - ▲ Moderate-risk patients
    - Amoxicilln 2 g PO 1 hour before procedure *or*
    - Ampicillin 2 g IV or IM 30 minutes before procedure
  - ▲ Moderate-risk patients allergic to penicillin
    - Vancomycin 1 g IV over 1-2 hours
    - Complete infusion within 30 minutes before starting procedure.
- ■ Approach to determining need for prophylaxis in mitral valve prolapse
  - ▲ Click with no murmur or presence of murmur unknown
    - If emergency procedure, prophylaxis
    - If not emergency, obtain echocardiogram (controversial opinion).
  - ▲ Mitral regurgitation shown by echocardiography, prophylaxis
  - ▲ No mitral regurgitation shown by echocardiography, no prophylaxis

INDEX

('i' indicates an illustration; 't' indicates a table)

R

Ranson criteria, acute pancreatitis severity, 680t

Rash
  causes, 241t
  cutaneous findings, 244t-246t
  descriptive terms, 240t
  differential diagnosis, 240, 242t-243t
  history, 242t-243t
  management, 243-244, 246-247
  risk assessment, 239-240
  symptoms, 242t-243t
  testing, 243, 244t-246t

Raynaud phenomenon, 509, 518, 520

Reactive arthritis, 526

Red blood cells (RBCs)
  destruction in splenomegaly, 256
  transfusion in anemia, 23
  transfusion therapy, 915t-916t

Red eye, 220, 222t, 223t-226t, 230

Reiter syndrome, 526

Renal biopsy, 454-455

Renal disorder
  anemia, 15t
  back pain, 28t, 32
  hematuria, 159t-160t
  HIV, 563t
  sepsis, 737

Renal failure. *See* Acute renal failure

Renal replacement therapies, 895
  continuous, 898-900
  intermittent, 896-898
  transplantation, 900

Renal tubular acidosis (RTA), 424, 425

Reptilase time (RT), 310t, 311

Respiratory acidosis, 418, 420t, 426-428
  causes, 427t

Respiratory alkalosis, 418, 420t, 428
  causes, 429t

Reticulocyte index (RI), 19

Retinal detachment, 228t, 231t

Retinitis, HIV, 593t-594t

Rheumatoid arthritis, 521-522
  complications, 523
  diagnosis, 523-524
  drug therapy, 525t, 907t
  management, 524
  presentation, 522

Rheumatologic disorder
  back pain, 28t, 32
  lower extremity pain, 202t, 204, 207-208, 210

Rigidity, abdominal pain, 2

Rocky Mountain Spotted Fever, 242t, 247

Romberg sign, 107

Roth spots, 617

Rumack-Matthew nomogram, 708, 709i

S

Sarcoidosis
  chest X-ray, 306i
  splenomegaly, 256

Scleritis, 230t, 334t

Scleroderma (limited), 521

Scleroderma (systemic), 518-519
  diagnosis, 520
  management, 520
  presentation, 519-520

Seizures. *See* Epileptic seizures

Sepsis
  cardiovascular failure, 736-737
  coagulopathy, 738
  definitions, 727
  diagnosis, 730-732, 731t
  epidemiology, 727-728
  gastrointestinal dysfunction, 737-738
  management, 732-739